OTOLARYNGOLOGY:
THE ESSENTIALS

D1640323

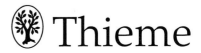
Thieme

OTOLARYNGOLOGY: THE ESSENTIALS

Edited by

Allen M. Seiden, M.D.
Professor
Department of Otolaryngology—Head and Neck Surgery
University of Cincinnati
Cincinnati, OH

Thomas A. Tami, M.D.
Professor
Department of Otolaryngology—
Head and Neck Surgery
University of Cincinnati
Cincinnati, OH

Robin T. Cotton, M.D.
Professor and Director
Department of Pediatric Otolaryngology
Children's Hospital Medical Center
University of Cincinnati
Cincinnati, OH

Myles L. Pensak, M.D.
Professor
Department of Otolaryngology—
Head and Neck Surgery
University of Cincinnati
Cincinnati, OH

Jack L. Gluckman, M.D.
Professor and Chairman
Department of Otolaryngology—
Head and Neck Surgery
University of Cincinnati
Cincinnati, OH

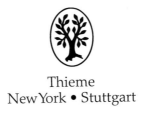

Thieme
New York • Stuttgart

Thieme New York
333 Seventh Avenue
New York, NY 10001

Editor: Esther Gumpert
Director of Production and Manufacturing: Anne Vinnicombe
Marketing Director: Phyllis Gold
Sales Manager: Ross Lumpkin
Chief Financial Officer: Peter van Woerden
President: Brian D. Scanlan
Medical Illustrators: Stacie Walker of Mazerac Design and Kerry G. Nicholson
Cover Designer: Kevin Kall
Compositor: Compset, Inc.
Printer: Maple-Vail Book Manufacturing Company

Library of Congress Cataloging-in-Publication Data

Otolaryngology: the essentials/ edited by Allen M. Seiden...[et al.].
    p. ;cm.
  Includes bibliographical references and index.
  ISBN 0-86577-854-X (alk. paper)
    1. Otolaryngology, Operative. I. Seiden, Allen M.
  [DNLM: 1. Otorhinolaryngologic Surgical Procedures. WV 168 0887 2001]
  RF51.O864 2001
  617.5'1—dc21   2001044346

Important note: Medical knowledge is ever-changing. As new research and clinical experience broaden our knowledge, changes in treatment and drug therapy may be required. The authors and the editors of the material herein have consulted sources believed to be reliable in their efforts to provide information that is complete and in accord with the standards accepted at the time of publication. However, in view of the possibility of human error by the authors, editors, or publisher of the work herein, or changes in medical knowledge, neither the authors, editors, publisher, or any other party who has been involved in the preparation of this work, warrants that the information contained herein is in every respect accurate or complete, and they are not responsible for any errors or omissions or for the results obtained from use of such information. For example, readers are advised to check the product information sheet included in the package of each drug they plan to administer to be certain that the information contained in this publication is accurate and that changes have not been made in the recommended dose or in the contraindications for administration. This recommendation is of particular importance in connection with new or infrequently used drugs.

Some of the product names, patents, and registered designs referred to in this book are in fact registered trademarks or proprietary names even though specific reference to this fact is not always made in the text. Therefore, the appearance of a name without designation as proprietary is not to be construed as a representation by the publisher that it is in the public domain.

Printed in the United States of America

5 4 3 2

TNY ISBN 0–86577–854–X
GTV ISBN 3–13–27821–8

CONTENTS

PREFACE

The speciality of otolaryngology—head and neck surgery has become increasingly diverse, making it difficult for clinicians to remain current, let alone to remain secure in their basic fund of knowledge. While several very detailed texts are available, these are cumbersome and more for specific reference than for broad review of general topics.

The present text was created to provide a more succinct and readable reference that still provides the essential basic science and clinical information relevant to most otolaryngologists. It is organized in a way that is designed to help a clinician retain this essential information.

The text is broken down into anatomical sections, and each section is in turn divided into chapters covering related anatomy and physiology (including embryology), relevant clinical tests that would be important for diagnosing problems pertaining to that particular area, congenital disorders, functional disorders, infectious and inflammatory disorders, neoplasms and cysts, and trauma. Information considered relevant but not neatly fitting into any of these aforementioned chapters is included in the final chapter of each section, which is aptly titled "Special Considera-

tions." All chapters are not needed for each section, but great care has been taken to make certain the information provided is complete.

In addition to these anatomical sections, several other topics are covered that were felt to be important to an overall review of otolaryngology—head and neck surgery, including flap reconstruction, aesthetic surgery, and skin lesions. These sections follow an individualized chapter format. Lastly, the final chapter lists and briefly characterizes all of the syndromes and eponyms with which on occasion an otolaryngologist may be confronted.

To further enhance retention, important pieces of information are pulled out from the text and highlighted. "Controversies" are those issues that continue to be disputed and for which there may be conflicting evidence. Opposing views are generally presented. "Pearls" are useful clinical tips that may facilitate a particular diagnosis, treatment, or surgical procedure. "Pitfalls" are findings that could potentially confound a particular diagnosis or lead to complications during a surgical procedure. "Special Considerations" are those facts that deserve careful emphasis in relation to a given topic.

We hope that this book will provide a readable yet comprehensive review source for otolaryngologists, residents, and all those with an interest in the specialty. We anticipate that its format will facilitate understanding and retention, and therefore we hope that it will be useful to most clinicians. It is a companion to Tami, Seiden, Pensak, Gluckman, and Cotton: *Otolaryngology: A Case Study Approach*, that takes these same basic facts and applies them to a clinical diagnosis.

Allen M. Seiden, M.D.
Thomas A. Tami, M.D.
Myles L. Pensak, M.D.
Robin T. Cotton, M.D.
Jack L. Gluckman, M.D.

CONTRIBUTORS

Andrew C. Campbell, M.D.
Campbell Facial Plastic Surgery
Sheboygan, WI

Robin T. Cotton, M.D., F.A.C.S., F.R.C.S.(C)
Professor and Director
Department of Pediatric Otolaryngology
Children's Hospital Medical Center
University of Cincinnati
Cincinnati, OH

Rick A. Friedman, M.D., Ph.D.
Clinician
House Ear Clinic
Scientist
House Ear Institute
Los Angeles, CA

Mark E. Gerber, M.D.
Assistant Professor
Department of Pediatric Otolaryngology
Northwestern University
Children's Memorial Hospital
Chicago, IL

Lyon L. Gleich, M.D.
Associate Professor
Department of Otolaryngology—Head and
   Neck Surgery
University of Cincinnati
Cincinnati, OH

Jack L. Gluckman, M.D.
Professor and Chairman
Department of Otolaryngology—Head and
   Neck Surgery
University of Cincinnati
Cincinnati, OH

Benjamin E. J. Hartley, M.B.B.S., B.Sc., F.R.C.S.
Consultant Pediatric Otolaryngologist
The Great Ormond Street Hospital
   for Children
London, United Kingdom

Robert W. Keith, B.A., M.A., Ph.D.
Professor of Otolaryngology (Audiology)
Department of Otolaryngology—Head and
   Neck Surgery
University of Cincinnati
Cincinnati, OH

Daniel J. Kelley, M.D.
Director, Head and Neck Oncology/
   Skull Base Surgery
Department of Otolaryngology and Head
   and Neck Surgery
Temple University School of Medicine
Philadelphia, PA

Bradley W. Kesser, M.D.
Fellow
House Ear Clinic
Los Angeles, CA

Greg R. Licameli, M.D.
Assistant Professor of Otology and Laryngology
Harvard Medical School
Cambridge, MA
Assistant Professor
Department of Otolaryngology
Childrens Hospital
Boston, MA

Judith Cjaza McCaffrey, M.D.
Assistant Professor of Otolaryngology—Head
  and Neck Surgery
Departments of Otolaryngology and
  Interdisciplinary Oncology
University of South Florida, H. Lee Moffitt
  Cancer Center
Tampa, FL

J. Scott McMurray, M.D., F.A.A.P.
Assistant Professor
Department of Surgery
Division of Otolaryngology—Head and Neck
  Surgery
University of Wisconsin Medical School,
  University of Wisconsin Hospital and Clinics
Madison, WI

Charles M. Myer III, M.D.
Professor
Department of Pediatric Otolaryngology
Children's Hospital Medical Center
University of Cincinnati
Cincinnati, OH

Tapan A. Padhya, M.D.
Assistant Professor
Department of Otolaryngology—Head and
  Neck Surgery
University of South Florida, H. Lee Moffitt
  Cancer Center
Tampa, FL

Myles L. Pensak, M.D.
Professor of Otolaryngology and Neurologic
  Surgery

Department of Otolaryngology—Head and
  Neck Surgery
University of Cincinnati
Cincinnati, OH

Louis G. Portugal, M.D.
Associate Professor and Director, Division of
  Head and Neck Surgery
Department of Otolaryngology—Head and
  Neck Surgery
University of Illinois at Chicago
Chicago, IL

Allen M. Seiden, M.D., F.A.C.S.
Professor
Department of Otolaryngology—Head and
  Neck Surgery
University of Cincinnati
Cincinnati, OH

Sally R. Shott, M.D.
Associate Professor
Department of Otolaryngology
University of Cincinnati
Department of Otolaryngology
Children's Hospital Medical Center
Cincinnati, OH

Kevin A. Shumrick, M.D.
Professor
Department of Otolaryngology—Head and
  Neck Surgery
University of Cincinnati
Cincinnati, OH

Yoram Stern, M.D.
Senior Lecturer
Department of Otolaryngology
Sackler Faculty of Medicine
Tel Aviv University
Schneider Children's Medical Center of Israel
Petah Tiqua, Israel

David L. Steward, M.D.
Assistant Professor
Department of Otolaryngology—Head and
  Neck Surgery
University of Cincinnati
Cincinnati, OH

Thomas A. Tami, M.D., FACS
Professor
Department of Otolaryngology—Head and
  Neck Surgery
University of Cincinnati
Cincinnati, OH

David L. Walner, M.D.
Lutheran General Children's Hospital
Park Ridge, IL
Assistant Professor

Department of Otolaryngology and
  Bronchoesophagology
Rush Presbyterian—St. Lukes Medical Center
Chicago, IL

Keith M. Wilson, M.D.
Associate Professor
Department of Otolaryngology—Head and
  Neck Surgery
University of Cincinnati
Cincinnati, OH

SECTION I

EAR

Chapter 1

ANATOMY AND PHYSIOLOGY

Rick A. Friedman

OUTER EAR

The pinnae of the adult are bilateral appendages consisting of elastic cartilage whose function is to provide sound localization. These structures develop from the six hillocks of His. The three anterior hillocks are derived from the first pharyngeal arch and the three posterior hillocks are derived from the second pharyngeal arch. The structures in the adult pinna derived from each hillock can be seen in Figure 1–1. The pinna normally rests at an angle of 30 degrees to the sagittal plane of the head. The growth of the pinna typically parallels that of the remainder of the head and neck until approximately 9 years of age, at which time the pinna is adult size.

SPECIAL CONSIDERATION

Preauricular pits, which are often seen congenitally and can create problems with recurrent infection, are not derived from pharyngeal arches, as are the pinna and external auditory canal. Rather, the most accepted theory as to their origin reflects a failure of fusion of two of the six hillocks of the first (mandibular) and second (hyoid) brachial arches that form the auricle.

The surface anatomy of the pinna is primarily determined by the contour of its underlying elastic cartilage framework. The skin of the lateral aspect of the pinna is tightly adherent to the contours of the cartilage, whereas that of the medial aspect of the pinna has a subcutaneous space, and therefore the skin is more mobile. The anatomy of the outer contour of the pinna is quite complex, as can be seen in Figure 1–1. There are several impressions on the lateral aspect of the pinna, including the triangular fossa, the scaphoid fossa, and the concha, which is divided by the crus of the helix into the cavum concha and the symba concha. The helix or curled outer edge of the pinna extends from the crus of the helix to the lobule. The antihelix begins as the superior and inferior crura and ends at the level of the antitragus. The tragus, the most anterior aspect of the pinna, is separated from the antitragus by the intertragal incisure. Similarly, the tragus is separated from the superiorly lying helical crus by the anterior incisure. The lobule, a noncartilaginous fibrofatty structure, lies at the inferior aspect of the pinna.

The pinna is attached to the lateral aspect of the cranium by its skin, cartilage, and a series of muscles and ligaments. The three extrinsic muscles of the pinna originate from the galea aponeurotica. The superior auricular muscle, the anterior auricular muscle, and the posterior

3

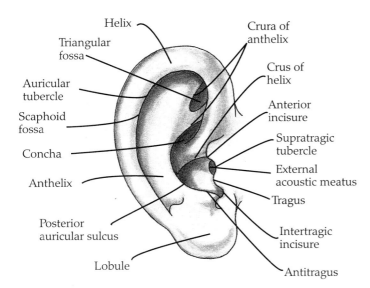

Helix
Triangular fossa
Auricular tubercle
Scaphoid fossa
Concha
Anthelix
Posterior auricular sulcus
Lobule
Crura of anthelix
Crus of helix
Anterior incisure
Supratragic tubercle
External acoustic meatus
Tragus
Intertragic incisure
Antitragus

FIGURE 1-1 The auricle.

auricular muscle are innervated by cranial nerve VII and insert into the pinna.

SPECIAL CONSIDERATION

Trauma to the pinna can result in auricular hematoma, which is a collection of blood beneath the adherent perichondrium on the lateral aspect of the pinna. Because of the sparcity of subcutaneous space, hematomas of the pinna disrupt the architecture of the lateral pinna and are quite obvious and painful. Blood supply to the cartilage provided by the perichondrium is disrupted, and can lead to remodeling and auricular deformity if not promptly treated.

The external auditory canal develops as a thickening of ectoderm from the first pharyngeal cleft. The ectodermal depression begins to invaginate medially. The mesoderm separating it from the tubotympanum is called the meatal plug. As this meatal plug resolves, the external auditory canal ectoderm comes into contact with the tubotympanic recess derived from endoderm and is separated only by a layer of connective tissue called the pars propria. The tympanic membrane is the area of contact between the meatal plug and the endoderm of the middle ear.

The adult external auditory canal measures approximately 2.5 cm in length and serves as a channel for the transmission of sound to the tympanic membrane. Its lateral one third consists of the elastic cartilage of the pinna. The medial two thirds of the external canal are osseous.

SPECIAL CONSIDERATION

The fissures of Santorini, typically two or three in number, are present in the cartilaginous external auditory canal. These fissures provide a potential route of spread for infection or neoplasm to the skull base and infratemporal fossa.

The skin of the outer third of the external auditory canal contains a variety of adnexal structures, including hair follicles, sebaceous glands, and modified apocrine glands, which secrete cerumen. The skin of the medial two thirds of the external canal is largely devoid of adnexal structures and is a very thin layer lying on the periosteum.

The pinna and external auditory canal serve to increase sound pressure levels at the tympanic membrane by their resonance properties. The pinna has two important acoustic components. The pinna adds approximately three decibels of gain intensity at 4000 Hz. The concha improves the transmission of sound at 5000 to 6000 Hz by approximately 10 decibels. The resonance properties of the ear canal can be likened to those of a pipe organ. Like a closed-end pipe, the maximum resonance occurs at approximately four times the length of the canal. This represents a wavelength of approximately 3500 Hz. The ear canal and the concha of the pinna act together for a net resonance at approximately 2700 Hz. This added gain falls well within the range of human speech.

MIDDLE EAR AND MASTOID

The middle ear is delineated laterally by the tympanic membrane, which is elliptical and slightly conical in shape. The apex of this cone lies at the umbo, which marks the inferior aspect of the manubrium, or the long process of the malleus. The adult tympanic membrane is angled approximately 140 degrees with respect to the superior wall of the external auditory canal. The vertical diameter of the tympanic membrane measures from 8.5 to 10 mm, and the horizontal diameter measures from 8 to 9 mm. The lateral or short process of the malleus can be seen well through the tympanic membrane.

The manubrium of the malleus is firmly attached to the tympanic membrane at the umbo and lateral process. There are anterior and posterior tympanic stria that extend from the lateral process of the malleus to the anterior and posterior tympanic spines. The area of the tympanic membrane above the stria is known as the pars flaccida or Shrapnell's membrane, and the area below is known as the pars tensa.

The pars tensa thickens peripherally to form the tympanic annulus. This annulus serves

> **PEARL...** Retraction pockets in the area of the pars flaccida often represent the tip of the iceberg and are generally large retraction pockets containing keratin. These have been termed primary acquired cholesteatomas.

to fasten the tympanic membrane in a groove known as the tympanic sulcus. The tympanic annulus and sulcus exist throughout the periphery of the pars tensa; however, they are both absent superiorly in the area of the notch of Rivinus, which anchors the pars flaccida.

The middle ear ossicles reside within the tubotympanic recess. This recess is derived from the first and second pharyngeal pouches. The malleus, the most lateral of the ossicles, is suspended within the middle ear by a series of ligaments and by its attachment to the tympanic membrane. The malleus consists of a head, neck, lateral process, anterior process, and long process, or manubrium.

The incus is attached to the malleus by the incudomalleal joint, a diarthrodial joint. The incus consists of a body, short process, long process, and lenticular process. The lenticular process articulates with the capitulum of the stapes at another diarthrodial joint. The third bone of the ossicular chain, the stapes, consists of a head, or capitulum, an anterior and posterior crus, and a base, or footplate.

Much of the ossicular chain is derived from the first and second pharyngeal arches. The first arch, or Meckel's cartilage, contributes to the head and neck of the malleus and the body and short process of the incus; the second arch cartilage, or Reichert's cartilage, contributes to the manubrium of the malleus and long and lenticular processes of the incus. The second arch also contributes to the suprastructure of the stapes. The base, or footplate, of the stapes is derived from the otic capsule.

The tympanic cavity, or middle ear cleft, in the adult measures approximately 15 mm in the vertical, anterior, and posterior dimensions. Its transverse dimension is somewhat hourglass shaped with a 6-mm width superiorly and a

4-mm width inferiorly, and a central constriction of approximately 2 mm in width. The middle ear cavity is pneumatized via the eustachian tube, which communicates with the nasopharynx. Posteriorly, the middle ear communicates with the mastoid antrum via the aditus ad antrum. The middle ear cavity can be considered a cuboidal space.

The floor of the cavity overlies the jugular bulb. The posterior aspect of the floor gives rise to the styloid eminence. The posterior wall or mastoid portion of the tympanic cavity is derived from Reichert's cartilage.

The posterior wall contains a series of eminences and recesses. The pyramidal eminence, which lies just medial to the descending facial nerve, emits the tendon of the stapedius muscle. The chordal eminence, which lies lateral to the pyramidal eminence and just medial to the tympanic membrane, houses a foramen called the iter chordae posterius through which the chordae tympani nerve gains access to the middle ear cleft. The facial recess is a depression that lies between the chordal eminence and the pyramidal eminence. The short process of the incus is the roof of this recess. Medial to the pyramidal eminence and posterior to the subiculum lies the tympanic sinus.

The facial recess can be accessed posteriorly through a posterior tympanotomy or a facial recess approach. The sinus tympani, as it lies medial to the facial nerve, can often be difficult to visualize. When anatomy permits, it can be approached through the retrofacial air cells just lateral to the posterior semicircular canal.

The superior wall of the tympanic cavity, or tegmen tympani, is a thin bony plate that overlies the undersurface of the temporal lobe dura. Suspensory ligaments for both the malleus and incus reside in this region. The anterior wall of the tympanic cavity, or protympanum, is composed of the vertical segment of the petrous carotid artery, the eustachian tube, and the semicanal of the tensor tympani muscle.

The medial wall of the tympanic cavity also contains a variety of prominences and recesses. The major prominence of the medial wall is the promontory or basal turn of the cochlea. The promontory is connected to the pyramidal process by a bridge of bone, the ponticulus. Descending vertically from the ponticulus and posterior to the round window niche is the subiculum. The two main depressions in the medial wall of the tympanic cavity are the oval window niche and the round window niche. Just above the oval window niche lies the horizontal segment of the facial nerve.

Between the third and seventh fetal months, four endothelial-lined sacs invaginate from the first brachial pouch, forming the tympanic cavity. These sacs consist of the saccus superior, saccus medius, saccus anticus, and saccus posticus. These sacs, and their secondarily formed mucosal folds, serve to compartmentalize the middle ear into a variety of spaces, the most notable of which, Prussak's space, lies lateral to the head and neck of the malleus and medial to the pars flaccida. It is this space that is involved early in primary acquired cholesteatoma.

The primary function of the middle ear cavity is to serve as an impedance matching system. The impedance matching improves the efficiency of sound energy transfer from the air-filled medium of the environment, including the external canal and middle ear, to the fluid-filled medium of the inner ear. Without the impedance match provided by the outer and middle ears, approximately 99.9% of sound energy would be reflected at the level of the oval window. There are two major components to this impedance matching system within the middle ear. The first component is the ratio of the areas of the tympanic membrane and the oval window, or stapes footplate. The ratio of the area of the tympanic membrane, which functionally is approximately 55 mm^2, to the area of the footplate, which is 2.3 mm^2, is 17:1. Sound pressure level is equal to the force divided by the surface area ($P = F/a$). Based on this formula, it can be seen that the pressure at the level of the oval window will be 17 times greater for a given force than the pressure at the tympanic membrane. This corresponds to an approximate gain of 26.5 decibels.

PEARL••• The tympanic membrane serves to block sound energy from simultaneously striking the oval and round windows. If this were to occur, sound waves would be instituted at the same time in opposite directions, resulting in cancellation. The phase differential or cancellation effect leads to an approximate 16 decibels of sound pressure level. For this reason, large perforations and those in the area of the round window niche are often associated with a higher degree of hearing loss.

A second impedance matching mechanism arises from the lever effect, or the difference in length of the long process of the malleus and the long process of the incus. The manubrium, the long process of the malleus, is approximately 1.3 times longer than the long process of the incus. This mechanical lever provides a gain of approximately 7.3 decibels.

Inner Ear

The inner ear develops embryologically from the ectoderm overlying the developing neuraxis. During approximately the third week of gestation, the otic placode begins to form and by close to 4 weeks of development, the otic pit has formed. The otocyst invaginates and becomes separate from the overlying ectodermal surface by approximately 30 days' gestation, at which time the endolymphatic duct begins to form. Over the ensuing weeks, the pars inferior, or cochlea and saccule, begins to form. Similarly, the pars superior, consisting of the semicircular canals and utricle, begins to canalize. By approximately 26 weeks of gestation, the inner ear is anatomically and functionally mature.

The osseous portion of the inner ear consists of the otic capsule, the densest bone in the body. It consists of the vestibule, which houses the saccule and utricle, the cochlea, with cochlear duct and the surrounding perilymphatic spaces, and the three semicircular canals. There are two aqueducts emanating from the inner ear. The vestibular aqueduct houses the endolymphatic duct, and the cochlear aqueduct provides communication between the subarachnoid space, in the area of the pars nervosa, and the scala tympani.

The vestibule is an irregularly shaped ovoid cavity with a medial to lateral diameter of approximately 4 mm. Along the medial wall, within the spherical recess, lies the saccule, and within the elliptical recess lies the utricle. The three semicircular canals communicate with the vestibule through five openings. These include the amputated ends of the superior, lateral, and posterior semicircular canals, as well as the nonampulated end of the lateral canal and the crus commune, which is a combination of the nonampulated ends of the superior and posterior semicircular canals. Anterior and inferior to the vestibule is the osseous cochlear cavity, which is shaped like a cone with its base directed medially and its apex directed anterolaterally. The cochlea makes 2 ½ turns around the central axis, known as the modiolus. The blood vessels and nerve fibers of the cochlea traverse this osseous framework. The osseous spiral lamina provides the medial attachment for the basilar membrane and Reissner's membrane. This serves to compartmentalize the cochlea, separating the cochlear duct, or the scala media, which contains endolymph, from the two perilymphatic spaces, which are adjacent to the endosteum of the otic capsule, the scala vestibule, and the scala tympani (Fig. 1–2). The helicotrema, at the apex of the cochlea, provides an avenue for the communication between the scala tympani and the scala vestibuli.

The membranous labyrinth is a series of epithelial-lined spaces that contain endolymph. The membranous labyrinth consists of the

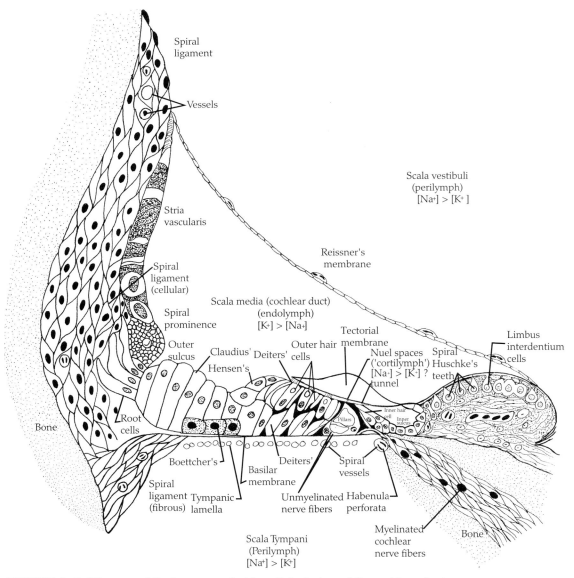

FIGURE 1–2 Diagram of the transverse (midmodiolar) view of the cochlear duct.

cochlear duct, the three semicircular ducts, and the saccule and the utricle. The cochlea communicates with the saccule via the ductus reuniens. The semicircular canals open directly into the utricle. The utricular duct and the saccular duct join to form the common endolymphatic duct, which travels through the vestibular aqueduct to the posterior cranial fossa ending as the endolymphatic sac. The endolymphatic sac resides within a fossa in the posterior petrous bone called the foveate impression. A slight covering of bone, the operculum, can be identified overlying a portion of the sac.

The cross-sectional anatomy of the cochlear duct reveals its intricate detail. Each turn of the cochlea is separated by the interscalar septum.

SPECIAL CONSIDERATION

In Mondini's dysplasia, there is often a defect of the interscalar septum between the second and beginning of the third turns, which leads to a scala communes or a common cavity deformity.

On the modiolar aspect of the cochlear duct, one can see the myelinated cochlear nerve fibers traveling within Rosenthal's canal. Overlying this is the spiral limbus, a condensation of the mesenchyme with an epithelial lining of its surface, the interdental cells. Continuing toward the lateral wall of the cochlear duct are the sulcus cells and the inner hair cell.

Immediately adjacent to the inner hair cell is the inner pillar cell; the space between is called the tunnel of Corti. The three outer hair cells are the next cells encountered. Adjacent to the outer hair cells and closer to the spiral ligament reside the Hensen cells, Claudius cells, and outer sulcus cells. The supporting cells of the outer hair cells are the Deiters cells, which lie beneath the outer hair cells and overlie the basilar membrane. On the lateral wall, the stria vascularis is evident with its high vascularity consistent with its function as a secretory organ for the endolymph. There is a high level of Na^+K^+ adenosine triphosphatase (ATPase) activity providing the high concentrations of

potassium necessary to maintain the endocochlear potential. The spiral ligament connects the basilar membrane to the lateral wall.

As previously described, the scala vestibuli and scala tympani contain perilymph with a sodium and potassium concentration similar to that of extracellular fluid. The scala media, on the other hand, contains endolymph with an intracellular-like fluid containing a very high potassium concentration (144 mEq per liter) and a low sodium concentration (13 mEq per liter). The scala media has a positive resting potential of approximately 80 mV, which is called the endocochlear potential. This endocochlear potential is maintained by the stria vascularis on the lateral wall of the cochlea. This steep electrochemical gradient for potassium is maintained by the specialized cells in the stria vascularis.

SPECIAL CONSIDERATION

Several forms of hereditary hearing loss involve abnormalities of the stria vascularis. In particular, pigmentary abnormalities that are associated with hearing loss, such as Waardenburg's syndrome type I, appear to result from a failure of melanocyte development in the stria vascularis. The role melanocytes play in generating the endocochlear potential is unknown at the present time; however, it is likely due to an endocochlear potential problem in these patients.

Acoustic energy, which is transmitted to the oval window, results in compression and rarefaction movements of the stapes footplate. This action is directly coupled to the perilymph of the scala vestibuli, which communicates ultimately with the scala tympani via the helicotrema. The sound energy is then released through the round window membrane at the termination of the scala tympani. The organ of Corti, which rests on the basilar membrane, is subject to shearing forces between the compression and rarefaction waves of the perilymph on Reissner's and the basilar membranes. It is the shearing forces between the tectorial membrane and the stereocilia of the hair cells that result in mechanotransduction of sound into electrical energy and an auditory nerve impulse.

The outer and inner hair cells have a number of morphologic and functional differences (Fig. 1–3). The spiral ganglion, which is composed of the cell bodies of the auditory nerve, has dendritic processes that synapse with the hair cells. These afferent fibers then synapse with secondary neurons in the cochlear nuclei. Of the approximately 50,000 auditory nerve fibers, 90% synapse with the inner hair cells (type I neurons). Each inner hair cell is innervated by only a few type I neurons. The other 5 to 10% of the auditory neurons innervate the outer hair cells and these are called type II neurons. The innervation pattern of the outer hair cells is much less selective.

The mechanical stimulation of the cochlea results from a traveling wave. It is the quality of the basilar membrane that dictates the regions of the cochlea that are tuned to high versus low frequencies. The basilar membrane in the basal regions of the cochlea is narrower and stiffer than that of the apical region. It is this physical quality that dictates the maximum amplitude of displacement of the basilar membrane in response to sound. High-frequency sounds tend to have their maximum displacement near the basal end of the cochlea, and low-frequency sounds have their maximum displacement in the apical regions of the cochlea, where the basilar membrane is wide and more compliant.

This theory of the transmission of sound is called the traveling wave theory. This traveling wave theory helps to explain the frequency selectivity of the inner ear; however, it does not explain the finely tuned nature of the transduction process.

It was once believed that the site of fine-tuning of the auditory system was at the level of the auditory nerve and the central nervous system. Recent evidence suggests that the fine-tuning is a result of a cochlear amplifier that is based in the outer hair cells. It appears that the outer hair cells have a contractile activity that appears to fine-tune the cochlear frequency response.

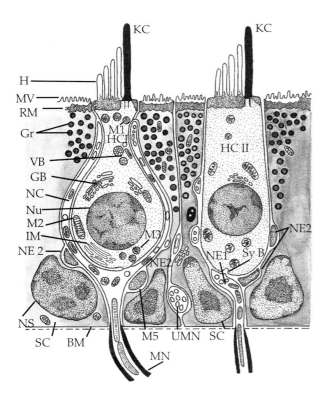

FIGURE 1–3 Types I and II vestibular hair cells. The flask-shaped type I cell (HC I) is surrounded by a nerve calyx (NC), which makes contact on its outer surface with granulated (presumably efferent) nerve endings (NE 2). Unmyelinated fibers (UMN) are extensions of myelinated fibers (MN), which lose their myelin sheaths as they pass through basement membranes. The type II sensory cell (HCII) is roughly cylindrical and is supplied by two nerve endings (NE 1 and NE 2), which can be seen on its basal end. Several groups of mitochondria (M_1–M_5) are found in the sensory cells and neural elements. Two kinds of hair project from the surfaces of sensory cells, stereocilia (H) and kinocilium (KC), a single kinocilium always being the longest on each cell. Supporting cells are easily distinguished from sensory cells by virtue of their large population of rather uniformly distributed granules (Gr).

The stereocilia of the hair cells are critical to the signal transduction process. Stereocilia are bundles of actin filaments that project from the apical surface of the hair cells. The outer hair cells are firmly embedded in the tectorial membrane, and the inner hair cells either have no obvious connection or are only loosely connected to the tectorial membrane. Each stereocilium is tethered to its neighbor by a tip link. These tip links serve to anatomically and functionally connect adjacent stereocilia, allowing them to move in unison. These tip links appear to have a critical role in the mechanotransduction process. Movement of the stereocilia toward the basal body results in the opening of mechanically gated channels allowing the influx of ions along an electrochemical gradient. Subsequent to this, voltage-gated calcium channels open, facilitating the release of neurotransmitters at the basal surface. Although tremendous progress is being made in the intricacies of sound transmission, there is much to be learned about this complex physiologic process.

The semicircular canals are three membranous tubes with a diameter of approximately 0.5 mm, each of which forms approximately two thirds of a circle with a diameter of approximately 6.5 mm. The three semicircular canals are aligned to form a coordinate system with horizontal canal and two vertical canals that are orthogonal to each other. The horizontal semicircular canal, with its two openings in the lateral wall of the utricle, makes a 30-degree angle with the horizontal plane.

At the anterior opening of the horizontal and superior semicircular canals and the inferior opening of the posterior canal, the membranous labyrinth enlarges to form the ampulla, in which a crest-like structure, the crista ampularis, resides. The hair cells are located on the surface of the crista with their cilia protruding and embedded in the cupula, which is a gelatinous mass of a composition similar to that of the otolithic membrane overlying the macula of the utricle and saccule. The hair cells within the crista ampularis are oriented so that all the stereocilia point in the same direction. Unlike the cochlea, which has no kinocilium, the hair cells of the vestibular labyrinth possess kinocilia that are the tallest of the cilia emanating from the apical surface of the hair cells. In the superior and posterior semicircular canal cristae, the kinocilia are directed away from the utricular orifice of the ampulla. In contrast, the kinocilia of the hair cells of the horizontal canal crista are directed toward the utricle.

The surfaces of the utricular and saccular maculae are completely covered by the otolithic membrane. Within this membrane are the otoconia, consisting of small calcium carbonate crystals with a density more than twice that of water. On the surface of the maculae of the saccule and utricle is an area known as the striola, a curved zone running through the center of each macula. The orientation of the stereocilia relative to the kinocilia is complex in these maculae but is symmetric about the striola.

The maculae of the utricle and saccule, with their otoconia, provide vestibular input regarding static gravitational pull and linear acceleration. In contrast, that of the semicircular canals provides information about angular accelerations. The work of Ewald in 1892 established the relationship between the planes of the semicircular canals, the direction of the flow of endolymph, and the direction of induced nystagmus. There were three important observations that became known as Ewald's laws: (1) Movements of the eye and head occur in the plane of the canal being stimulated, and the slow phase of nystagmus occurs in the direction of endolymphatic flow. (2) Movement of the endolymph toward the ampulla or ampulopeatal flow in the horizontal canal results in a stimulatory effect. (3) Movement of the endolymph away from the ampulla or ampulofugal flow in the superior and posterior canals causes stimulation of the vestibular nerve fibers. Ultimately it was determined that movement of the stereocilia toward the kinocilium resulted in an excitatory stimulus, and movement in the opposite direction resulted in an inhibitory stimulus.

SUGGESTED READINGS

Baxter A. Dehiscence of the fallopian canal. An anatomical study. *J Laryngol Otol* 1971;85:587.

De Vries H. The mechanics of the labyrinth otoliths. *Acta Otolaryngol* 1950;38:262.

Ewald R. *Physiologische Untersuchungen uber das Endorgan des Nervous Octavus.* Wiesbaden, Germany: Bergmann; 1892.

Proctor B. The development of the middle ear spaces and their surgical significance. *J Laryngol Otol* 1964;78:631.

Ramprashad F, Landolt JP, Money KE, Laufer J. Dimensional analysis and dynamic response characterization of mammalian peripheral vestibular structures. *Am J Anat* 1984;169:295.

Rogers BD. Anatomy, embryology, and classification of auricular deformities. In: Tanzer RC, Edgerton MT, eds. *Symposium on Reconstruction of the Auricle.* Vol 10. St Louis: CV Mosby; 1974.

Wever EG, Lawrence M. *Physiological Acoustics.* Princeton, NJ: Princeton University Press; 1954.

Chapter 2

CLINICAL TESTS

Robert W. Keith

This chapter briefly summarizes the most important aspects of audiologic diagnosis, including terminology and the basic diagnostic approach to type and degree of hearing impairment. Although the anatomy of the ear is covered in greater detail in the previous chapter, the following brief review of anatomy serves to set the stage for the discussion of testing. An outline of balance disorders testing is also provided.

ANATOMY OF THE COCHLEA

The cochlea is a pea-sized structure embedded in the temporal bone of the skull. It is a helix of about 2.5 turns and would be 34 mm long if unrolled. It consists of three fluid-filled canals:

1. *Scala vestibule:* At the base of this canal, the stapes transmits sound via the oval window.
2. *Scala tympani:* This is connected to the scala vestibule at the cochlear apex by a small hole (helicotrema). At the base, this canal terminates with the round window. The scala vestibule and scala tympani are both filled with perilymph, a normal extracellular fluid with low levels of potassium.
3. *Scala media:* This space is between the other two canals but is isolated from them by two membranes. It contains endolymph, which has high levels of potassium (K).

ANATOMIC FRAMES OF REFERENCE

The base is the end in contact with the stapes. The other end (top of the spiral) is the apex. "Inner" is toward the center of the spiral (modiolus), while "outer" is away from the center. The scala vestibule is "up" and the scala tympani "down."

ANATOMY OF THE ORGAN OF CORTI AND HAIR CELLS

The organ of Corti lies on the basilar membrane and contains parallel rows of hair cells. There are three rows of outer hair cells and one row of inner hair cells. Each ear has approximately 3500 inner hair cells and 12,000 outer hair cells. Hair cells are mechanosensitive: they detect movement, which affects their release of neurotransmitter. Movement is detected by the roughly 100 stereocilia at the apical end of each hair cell. The stereocilia are embedded in or positioned near an overlying (tectorial) membrane.

OVERVIEW OF SOUND TRANSDUCTION IN THE COCHLEA

At the oval window, the stapes pushes in and pulls out once per cycle of the sound wave. At a given point along the basilar membrane, the following five events also happen during one phase of each cycle: (1) The basilar membrane is pulled upward. (2) Bundles of hair cell stereocilia are displaced in the outer direction. (3) K+ channels in the stereocilia open. (4) The hair cells depolarize as K+ enters from the endolymph through the channels. (5) The depolarized hair cells release additional neurotransmitter onto auditory nerve fibers. During the other phase of each cycle, the same five events occur with opposite polarity (membrane goes downward, hair cells hyperpolarize, etc.). Thus all five of these events oscillate at the frequency of the stimulus tone. For each of these events, the amplitude increases with increasing sound pressure.

With each cycle of a pure tone the stapes pulls and then pushes on the oval window. The result is a pressure wave that displaces the basilar membrane. A traveling wave develops along the length of the basilar membrane with maximum displacement related to the primary frequency of the stimulus (Fig. 2–1). The maximum displace-

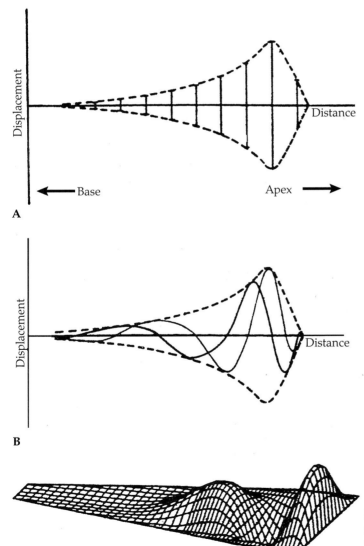

A

B

C

FIGURE 2–1 A traveling wave moving along the length of the basilar membrane has a maximum displacement related to the primary frequency of the stimulus.

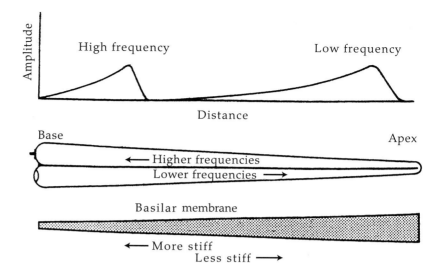

FIGURE 2–2 Tonotopic organization is preserved throughout the auditory system from cochlea to cortex.

ment of the basilar membrane is greatest near the base for high-frequency tones and near the apex for low frequencies (Fig. 2–2). This tonotopic organization is preserved throughout the auditory system from the cochlea to the cortex.

ACOUSTICS

The frequency of pure tones is expressed in hertz (Hz), formally known as cycles per second.

Intensity is expressed in decibels (dB). The decibel is a unit for expressing the ratio between two sound pressures; it is one tenth of a Bel. Important aspects of the decibel include the following: (1) it involves a ratio; (2) it involves a logarithm; (3) it is therefore nonlinear; (4) it is expressed in terms of various reference levels, which must be specified; and (5) it is a relative unit of measure. The formula for expressing dB sound pressure level is dB SPL = $20 \log_{10} P/P_o$, where P = sound pressure (in force/area, e.g., newtons/m² and P_o = reference pressure (20 μN/m²).

Common sound level references include the following:

▼ dB SPL: decibel sound pressure level
▼ dB HL: decibel hearing level is the number of decibels above an average normal threshold for a given signal. This is the notation used on the audiogram. The hearing-level dial of an audiometer is calibrated in dB HL.

▼ dB SL: decibel sensation level is the number of decibels above the hearing threshold of a given listener for a given signal. This unit is useful in expressing the level above audiometric threshold that certain diagnostic tests are administered, for example, the word discrimination score.

AUDITORY PERCEPTION

The psychophysical principles of audition include the following:

1. Pitch is related to the frequency of the signal. Pitch abnormalities (diplacusis) are symptomatic of certain cochlear disease processes.

2. Loudness is related to the intensity of the signal. Loudness abnormalities (auditory recruitment and decruitment) are related to lesions of the cochlea and auditory nerve, respectively.

   Any dynamic range of 60 dB or less is a sign of the presence of auditory recruitment. Decruitment is defined as a less than normal growth in loudness of a signal as the intensity is increased. Patients with auditory nerve deafness and decruitment show discomfort thresholds beyond the limits of the audiometer, that is, greater than 110 dB HL.

3. Duration is related to the length of time the signal is presented. The normal ear inte-

grates energy at auditory threshold over the first 200 milliseconds (msec). That is, a signal of 20 msec will require greater signal intensity to hear the tone than one of 200 msec. Occasionally temporal processing disorders that originate at brainstem or cortical levels are found in persons with central auditory processing disorders.

THRESHOLD OF HEARING

A young person with no history of otologic disease or noise trauma can hear frequencies from about 20 to 20,000 Hz. The threshold of audibility curve reported in the decibel sound pressure level (SPL) indicates that the absolute threshold for hearing varies with frequency. The ear is more sensitive to sounds in the frequency range between 1000 and 4000 Hz, and less sensitive to sounds at higher and lower frequencies.

The threshold of audibility curve is converted from dB SPL to dB hearing level (HL) for clinical purposes. The normal threshold for hearing measured in dB HL is 0 dB HL over a frequency range of 125 to 8000 Hz. Hearing thresholds are poorer as persons age, with a gradual decline in hearing for frequencies above 2000 Hz. Other typical patterns of hearing loss include the notch-shaped audiogram with the primary deficit at 3000 to 6000 Hz associated with noise trauma hearing loss. Meniere's disease typically results in a fluctuating low-frequency sensorineural hearing loss, and acoustic tumors show a unilateral high-frequency hearing loss with poor word discrimination.

ASSESSMENT OF HEARING

The measurement of hearing has several purposes:

▼ Quantitative assessment of hearing: describing the magnitude of hearing loss
▼ Site of lesion testing within the auditory system
▼ Habilitation of the hearing impaired, including selection and fitting of hearing aids
▼ Monitoring hearing levels for prevention of hearing loss with patients on ototoxic medication
▼ Monitoring the effectiveness of hearing conservation programs in industry
▼ Medical legal and compensation examination

THE HISTORY OF AUDIOMETRY

Pure-tone audiometry has developed from the basic principles of the tuning-fork tests that were introduced during the 1800s. These tests were named after the men who first described them and include the Weber test introduced in 1834, the Rinne test in 1855, and the Schwabach test in 1885. The principles of these tests are at the foundation of interpreting modern pure-tone audiometric tests.

The Weber test is most useful when a unilateral hearing loss is present. This test is conducted by placing the stem of a vibrating tuning fork on the midline of the patient's skull. The patient is asked to indicate the ear in which the sound is heard. Localization of the sound toward the poorer hearing ear indicates the presence of a conductive hearing loss on that side. Localization to the better ear indicates that the hearing loss in the opposite ear is sensorineural.

The Rinne test is conducted by comparing the loudness of sound presented by air and bone conduction. If bone conduction (BC) is heard louder or longer than air conduction (AC) (a negative Rinne), a conductive hearing loss is present. A sensorineural loss is present if air conduction is heard louder or longer than bone conduction (a positive Rinne) and the Weber test lateralizes to the opposite ear. The higher the frequency at which a negative Rinne (BC > AC) is obtained, the greater the conductive hearing loss.

PITFALL••• One of the biggest problems with the Rinne test occurs when the examiner fails to recognize that the sound emanating from the stem of a tuning fork will be conducted by the bones of the skull to both cochlea. Therefore, a patient with a "dead" ear can easily hear the sound in the better ear by cross conduction of the bone-conduction stimulus. This phenomenon is called crossover. When unrecognized crossover occurs, the examiner will report a negative Rinne (BC > AC), indicating the presence of a conductive hearing loss, when in fact a false-negative Rinne has occurred. To avoid crossover, it is necessary to mask the nontest ear with noise.

The Schwabach test was used to determine whether the patient's hearing by bone conduction was normal or impaired. The test is conducted by presenting a bone-conducted sound to the patient's mastoid process. When the patient no longer hears the sound, the tuning fork is moved quickly to the examiner's mastoid. Assuming that the examiner's bone-conduction hearing is known, the Schwabach test determines whether the patient's bone-conduction hearing is better than, equal to, or worse than the examiner's and is therefore normal or impaired.

Another tuning-fork test with audiologic implications is the Bing test for the occlusion effect. With a sounding tuning fork in the midline position, the examiner gently occludes the patient's external auditory canal with a finger. When middle ear function is normal, the occlusion of the ear canal results in an increase in loudness of the tuning fork with a shift of the sound toward the occluded ear. When there is a greater than 5- to 10-dB conductive hearing loss present, occluding the external canal will have no noticeable effect.

Using tuning-fork tests, the examiner can determine, within certain limitations, whether the patient's hearing loss is conductive or sensorineural, and whether a hearing loss by bone conduction exists. There are, however, many problems inherent in their use, and results can be variable. One difficulty with the Weber test is that some children and adults find it difficult to report where they hear a tone. In addition, patients who have long-standing unilateral sensorineural hearing loss have lost the ability to localize sound and are apt to give tuning-fork results that are inconsistent with their hearing losses.

PURE TONE AUDIOMETRY

The audiogram is a graph of a person's hearing threshold levels reported in dB HL as a function of frequency in Hz. Pure tone signals are presented at the octave frequencies between 250 and 8000 Hz and also at 3000 Hz. A patient is asked to respond to the quietest sound that can be heard. The threshold of hearing is defined as the minimum effective sound pressure of a signal that is capable of evoking an auditory sensation. In audiometry, threshold is recorded as the intensity of a tone at which the patient will respond approximately 50% of the time.

Air-conduction thresholds are measurements made using earphones from an audiometer. The hearing sensitivity of the entire auditory system is tested. Sound travels through the outer and middle ear to the cochlea and auditory nerve on the way to the brainstem and auditory cortex.

The air-conduction pure tone average (PTA) is the average of the hearing levels at frequencies 500, 1000, 2000 Hz—the speech frequency region. Some authors include 3000 Hz in the PTA because of the special importance of hearing at that frequency for understanding speech.

Bone conduction is the measurement made with a vibrating oscillator that tests the hearing sensitivity of the inner ear and auditory structures medial to the inner ear. The bone-conduction vibrator is usually placed on the mastoid process.

The air–bone gap is the difference between the air-conduction threshold and bone-conduction threshold at a test frequency in the same ear. Air-conduction thresholds that are poorer than bone thresholds by 10 dB or more indicate that sound transmission through the middle ear is impaired. The size of the air–bone gap indicates the degree of conductive hearing loss. A negative Rinne tuning-fork finding (BC > AC) is equivalent to the audiometric finding of an air–bone gap. No air–bone gap is found in a sensorineural hearing loss (cochlear and/or eighth nerve pathology).

MASKING

When the possibility of crossover exists during pure-tone testing, masking is introduced into the nontest ear to rule out a response from that side. It is best to assume that a bone-conduction signal stimulates both cochlea simultaneously and that masking is required whenever an air–bone gap is observed. During air-conduction testing, it is best to assume that the signal reaches the opposite cochlea by transmission through the bones of the skull. Therefore, it is necessary to mask when the air-conduction threshold of the test ear exceeds the bone-conduction threshold of the nontest ear by 40 dB or more when standard earphones are used. The use of insert earphones extends the intra-aural attenuation to approximately 70 dB or more, reducing the need for masking and improving test validity. The amount of masking used in any situation is determined by many factors. Narrow band noise is the only acceptable masker for pure-tone testing.

SPEECH AUDIOMETRY

The *speech reception threshold* (SRT) intensity, reported in dB HL, is the threshold at which speech can be understood. The SRT is determined using spondee words, which are two-syllable words with equal stress on each syllable (e.g., hotdog, cowboy, outside).

The *speech awareness threshold* (SAT) is the lowest intensity reported in dB HL at which speech is detected but not understood. SATs are usually obtained if an SRT cannot be determined because of poor word recognition ability.

Word recognition is the ability to discriminate single words presented at a comfortable listening level. The score is the percentage of words correctly identified from a list of 50 phonetically balanced words presented at 40 dB above the SRT (40 dB SL). This was previously called the speech discrimination test.

Most word recognition tests consist of lists of 50 monosyllables representing familiar words that are equally difficult to understand. Undistorted word recognition tests presented in quiet at comfortable loudness levels are not sensitive measures of disorders of the auditory system. Nevertheless, word recognition test results can be useful for diagnostic purposes.

In general, patients with normal hearing and a purely conductive loss have high word recognition scores, between 96 and 100%. Patients with high-frequency or mild flat cochlear hearing loss can also be expected to yield high discrimination scores. Usually, the greater the cochlear hearing loss, the poorer the word recognition score with the degree of discrimination compatible with the magnitude and slope of the pure tone hearing loss. A neural lesion, on the other hand, will often yield word recognition scores that are relatively poorer than may be expected on the basis of examining the pure-tone thresholds.

> **PEARL...** As a diagnostic guideline, word recognition scores that are poorer than predicted from pure-tone thresholds should alert the examiner to the possible presence of a retrocochlear lesion. In these cases additional diagnostic testing to include acoustic reflex threshold and decay and auditory evoked potentials should be administered.

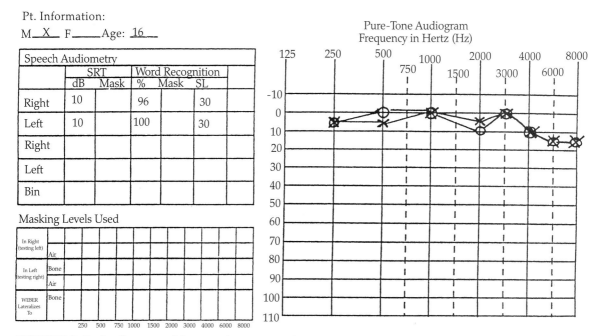

FIGURE 2–3 Audiogram with normal pure-tone thresholds, speech reception thresholds, and word discrimination score.

Figure 2–3 shows an audiogram with normal pure-tone thresholds, speech reception thresholds, and word discrimination score.

One simple measurement of auditory recruitment is the *loudness discomfort level* (LDL) for speech. The test is administered by increasing the intensity of speech while querying the patient about its loudness. The objective is to identify the level at which speech is uncomfortably loud and further increases would be painfully loud. The difference between the patient's SRT and LDL is an indication of the dynamic range for speech. The narrower the range, the greater the evidence of auditory recruitment.

ACOUSTIC IMMITTANCE TESTING

Tympanometry is the measurement of tympanic membrane mobility as a function of pressure changes in the ear canal. A *tympanogram* is its graphic representation, with pressure plotted on the horizontal axis and compliance on the vertical axis. There are three general findings of tympanometry (Fig. 2–4). Jerger labeled these as types A, B, and C, although these terms are not in general use at this time.

A normal notch-shaped tympanogram with maximum compliance (shown by the peak) at +25 to −150 mm H_2O (type A) indicates normal middle ear pressures, implying that eustachian tube function is normal. This finding does not rule out middle ear abnormalities such as stapes ankylosis from otosclerosis.

A broad, flat tympanogram with no point of maximum compliance (type B), assuming that otologic examination finds no evidence of impacted cerumen, polyp, foreign body, or other material filling the external auditory meatus, is consistent with fluid in the middle ear (otitis media, blood, or cerebral spinal fluid are examples depending on the patient history). A flat tympanogram with a large physical volume test indicates the presence of a perforation or patent pressure equalization (PE) tube.

A rounded tympanogram with middle ear pressures more negative than −150 mm H_2O (type C) implies compromised eustachian tube function. Otologic examination would typically find a retracted tympanic membrane (TM) with the possibility of a meniscus or bubbles indicating the presence of fluid in the middle ear.

The *physical volume test* (PVT) is a measurement of the volume of the external auditory

Tympanometry

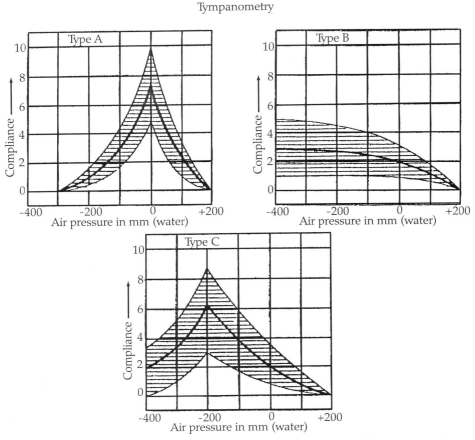

FIGURE 2-4 Three general findings in tympanometry: type A with normal notch-shaped tympanogram and maximum compliance at +25 to −150 mm H₂O; type B, broad flat tympanogram with no point of maximum compliance; and type C, rounded tympanogram with middle ear pressures more negative than −150 mm H₂O.

canal measured in cubic centimeters equivalent volume of air. The PVT depends on the age of the patient. In adolescents and adults, a PVT of >1.5 cc with a flat tympanogram is consistent with the presence of a TM perforation.

Compliance is a measurement of the stiffness or mobility of the middle ear system. Compliance is reported in cubic centimeters equivalent volume of air or in decapascals.

The *acoustic reflex (AR) test* is a measurement of the threshold of contraction of the stapedius muscle to an acoustic signal of high intensity. This test is used to evaluate the function of the cochlea, the ascending auditory nerve, and the brainstem reflex arc including the descending pathways to the facial nerve. Ipsilat-

eral stimulation results in bilateral stimulation of the stapedius muscles.

The AR threshold occurs between 70 and 90 dB HL in the normal ear, which is also 70 to 90 dB SL. An acoustic reflex threshold at less than 40 dB SL in an ear with sensorineural hearing loss indicates the presence of auditory recruitment.

Acoustic reflex decay is a test for excessive adaptation of the acoustic reflex through prolonged acoustic stimulation. Adaptation is defined as relaxation of the stapedius muscle in the presence of continuous stimulation. Acoustic reflex decay is present when adaptation exceeds 50% in 10 seconds, suggesting retrocochlear pathology including an acoustic nerve tumor.

SITE-OF-LESION TESTS

The *auditory brainstem response test* (ABR) entails recording small neuroelectric potentials originating from the auditory nerve to the high brainstem. Obtained through the use of an averaging computer, five waves occurring in the first 10 msec following the stimulus are used clinically, while the sixth wave is ignored for clinical purposes. Labeled waves I through V, the source of the potentials can be easily remembered through the mnemonic ECOLI (Fig. 2–5):

> E = eighth nerve—waves I and II
> C = cochlear nucleus—wave III
> O = olivary complex—wave IV
> L = lateral lemniscus—wave V
> I = inferior colliculus—wave VI

Using standard circumaural earphones, the latency of each wave is approximately 0.5 msec longer than its label; for example, wave I is 1.5 msec, wave II is 2.5 msec, etc. The standard deviation of each wave is approximately 0.2 msec.

The clinical uses of ABR include the following:

1. Neurologic: to determine site of lesion within the auditory pathways of the auditory nerve and brainstem. For example, a wave V interaural latency difference of >0.2 to 0.3 msec (when hearing is symmetrical) indicates the possibility of a retrocochlear lesion in the ear with the prolonged finding.
2. Audiometric: to determine estimates of hearing sensitivity in neonates, infants, and others unable to cooperate during routine audiometry. Click stimuli provide estimates of hearing in the 2000- to 4000-Hz range, and tone bursts (tone pips) provide low-frequency information.

Electrocochleography (ECoG) is a special evoked potential test that measures the summation potential (SP)/action potential (AP) ratio from the cochlea. An SP/AP ratio >0.5 is consistent with a diagnosis of endolympathic hydrops in patients with Meniere's disease.

Otoacoustic emissions (OAEs), called cochlear echoes, are literally small echoes from hair-cell activity within the cochlea in response to acoustic stimulation. The healthy cochlea responds with these echoes every time it processes sound; damaged cochleas do not. OAEs are frequently used for infant hearing screening and to monitor the status of the cochlea due to noise exposure or ototoxic medications. The OAE is present if hearing is equal or better than 30 dB HL and absent if a hearing loss exceeds 30 dB HL.

Electronystagmography (ENG) is a test that measures eye movements of the dizzy patient. The ENG can help localize between peripheral vestibular and central nervous system (CNS) pathology.

Central auditory testing is used to identify central auditory processing disorders (CAPDs) that can be defined as the impaired ability to attend, discriminate, comprehend, and remember auditory information despite normal hearing sensitivity. CAPD results from CNS dysfunction. Symptoms of CAPD are often more pronounced with competing speech, speech in noise, or other poor acoustic environments. CAPD in children can result in poor performance in the classroom. Adults with CAPD

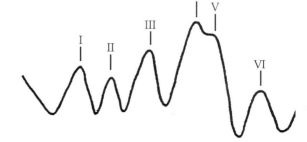

FIGURE 2–5 Normal auditory brainstem response (ABR) with six waves from five different anatomic sites.

often have difficulty in vocational and social situations. The test battery used to identify CAPD consists of a battery of sensitized speech tests that include filtered words, speech in noise, and competing words and sentences.

ASSESSMENT OF HEARING HANDICAP

In the assessment of hearing handicap the terms *hearing impairment, handicap,* and *disability* convey different meanings. Hearing impairment means a deviation in auditory structure or function. Hearing handicap means the disadvantage imposed by a hearing loss on a person's daily communication. Hearing disability is the determination of compensation for the loss of function caused by a hearing impairment that is sufficient to cause a hearing handicap. In general, the size of the hearing disability award should be in direct proportion to the extent of the hearing handicap.

For purposes of discussing test results with patients, many clinicians use adjective descriptions to designate the magnitude of the hearing impairment. These terms are not standardized and do not take into account word recognition ability and other factors. A commonly used scale is as follows:

▼ Normal hearing = 0 to 20 dB HL
▼ Mild loss = 21 to 40 dB HL
▼ Moderate loss = 41 to 55 dB HL
▼ Moderately severe loss = 56 to 70 dB HL
▼ Severe loss = 71 to 90 dB HL
▼ Profound loss = >90 dB HL

A mild to moderate hearing loss will usually cause noticeable difficulty in communication for adults, and it can have a serious effect on speech and language development in children.

Persons with a severe hearing loss can rarely understand or hear speech well enough to communicate without visual cues or amplification.

For persons with a profound hearing loss, communication is usually nonauditory, and they are sometimes candidates for cochlear implants.

Many different formulas have been used for assigning percentage loss of hearing handicap for disability determination. The American Academy of Otolaryngology–Head and Neck Surgery (AAO-HNS) recommends a formula based on the patient's average hearing level for thresholds at 500, 1000, 2000, and 3000 Hz. The monaural percentage loss is computed by taking that average minus 25 dB (the low "fence" where handicap presumably begins) multiplied by 0.015 (1.5%).

AUDIOMETRIC INDICATORS OF SITE OF LESION IN THE AUDITORY SYSTEM

Typically, patients with conductive lesions have an air–bone gap and normal word recognition. If eustachian tube function is abnormal, the patient will have an abnormal tympanogram.

Patients with cochlear lesions have a loss of word discrimination that is reduced proportionately to the degree of hearing loss, and the presence of auditory recruitment. Patients with cochlear hearing loss also have a normal tympanogram with acoustic reflexes at low sensation levels (SLs). They do not show acoustic reflex decay, they have absent OAEs, and they have normal ABRs unless the hearing loss exceeds 70 dB HL.

Patients with a unilateral acoustic tumor show a unilateral high-frequency sensorineural hearing loss, disproportionately reduced word recognition ability when compared to the degree of hearing loss, and decreased word recognition ability at high stimulus intensities. The latter is called "performance-intensity word recognition rollover functions" (known as PB rollover) and is obtained by testing for a word recognition score at the most comfortable listening level (MCL) and again at a high intensity (e.g., 90 dB HL). Performance decrements are commonly observed at high intensities when eighth nerve and brainstem lesions are present. Patients with cochlear lesions show little or no PB rollover.

> **PEARL...** Any unexplained unilateral high-frequency sensorineural hearing loss with reduced word recognition scores should be investigated to rule out the possibility of acoustic neuroma.

Patients with auditory nerve lesions also show decruitment, abnormally rapid auditory adaptation, a normal tympanogram, and elevated acoustic reflex thresholds with acoustic reflex decay or absent acoustic reflexes. They also show abnormal auditory brainstem responses with prolonged latency of response or absent waveforms.

HEARING AIDS

Selection and fitting of hearing aids can be achieved on patients with all types and degrees of hearing loss. Any age patient (infant to geriatric) can be fit with hearing aids. Counseling patients on realistic expectations with the hearing aid and on proper care and use is vital to successful hearing aid use. The basic function of a hearing aid is to amplify sound at the frequencies where hearing loss is present. If a patient has poor word recognition, a hearing aid will not improve the understanding ability but will amplify sounds so they can be heard.

Types and styles of hearing aids include behind-the-ear hearing aids (BTE), in-the-ear hearing aids (ITE), in-the-canal hearing aids (ITC), and completely-in-the-canal hearing aids (CIC). Eyeglass hearing aids and body aids are infrequently seen.

Hearing aid technology has improved greatly over the past 10 years. The type of circuitry inside the hearing aid is most important, but different technologies can be fit into any size hearing aid:

▼ Conventional technology: The hearing aid is manufactured with circuitry inside that is specific for the hearing loss. There is little flexibility available with this type of circuitry.

▼ Programmable: A computer is used to program the hearing aid, resulting in substantial flexibility. If a patient's hearing loss changes, the hearing aid can be reprogrammed to fit the current need.

▼ Digital: This type of programmable hearing aid changes the acoustic signal into a digital signal, with subsequent improvement in sound quality and noise reduction. This is the most advanced hearing aid on the market,

and is therefore more expensive than the other types.

Recent hearing aids are minicomputers that sample and process sound >40,000 times per second. They selectively amplify sounds of greater hearing loss. They have automatic volume control that amplifies more in quiet surroundings and less in loud backgrounds. They provide excellent hearing results compared to old-style conventional hearing aids.

> **PEARL...** It is important to remember that a majority of hearing aid users have a sensorineural hearing loss. There is no truth to the old saying that people with sensorineural hearing loss cannot benefit from a hearing aid.

BALANCE ASSESSMENT

The first approach to balance assessment is taking a history that includes the patient's report of balance problems. Factors include:

1. Vertigo: a sense of movement, usually rotatory in nature—a true spinning sensation

2. Unsteadiness: a loss of equilibrium described as "almost falling" or "my balance is off"

3. Light-headedness: a feeling often related to quick positional changes

4. Dizziness: a disturbed sense of relationship to space

The onset of the balance disorder, the frequency and duration of symptoms, and whether they are episodic or constant are important to the clinical diagnosis. In addition, it is necessary to obtain information on associated otologic complaints, previous otologic surgery, head trauma, straining, and diving. The patient's history of medications including use of ototoxic/vestibulotoxic medicine should be obtained. A medical history to evaluate diabetes, thyroid disease, cardiovascular disease, eye disease, and infectious disease should be obtained. Finally, the patient is evaluated for CNS symptoms such as loss of consciousness, seizure, confusion, memory loss, peripheral weakness, numbness, dysphagia, blurred or loss of vision.

The otolaryngologist's goal is to distinguish between peripheral and central causes of balance problems.

SPECIAL CONSIDERATION

Balance is controlled by visual, vestibular, and proprioceptive systems, and all need to be considered in the evaluation of balance disorders.

CLINICAL TESTS

Clinical tests include the Romberg, in which the patient stands with feet together, arms folded across the chest, and eyes closed. The test may be made more difficult by having the patient extend the arms and stand in a tandem position. Patients with acute unilateral labyrinthine lesions sway and fall toward the damaged side.

Tandem walking is performed with eyes open, heel-to-toe walking. This is primarily a test of cerebellar function because vision compensates for chronic vestibular and proprioceptive deficits. Tandem walking with eyes closed provides a better test of vestibular function as long as cerebellar and proprioceptive function are intact. The patient will fall toward the damaged side.

Past pointing is evaluated with eyes closed and an extended arm. The patient then attempts to point from finger to nose. Consistent deviation to one side is past pointing. Patients with acute peripheral vestibular damage past point toward the side of the loss.

Examination for eyes-open spontaneous nystagmus is conducted both with and without Froenzel lenses.

PEARL••• Eyes-open nystagmus connotes central nervous system disease unless the patient has experienced recent acute vestibular disease or loss of vestibular function.

ELECTRONYSTAGMOGRAPHY

Electronystagmographic (ENG) examination includes the following:

1. Eye movement tests
   a. saccade: rapid eye movements made to bring a target onto the fovea
   b. smooth pursuit: pendular tracking
   c. gaze: fixation on a target 20 to 30 degrees to the right and left for at least 30 seconds
2. Positioning tests: slowly positioning the patient with supine, right lateral, and left lateral positions
3. Positional testing (Dix Hallpike maneuver): with the head turned to the extreme right/left the patient is quickly moved back to a head hanging position for 60 seconds. The test is repeated to the opposite side. The classic finding of benign paroxysmal positioning vertigo (BPPV), which is an end-organ disease (cupulolithiasis) includes brief down-beating nystagmus, accompanied by vertigo, that fatigues (is not present) on repeated positioning.

During caloric testing each ear is irrigated with 250 mL of water at 30° and 40°C for 40 seconds (with several minutes' rest between each stimulus). The caloric stimulus results in a brisk eye movement that has a slow (vestibular) phase and fast (central correcting) phase. Nystagmus is said to be in the direction of the fast phase (clinical consensus). The direction of eye movement can be remembered with the mnemonic COWS: cold opposite, warm same. That is, eye movement is away from the cold stimulus and toward the warm stimulus. Velocity of eye movement is calculated and compared from side to side. A "weaker" caloric response on one side of 20% or greater is interpreted as a peripheral vestibular lesion on that side. Because of the anatomy of the system, caloric examination tests only the horizontal semicircular canal. A summary of ENG abnormalities is shown on Table 2–1.

PITFALL••• ENG testing is invalidated if the patient is taking vestibular suppressants or has been drinking alcohol.

TABLE 2–1 SUMMARY OF ELECTRONYSTAGMOGRAPHY (ENG) ABNORMALITIES

Test and Abnormality	Location of Lesion
Saccade test	
Multiple-step saccades	Always CNS (cerebellar system)
Hypermetric saccades	Always CNS (cerebellar system)
Internuclear opthalmoplegia	Always CNS (medial longitudinal fasciculus)
Slowing	Always CNS
Gaze test	
Spontaneous nystagmus, by visual fixation	Usually peripheral vestibular system (ear suppressed in opposite direction of nystagmus)
Spontaneous nystagmus, not suppressed by visual fixation	Always CNS
Unilateral gaze nystagmus	Always CNS
Bilateral gaze nystagmus	Always CNS
Congenital nystagmus	Always CNS (benign)
Square wave jerks	Always CNS (cerebellar system)
Periodic alternating nystagmus	Always CNS
Rebound nystagmus	Always CNS (cerebellar system)
Downbeating nystagmus	Always CNS (cerebellum or lower brainstem)
Upbeating nystagmus	Always CNS (cerebellum or medulla)
Tracking test	
Saccadic pursuit	Always CNS
Disconjugate pursuit	Always CNS
Optokinetic test	
Weak response	
Unilateral	Always CNS
Bilateral	Always CNS
Positional test	
Positional nystagmus, suppressed by visual fixation	
Direction-fixed	Peripheral vestibular system (either ear) or CNS
Direction-changing in different head positions	Peripheral vestibular system (either ear) or CNS
Direction-changing in single head position	Always CNS
Positional nystagmus, not suppressed by visual fixation	Always CNS
Hallpike maneuver	
Benign paroxysmal positional nystagmus	
Unilateral	Usually peripheral vestibular system (undermost ear)
Bilateral	Usually peripheral vestibular system (both ears)
Any other nystagmus	Usually CNS

Continued on p. 26

TABLE 2–1 SUMMARY OF ELECTRONYSTAGMOGRAPHY (ENG) ABNORMALITIES (*Continued*)

Test and Abnormality	Location of Lesion
Caloric test	
Unilateral weakness	Always peripheral vestibular system (weak ear)
Directional preponderance	Peripheral vestibular system (either ear) or CNS
Bilateral weakness	Usually peripheral vestibular system (both ears)
Failure of fixation suppression	Always CNS
Caloric inversion	Always CNS
Caloric perversion	Always CNS

CNS, central nervous system.

PLATFORM POSTUROGRAPHY AND ROTATIONAL CHAIR TESTS

There are other computerized methods of assessing balance function with sway platform posturography and rotational chair testing. These tests are not in general use, however, and are nonspecific for end-organ or CNS abnormality. One benefit of sway platform posturography is that it simultaneously assesses visual, vestibular, and proprioceptive systems. The test is especially helpful in testing older patients with balance problems who do not have specific vestibular or CNS abnormalities but are at risk for falling.

Some interpretation tidbits are as follows:

▼ All abnormalities on the oculomotor tests, for example, saccades, gaze, and smooth pursuit, indicate CNS disease, not peripheral vestibular lesions.

▼ Eyes-open nystagmus is always a CNS disease unless a recent acute peripheral vestibular lesion exists.

▼ A clinically significant difference on caloric testing is 20%, called a "unilateral weakness" or sometimes "canal paresis."

▼ Failure of fixation suppression during caloric testing is a sign of CNS disease.

▼ Positive Hallpike maneuver assists in the diagnosis of benign paroxysmal positioning vertigo (BPPV) that is shown by delayed nystagmus and vertigo, and fatigues on repositioning . . .

▼ There are two theories of the causes of BPPV: (1) canalithiasis, with otoconia floating freely in the endolymph of the canal that move the cupula and fire the neurons of that semicircular canal; and (2) cupulolithiasis, where fragments of otoconia adhere to the cupula, making the ampula gravity-sensitive, increasing the density of the cupula, producing inappropriate deflection of the cupula in certain head positions resulting in vertigo, nystagmus, and nausea.

▼ Symptoms of Meniere's disease include episodic vertigo lasting 45 minutes to hours, roaring tinnitus, low-frequency fluctuating hearing loss, and a feeling of fullness or pressure in the ear.

▼ Episodic vertigo lasting for seconds and associated with looking up or down is compatible with BPPV.

▼ The cerebellar clamp is effective after approximately 3 days so that persons with acute unilateral vestibular lesions begin to compensate in that time period.

▼ Any unexplained unilateral high-frequency sensorineural hearing loss needs to be followed to rule out a possible eighth nerve tumor.

SUGGESTED READINGS

American Academy of Otolaryngology and American Council of Otolaryngology. Guide for the evaluation of hearing handicap. *JAMA* 1979;241:2055.

American-Speech-Language-Hearing Association. On the definition of hearing handicap. *ASHA* 1981;23:293.

Baloh, RW. *Dizziness, Hearing Loss and Tinnitus: The Essentials of Neurotology.* Philadelphia: FA Davis; 1984.

Glasscock M, Cueva RA, Thedinger BA. *Handbook of Vertigo.* New York: Raven Press; 1990.

Hall JW, Mueller HG. *Audiologists' Desk Reference, vol I: Diagnostic Audiology Principles, Procedures and Protocols.* San Diego: Singular Publishing Group; 1997.

Hefner ST. *The Audiogram Workbook.* New York: Thieme; 1998.

Jacobson GP, Newman CW, Kartush JM. *Handbook of Balance Function Testing.* Baltimore: Mosby Year Book; 1993.

Møller AR, Jannetta PJ. Neural generators of the brainstem auditory evoked potentials. In: Nodar RH, Barber C, eds. *Evoked Potentials II: The Second International Evoked Potentials Symposium.* Boston: Butterworth; 1984:137–144.

Roeser RJ. *Roeser's Audiology Desk Reference: A Guide to the Practice of Audiology.* New York: Thieme; 1996.

Chapter 3

CONGENITAL DISORDERS

Rick A. Friedman

There are a multitude of developmental pathways in operation during the period of temporal bone morphogenesis. Thus it is no wonder that there are a number of congenital disorders affecting the many complex structures in this region. Abnormal development of temporal bone structures can result in conductive hearing loss, sensorineural hearing loss, facial nerve dysfunction, or any combination of these. Aberrancies in development can result from chemical teratogens, prenatal or perinatal infectious diseases, or abnormalities of gene expression or function. Modern scientific methodologies are shedding new light on the molecular mechanisms behind many of these problems. For example, molecular genetics has helped to identify single genes responsible for the normal development of the inner, middle, and outer ear, structures once thought to arise independently.

CONGENITAL DEAFNESS

An estimated 50% of congenital inner ear diseases are genetically acquired. With recent advances in technology has come a tremendous increase in the number of available genetic markers. Improved mapping resolution combined with advances in phenotypic identification has led to the chromosomal mapping and,

in a few instances, the molecular characterization of several forms of inherited deafness. See Chapter 91 for more information on congenital deafness syndromes.

AURAL ATRESIAS

Aural atresias are characterized by aplasia or hypoplasia of the external auditory canal (EAC) and tubotympanum. Abnormalities of the pinna (microtia) are frequently associated with aplasias or hypoplasias of the middle ear. These developmental abnormalities are often sporadic and isolated but can be part of a syndrome such as Treacher Collins, Nager, or Goldenhar. Aural atresia occurs in approximately 1 in 10,000 to 20,000 live births. Unilateral atresia is three times more common than bilateral atresia, and the atresias are most commonly osseous. Cartilaginous atresias also occur, resulting in complete soft tissue occlusion or canal stenosis.

PEARL... Although EAC stenosis may not be associated with hearing loss, stenoses of less than 2-mm diameter are frequently associated with EAC cholesteatomas requiring surgical therapy.

SPECIAL CONSIDERATION

Aural atresias are most common in males and most often involve the right ear. Although some cases of atresia are associated with normal pinnae, the vast majority demonstrate microtia. In general, the severity of the microtia correlates with the severity of the atresia of both the EAC and the middle ear. Aberrancies of the path of the facial nerve are also more often associated with more severe microtias and occur in approximately 25%.

The pinna arises from the first and second branchial arches, the so-called hillocks of His (Table 3–1). Its development is completed by approximately the third month of gestation. The EAC is derived from the first branchial cleft and develops by invagination of the ectoderm into the underlying plug of mesenchymal tissue. This process is completed by 7 months of gestation.

The middle ear cleft (tubotympanum) arises from the first and second branchial pouches. Through a process of invagination and mesenchymal dissolution, the middle ear cleft mucosa expands and ultimately contacts the epithelium of the EAC, forming the tympanic membrane.

The mesenchymal tissue of the ossicular chain is derived from the first and second branchial arches, Meckel's and Reichert's cartilage, respectively. Meckel's cartilage forms the head, neck, and lateral process of the malleus, as well as the body and short process of the incus.

TABLE 3–1 DEVELOPMENT OF THE AURICLE

First Branchial Arch	Second Branchial Arch
First hillock—tragus	Fourth hillock—antihelix
Second hillock—helical crus	Fifth hillock—antitragus
Third hillock—helix	Sixth hillock—lobule and lower helix

Reichert's cartilage contributes to the long process of the malleus and the long and lenticular processes of the incus. The suprastructure of the stapes is derived from second arch mesenchyme; however, the footplate originates from the otic capsule. The ossicular chain is usually developed by the fourth month and the mesenchyme surrounding the ossicular chain has almost completely disappeared by the eighth month.

PEARL... Facial nerve anatomy can be anomolous in cases of temporal bone hypoplasias and atresias. This abnormality often manifests as an abnormally acute angle at the second genu (60 degrees rather than the normal 120 degrees). Additionally, congenital absence of the oval window is typically associated with an aberrant facial nerve course. In these cases the facial nerve is found more inferiorly, often overlying the promontory.

After careful examination of a newborn with aural atresia, an assessment of auditory function should be made with auditory brainstem response audiology.

SPECIAL CONSIDERATION

Sensorineural hearing loss is associated with atresia in about one quarter to one-half of cases. Unilateral atresias with normal hearing in the uninvolved ear do not require amplification. Bilateral atresia cases should be fitted with bone conduction hearing aids at the earliest possible date.

Classification schemes for aural atresias have been developed to guide surgical management. The first of these was developed in 1955 by Altmann. This classification scheme has recently been expanded upon by De La Cruz and considers minor and major malformations based on the following: (1) mastoid pneumatization, (2) anatomy of the oval window niche, (3) course of the facial nerve, and (4) anatomy of the inner ear. Minor malformations are those demonstrating favorable anatomy for each of the four criteria.

Schuknecht's classification is based on both clinical and surgical observations. Jahrsdoerfer et al have created a 10-point grading system for guiding surgical management and predicting postoperative success (Table 3–2). These authors feel a score of eight or better portends the greatest likelihood of surgical success. These classification systems require high-resolution computed tomography (CT) scans of the temporal bone.

PEARL••• Most investigators do not recommend obtaining these scans until the child is nearing the age of surgical candidacy (approximately age 6, after auricular reconstruction).

TABLE 3–2 GRADING SYSTEM OF CANDIDACY FOR SURGERY OF CONGENITAL AURAL ATRESIA

Parameter	Points
Stapes present	2
Oval window open	1
Middle ear space	1
Facial nerve normal	1
Malleus-incus complex present	1
Mastoid well pneumatized	1
Incus-stapes connection	1
Round window normal	1
Appearance of external ear	1
Total available points	10

Rating	Type of Candidate
10	Excellent
9	Very good
8	Good
7	Fair
6	Marginal
≤5	Poor

From Jahrsdoerfer RAQ, Yeakley JW, Aguilar EA, et al. Grading system for the selection of patients with congenital aural atresia. *Am J Otol* 1992; 13:6–12. Reprinted by permission of *Otology and Neurotology,* formerly the *American Journal of Otology.*

Congenital aural atresias may be associated with cholesteatoma. For example, patients with Schuknecht's type A or B are at risk for canal cholesteatomas. Patients with canal stenoses or atresias of less than 2-mm diameter are at significant risk for cholesteatomas of the EAC. Furthermore, middle ear and mastoid cholesteatomas have been identified in approximately 14% of atresias.

The success of atresiaplasty has come with tremendous refinements in tympanoplasty, canaloplasty, and meatoplasty. Surgical approaches can be divided into anterior, transmastoid, and modified anterior. All patients undergo general anesthesia without muscle relaxants. The facial nerve monitor is employed in every case.

A standard postauricular incision is performed with care not to expose the costal cartilage auricular graft. After incision of the periosteum, it is elevated to expose the mastoid posteriorly and the temporomandibular joint anteriorly.

SPECIAL CONSIDERATION

During surgical reconstruction care must be taken to avoid injury to an aberrantly located facial nerve.

Temporalis fascia is harvested in the usual fashion.

The anterior approach begins with careful drill dissection at the level of linea temporalis just posterior to the glenoid fossa. The dissection is carefully continued with a diamond burr until the epitympanum and ossicular mass are identified. An ear canal of approximately 1.5 times normal is created with the diamond burr. A 6 cm × 6 cm split-thickness skin graft (0.012 inch) harvested from the abdomen is used to line the newly created canal after the tympanic membrane graft has been placed. It is important to stent the external canal and meatoplasty to prevent stenosis. The modified anterior approach is used in patients with thick atresia plates. In this technique, a small posterior antrotomy is performed in an effort to identify the lateral semicircular canal for orientation. The remainder of the procedure is as described above.

The transmastoid technique involves beginning more posteriorly and creating a mastoid cavity. This technique has largely been supplanted by the anterior approach.

The results of atresiaplasty depend largely on patient selection. In properly selected patients, one should expect an air–bone gap of less than 30 dB in approximately 70% of patients.

> **PITFALL•••** The most common reason for failure is tympanic membrane graft lateralization.

Other potential complications include restenosis, sensorineural hearing loss, and facial nerve paralysis.

CONGENITAL CHOLESTEATOMA

Cholesteatomas are classified as acquired and congenital. The vast majority of cholesteatomas are acquired. Some authors feel the incidence of congenital cholesteatoma may be higher than reported; however, it remains an infrequent diagnosis.

Congenital cholesteatomas appear to arise from epithelial rests within the embryonic middle ear cleft. These rests fail to resolve in some individuals and result in the proliferation of squamous epithelium within a matrix. Another theory on the pathogenesis of these cholesteatomas suggests that some cases may result from seeding of the inner ear with skin cells circulating in the amniotic fluid.

By definition, congenital cholesteatomas arise in ears with no prior history of chronic otitis media. It is for this reason that they are often identified serendipitously usually during the placement of ventilation tubes. They are typically not associated with hearing loss early in their course. Those that continue to grow unrecognized ultimately come to our attention because of the conductive hearing loss associated with ossicular erosion.

The embryonic epithelial rests are most often identified in the anterior mesotympanum, anterior to the malleus. It is for this reason that the otomicroscopic appearance is one of a whitish mass in the anterosuperior quadrant of the tympanic membrane. Larger cholesteatomas can be found to involve the middle ear and mastoid more diffusely.

Congenital cholesteatomas must be differentiated from simple epithelial pearls within the tympanic membrane. This can often be done in the office but can be clarified by examination under anesthesia and/or radiographic imaging. Other benign and malignant tumors of the middle ear must be considered prior to surgical management.

The surgical management of congenital cholesteatomas depends on their origin and extent. Small anterosuperiorly placed cholesteatomas whose entire extent can be seen through the tympanic membrane can be managed through a transcanal or postauricular approach and a superiorly based tympanotomy flap.

> **PEARL•••** Those patients with more extensive involvement should undergo preoperative imaging to assist in patient and parent preparation and operative planning. Noncontrast, high-resolution CT scans of the temporal bone, in both axial and coronal plains, provide excellent detail for preoperative evaluation.

More extensive cholesteatomas are managed by standard tympanomastoidectomy techniques. Many surgeons prefer a staged intact canal wall approach. Because of the high rate of residual disease, a staged approach, with reexploration in 6 to 7 months, is essential in patients with extensive disease.

SUGGESTED READINGS

Altmann F. Congenital atresia of the ear in man and animals. *Ann Otol Rhinol Laryngol* 1955; 64:824–858.

De La Cruz A, Linthicum FH, Luxford WM. Congenital atresia of the external auditory canal. *Laryngoscope* 1985;95:421–427.

Grundfast KM, Camilon F. External auditory canal stenosis and partial atresia without associated anomalies. *Ann Otol Rhinol Laryngol* 1986;95:505–509.

Harada O, Ishii H. The condition of the auditory ossicles in microtia: findings in 57 middle ear operations. *Plast Reconstr Surg* 1972;50: 48–53.

House HP. Management of congenital ear canal atresia. *Laryngoscope* 1953;63:916–946.

Jahrsdoerfer RA, Cole RR, Gray LE. Advances in congenital aural atresia. *Adv Otolaryngol Head Neck Surg* 1991;5:1–15.

Jahrsdoerfer RAQ, Yeakley JW, Aguilar EA, et al. Grading system for the selection of patients with congenital aural atresia. *Am J Otol* 1992; 13:6–12.

Schuknecht HF. Congenital aural atresia and congenital middle ear cholesteatoma. In: Nadol JB, Schuknecht HF, eds. *Surgery of the Ear and Temporal Bone.* New York: Raven Press; 1993:263–274.

Chapter 4

FUNCTIONAL DISORDERS

Bradley W. Kesser and Rick A. Friedman

HEARING LOSS

In the strict sense, functional hearing loss may refer to pseudohypacusis; that is, the patient complains of hearing loss when there is none. Motivation for pseudohypacusis may include the desire for attention, legal issues, disability reimbursement, or malingering. This type of functional hearing loss is not discussed here, but a good review of pseudohypacusis and how to evaluate and "catch" patients falsifying hearing loss may be found in Qiu et al.

For the purposes of this chapter, functional hearing loss means organic hearing loss, that is, true pathology. Any discussion of hearing loss and its evaluation must address the nature or the mechanism of the hearing loss—conductive or sensorineural. This chapter briefly addresses both types of hearing loss and discusses their evaluation and treatment.

A conductive hearing loss is any loss that results from an inability of the ear to bring, or conduct, sound energy to the inner ear. Sound energy is simply compression and rarefaction of air molecules. Sound travels in waves, as the leading edge of the sound wave consists of compressed air molecules. Behind the compression, the molecules are widely dispersed, called rarefaction. The sound waves are collected by the auricle and directed into the external auditory canal where they travel down the canal and move or vibrate the tympanic membrane. Vibration of the tympanic membrane causes the middle ear ossicular chain to vibrate—malleus to incus to stapes. The stapes acts as a piston; it moves up and down (or side to side for proper orientation).

Movement of the stapes footplate at the oval window sends a fluid wave into the vestibule and into the cochlea. The middle ear conductive mechanism therefore converts sound energy (in the form of sound waves) into mechanical energy (in the form of movement of the middle ear bones). Any abnormality or pathology up to this point will result in a conductive hearing loss—an inability of the outer and middle ear to "conduct" sound to the inner ear.

A conductive hearing loss may be as simple as a cerumen impaction or may be as complex as a subtle ossicular deformity. Several causes of conductive hearing losses are shown in Table 4–1.

From this point, the mechanical energy of the fluid wave inside the inner ear causes displacement of the delicate hair cells along the basilar membrane. Movement of hair cells causes ions to move across natural gradients, or differences in concentrations. The flow of ions sets up a potential—the electrical signal. The electrical signal travels along bipolar neurons whose cell bodies are located in the modiolus. Their axons compose the cochlear nerve, and terminal

TABLE 4–1 CAUSES OF CONDUCTIVE HEARING LOSS

Cerumen impaction

Otitis externa

Osteoma/exostoses of the external auditory canal

Otitis media (acute or chronic)

Tympanic membrane perforation

Middle ear mass

Cholesteatoma

Adenoma

Neuroma

Plasmacytoma

Glomus tumor (jugulare or tympanicum)

Carcinoma

Ossicular erosion from chronic otitis media, cholesteatoma

Temporal bone trauma (generally, longitudinal fractures)

Hemotympanum

Disruption of the ossicular chain

Otosclerosis

Tympanosclerosis

Congenital aural atresia (congenital absence of the ear canal and tympanic membrane with fixation of the ossicles)

TABLE 4–2 COMMON CAUSES OF SENSORINEURAL HEARING LOSS

Presbycusis

Noise-induced hearing loss

Ototoxicity

Meniere's disease

Auditory neuropathy

Acoustic neuroma (vestibular schwannoma)

Autoimmune sensorineural hearing loss

Viral labyrinthitis (including idiopathic sudden sensorineural hearing loss)

Bacterial labyrinthitis

Otosyphilis

Perilymph fistula

Temporal bone trauma (generally a transverse fracture through the otic capsule)

Enlarged vestibular aqueduct syndrome

Syndromic hereditary hearing loss (e.g., Waardenburg's, Usher's)

Nonsyndromic hereditary hearing loss

Congenital inner ear anomalies (e.g., Mondini's deformity)

boutons end in the cochlear nucleus where the first synapse is made. From the cochlear nucleus, the signal travels to higher brain centers.

The inner ear, therefore, converts mechanical energy into electrical energy that travels along neurons to the brain. Any pathology or disruption of this delicate system—inner ear to brainstem—results in a sensorineural hearing loss. Different causes of sensorineural hearing losses are shown in Table 4–2.

The term *sensorineural* implies two components to this delicate inner ear system—sensory and neural. The sensory component refers to the hair cells, as they are sensory end organs. They are the receptors for the hearing organ. The neural component refers to the cochlear nerve and nucleus. Dysfunction in either of these structures results in a sensorineural loss. Years ago, scientists were not able to separate these two components. With the introduction of otoacoustic emissions (OAEs), we can now differentiate a sensory loss from a neural loss.

SPECIAL CONSIDERATION

The presence of otoacoustic emissions signals functioning hair cells; absence of OAEs implies impairment in the hair cells themselves (a purely sensory loss).

Treatment for sensory versus neural hearing loss is no different, so OAEs have limited clinical applicability.

PATIENT EVALUATION

The history of the hearing loss is the first step in patient evaluation. When did the hearing loss start? Is the onset of hearing loss sudden or gradual? Is the hearing loss accompanied by associated symptoms of otorrhea, dizziness, otalgia, tinnitus, pressure, etc.? Is there a family history of hearing loss? A history of noise exposure or ototoxic medication? How is the patient's general health? What medications is the patient taking?

The physical examination includes otoscopy, a general otolaryngologic exam, and tuning fork tests. Tuning forks will help sort out whether the loss is conductive or sensorineural. On the Weber exam, a conductive loss lateralizes to the affected ear; a sensorineural loss lateralizes to the contralateral ear. The Rinne test pits bone conduction against air conduction by holding the fork behind the ear on the mastoid and asking the patient if the tone is louder behind the ear on the bone or in front of the ear through the air. Louder on the bone signifies a conductive loss—the middle ear is not efficiently conducting the sound waves to the inner ear. Finally, the audiometric exam is absolutely crucial. In cases of conductive hearing losses, the patient will have an air–bone gap, which is defined as a difference in hearing level between air conduction and bone conduction. Sensorineural losses will show air and bone conduction on the same line.

SENSORINEURAL HEARING LOSSES

Presbycusis

Perhaps the most common cause of sensorineural hearing loss, presbycusis affects millions of Americans each year. The pathophysiology of presbycusis is unknown, but is thought to be a progressive loss of hair cells in the cochlea. Presbycusis generally manifests initially as a high-frequency loss with progressive losses into the lower frequencies. Complete deafness from presbycusis is rare. Treatment at this time consists of hearing amplification.

Noise-Induced Hearing Loss

Exposure to loud noises over an extended period of time results in an audiogram with a characteristic "notch" or loss at 4000 Hz. As the hearing loss progresses, the notch widens to encompass higher and lower frequencies. Screening for noise exposure (military service, gun shooting, rock concerts, factory work, aircraft flying), especially ongoing noise exposure, is very important in the history. Occupational

TABLE 4–3 OCCUPATIONAL SAFETY AND HEALTH ADMINISTRATION (OSHA) GUIDELINES ON OCCUPATIONAL NOISE EXPOSURE—PERMISSIBLE NOISE EXPOSURES

Duration Per Day (Hours)	Sound Level (dB)
8	90
6	92
4	95
3	97
2	100
1.5	102
1	105
0.5	110
<0.25	115

hearing loss is also important to document, as the Occupational Safety and Health Administration (OSHA) has established guidelines and recommendations for minimizing occupational noise exposure (Table 4–3). Hearing protection (inserts or earmuffs) is critical for these patients; hearing rehabilitation is limited to standard amplification.

Ototoxicity

Screening for exposure to ototoxic medications is also an important part of the history. Patients with a history of malignancy may have been put on a platinum-based regimen and suffered high-frequency sensorineural loss. A list of potentially ototoxic medications is given in Table 4–4. Hearing rehabilitation involves discontinuing or changing the medication if the patient is

TABLE 4–4 COMMON OTOTOXIC MEDICATIONS

Aminoglycoside antibiotics

Macrolide antibiotics (erythromycin)

Vancomycin

Platinum-based chemotherapeutic agents (cisplatin, carboplatin)

Quinine

Salicylates (aspirin)

Loop diuretics (furosemide, bumetanide)

continuing to take it, and standard hearing amplification if the hearing is still serviceable.

Meniere's Disease

Hearing loss in Meniere's disease is characteristically low frequency early in the disease. Later in the course, the audiogram becomes flat with a moderate to severe sensorineural loss. Of course, in Meniere's disease the hearing loss is accompanied by episodes of vertigo, tinnitus, and often a pressure or fullness in the affected ear. Medical treatment is both symptomatic and directed, with antiemetics and antihistamines for the nausea and dizziness, and diuretics aimed at restoring the natural fluid balance in the inner ear.

Surgery for Meniere's disease has also been successful. Patients with Meniere's disease are most incapacitated by dizziness. The endolymphatic sac procedures are designed to open the natural drainage pathway for labyrinthine fluid. Ablative procedures destroy the labyrinth when the hearing is poor (labyrinthectomy), or section the vestibular nerve to interrupt vestibular input to the brain while preserving hearing input. For a more complete review of Meniere's disease and its treatment, see LaRouere (1996).

Acoustic Neuroma

Patients with acoustic neuromas present with an asymmetric sensorineural hearing loss. Acoustic neuromas can also be associated with tinnitus and subtle balance problems.

> **PEARL...** Any patient with an asymmetric sensorineural hearing loss, especially when the speech discrimination is out of proportion to the pure tone average (poorer speech discrimination), should be screened for a retrocochlear lesion. Magnetic resonance imaging (MRI) with gadolinium contrast is the gold standard examination.

Sudden Sensorineural Hearing Loss

Very rarely, patients will experience a sudden loss of hearing with no explanation or prodrome. An audiogram confirms the hearing loss.

Imbalance, dizziness, tinnitus, and aural fullness will sometimes accompany the hearing loss. It may occur after an upper respiratory infection or other illness. Idiopathic sudden sensorineural hearing loss is a diagnosis of exclusion. The pathophysiology is thought to result from a viral infection, but a vascular event ("mini-stroke" of the ear) is another possibility.

Certain screening examinations must be undertaken to rule out other causes. These include MRI with contrast to rule out acoustic neuroma and perhaps screening blood work such as microhemagglutination–*Treponema pallidum* (MHA-TP), erythrocyte sedimentation rate, rheumatoid factor, and antinuclear antibodies to rule out leutic or autoimmune (and otherwise treatable) causes.

In the absence of a clear etiology, we recommend a course of steroids (generally prednisone starting at 1 to 2 mg/kg and tapering over 2 weeks).

> ## CONTROVERSY
>
> The role of antivirals (acyclovir, Famvir) is controversial.

Many patients do recover some hearing with idiopathic sudden sensorineural hearing loss; vestibular symptoms, if present, will resolve.

CONDUCTIVE HEARING LOSSES

In most cases, the etiology of a conductive hearing loss can be determined on the basis of the physical and otoscopic examinations.

Cerumen Impaction

Removal of the impacted wax can be rewarding for both physician and patient. A "cure" for hearing loss is rare and gratifying. But patients should be cautioned never to use Q-tips in their ears!

Otitis Externa

Patients with otitis externa generally complain of otalgia with otorrhea with some hearing loss. These symptoms often follow manipulation/

trauma to the ear (with Q-tips) or water exposure. Pain with auricular manipulation and an erythematous, edematous canal full of debris are the classic signs. Treatment is local—debridement and cleansing of the external canal and topical antibiotic drops. The inflammation will settle down in a matter of days, and the hearing loss will resolve.

Other diseases of the external auditory canal can cause hearing loss. New bone growth in the form of exostoses or osteomas can grow to obstruct completely the canal and prevent sound waves from reaching the tympanic membrane. Surgery in needed to remove this bone growth and prevent canal cholesteatoma formation.

> **PEARL...** Cancers of the canal can present with hearing loss and a draining ear refractory to medical management. Any such ear must be biopsied to rule out carcinoma.

Otitis Media

Fluid behind the tympanic membrane, whether serous or purulent, will cause hearing loss as a result of the inability of the eardrum and ossicular chain to vibrate properly. Diagnosis is made on physical exam; treatment is aimed at cooling down an acute, infectious process and maximizing eustachian tube function to allow the body to reabsorb this fluid. Trials of steroid nasal sprays, decongestants, and expectorants are warranted before surgical intervention.

Myringotomy can be performed in the office on an adult or in the operating room on a child. Suctioning the fluid in the middle ear space with or without placement of a ventilation tube will allow the middle ear space to aerate and improve middle ear function.

Chronic Otitis Media

A number of conditions associated with chronic otitis media may result in a conduction hearing loss. Perforation of the eardrum interrupts the conduction of sound to the inner ear. Cholesteatoma can erode the ossicles and cause ossicu-

lar discontinuity, leading to a maximal conductive hearing loss (about 60 dB). The most common area of erosion is the incudostapedial joint, which can be seen in the posterior-superior quadrant of the middle ear space.

> **PEARL...** In the presence of a tympanic membrane perforation, a conductive hearing loss of greater than 30 to 35 dB should suggest the possibility of associated ossicular disruption.

Surgery to remove the cholesteatoma, patch the eardrum, and restore the ossicular chain can be performed to make the ear clean and dry and to rehabilitate the hearing. For an excellent discussion of the surgical management of chronic otitis media, see Sheehy and Brackmann (1994).

Otosclerosis

Patients who are found to have a conductive loss in the presence of a clean, dry ear with an intact tympanic membrane are candidates for exploratory tympanotomy. The most likely finding at surgery is a fixed stapes, the result of otosclerosis. Otosclerosis is characterized by new bone growth around the footplate of the stapes. This new bone fixes the footplate, preventing its proper vibration and ability to generate the fluid wave into the cochlea. Surgeons can restore hearing through an operation (the stapedectomy or stapedotomy). The operation involves removing the stapes and the footplate or creating a small window (fenestra) in the footplate and placing a prosthesis from the incus to the oval window. Good candidates for the stapes operation are those patients who reverse their tuning-fork exam (i.e., report that bone conduction is louder than air conduction on the Rinne test) with both the 512-Hz and 1024-Hz forks.

Middle Ear Mass

A patient with a mass in the middle ear will present with a conductive hearing loss secondary to interference with the ossicular chain. Many times, the mass can be seen through the tympanic membrane on otoscopy. Patients with glomus tumors will also have pulsatile tinnitus. Middle ear masses include congenital cholesteatoma, glomus tympanicum or jugulare, middle ear adenoma or adenocarcinoma, osteoma, neuroma (facial nerve or Jacobson's nerve), high jugular bulb, aberrant carotid artery, lymphoma, plasmacytoma, and others. We recommend an imaging study, usually high-resolution temporal bone computed tomography (CT) scanning, prior to any biopsy or surgical intervention for a middle ear mass with an intact tympanic membrane. Imaging will then guide further workup or surgical approach.

CONCLUSION

History, otoscopic examination, and audiometric testing are the key ingredients in evaluating the patient who presents with hearing loss. The first branch point in the workup must be to determine whether the patient has a conductive or sensorineural loss. From that point, key elements of the history and physical will guide the diagnosis and/or further workup. Many surgical procedures in otology/neurotology are very rewarding for patients and surgeons, as they attempt to restore hearing. It is our judgment that decides who will benefit from which intervention. Thorough knowledge of the different causes of hearing loss will enable us to serve our patients with the very best care.

DIZZINESS

The patient who presents to the otolaryngologist–head and neck surgeon with the chief complaint of dizziness can be frustrating and challenging. The key to the diagnosis lies in the history. A very focused and precise history will lead the otolaryngologist down the path to the correct diagnosis and to effective treatment.

THE HISTORY

Taking the history is the most important part of the patient encounter. A few pointed questions will nail down the nature of the dizziness. Keeping the patient focused on the question at hand and being as precise as possible will keep matters clear in the physician's mind and prevent patient rambling. The history should answer the fundamental question, Is this patient's dizziness otogenic?

Before asking about the character of the dizziness, the first question we ask is about the onset of the dizziness. This is a fairly straightforward question that doesn't make the patient define dizziness right away. Is the process acute, subacute, or chronic? Also, does the dizziness come in "waves," "attacks," or "spells?" Or was there a single major attack that has improved to some extent? Dizziness of peripheral vestibular origin tends to come in attacks or spells. Duration of the attack is the next logical follow-up question. Dizziness lasting seconds probably has a different etiology from dizziness lasting hours or days or even constant. Frequency of attacks is our next question: "Do these spells come once a week, three times a day, etc.?"

At this point, the nature of the dizziness is addressed. A patient may describe different kinds of dizziness (true vertigo with imbalance as well as some light-headedness) and may be confused by the frequency and duration questions. Now is the time to nail down as precisely as possible the nature of the dizziness. Is it true vertigo? ("Does the room spin during an attack? Do your eyes flicker? Does it feel like the sensation you experienced when you were a child and turned round and round and then stopped and watched the world spin in front of your eyes?") Yes to these questions indicates true vertigo, which is usually of peripheral vestibular origin. Once the nature of the dizziness is established, it may be easier to get a handle on how often the severe attacks of room-spinning dizziness occur (frequency) and how long they last (duration). Sometimes the attacks are preceded or followed by light-headedness or imbalance; it is important to make this distinction. Symptoms of imbalance are also important to document: Does the patient bump into walls, feel more clumsy, have to hold on to something to ambulate? True imbalance may or may not be of peripheral vestibular origin.

Next, ask about associated symptoms. Does the patient experience aural symptoms—fullness, pressure, tinnitus, hearing loss, otorrhea, or otalgia? Do these symptoms precede, accompany, or follow the dizzy spells? Is the patient nauseated and does he actually vomit? Is there significant fatigue or a feeling of being "wiped out" after an attack? Does anything bring on an attack (e.g., turning the head to one side, rolling over in bed, allergy attack, lifting the head off the pillow, or standing up)? Does anything avert or relieve an attack (taking meclizine, lying still, closing the eyes)?

Finally, how disabling is the patient's dizziness? Can he drive a car? Does he fear going outside? All of these questions are designed to assist the physician and patient in differentiating between peripheral and central vertigo (Table 4–5) and arriving at a proper diagnosis; the more precise and focused the history, the easier and more accurate the diagnosis. Time spent taking an exact history is worth the reward of a proper diagnosis and treatment plan.

PHYSICAL EXAMINATION

The physical examination may help uncover the nature of the dizziness. Always perform an otoscopic examination to make sure there is no evidence of chronic otitis media with a possible labyrinthine fistula. Fluid behind an intact tympanic membrane may be perilymph—a fistula test may give you the diagnosis (see below).

Extraocular motility testing should be performed to examine for spontaneous nystagmus.

TABLE 4–5 FEATURES IN THE HISTORY THAT HELP DISTINGUISH BETWEEN PERIPHERAL AND CENTRAL CAUSES OF VERTIGO

	Peripheral	*Central*
Imbalance	Mild-moderate	Severe
Nausea and vomiting	Severe	Variable; may be minimal
Auditory symptoms	Common	Rare
Neurologic symptoms	Rare	Common
Compensation	Rapid	Slow

Peripheral vestibular lesions will manifest nystagmus with the fast-beating component in the same direction regardless of direction of gaze. The fast-beating component will actually change direction when the gaze is turned if the lesion is central.

PEARL... The mnemonic COWS (cold opposite, warm same) is very helpful when evaluating nystagmus. "Cold" lesions (remember the fast component beats opposite the affected ear in a cold lesion) include any sudden unilateral loss of vestibular function (e.g., during an attack of Meniere's disease, a "viral" labyrinthitis, or postoperative acoustic neuroma resection, vestibular nerve section, or labyrinthectomy). Toxic or bacterial labyrinthitis causes "warm" lesions.

The head thrust test is another helpful test. The examiner asks the patient to maintain visual fixation on a stationary point while he moves the head rapidly from right to left or left to right in the horizontal plane. A normal response consists of smooth eye movement in the direction opposite the head movement that begins at an almost undetectable latency after the onset of head movement. A response indicative of vestibular hypofunction in the ear toward which the head is being moved is identified when the initial eye movement is low in amplitude. Several rapid eye movements that appear similar to saccades in the direction opposite the head movement then occur at periods from 100 to 200 msec after onset of the head thrust. These rapid eye movements are used to reestablish fixation on the target and are reflective of peripheral vestibular pathology.

Cerebellar dysfunction will result in disdiadochokinesis on tests of rapidly alternating movements. Dysmetria on finger-to-finger and finger-to-nose testing is also indicative of cerebellar dysfunction. Romberg and tandem Romberg testing may also pick up central and/or peripheral vestibular dysfunction.

The following is by no means an exhaustive list or discussion, but presents several of the more common etiologies of patients' dizziness. Again, the diagnosis lies in the history.

ETIOLOGY

Benign Paroxysmal Positional Vertigo (BPPV)

Attacks of true vertigo in these patients follow characteristic head movements, usually in one particular direction. Patients most often notice the vertigo when turning over in bed. The true vertigo lasts only about 15 to 30 seconds and goes away on its own. There is a latency period—a brief second or two when patients are asymptomatic after the head movement, and then the vertigo begins. The attacks are usually too short to induce nausea or vomiting, and ear symptoms are rare. Patients may have one or many attacks in a single day, and a particular series of attacks can occur over days to weeks.

SPECIAL CONSIDERATION

The Dix-Hallpike maneuver (rapidly moving the patient from an erect sitting position to a supine position with the head hanging) in the office will induce a characteristic rotatory nystagmus with the head hanging down and toward the affected ear.

The pathophysiology of BPPV, the most common type of vertigo, is thought to arise from displacement of an otolithic crystal from the macula of the utricle or saccule into the posterior semicircular canal. With head movement in the affected direction, the crystal sets in motion an abnormal fluid wave in the posterior canal that causes asymmetric vestibular input into the brain. This asymmetry results in the patient's vertigo that lasts only 15 to 30 seconds until the fluid wave is damped out.

Treatment consists of reassurance—these attacks are not serious and are not indicative of a "brain tumor" or other serious pathology. The attacks will go away but it is impossible to predict when. Epley maneuvers can also be done in an attempt to reposition the particle back into the vestibule.

Meniere's Disease

Patients with Meniere's disease suffer attacks of room-spinning dizziness, nausea with or without vomiting, aural fullness/pressure, tinnitus, and fluctuating hearing loss. The attacks of vertigo can last hours, and patients feel wiped out and exhausted after the attack. The tinnitus is often described as a roaring or rushing sound, loudest during the acute attack. Physical exam may be completely normal, but an audiogram will classically show a low-frequency sensorineural loss. Patients may have low-grade tinnitus or aural fullness between attacks but are generally not dizzy.

The diagnosis is often one of exclusion, as the asymmetry of symptoms between ears often leads to blood work (erythrocyte sedimentation rate, fluorescent treponemal antibody test, rheumatoid factor, antinuclear antibody test, and thyroid studies) to rule out other potentially treatable causes and an MRI with contrast to rule out an acoustic neuroma. The diagnosis ultimately lies in the history.

Treatment of Meniere's disease offers both medical and surgical options. Patients refractory to medical therapy (diuretics, vestibular suppressants, antiemetics) go on to surgery. Surgical options include decompression of the endolymphatic sac with or without drainage/shunting and destructive procedures such as vestibular nerve section (with serviceable hearing in the ear) and labyrinthectomy (for patients with severe or profound hearing loss). The last two surgical options ablate the peripheral vestibular input to the brain, thereby eliminating the abnormal signal generated by the peripheral vestibular end organ. The two procedures have greater than a 92% success rate in relieving the most disabling symptom of Meniere's disease—vertigo.

Perilymphatic Fistula

Intermittent vertigo lasting seconds to minutes can also be caused by a leak of perilymph around the oval window into the middle ear. A perilymph fistula may or may not be accompanied by hearing loss. Symptoms are often exacerbated by changes in atmospheric pressure or Valsalva's maneuver. A history of head trauma or acoustic trauma may precede symptoms.

Physical exam helps most with this diagnosis. Clear fluid may be evident behind an intact tympanic membrane.

> **PEARL...** The patient will experience dizziness and may have nystagmus when applying positive and negative pressure to the external canal on pneumatic otoscopy (fistula test with Hennebert's symptom and sign).

The only true way to make the diagnosis comes at exploratory tympanotomy, and even that can be difficult at times.

Acute Vestibular Neuronitis

Sudden onset of severe room-spinning vertigo often accompanied by nausea and vomiting is the initial presentation of acute vestibular loss. The dizziness may or may not be accompanied by aural symptoms. The dizziness generally abates over the course of several hours to a day, but the patient is left with imbalance and dysequilibrium. The imbalance can go on for days—vestibular function will either recover and the patient will return to baseline, or vestibular function will be lost, and the patient must compensate, which can take days to weeks.

Treatment is supportive (meclizine, phenergan, diazepam) during the acute phase with vestibular exercises with or without vestibular rehabilitation over the subacute phase. Reassurance is very important to these patients. Electronystagmography (ENG) testing is helpful in documenting (residual) vestibular function. Some patients retain partial vestibular function and will actually do better after complete unilateral ablation (vestibular nerve section) of vestibular function.

Acoustic Neuroma

Tumors of the eighth cranial nerve can present with dizziness and imbalance. Patients may also have an asymmetric sensorineural hearing loss and (unilateral) tinnitus. Acoustic neuromas generally do not present with attacks of vertigo—the imbalance is more subtle as the contralateral ear and brain compensate over time for gradual loss of balance function on the tumor side. Nevertheless, acoustic neuromas must be considered in the differential diagnosis of the patient presenting with dizziness or unsteadiness or imbalance.

> **PEARL...** MRI with gadolinium contrast is the gold standard in diagnosing these tumors. A history of dizziness or imbalance with an asymmetric sensorineural hearing loss is a clear indication for an MRI with contrast.

Chronic Otitis Media

The diagnosis of labyrinthine fistula must be considered in any patient with a tympanic membrane perforation, cholesteatoma, or purulent otorrhea, and the acute onset of vertigo with or without hearing loss. High-resolution CT scanning is helpful in documenting extent of disease. Treatment is surgical and beyond the scope of this chapter.

Vascular Causes

Orthostatic hypotension can result from hypovolemia, overmedication for hypertension, autonomic instability/neuropathy as seen in diabetics, and carotid artery atherosclerosis. It is important to screen the medical history. Recent addition or change in blood pressure medication is a common cause of orthostasis. History of diabetes, peripheral vascular disease, and/or stroke (see following text) is noteworthy. Dizziness in this context is not vertiginous and often comes on when standing or raising the head. Patients describe more of a "light-headed" or "swimmy" sensation without true room-spinning vertigo. Symptoms last only a few seconds to a minute and go away. Physical exam may show orthostatic hypotension when blood pressure and pulse are taken with the patient lying down, sitting, and standing. A carotid bruit may be present.

Claudication of the posterior cerebral circulation, for example vertebrobasilar insufficiency, can also cause dizziness. This results from temporary hypoxia of the brainstem. Dizziness comes on when moving the head on the neck or neck on the shoulders; stretching the cervical vertebrae can pinch off the vertebral arteries. Dizziness is usually brief, lasting seconds to minutes, and resolves with holding the head erect or lying down. Other posterior circulation symptoms may also be present, including facial numbness, diplopia, and decreased visual acuity. Carotid and vertebral artery duplex scanning aid in diagnosis.

Posterior circulation stroke must be considered in the elderly patient presenting with acute vestibular symptoms. Wallenberg's syndrome is caused by occlusion of the posterior inferior cerebellar artery with resultant infarction of the lateral medulla. Symptoms include vertigo, nausea, vomiting diplopia, dysarthria, and ipsilateral loss of pain and temperature sensation in the face with contralateral loss of pain and temperature sensation in the trunk and extremities.

PEARL••• Head CT is extremely important in patients presenting with an acute vestibular syndrome, headache, and a history of hypertension, stroke, or vascular disease. CT scanning documents extent of the injury and the presence of a hemorrhagic stroke or cerebellar swelling that may compress the brainstem secondary to a noncommunicating hydrocephalus. This condition requires prompt neurosurgical consultation.

Multiple Sclerosis

Multiple sclerosis is a degenerative neurologic disease characterized by destruction of myelin. It has a tendency to attack young adults; the hallmark of the diagnosis rests on a history of neurologic deficits that remit and relapse over time with evidence of more than one discrete lesion of the central nervous system. Symptoms vary greatly but can include weakness or numbness in one or more limbs, optic neuritis (the rapid evolution of partial or total loss of vision in one eye often accompanied by pain), transverse

myelitis (rapidly evolving paraparesis, sensory level on the trunk, and bilateral Babinski signs), nystagmus, and ataxia. Cerebellar ataxia features include intention tremor, scanning speech, and rhythmic instability of the head and trunk with incoordination. Nystagmus, scanning speech, and intention tremor compose Charcot's triad. Diagnosis is made by MRI and lumbar puncture. Enhancing plaques are seen on MRI; oligoclonal bands are noted on cerebrospinal fluid evaluation. Referral to a neurologist is the most appropriate management. Although rare, multiple sclerosis should be kept in the back of the mind, especially when evaluating the young patient with dizziness and cerebellar findings.

CONCLUSION

A systematic, organized, and precise approach to the patient with dizziness is the key to diagnosing the problem. The etiology is often inferred from the history. The overriding question is whether or not the patient's dizziness is of peripheral vestibular origin. Physical exam is important to document the status of the ears, cerebellar function, and other posterior circulation/cranial nerve findings. Helpful diagnostic tests include MRI and CT scanning, electronystagmography, and vascular studies. With the proper diagnosis, appropriate treatment strategies can then be implemented.

SUGGESTED READINGS

Adams RD, Victor M, Ropper AH. Multiple sclerosis and allied demyelinative diseases. In: Adams RD, Victor M, eds. *Principles of Neurology*, 6th ed. New York: McGraw-Hill; 1997: 902–927.

Arenberg IK, Silverstein H, Garcia-Ibanez E, Vander Ark G. Primary surgery for Meniere's disease: destructive surgery versus conservative surgery. *Am J Otol* 1986;7:4.

Baloh RW. Differentiating between peripheral and central causes of vertigo. *Otolaryngol Head Neck Surg* 1998;119:55–59.

Epley JM. The canalith repositioning procedure for treatment of benign paroxysmal positional vertigo. *Otolaryngol Head Neck Surg* 1992;107:399–404.

Gacek RR. The surgical management of labyrinthine fistula in chronic otitis media with cholesteatoma. *Ann Otol Rhinol Laryngol* 1974;83 (suppl 10):3–19.

Gacek RR, Gacek MR. Comparison of labyrinthectomy and vestibular neurectomy in the control of vertigo. *Laryngoscope* 1996; 106: 225–230.

Gillespie MB, Minor LB. Prognosis in bilateral vestibular hypofunction. *Laryngoscope* 1999; 109:35–41.

Hotson JR, Baloh RW. Acute vestibular syndrome. *N Engl J Med* 1998;339:680–685.

LaRouere MJ. Surgical treatment of Meniere's disease. *Otolaryngol Clin North Am* 1996;29: 311.

Meyerhoff WL, Marple BF. Perilymphatic fistula. *Otolaryngol Clin North Am* 1994;27:411–426.

Qiu WW, Stucker FJ, Yin SS, Welsh LW. Current evaluation of pseudohypacusis: strategies and classification. *Ann Otol Rhinol Laryngol* 1998;107:638.

Sheehy JL, Brackmann DE. Cholesteatoma surgery: management of the labyrinthine fistula—a report of 97 cases. *Laryngoscope* 1979; 83:1594–1621.

Sheehy JL, Brackmann DE. Surgery of chronic otitis media. In: English GM, ed. *Otolaryngology,* vol 1. Philadelphia: JB Lippincott; 1994:1.

Stokroos RJ, Albers FWJ, Tenvergert Em. Antiviral treatment of idiopathic sudden sensorineural hearing loss: a prospective, randomized double-blind clinical trial. *Acta Otolaryngol* 1998; 118:488.

Chapter 5

Infectious and Inflammatory Disorders

Bradley W. Kesser and Rick A. Friedman

Infectious and inflammatory diseases of the ear can affect the outer (Table 5–1), middle (Table 5–2), and inner (Table 5–3) ear. Otitis media is the most common diagnosis of patients who make office visits to physicians in the United States. In addition, bilateral myringotomy with placement of ventilation tubes is the most common surgical procedure performed in the United States, where an estimated 1.05 million tympanostomy tube procedures are performed annually. Otitis media with effusion (OME) incurs approximately $5 billion annually in direct and indirect costs. Given the magnitude of the disease and its impact on our society as well as conflicting reports over the most appropriate and cost-effective management of the problem, consensus on the treatment of OME has been difficult to achieve.

CONTROVERSY

Attempts have been made to devise an algorithm for the management of OME in young children, but these guidelines have been met with criticism.

Reviewed herein are the terminology, epidemiology, pathophysiology, and treatment—both medical and surgical—of the more common inflammatory diseases of the ear.

OUTER EAR

ACUTE OTITIS EXTERNA

Severe ear pain, especially with manipulation of the auricle or any attempt at an otoscopic examination, is the hallmark of otitis externa (also called swimmer's ear because it is often brought on by getting water in the ears). Other symptoms include itching, hearing loss, and fullness. The canal skin is erythematous, edematous, and exquisitely tender. Squamous debris and purulence are often found in the canal, if it is not swollen shut. The most common offending organism is *Pseudomonas;* cultures are rarely taken.

The infection is usually caused by a break in the normal protective barrier of the canal skin. Q-tip use leads to a small abrasion or laceration of the canal skin, which allows bacteria to take hold in the thin subcutaneous tissue/periosteum. The warm, moist environment of the ear canal allows bacteria to multiply and to cause the acute infection. Water in the ear canal optimizes conditions for bacteria.

Otitis externa may also develop as a sequela of chronic suppurative otitis media. Purulent drainage through a tympanic membrane perfo-

TABLE 5–1 INFLAMMATORY DISEASES OF THE OUTER EAR

Acute otitis externa

Necrotizing otitis externa

Otomycosis

Herpes zoster oticus (Ramsay Hunt)—also affects inner ear

Chondritis/perichondritis

Relapsing polychondritis

Chronic eczematoid dermatitis

Leprosy

Chondrodermatitis nodularis chronicum helicis

TABLE 5–3 INFLAMMATORY DISEASES OF THE INNER EAR

Acute labyrinthitis

Serous labyrinthitis

Petrous apicitis

Vestibular neuronitis

Cogan's disease

Autoimmune inner ear disease

Syphilis (luetic ear disease)

ration leads to secondary inflammation and infection of the ear canal. Treatment with both topical (for the external infection) and systemic (for the middle ear infection) antibiotics is often necessary.

Treatment of acute otitis externa consists of meticulous aural hygiene—debridement and cleansing in the office—followed by ototopical therapy, usually consisting of a combination antibiotic and steroid preparation. In truth, all of the commercially available eardrops are comparable, although an alcohol-based preparation (i.e., a solution) should not be used in the presence of a tympanic membrane perforation.

SPECIAL CONSIDERATION

There has been no evidence to show that these drops can otherwise cause sensorineural hearing loss in the presence of a perforation in humans.

TABLE 5–2 INFLAMMATORY DISEASES OF THE MIDDLE EAR

Acute otitis media

Otitis media with effusion

Chronic otitis media

Tympanosclerosis

Wegener's granulomatosis

Tuberculous otitis media

The canal that is swollen shut requires placement of a wick so that the topical antibiotic can reach the medial canal. Frequent cleanings may be necessary, and the patient should be followed every few days until the acute infection has quieted. The more thoroughly the otolaryngologist is able to clean the ear in the office, the faster the resolution. Pain medicine will also bring some relief to these patients. Q-tip use is absolutely forbidden; the patient is instructed to keep water out of the ears. Relief usually comes within 2 to 3 days.

NECROTIZING OTITIS EXTERNA

Any patient with acute otitis externa should be questioned about medical history of diabetes, HIV/AIDS, and any other potentially immunocompromised state. A patient with such a history is at risk for necrotizing otitis externa, once called malignant otitis externa and also referred to as skull base osteomyelitis. The diagnosis is made based on history and physical findings—persistent otalgia for longer than 1 month, persistent, purulent otorrhea with granulation tissue or exposed bone of the ear canal, immunocompromised state or diabetes, and cranial nerve involvement. The most common cranial nerves affected are VII, X, and XI.

PEARL... Otolaryngologists should keep a high index of suspicion in any diabetic or immunocompromised patient with otitis externa.

Treatment of necrotizing otitis externa consists of intravenous antibiotics active against the most common offending organisms, *Pseudomonas, Proteus,* and *Klebsiella.* Cultures should be taken. Recommended antibiotics include ticarcillin/clavulanate, ciprofloxacin, an aminoglycoside, ceftazidime (third-generation cephalosporin), or imipenem. The ear should be meticulously cleaned daily, and the physical examination followed. Ototopical drops are also started.

Temporal bone computed tomography (CT) scanning is the radiologic study of choice as it best demonstrates bone erosion and/or destruction. Some authors have recommended nuclear medicine studies to follow the course of the disease. Gallium scanning lights up areas where gallium has been taken up by polymorphonuclear leukocytes (PMNs)—sites of active infection; it will not show the extent of osteomyelitis. Technetium scanning is complementary, as it gives excellent information about bone function and osteoblastic activity—sites of acute and chronic osteomyelitis. The technetium scan is useful to make the diagnosis of necrotizing otitis externa; the gallium scan is helpful in following the disease process. With treatment response, the gallium scan will revert back to normal; the technetium scan will lag behind for months.

Most patients will respond to aggressive medical therapy; some will continue to have pain and granulations and may develop cranial neuropathy. Surgical treatment is aimed at the removal of infected tissue and osteomyelitic bone. Decompression of the descending facial nerve may also speed facial nerve recovery.

Morbidity in necrotizing otitis externa is significant. Extension of infection may produce additional lower cranial nerve neuropathies, dural vein thrombosis, meningitis, brain abscess, and even death. Successful treatment involves early diagnosis with a high index of suspicion, aggressive medical care, including intravenous and topical antibiotics, vigorous aural hygiene, and control of diabetes or any other predisposing condition. Cessation of treatment relies on clinical judgment with resolution of cranial neuropathies and quiescence of the inflammatory response and granulation tissue in the ear canal.

OTOMYCOSIS

Fungal infection of the ear canal may occur as a result of chronic ototopical drop use or as a superinfection of chronic bacterial infection. Antibiotic drops kill the normal flora of the ear canal and allow fungal overgrowth. Diagnosis is made on otoscopic examination—white, gray, or black fungal spores are seen in the canal. *Aspergillus* is the most common species. Patients often complain of itchiness without pain.

As with otitis externa, the key to treatment is cleaning. Once cleaned, the canal can be painted with gentian violet, a drying agent. Other effective preparations include cresylate (but not in the presence of a perforation), boric acid powder, and chloromycetin, sulfanilamide, and fungizone (CSF) powder. Acidifying solutions such as aluminum sulfate-calcium acetate (Domeboro) are also effective.

HERPES ZOSTER OTICUS

Burning ear pain followed in a few days by a vesicular eruption involving the pinna and ear canal characterize herpes zoster infection. The infection can also involve the facial nerve and cause a temporary facial paresis (Ramsay Hunt syndrome). The vesicles eventually crust and weep; treatment includes drying agents such as powders or hydrogen peroxide as well as an antiviral (acyclovir, valcyclovir, famcyclovir) and steroid for facial nerve weakness.

CHONDRITIS/PERICHONDRITIS

Infection of the perichondrium and/or cartilage of the auricle is usually caused by *Pseudomonas. Staphylococcus* can also cause infection of the auricular skin with extension into the perichondrium. Trauma, both surgical and environmental (bites, earrings, accidents), introduces pathogenic organisms. Infection from the external canal can also progress to involve the auricle. The ear is indurated, painful, and erythematous with loss of the cartilaginous prominences and contour. The skin weeps serous or purulent exudate.

Treatment involves debridement with topical and oral antibiotics. Antipseudomonas antimicrobials (ciprofloxacin) are appropriate. Failure to respond to these measures along with spread of the infection to the surrounding soft tissues warrants more aggressive debridement and intravenous antibiotics. Cultures should also be taken. Infection resulting in cartilage necrosis should be surgically debrided in the operating room. Local skin flaps should be advanced over small drains for coverage. The risk of such an infection is loss of the entire auricle; staying one step ahead of the disease will prevent significant tissue loss.

RELAPSING POLYCHONDRITIS

Thought to be an autoimmune disorder, relapsing polychondritis is characterized by episodic inflammation of the cartilages of the head and neck, including auricular, nasal, laryngeal, tracheal, and bronchial. Symptoms during flare-ups include fever, pain, erythema, edema, anemia, and elevated erythrocyte sedimentation rate. Mortality is secondary to respiratory obstruction and airway collapse from cartilage destruction. Because the initial presentation may be limited to the ear, an index of suspicion for this disease is necessary. Biopsy of auricular cartilage may show inflammatory cells, necrosis, or fibrosis. Treatment is with corticosteroids; rheumatologic referral is also indicated.

CHRONIC ECZEMATOID DERMATITIS

Patients with chronic eczema can be very difficult to treat. They have severe itchiness of the ear canal and often use Q-tips to relieve symptoms.

> **PEARL...** Q-tip use only sets up a pattern of further skin irritation and increased itchiness. Eventually, the Q-tip will cause a secondary acute otitis externa.

Nevertheless, dermatitis of the ear canal can be treated and helped.

As mentioned, itchiness is the number one complaint. Some patients may have drainage, and in fact there may be some desquamated epithelium and debris in the canal that needs cleaning. The canal skin can be erythematous but is generally not edematous. Pain is not a feature. The condition is caused by irritation (local factors, genetic predisposition, etc.) of the canal skin, resulting in the rapid turnover of the surface epithelium, hence the often prolific desquamation.

Treatment consists of aural hygiene in the office, water precautions, keeping all foreign bodies out of the ear (especially Q-tips), and topical medication. A drop or two of baby oil or mineral oil two to three times a week may be all that is necessary. Microscopic application of triamcinolone ointment in the office has proven helpful to these patients. Other topical steroids, including triamcinolone lotion and hydrocortisone, can also be tried. Seborrhea can be treated with any of the dandruff shampoo products, including any with selenium sulfide. The disease course waxes and wanes, and patients come in during acute exacerbations.

MIDDLE EAR

Otitis media, in its broadest sense, refers to any inflammatory process in the middle ear. The etiology of the inflammation can be (and usually is) infectious in nature, but it can also involve rarer systemic inflammatory diseases (e.g., Wegener's granulomatosis). The inflammation can be marked by the presence or absence of an effusion, or fluid in the middle ear space. The fluid can be serous (thin, watery, often golden), purulent (pus), or mucoid (thick, viscid, "glue").

ACUTE OTITIS MEDIA

Acute otitis media (OM) refers to an inflamed middle ear mucosa and tympanic membrane. An effusion may or may not be present; if present, the fluid is purulent. The tympanic membrane appears dull, erythematous, and inflamed; normal landmarks are lost. The membrane will bulge with an effusion behind it.

In infants and children, acute otitis media without effusion is usually caused by the same organisms that are isolated from acute OME. Acute OME occurs most frequently in infants. Redness with or without bulging of the tympanic membrane, fever, irritability, and pain are the cardinal signs and symptoms. The older child with acute OME will have a red tympanic membrane and middle ear effusion, but may not have pain or fever. The middle ear effusion is generally purulent.

For the single episode of acute OM, antimicrobial therapy targets the most common offending pathogens, *Streptococcus pneumoniae, Haemophilus influenzae,* and *Moraxella catarrhalis.* A 10-day course of amoxicillin is recommended as first-line empiric therapy. Studies have shown a rise in the β-lactamase–producing organisms, *H. influenzae* and *M. catarrhalis.* β-lactamase renders the organism that produces it resistant to penicillin (and ampicillin).

SPECIAL CONSIDERATION

Persistent or recurrent acute OM may be secondary to a β-lactamase–producing organism and requires a broader spectrum antibiotic; good choices in this setting include cefuroxime, erythromycin-sulfisoxazole, trimethoprim-sulfamethoxazole, or amoxacillin-clavulanate. Antipyretics (but not aspirin) are also indicated for children with acute OM.

A child (or adult) with an infectious complication of otitis media demands more agressive therapy, including intravenous antibiotics and possibly surgical intervention. Complications of otitis media are listed in Tables 5–4 and 5–5. Management of these complications is beyond the scope of this chapter.

Children with recurrent acute OM may exhibit normal middle ear examinations between episodes or may retain persistent effusions, and fall into the category of chronic OME. The goal

TABLE 5–4 INTRATEMPORAL COMPLICATIONS OF OTITIS MEDIA

Labyrinthitis
Petrous apicitis
Facial nerve paresis/paralysis
Sensorineural hearing loss
Coalescent mastoiditis
Labyrinthine fistula

of any treatment of the patient with recurrent acute OM is the long-term prevention of further episodes of OM. Two modalities have been proposed: (1) antimicrobial prophylaxis and (2) ventilation tube placement. Antimicrobial prophylaxis involves placing the patient on a low-dose daily antibiotic to prevent further infections. Many trials using many different regimens have shown efficacy in the prevention of recurrent acute OM. Children with multiple episodes of acute OM can be treated with long-term, low-dose chemoprophylaxis before surgical therapy is considered. Antibiotic prophylaxis has especially been recommended for high-risk children during the winter season and/or during an upper respiratory infection (URI) (amoxicillin 20 mg/kg qhs or sulfisoxazole 50 to 75 mg/kg qhs).

Placement of tympanostomy tubes is also effective treatment in the prevention of recurrent acute OM. Many authorities accept four episodes of acute otitis media in 6 months as a criterion for tympanostomy tube placement. Failure of antibiotic prophylaxis is also a clear indication. Gebhart was the first to demonstrate a reduction in the number of new episodes of

TABLE 5–5 INTRACRANIAL COMPLICATIONS OF OTITIS MEDIA

Meningitis
Epidural abscess
Subdural abscess
Brain abscess
Lateral sinus thrombosis
Otitic hydrocephalus

acute OM following the insertion of tympanostomy tubes. Parents often tire of frequent courses of antibiotics (or the daily use of prophylaxis) and may favor surgical treatment. The child who develops acute OM after withdrawal of prophylaxis is also a surgical candidate.

OTITIS MEDIA WITH EFFUSION (OME)

Otitis media with effusion simply refers to fluid in the middle ear without signs or symptoms of ear infection. Asymptomatic middle ear effusion (OME) can be classified as acute (<3 weeks), subacute (3 weeks to 3 months), or chronic (COME) (>3 months). Note that acute and chronic refer to the temporal course of the disease, not to severity. Synonyms of OME include secretory OM, nonsuppurative OM, or serous OM; the most commonly used is OME.

Epidemiology

Studies by Teele et al have found that 13% of children in their study groups had at least one episode of acute otitis media by age 3 months; that percentage increased to 67% by 12 months. By age 3, 46% of children had three or more episodes of acute otitis media. The highest incidence of acute OM was found in children 6 to 11 months. The majority of children with multiple recurrences of otitis media have their first episode before the age of 12 months.

An episode of acute otitis media is a significant risk factor for the development of otitis media with effusion. A number of investigators have documented persistent middle ear effusion following a single episode of acute OM. Middle ear effusion has been shown to persist following an episode of acute OM for 1 month in 40% of children, 2 months in 20%, and 3 or more months in 10%.

Risk Factors

Risk factors for OME include male gender, recent URI, bottle feeding, cigarette smoke in the house, increased number of siblings in the house, and probably the most important—day care.

> ## SPECIAL CONSIDERATION
>
> Children in a public day-care facility have a fivefold increase in OM at age 2 years compared with children in home care.

White Americans and Hispanics are more susceptible than African Americans; Native Americans and Eskimos are at greater risk.

Skeletal and anatomic factors also predispose to OME. Cleft palate—either overt or submucous—is a significant risk factor. Other craniofacial anomalies including Treacher Collins, Apert's, the mucopolysaccharidoses, and Down syndrome put children at greater susceptibility to middle ear disease, presumably due to immaturity, dysfunction, and anatomic course of the eustachian tube.

Children with immunodeficiencies are also at greater risk. Immunoglobulin G (IgG) subclass deficiencies, acquired immunodeficiency syndrome (AIDS), complement deficiencies, and immunosuppression secondary to medication all predispose to otitis media. Ciliary dysfunction and cystic fibrosis are also known risk factors.

Microbiology

Bluestone et al (1992) obtained aspirates of middle ear effusions by tympanocentesis in infants and children with acute OM or OME; 35% of aspirates from ears with acute OM grew *S. pneumoniae*, 23% grew *H. influenzae*, and 14% grew *M. catarrhalis*. *S. pneumoniae* remains the most common bacterium causing acute OM. Introduction of the pneumococcal vaccine may significantly reduce the incidence of pneumococcal disease, including otitis media.

The asymptomatic middle ear effusion (OME) was previously thought to be sterile. Post et al (1995) found that 77% of middle ear effusions had evidence of the three major organisms by PCR (with or without being culture-positive), whereas only 28% were

SPECIAL CONSIDERATION

Newer, more sensitive cultures as well as the introduction of polymerase chain reaction (PCR) testing has shown bacteria and bacterial DNA in asymptomatic middle ear effusions.

culture-positive. The most common bacteria were *H. influenzae* (54.5%), *M. catarrhalis* (46.4%), and *S. pneumoniae* (29.9%). In infants younger than 6 weeks of age, gram-negative bacilli cause about 20% of acute otitis media episodes. The incidence of β-lactamase–producing bacteria *(H. influenzae)* is on the rise.

Treatment

There has been much debate on the optimal treatment for OME. As mentioned, 10% of children with acute OM will have persistent middle ear effusion 3 months or longer after resolution of the acute infection. Because most children clear their effusion within 1 to 2 months, these patients need no further therapy. The minority who retain fluid in the middle ear longer than 3 months, however, are at risk for other sequelae, including hearing loss, language delay, vertigo or unsteadiness, tympanic membrane changes (including atelectasis and/or retraction pockets), further middle ear pathology (including ossicular problems and adhesive otitis), and discomfort with nighttime wakefulness and irritability.

A number of treatment strategies have been proposed for COME: antimicrobial therapy, steroids, antihistamines/decongestants, tympanostomy tubes with or without adenoidectomy, and mastoidectomy.

Antimicrobial Therapy

More sensitive techniques (e.g., PCR) for examining middle ear effusions have demonstrated bacterial DNA in middle ear effusions once thought "sterile" or culture-negative. Prolonged antibiotic therapy theoretically eradicates the organism and eliminates the chronic source

of effusion. Studies have shown the efficacy of antibiotics in OME. According to the clinical practice guideline, Managing Otitis Media with Effusion in Young Children (Stool et al, 1994), antimicrobial therapy is an appropriate treatment option in the child (age 1 to 3) with OME up to 3 months after documentation of effusion. The patient with persistent effusion at 3 months should then undergo hearing evaluation; a 20-dB or worse bilateral hearing level is then an indication for tympanostomy tube insertion.

CONTROVERSY

Despite studies showing the efficacy of antibiotics in OME, both theoretical and practical arguments can be made against their use in COME.

Clinical experience indicates that the utility of antibiotics is reduced as the number of treatment courses increases. Children receiving four or more courses of antibiotics over a 3- to 4-month period are most likely not going to resolve their effusion with medical management. Other adverse effects of prolonged antimicrobial therapy include development of anaphylaxis and allergic reactions, hematologic disorders, and the emergence of resistant organisms, a serious worldwide problem best demonstrated by the development of resistance to penicillin by *S. pneumoniae*. Finally, Rosenfeld and Post (1992) found through a large meta-analysis of existing studies that the benefit of antimicrobial therapy in COME is slight.

Antihistamines/Decongestants

Antihistamine/decongestant combinations or monotherapy have not been shown to be of benefit in the treatment of COME. The Agency for Health Care Policy and Research (AHCPR) guideline does not recommend these agents for COME.

Corticosteroid Therapy

Steroid therapy for COME has been controversial. Lambert (1986) found no difference in outcomes between the steroid group and the control group with COME. At this time, the AHCPR guideline does not recommend steroid therapy for COME.

Surgical Therapy

Armstrong (1954) introduced ventilation tube placement in 1954 as treatment for OME. The ventilation tube acts as an artificial eustachian tube, aerating the middle ear and equilibrating middle ear pressure with atmospheric pressure. The pathophysiology of COME involves both eustachian tube dysfunction and reflux of nasopharyngeal organisms. Ventilation tubes are aimed at correcting the former.

Children with tubes in place can still get otitis media; however, the acute infection will not be painful as the infected effusion is allowed to pass through the tube and out of the middle ear. The effusion will also not be associated with hearing loss; correction of hearing loss is one of the most important goals of surgical therapy. Tube insertion with or without adenoidectomy has been shown to improve conductive hearing loss secondary to OME and to decrease the amount of time spent with middle ear effusion. The AHCPR guideline recommends tube insertion for the 1- to 3-year-old child with a 3-month or longer history of OME and a 20-dB or worse bilateral hearing loss. In practice, however, tube insertion is performed on a more frequent basis than the recommendations would allow; the guidelines have a "serious bias toward nonsurgical treatment" (Healy, 1994). Placement of tubes is often a clinical judgment based on experience and addressed on a case-by-case basis.

Adenoidectomy

Nasopharyngeal reflux of secretions and microorganisms into the middle ear plays a large role in the pathophysiology of COME. As such, adenoidectomy is designed to remove the source of the infecting microorganisms. Three landmark studies have demonstrated the efficacy and low morbidity associated with adenoidectomy for COME (Gates et al, 1987; Maw, 1983; Paradise et al, 1990). Adenoidectomy is ef-

fective treatment for COME and significantly reduces its morbidity. Its effect is independent of adenoid size. In fact, it is argued that the small, "smoldering" adenoid chronically harbors bacteria and is a major contributor to OME.

> **PEARL...** The decision for adenoidectomy should be based on the severity and persistence of the middle ear disease, not the size of the adenoid.

Nasal obstruction with adenoid hypertrophy stands alone as an indication. Given the increased cost and slightly increased risk to the patient, Paradise and Bluestone (1988) have argued for adenoidectomy only in recurrent cases. We also recommend adenoidectomy for recurrent cases—cases where the child (over 4 years) needs a second set of tubes.

Mastoidectomy

Rarely, mastoidectomy is required for COME. The continuously draining ear with secretory tissue in the mastoid (serous mastoiditis) will most benefit from opening the aditus ad antrum and facial recess to increase aeration of the middle ear/mastoid air cell system. Removal of secretory tissue or granulation tissue will also improve symptoms. Because of the rare necessity for mastoidectomy in COME, no systematic study has been undertaken to prove its efficacy. The decision to proceed with mastoid surgery is based on clinical experience and judgment.

CHRONIC OTITIS MEDIA (COM)

The designations "suppurative and nonsuppurative" and "with and without cholesteatoma" are a bit artificial, as we consider any pathology of the middle ear with a tympanic membrane perforation as "chronic otitis media." The adjective *suppurative* simply refers to the presence of otorrhea. Chronic otitis media can also be with or without cholesteatoma; nevertheless, it all falls under the term *chronic otitis media*.

This disease process ranges from the simple dry tympanic membrane perforation to the extensive draining cholesteatoma. Cholesteatoma refers to skin in the middle ear space. This skin becomes intermittently infected, and the ear drains. The pathophysiology of cholesteatoma and its potential for damage, including bone erosion, is complex. Skin is introduced into the middle ear through trauma, iatrogenic causes (e.g., tympanostomy tube), and eustachian tube dysfunction. As long as the skin can be cleaned and debrided, cholesteatoma may not cause trouble. When the skin grows into a pocket and is not able to be evacuated after sloughing, cholesteatoma can grow and erode bone. Infection and moisture hasten this process.

Diagnosis of COM is made on history and physical examination. A history of otorrhea, hearing loss, ear infections, or trauma is a good clue to the diagnosis. Otoscopic examination should be done with the microscope to appreciate fully the anatomy and pathology. Cholesteatoma can often be seen in the pars flaccida, posterosuperior ear canal, or through the tympanic membrane.

> **PEARL...** If there is any question between cholesteatoma and tympanosclerosis (see following text), pneumatic otoscopy will aid in diagnosis: tympanosclerosis will move with the drum (it is part of the drum); cholesteatoma will not.

An audiogram will show conductive hearing loss if there has been ossicular erosion or interference with ossicular conduction.

The bacteriology of chronic suppurative OM with or without cholesteatoma is different from acute and chronic OME. Most frequently isolated bacteria include *Pseudomonas aeruginosa* (most common), *Staphylococcus aureus*, *Corynebacterium, Klebsiella pneumoniae,* and anaerobes. Given better culture techniques, anaerobes have been increasingly isolated from chronic suppurating ears; these organisms include *Bacteroides* spp., *Peptococcus* spp., *Peptostreptococcus* spp., and *Propionibacterium acnes.*

Treatment of COM is surgical—tympanoplasty with or without mastoidectomy. It is preferable but not essential to dry the ear before surgery. The technique of tympanoplasty with mastoidectomy is best reviewed in Sheehy and Brackmann (1994).

IDIOPATHIC HEMOTYMPANUM (IH)

The clinical hallmark of idiopathic hemotympanum is the dark-blue appearing tympanic membrane. There is usually no antecedent history of trauma, but trauma can induce this condition. Long-standing cases of chronic OME that develop granulomatous deposits in the middle ear and mastoid can lead to IH. Symptoms of IH are those of OME—hearing loss with a plugged or pressure sensation in the ear. IH is more common in adults. A dark-blue appearing TM is apparent—fluid at myringotomy is dark brown and syrupy in consistency. Histologically, cholesterol crystals are seen, hence the pathologic term *cholesterol granuloma.* It is theorized that a small mucosal hemorrhage in the absence of adequate ventilation and drainage results in deposition of hemosiderin, iron, and blood breakdown products into the submucosa. Three etiologic factors are thought to be responsible: interference with drainage, hemorrhage, and obstruction of ventilation.

The contents of the hemorrhage can then be walled off, with resultant cyst development. The cyst then slowly expands causing bone thinning and erosion. These cholesterol cysts can take an aggressive course with bone erosion and osteitis. Treatment can entail observation alone with serial magnetic resonance imaging (MRI) scanning or surgical drainage.

TYMPANOSCLEROSIS

Tympanosclerosis appears as a hard white plaque in the eardrum. It is thought to arise from hemorrhage within the layers of the drum. It can be limited to the membrane only or can involve extensively the entire middle ear space, causing ossicular fixation and conductive hearing loss. The pathophysiology is fibrosis.

Diagnosis is made on history and physical examination. Patients may not have otorrhea but will present with hearing loss, or tympanosclerosis may be an incidental finding. The drum may be intact. Otoscopic exam will often show the plaques within the tympanic membrane; pneumatic otoscopy confirms the diagnosis. Audiogram may show significant conductive hearing loss. Tuning-fork testing will confirm the nature of the hearing loss and thus should always be performed.

Treatment again is observation or surgery. Certainly no treatment is necessary in the absence of symptoms; tympanosclerosis by itself within the eardrum requires no further therapy. Patients are informed that there is some "scarring" on the drum, but that it will not cause any problem. Significant hearing loss, on the other hand, may warrant exploratory tympanotomy and/or tympanoplasty with removal of plaques from the ossicles and oval window area. This can often be done transcanal. The disease process is not dangerous, and if the patient desires, a hearing aid may be the only rehabilitation necessary.

WEGENER'S GRANULOMATOSIS

Wegener's granulomatosis can manifest as chronic bilateral serous otitis media in an adult patient. It can cause facial nerve paralysis and conductive hearing loss. It can also cause sensorineural hearing loss secondary to vasculitis of the stria vascularis. External ear involvement can also occur resulting in diffuse, brawny erythema and edema of the auricle. Significant renal (hematuria) and pulmonary (dyspnea, shortness of breath) histories should be sought. Initial workup includes chest X-ray, urinalysis, complete blood count (CBC), and erythrocyte sedimentation rate (ESR). The diagnosis is made by a serum cellular antineutrophil cytoplasmic antibody (c-ANCA) test or with tissue biopsy; involved nasal mucosa, lung, or kidney are the preferred sites. Vasculitis and necrotizing granulomas are the histopathologic findings. Cyclophosphamide and steroids are the cornerstones of treatment, in consultation with a rheumatologist. Tympanostomy tube placement will temporize hearing loss until the disease is brought under control. Index of suspicion is the key to this diagnosis.

TUBERCULOUS OTITIS MEDIA

Hematogenous and lymphatic spread of infection from pulmonary disease or possibly ascending infection from the nasopharynx into the eustachian tube accounts for otitis media caused by *Mycobacterium tuberculosis*. Tuberculous otitis media in the absence of active pulmonary infection is rare.

> **PEARL•••** Tuberculous infection of the middle ear generally causes multiple small tympanic membrane perforations with painless clear otorrhea.

The perforations may coalesce to form one large total perforation. Ossicular destruction results in conductive hearing loss. Facial nerve involvement with facial paresis is common and reversible with antituberculous medication. Middle ear mucosa appears polypoid or granular; bony sequestra may form.

Diagnosis is based on a positive tuberculin skin test and more importantly, demonstration of acid-fast bacilli in the otorrhea or on tissue stain. Actual culture is inconsistent, unreliable, and may take as long as 6 weeks to grow. First-line treatment is medical, with antituberculous antibiotics. Surgical therapy may be necessary to debride bony sequestra. Once the acute infection is quieted, the ear may be treated as any COM ear, with techniques of tympanoplasty with or without ossicular reconstruction applicable.

INNER EAR

LABYRINTHITIS

Acute infection of the inner ear may be serous or purulent, viral or bacterial. Purulent (suppurative) bacterial labyrinthitis results from cholesteatomatous invasion of the otic capsule or by spread of infection from the subarachnoid space through the cochlear aqueduct during acute bacterial meningitis. Organisms responsible for infection are those associated with the primary infection—*S. pneumoniae, H. influenzae,* and *M. catarrhalis* in cases of bacterial meningitis, and *P. aeruginosa* and *P. mirabilis* in cases of COM.

The patient can be quite toxic, with mental status changes, vertigo, fever, headache, and hearing loss. Suppurative labyrinthitis with subsequent meningitis can be fatal. The patient should be stabilized with intravenous fluids and antibiotics. Broad-spectrum antimicrobial therapy aimed at the most likely offending organisms and imaging studies (CT as first-line study) are instituted immediately.

SPECIAL CONSIDERATION

Steroids are also given to children with bacterial meningitis, as they have been shown to reduce the morbidity (including hearing loss) of bacterial meningitis.

Once the patient is stabilized, surgical intervention (tympanoplasty with mastoidectomy) is indicated for COM. An audiogram should be obtained at some point (preferably prior to surgery) to document hearing loss. Hearing and vestibular loss in the setting of suppurative labyrinthitis are permanent.

Serous labyrinthitis can also follow or accompany acute and chronic otitis media. Toxins, metabolic products of bacteria, or host inflammatory cytokines from the middle ear infection are introduced into the inner ear either through the round window membrane or through erosion with fenestration of a semicircular canal (usually the lateral canal) by cholesteatoma. Patients are vertiginous, with nystagmus, hearing loss, nausea, and occasionally fever. Prompt institution of intravenous antibiotics and control of the middle ear disease (through myringotomy in cases of acute otitis media or tympanoplasty with mastoidectomy in cases of COM) will quiet the middle and inner ear inflammatory reaction, usually without permanent sequelae. Management of labyrinthine fistula is beyond the scope of this chapter; for a good reference, see Sheehy and Brackmann (1979).

A number of viruses have been implicated in viral labyrinthitis, including rubella and cytomegalovirus (CMV) in congenital hearing loss; measles, mumps, and varicella-zoster virus can cause postnatal hearing loss.

SPECIAL CONSIDERATION

The incidence of congenital CMV infection is greater than that of any other virus, and CMV is the most common cause of viral-induced congenital deafness.

Early identification of hearing loss in children, especially newborn screening in high-risk children is mandatory. Serial auditory brainstem response testing and otoacoustic emissions are used to follow and document hearing as the child develops. Unfortunately, neither medication nor surgery is able to return hearing after such an inner ear insult. Hearing rehabilitation, including conventional amplification and cochlear implantation, is implemented as early as possible. Research into hair cell regeneration will pave the way for "curing" sensorineural hearing loss.

LUETIC EAR DISEASE

Syphilitic infection of the inner ear comes in two forms, congenital and acquired. Congenital infection with the spirochete *Treponema pallidum* can be early (infantile) or late (tardive). Early congenital syphilis is generally fatal, and the labyrinthine manifestations are secondary to the systemic disorders.

Late congenital syphilis can present with both vestibular and auditory symptoms. Sudden symmetric sensorineural hearing loss in a child should be evaluated for syphilis, especially in the presence of the classic signs of congenital syphilis: Hutchinson's teeth, mulberry molars, interstitial keratitis, snuffles, and bossing of the skull. Laboratory testing is discussed below. Clinical history of congenital luetic ear disease may also be that of a 25- to 35-year-old with bilateral, asymmetric, fluctuating sensorineural hearing loss with sudden onset and variable progression. Episodic tinnitus and vertigo may also be present.

In acquired syphilis, sensorineural hearing loss can develop in the primary, secondary, latent, and tertiary stages of the disease.

Histopathology of luetic labyrinthitis shows endolymphatic hydrops; patients present with sensorineural hearing loss often accompanied by vestibular symptoms. Hearing loss can be symmetric or asymmetric, may fluctuate, and may progress to a profound loss.

> **PITFALL...** There is no pathognomonic constellation of symptoms for luetic otitis; clinical presentation can be widely varied, and is similar to Meniere's disease.

Early-stage sensorineural hearing loss tends to be low frequency, with a flat audiometric pattern in later stages of the disease. Most patients do have episodic vestibular symptoms.

Physical examination is significant for the hearing loss and imbalance; otoscopy is normal. Hennebert's sign (induction of nystagmus with changes in ear canal pressure applied with pneumatic otoscopy) and Tullio's sign (vertigo and nystagmus induced by loud noise) may or may not be present.

Recommended serologic testing includes either the fluorescent treponemal antibody absorption test (FTA-ABS) or the microhemagglutination assay for *T. pallidum* antibodies (MHA-TP). These tests should be used for otologic diagnosis; the less sensitive Venereal Disease Research Laboratory (VDRL) and rapid plasma reagent (RPR) tests are not recommended. In a population of adults with unexplained sensorineural hearing loss, 6.5% had a positive FTA-ABS compared with a 2% prevalence in the control population; 7% of patients with symptoms of Meniere's disease were positive.

Penicillin G has the greatest antitreponemal activity; treatment recommendations for luetic otitis include 2.4 million units of benzathine penicillin intramuscularly for early-stage disease. Late-stage disease is treated with a 3-week course of 1.8 million units of procaine penicillin IM daily with 500 mg of probenicid po every 6 hours followed by a 3-month course of 2.4 million units of benzathine penicillin G IM every week. Prednisone 80 mg daily is also given for 1 month, followed by a tapering course to reduce the inflammatory reaction and injury as the spirochete is eliminated.

PETROUS APICITIS

Petrous apicitis is a rare complication of otitis media. Gradenigos' syndrome—retroorbital pain, purulent otorrhea, and sixth nerve palsy—is the hallmark of acute infection of the petrous apex. CT and MRI scanning are complementary in the diagnosis of the disease process. Intravenous antibiotics are begun as soon as possible; surgical intervention is often required to drain a loculated infection in the petrous apex.

VESTIBULAR NEURONITIS

The diagnosis of vestibular neuronitis is made primarily based on the patient's history. The classic story is that of a sudden, severe attack of room-spinning dizziness (vertigo) lasting several hours to days, accompanied by nausea, vomiting, and severe imbalance. There may be tinnitus, but not hearing loss. As the acute attack subsides, the patient is still left with significant imbalance that lasts for days to weeks, is worse at night, and worse with sudden or sharp turns of the head or body. Early on, any movement will aggravate the dizziness.

The insult represents an acute unilateral loss of vestibular function; the patient can take months to compensate. The diagnosis can be difficult to differentiate from Meniere's disease, but Meniere's patients do not get the imbalance following an attack; hearing loss is significant in patients with Meniere's. Meniere's patients will also have several attacks; vestibular neuronitis is a single attack that lasts longer than the typical Meniere's attack.

Physical exam may show an anxious, diaphoretic patient. Spontaneous nystagmus is usually present, but other cranial nerve or cerebellar findings are absent. The Romberg test may be positive. An audiogram should be obtained to document hearing status. Electronystagmography (ENG) will show unilateral peripheral vestibular loss.

Treatment of vestibular neuronitis is supportive. Reassurance is very important to these patients, as they often do not comprehend what is happening and invariably think the worst. Intravenous fluids for rehydration may be necessary. Vestibular suppressants (diazepam, meclizine, or other antihistamine) are used sparingly as they may interfere with central compensation. They are necessary early in the disease, but should be quickly tapered down. Antiemetics are also helpful. Patients generally compensate within several months; vestibular exercises hasten the process.

COGAN'S SYNDROME

Cogan's syndrome is the prototype of immune-mediated inner ear disease. Nonsyphilitic ocular inflammation and audiovestibular dysfunction are thought to be secondary to an autoimmune phenomenon. Patients typically have interstitial keratitis, but can also have scleritis, uveitis, or conjunctivitis (atypical Cogan's). Bilateral fluctuating sensorineural hearing loss, episodic vertigo, tinnitus, and aural pressure, similar to Meniere's disease, characterize the ear symptoms; they can precede or follow eye symptoms. Temporal bone histopathology has documented atrophy of the organ of Corti, fibrosis, osteoneogenesis, and plasma cell and lymphocytic infiltration.

Topical corticosteroids for ocular disease are the preferred treatment; oral corticosteroids are the treatment of choice for audiovestibular symptoms. Steroids can stabilize and even recover hearing. The audiogram should be followed, and short bursts of steroids are helpful during exacerbations of the disease, although the hearing loss is relentless.

AUTOIMMUNE INNER EAR DISEASE

McCabe (1979) originally reported on a group of patients with bilateral, asymmetric sensorineural hearing loss that was progressive over the course of weeks to months. Some patients experienced vestibular symptoms. He treated these patients with immunosuppressive therapy with marked improvement in their hearing. He theorized that these patients suffered from an autoimmune-mediated injury to the inner ear and that this injury was reversible. Subsequent reports have substantiated his findings, and there are now laboratory tests that can be used to confirm a presumptive diagnosis—the lymphocyte transformation test and Western blot immunoassay. The diagnosis is essentially a clinical one. Patients tend to be middle-aged women; history of other autoimmune or immune-mediated disorders supports the diagnosis.

An empiric trial of steroids is warranted in such a patient with the typical clinical history. Recommendations are for prednisone 1 mg/kg/day for 1 month followed by a tapering dose. Recovery of hearing or resolution of symptoms following an empiric course of oral steroids also makes the diagnosis. Some clinicians have used cyclophosphamide to block the immune response, but we do not recommend this for first-line therapy. Plasmapharesis has also been tried.

SUGGESTED READINGS

Armstrong BW. A new treatment for chronic secretory otitis media. *Arch Otolaryngol* 1954; 69:653–654.

Bluestone CD, Klein JO. Otitis media: a spectrum of diseases. In: Lalwani AK, Grundfast KM, eds. *Pediatric Otology and Neurotology.* Philadelphia: Lippincott-Raven; 1998:233–240.

Bluestone CD, Stephenson JS, Martin LM. Ten-year review of otitis media pathogens. *Pediatr Infect Dis J* 1992;11(8 suppl):S7–11.

Darmstadt GL, Harris JP. Luetic hearing loss: clinical presentation, diagnosis, and treatment. *Am J Otolaryngol* 1989;97:409.

Gates GA. Cost-effectiveness considerations in otitis media treatment. *Otolaryngol Head Neck Surg* 1996;114:525–530.

Gates GA, Avery CA, Prihoda TJ, Cooper JC. Effectiveness of adenoidectomy and tympanostomy tubes in the treatment of otitis media with effusion. *N Engl J Med* 1987;317: 1444–1451.

Gates GA, Muntz HR, Gaylis B. Adenoidectomy and otitis media. *Ann Otol Rhinol Laryngol* 1992;101:24–32.

Gebhart DE. Tympanostomy tubes in the otitis media prone child. *Laryngoscope* 1981;91: 849–866.

Grundfast KM. Management of otitis media and the new Agency for Health Care Policy and Research Guideline. *Arch Otolaryngol* 1994;120:797–798.

Gulya AJ. Infections of the labyrinth. In: Bailey BJ, ed. *Head and Neck Surgery–Otolaryngology.* Philadelphia: JB Lippincott; 1993:1769–1781.

Healy GB. Managing otitis media with effusion in young children: a commentary. *Arch Otolaryngol* 1994;120:1049–1050.

Henderson FW, Giebink GS. Otitis media among children in day care: epidemiology and pathogenesis. *Rev Infect Dis* 1986;8:533–538.

Hughes GB, Moscicki R, Barna B, San Martin J. Laboratory diagnosis of immune inner ear disease. *Am J Otol* 1994;15:198–202.

Karma PH, Penttila MA, Sipila MM, Kataja MJ. Otoscopic diagnosis of middle ear effusion in acute and non-acute otitis media. *Int J Pediatr Otorhinolaryngol* 1989;17:37–49.

Kleinman LC, Kosecoff J, Dubois RW, Brook RH. The medical appropriateness of tympanostomy tubes proposed for children younger than 16 years in the United States. *JAMA* 1994; 271:1250–1255.

Kovatch AL, Wald ER, Michaels RH. β-Lactamase producing *Branhamella catarrhalis* causing otitis media in children. *J Pediatr* 1983;102:261–264.

Lambert PR. Oral steroid therapy for chronic middle ear effusion: a double-blind crossover study. *Otolaryngol Head Neck Surg* 1986;95: 193–199.

Lebel M, Freij B, Syrogiannopoulos G, et al. Dexamethasone therapy for bacterial meningitis: results of two double-blind placebo-controlled trials. *N Engl J Med* 1988;319:964–971.

Lowhagen G-B, Rosenhall U, Andersson M, et al. Central nervous system involvement in early syphilis. *Acta Derm Venereol (Stockh)* 1983;63:530.

Mandel EM, Rockette HE, Bluestone CD, et al. Efficacy of amoxicillin with and without decongestant-antihistamine for otitis media with effusion in children. *N Engl J Med* 1987; 316:432–437.

Maw AR. Chronic otitis media with effusion (glue ear) and adenotonsillectomy: a prospective randomized controlled study. *BMJ* 1983; 287:1586–1588.

McCabe BF. Autoimmune sensorineural hearing loss. *Ann Otol Rhinol Laryngol* 1979;88: 585–589.

Papastavros T, Giamarellou H, Varlejides S. Role of aerobic and anaerobic microorganisms in chronic suppurative otitis media. *Laryngoscope* 1986;96:438–442.

Paradise JL, Bluestone CD. Adenoidectomy and chronic otitis media [letter]. *N Engl J Med* 1988;318:1470–1471.

Paradise JL, Bluestone CD, Rogers KD, et al. Efficacy of adenoidectomy for recurrent otitis media in children previously treated with tympanostomy tube placement. *JAMA* 1990; 263:2066–2073.

Perrin JM, Charney E, MacWhinney JB Jr, et al. Suifisoxazole as chemoprophylaxis for recurrent otitis media. *N Engl J Med* 1974;291: 664–667.

Post JC, Preston RA, Aul JJ, et al. Molecular analysis of bacterial pathogens in otitis media with effusion. *JAMA* 1995;273:1598–1604.

Rosenfeld RM, Post JC. Meta-analysis of antibiotics for treatment of otitis media with effusion. *Otolaryngol Head Neck Surg* 1992;106: 378–386.

Schappert SM. Office visits for otitis media: United States, 1975–90. *Vital Health Stat* 1992;214:1.

Schwartz RH, Rodriguez WJ, Grundfast KM. Duration of middle ear effusion after acute otitis media. *Pediatr Infect Dis J* 1984;3:204–207.

Sheehy JL, Brackmann DE. Cholesteatoma surgery: management of the labyrinthine fistula: a report of 97 cases. *Laryngoscope* 1979;89:78.

Sheehy JL, Brackmann DE. Surgery of chronic otitis media. In: English, ed. *Otolaryngology*, vol 1. Philadelphia: JB Lippincott; 1994: 1–87.

Shurin PA, Pelton SI, Turczyk VA, et al. Persistence of middle ear effusion after acute otitis media. *N Engl J Med* 1979;300:1121–1123.

Stool SE, Berg AO, Berman S, et al. *Managing Otitis Media with Effusion in Young Children: Quick Reference Guide for Clinicians.* AHCPR publication no. 94-0623. Rockville, MD: Agency for Health Care Policy and Research, Public Health Service, U.S. Dept. Health and Human Services; 1994.

Teele DW, Klein JO, Rosner B. Epidemiology of otitis media in children. *Ann Otol Rhinol Laryngol* 1980;89(suppl 68):5–6.

Teele DW, Klein JO, Rosner B, and the Greater Boston Otitis Media Study Group. Middle ear disease in the practice of pediatrics: burden during the first five years of life. *JAMA* 1983;249:1026–1029.

Teele DW, Klein JO, Rosner BA, and the Greater Boston Otitis Media Study Group. Epidemiology of otitis media during the first seven years of life in children in Greater Boston: a prospective cohort study. *J Infect Dis* 1989; 160:83–94.

Varsano I, Volovitz B, Mimouni F. Sulfisoxazole prophylaxis of middle ear effusion and recurrent acute otitis media. *Am J Dis Child* 1985; 139:632–635.

Chapter 6

NEOPLASMS AND CYSTS

Rick A. Friedman

The outer, inner, and middle ear are composed of a variety of specialized tissues. The structures of the ear are derived from the three embryonic layers including the ectoderm, mesoderm, and endoderm. As such, a variety of tumors of these epithelial and connective tissue layers may arise. Until very recently, the inner ear was felt to be a privileged site in regard to neoplasms. As this chapter discusses, no part of the ear is considered free from the risk of primary or metastatic tumor.

BENIGN NEOPLASMS OF THE EAR

KERATOACANTHOMA OF THE EXTERNAL EAR

A keratoacanthoma is a benign squamous epithelial neoplasm that arises on sun-exposed areas of the skin. These tumors are characterized by rapid development, followed by rapid involution and regression. They are often noted for their crater-like appearance during involution.

These tumors are seen most commonly later in life, during the sixth and seventh decades, and they appear to affect males more often than females. Approximately 10% of these lesions occur on the pinna.

PITFALL... These lesions typically begin as red papules and demonstrate rapid enlargement over a few week period, culminating in an exophytic nodule that on appearance may simulate squamous cell carcinoma.

This stage of rapid proliferation is often followed by a plateau period lasting up to several months. This plateau period is followed by the rapid phase of involution often with complete regression leading to only mild scar formation.

The etiology of this disorder is unknown, but likely results from sun damage. These lesions must be differentiated from squamous cell carcinoma and this can often be done by looking at the nuclear-to-cytoplasmic ratio and/or areas of vascular or perineural invasion. The suggested treatment of these lesions is complete surgical excision, which is often curative. In a very small percentage of these cases, keratoacanthoma may recur.

CERUMEN GLAND ADENOMA

Cerumen gland adenomas are benign tumors of cerumen-secreting modified apocrine glands that are located in the lateral third of the external auditory canal. *Ceruminoma* is a term often used to describe these tumors. Cerumenal gland neoplasms are extremely uncommon; however, they represent one of the more common tumors of the external auditory canal. These tumors can be benign or malignant. The malignant varieties include adenocarcinoma and adenoid cystic carcinoma.

These tumors affect males more often than females and are most frequently seen in the fifth and sixth decade of life. Symptoms of these tumors are a slow-growing external canal mass resulting in hearing loss and occasionally otitis externa due to a canal obstruction. Ulceration of these lesions is extremely uncommon, and, if it is seen, one should suspect a malignancy. The differential diagnosis of these neoplasms includes neoplasms of the parotid gland that have gained access to the external auditory canal through the fissures of Santorini. The treatment for benign lesions is complete surgical excision, which is often curative.

BENIGN NEOPLASMS OF THE MIDDLE EAR AND TEMPORAL BONE

MIDDLE EAR ADENOMA

The submucosa of the middle ear contains many secretory glands. As such, the middle ear is a potential site for the development of benign glandular neoplasms or adenomas. Middle ear adenomas are considered extremely rare. Any portion of the middle ear may be affected including the eustachian tube, the mastoid air cells, and the tympanic cavity. These lesions most often present with unilateral conductive hearing loss due to impingement upon the ossicular chain. These lesions are often readily identified on microscopic otologic examination, revealing a bland-appearing middle ear space. Radiographically, these lesions often appear rounded without evidence of bone erosion.

The differential diagnosis of this lesion includes malignant glandular neoplasms of the middle ear and neuromas of the facial nerve, among others. Additionally, adenomas with neuroendocrine features, called carcinoid tumors of the middle ear, do occur and can be dif-

ferentiated histologically. The treatment of these tumors is complete surgical excision. This often requires a tympanomastoid approach.

JUGULOTYMPANIC PARAGANGLIOMA

The first descriptions of "swellings" or "ganglions" associated with the tympanic nerve appeared in the mid- and late 1800s. It was not until 1941 that, in his address to the American Association of Anatomists, Guild (1953) described the "presence of a previously unrecognized structure," which he called the "glomus jugularis" or jugular body. In his first report, he described glomus formations along the course of Jacobson's nerve from its beginning near the adventitia of the jugular bulb to the cochlear promontory. Soon thereafter he noted these formations along the course of Arnold's nerve from the skull base into the mastoid canaliculus and fallopian canal.

Biology

The chief cells, the principal cells of paraganglionic tissue, are derived from the neural crest and migrate in close association with the ganglia of the sympathetic nervous system.

SPECIAL CONSIDERATION

The term *glomus* was applied because of an original belief that the chief cell was derived from specialized pericytes as seen in true arteriovenous (glomus) complexes. This theory is no longer felt to be true; hence, the correct terminology is paraganglia.

Tumors of the paraganglia, paragangliomas, can be divided into two main groups: adrenal and extra–adrenal. Extraadrenal paragangliomas are associated with sympathetic ganglia in the abdomen, chest, retroperitoneum, and mediastinum. Classification of paragangliomas of the head and neck (branchiomeric) is based on their anatomic location and includes the carotid body and jugulotympanic, vagal, laryngeal, nasal, and orbital paragangliomas. The most common location in the head and neck is the carotid body, followed by the jugulotympanic region.

Paragangliomas display a characteristic histologic pattern. Light microscopy demonstrates clusters of chief cells (zellballen) and sustentacular cells, with abundant small blood vessels and unmyelinated nerve fibers presumably derived from the glossopharyngeal nerve.

The main focus of this section is on the management of paragangliomas arising within the temporal bone, the so-called jugulotympanic paragangliomas. This group of paragangliomas includes those of the jugular bulb region (jugulare) and the tympanic cavity (tympanicum). These tumors are considered the most common tumors of the middle ear and the second most common tumors of the temporal bone after acoustic neuromas. The majority of these tumors arise in the jugular bulb.

Clinical Characteristics

Paragangliomas appear to be most common in Caucasians, although there is no clear cut racial predilection. These tumors occur more commonly in women, and, although they have been described in patients as young as 6 months and as old as 88 years, they are typically identified in the fourth or fifth decades of life. A hereditary component to some tumors has been seen with an autosomal-dominant mode of transmission.

Paragangliomas demonstrate a slow and insidious pattern of growth. The time to onset of symptoms depends on the site of origin of the tumor. However, there are typically few symptoms until the lesion is far advanced.

Otologic symptoms are by far the most common presenting complaints and consist of pulsatile tinnitus and conductive hearing loss. Tympanicum tumors present earlier than those of the jugular bulb region due to earlier involvement of the umbo with resultant transmission of pulsations and subsequent conductive hearing loss.

Paragangliomas rarely metastasize and most often spread along paths of least resistance. They tend to migrate their way through the temporal bone via vascular channels, naturally occurring fissures and formina, and, most importantly, along air cell tracts.

Neurologic deficits are the second major group of symptoms and signs often appearing after considerable tumor growth. The incidence of cranial nerve involvement by tumor is approximately 37% and that of intracranial extension is 15%.

Tumors originating in the jugular bulb, or those from the middle ear that extend inferiorly to involve this region, make themselves apparent by their compression of cranial nerves IX, X, XI, and XII either at the jugular foramen and hypoglossal canals (Vernet's and Collet-Sicard syndromes) or in the carotid sheath after extension into the parapharyngeal space. Involvement of the internal carotid artery either in the neck or in the petrous portion of the temporal bone can lead to Horner's syndrome by involvement of the sympathetic plexus.

Radiologic Diagnosis

Radiologic evaluation is essential for the proper diagnosis and management of jugulotympanic paragangliomas. Techniques such as plain films of the mastoid and polytomography have been supplanted by high-resolution computed tomography (HRCT) and magnetic resonance imaging (MRI). Furthermore, unless the tumor is embolized or envelops much of the internal carotid artery, HRCT and MRI obviate the need for angiography.

HRCT scans in the axial and coronal planes, including soft tissue and bone algorithms,

PEARL••• The signs and symptoms have been placed into three groups based on the tumor characteristics and location: (1) those due to the presence of tumor in the middle ear—conductive hearing loss, aural polyp, and aural discharge; (2) those due to the vascularity of the tumor—pulsatile tinnitus, aural bleeding, and a positive Brown's or Aquino's sign; the former consists of cessation of tumor pulsation and tumor blanching with positive pressure on pneumotoscopy, and the latter consists of cessation of tumor pulsation with ipsilateral carotid artery compression; and (3) those that suggest tumor extension to vital structures—sensorineural hearing loss, vertigo, aural pain, and cranial neuropathy.

provide information critical to the differential diagnosis and approach to management of these tumors. HRCT supplements clinical otoscopy in defining the extent of tumor beyond the microscopically visible limits of the tympanic annulus, and it aids in the differentiation of tumors from vascular anomalies.

MRI is superior to HRCT in its ability to characterize the vascular nature of tumors involving the jugular bulb and skull base without the use of contrast and without the artifact from the petrous bone typically seen on CT. MRI displays the important relations of the tumor to the surrounding great vessels, including venous invasion. T1-weighted images, with and without contrast, display the highly vascular nature of the tumor matrix, and T2-weighted images provide excellent soft tissue contrast.

PEARL••• For lesions larger than 2 cm, T2-weighted MRI images often display the "salt and pepper" appearance characteristic of paragangliomas.

Differential Diagnosis

When considering the differential diagnosis of paragangliomas, we must consider two different presentations: (1) intratympanic vascular masses and (2) lesions of the skull base *artery* and *transdural* tumors are far more extensive and require an infratemporal fossa approach and excision of the intracranial component.

Radiation Therapy

The role of radiation therapy in the treatment of jugulotympanic paragangliomas is quite controversial. Many reports have appeared in the old and recent literature reporting tumor control rates of 70 to 90% with radiation as primary, adjunctive, or salvage therapy. The doses given in these studies are between 3500 and 5000 cGy. The primary effect of radiation therapy appears to be on the vascular and stromal elements of the tumor, with little effect on the tumor cells. Viable tumor cells remain after radiation, and tumors have been known to recrudesce after more than a decade. With the advent of microsurgical techniques, there are few specific indications for radiation therapy. This form of treatment is recommended for elderly patients with symptomatic tumors or for patients who are unsuitable for, or unwilling to undergo, surgical resection.

MALIGNANT NEOPLASMS OF THE EAR AND TEMPORAL BONE

BASAL CELL CARCINOMA

Basal cell carcinomas are the most common cutaneous malignancies in humans. They are characterized by their slow-growing locally infiltrative nature and involve the skin and the subcutaneous adnexal tissue. They are more common in males than females and typically occur later in life. Sun-exposed areas of the head and neck are more frequent sites of occurrence, but the most common locations include the nose, the periorbital region, the nasal-labial area, and the periauricular area. Basal cells of the external auditory canal are unusual. Certain biologically aggressive basal cell carcinomas can be very destructive and involve the external canal, the auricular cartilage, and even the temporal bone.

The genetic basis for basal cell carcinoma has recently been elucidated. In particular, an autosomal-dominant disorder called nevoid basal cell carcinoma syndrome has been identified at the molecular level. These patients develop multiple basal cell carcinomas and have associated palmar and plantar pitting, odontogenic keratosis of the jaw and ribs, and neurologic abnormalities.

There are a variety of histologic patterns of basal cell carcinoma, the most significant and aggressive of which include the causing caudal cranial nerve deficits. Radiographic imaging is an essential aid to the differential diagnosis, with HRCT the preferred modality for the former and MRI for the latter.

> **PITFALL...** Vascular anomalies of the middle ear may present in a fashion identical to that of an intratympanic paraganglioma. The principal anomalies include the aberrant or laterally displaced internal carotid artery, the dehiscent or high-riding jugular bulb, and the congenital or acquired intratympanic carotid artery aneurysm.

The differential diagnosis of jugular foramen masses includes a variety of benign and malignant neoplasms and is beyond the scope of this chapter. In brief, schwannomas of cranial nerves IX, X, XI, and XII and meningiomas can all present with caudal cranial nerve deficits. A variety of primary and metastatic lesions of the skull base can also lead to caudal cranial nerve deficits. Here, too, radiography is essential to the differential diagnosis.

Tumor Classification and Selection of Surgical Approach

Numerous classification schemes have been devised for the clinical characterization of paragangliomas. These schemes are largely based on anatomic location and tumor extent. The classification described by De la Cruz (Brackmann, 1994) has been extremely useful in the treatment planning of these tumors. In this classification scheme, tumors are described by their anatomic extent and each group of tumors has a corresponding operative approach.

Tympanic tumors are those arising in the middle ear and confined entirely to the mesotympanum. The complete extent of the tumor is visible through the tympanic membrane; hence, tumor excision can be performed through a transcanal approach. In contrast, a *tympanomastoid* tumor arises from the middle ear but has extended into the posterior tympanum or the hypotympanum beyond the visible confines of the tympanic annulus. Radiographically, these tumors do not involve the jugular bulb, and they can be excised through a mastoid-extended facial recess approach.

Jugular bulb tumors are confined to this region and may extend to the middle ear and mastoid. They do not involve the carotid artery or the intracranial compartment. These tumors are excised through the mastoid-neck approach. Large tumors may require limited rerouting of the facial nerve to the second genu.

The management of basal cell carcinoma of the pinna is very much like that in other areas of the head and neck. Morphea or sclerosing and keratotic types require aggressive management.

> ## SPECIAL CONSIDERATION
>
> The pinna is considered one of the areas of high risk for recurrence as there are embryonic fusion planes in and around the pinna. For this reason it is recommended that Mohs' surgical approach be undertaken to clear margins.

Several modes of therapy exist including simple excision, electrodesiccation and curettage, and radiation; however, cure rates appear to be better with the Mohs' surgical technique.

For basal cell carcinomas of the external canal and/or temporal bone, more complicated surgical excision is required, often necessitating lateral temporal or subtotal temporal bone resection. Basal cell carcinoma must be differentiated from another form of cancer that can involve the pinna, called Merkel's cell carcinoma. This is also known as a neuroendocrine carcinoma of the skin. This rare lesion is most common in the seventh and eighth decades of life and is characterized by poorly differentiated malignant small cells in the dermis and subcutaneous tissues. The margins of this tumor are often poorly defined and there is a high rate of regional lymph node involvement. Recommended therapy is wide local excision with lymph node dissection when helpful.

SQUAMOUS CELL CARCINOMA OF THE EAR AND TEMPORAL BONE

Squamous cell carcinoma represents the most common malignant neoplasm of the external auditory canal, middle ear, and temporal bone.

This lesion likely results from actinic damage; however, there seems to be an association with chronic otitis media. Squamous cell carcinoma of the ear and temporal bone affects males more commonly than females and is seen in later life.

> **PEARL•••** Patients often present with a nonhealing ulcer, many times mistaken for chronic otitis externa, and treated as such.

It is important that all primary care physicians recognize that simple otitis externa responds to medical treatment relatively rapidly. When pain persists and granulation tissue is present for a prolonged period of time, a biopsy should be performed.

Imaging studies of the temporal bone must be obtained to evaluate soft tissue and bony involvement. HRCT scan of the temporal bone provides the most information regarding bone destruction and the extent of invasion into the middle ear and mastoid. MRI can help define the relationship of the tumor to vascular structures of the skull base and extension of the tumor intracranially. Physical examination, in concert with radiographic studies, allows appropriate staging and provides the framework for therapeutic intervention.

Although a basic surgical tenet is en-bloc resection of carcinoma, the management of carcinomas of the temporal bone utilizing this approach places the patient at significant risk of morbidity and intraoperative mortality. As such, a graduated approach to tumor management has been described. The procedure begins with a wide postauricular incision and lateral temporal bone resection. After removal of the external auditory canal with the tympanic membrane, malleus, and incus, the further extent of the lesion can be assessed and the appropriate temporal bone drilling can be performed until normal-appearing bone is identified. After completion of the resection, the middle ear cavity can be lined with a split-thickness skin graft and in cases requiring postoperative radiation therapy, consideration for a vascularized flap to prevent osteoradionecrosis is essential.

Patients with intracranial extension or circumferential involvement of the petrous portion of the internal carotid artery should be considered for palliative rather than curative treatment options. Patients with involvement of the middle ear and mastoid should undergo combined therapy. In general, the prognosis for early stages is good; however, patients with tumors involving the middle ear and mastoid bone historically have poor long-term prognoses.

SUGGESTED READINGS

Aquino J. Glomus jugulare tumors. *Arch Otolaryngol* 1957;65:263.

Batsakis JG. Adenomous tumors of the middle ear. *Ann Otol Rhinol Otolaryngol* 1989;98:749–752.

Benecke JE, Noel FL, Carberry JN, House JW, Patterson M. Adenomatous tumors of the middle ear and mastoid. *Am J Otol* 1990;11:20–26.

Brackmann DE, Arriaga MA. Surgery for glomus tumors. In: Brackmann DE, Shelton C, Arriaga MA, eds. *Otologic Surgery*. Philadelphia: WB Saunders; 1994:579–594.

Brackmann DE, House WF, Terry R, Scanlan RL. Glomus jugulare tumors: effect of irradiation. *Trans Am Acad Ophthalmol Otolaryngol* 1972;76:1423.

Brown LA. Glomus jugulare tumor of the middle ear: clinical aspects. *Laryngoscope* 1953;63:281.

Cole JM, Beiler D. Long-term results of treatment for glomus jugulare and glomus vagale tumors with radiotherapy. *Laryngoscope* 1994;104:1461.

Dehner LP, Chen KTK. Primary tumors of the external middle ear: benign and malignant glandular neoplasms. *Arch Otolaryngol* 1980;106:13–19.

de Jong AL, Coker NJ, Jenkins HA, Goepfert H, Alford BR. Radiation therapy in the management of paragangliomas of the temporal bone. *Am J Otol* 1995;16:283.

Glenner GG, Grimley PM. Tumors of the extra-adrenal paraganglion system (including chemoreceptors). In: Glenner GG, ed. *Atlas of Tumor Pathology*, 2nd series, fascicle 9. Washington, DC: Armed Forces Institute of Pathology; 1974:1.

Goodwin RE, Fisher GH. Ketatocanthoma of the head and neck. *Ann Otol Rhinol Otolaryngol* 1980;89:72–74.

Guild SR. The glomus jugulare, a nonchromaffin paraganglion, in man. *Ann Otol Rhinol Laryngol* 1953;62:1045.

Gulya AJ. The glomus tumor and its biology. *Laryngoscope* 1993;103(suppl 60):3.

Kinney SE, Wood BG. Malignancies of the external ear canal and temporal bone: surgical techniques and results. *Laryngoscope* 1987;97:158.

Krause W. Die glandula tympanica des menschen. *Centralbl Med Wissensch* 1878;16:737.

Mendenhall WM, Parsons JT, Stringer SP, Cassisi NJ, Singleton GT, Million RR. Radiotherapy in the management of temporal bone chemodectoma. *Skull Base Surg* 1995;5:83.

Valentin G. Ueber eine gangliose anschwellung in der Jacobsonchen anastomose des menschen. *Arch Anat Physiol Wissensch Med* 1840;89:287.

Wenig BM. Neoplasms of the ear. In: Wenig BM, ed. *Atlas of Head and Neck Pathology.* Philadelphia: WB Saunders; 1993:368.

Chapter 7

TRAUMA

Rick A. Friedman

The ear and temporal bone are uniquely vulnerable to injury throughout life. The prominence of the pinna places it at risk for blunt and sharp trauma, and the delicate structures of the middle ear and otic capsule are readily injured by direct or indirect trauma. This chapter reviews the diagnosis and management of a variety of injuries to the ear and temporal bone.

AURICULAR HEMATOMA

Blunt trauma, lacerations, avulsions, and burns can result in significant auricular deformity. Auricular hematoma typically results from direct blunt trauma to the external ear. Although physical contact in a variety of sports may lead to auricular hematoma, high school and collegiate wrestling are the most common sources of this injury.

Patients with auricular hematoma typically present with a soft, fluctuant mass on the outer surface of the pinna. The hematoma most often accumulates in the scaphoid fossa, the triangular fossa, or the concha. In addition to the pain of the blow, the patients often have a feeling of warmth in the involved pinna from the accumulated blood.

The pathophysiology of the acute injury can be explained by the local anatomy. The skin overlying the anterior surface of the pinna is adherent to the underlying perichondrium. Unlike the posterior surface, which can withstand a shearing force due to a layer of subcutaneous loose connective tissue, the full impact of the blow to the anterior surface is transmitted directly to the adherent perichondrium and cartilage.

Left untreated, a so-called cauliflower ear will develop. Many theories on the pathogenesis of this entity have been put forth. In a convincing set of experiments, Ohlsen et al (1975) demonstrated that blood placed in the subcutaneous tissue of a rabbit's ear, between the skin and perichondrium, resolved without deformity. A similar deposit of blood placed between the auricular cartilage and its overlying perichondrium resulted in the accumulation of chondrocytes, chondroneogenesis, and a cauliflower ear. It is, therefore, imperative to efficiently and expeditiously treat these injuries.

The treatment of auricular hematoma is aimed at evacuation of the blood and the prevention of its reaccumulation. Many forms of therapy have been described including simple aspiration, incision and drainage, aspiration or incision followed by bolster placement, suction drainage, and posterior transcartilaginous incision. It is clear that aspiration alone results in a high rate of treatment failure. Giffin (1985) described incision of the auricle anteriorly in a cosmetic location, followed by evacuation of the hematoma, excision of the newly formed fibrocartilage and overlying perichondrium, and placement of cotton bolsters. Schuller et al (1989) described a technique of evacuation by incision and drainage followed by the immediate placement of a pressure dressing consisting of molded dental rolls secured with through-and-through sutures. This technique allows the athlete to return to activity immediately. In those patients treated in this fashion for a 14-day period, no recurrences of hematoma or subsequent auricular deformity were encountered.

AURICULAR BITE WOUNDS

Approximately one million animal bite victims seek medical attention each year, and the majority of them are in the pediatric population. Dogs are responsible for the large majority of these injuries. Although far less common, human auricular bite wounds occur with some frequency secondary to either rough play or assault. In a review of bite wounds in children, Brook (1987) described the microbiology of 21 animal bites and 18 human bites. Six of the 39 wounds occurred on the head and neck. Mixed aerobic and anaerobic flora were most commonly cultured from the wounds of both animal and human bites. The most frequent isolates from animal bites were, in descending order, *Staphylococcus aureus, Pasteurella multocida,* and anaerobic cocci. The most frequent isolates from human bites were *S. aureus,* gamma-hemolytic streptococci, anaerobic cocci, *Fusobacterium* spp., and *Bacteroides* spp. *P. multocida* and *Pseudomonas fluorescens* were notably absent in human wounds in contrast to animal wounds. Furthermore, 41% of the 39 wounds in Brook's study contained β-lactamase–producing organisms.

No single antimicrobial eradicates all of the pathogens responsible for bite wound infections. Treatment should be directed at specific isolates through appropriate bacterial cultures. Penicillin and ampicillin are the best agents for the treatment of *P. multocida* and other oral flora. *S. aureus* and a large percentage of *Bac-*

teroides spp. are resistant to penicillins. The combination of amoxicillin and clavulanic acid is very effective against most uncomplicated animal and human bite wounds.

Early treatment of all bite wounds is essential for the prevention of infection and to achieve an optimal cosmetic result. Stucker et al (1990) described their comprehensive management of bite wounds. Their treatment begins with immediate jet lavage, debridement of all devitalized tissue, and intravenous antibiotics (Timentin). The decision regarding method and timing of repair depends on the site and severity of the wound, the source of the wound, and the time elapsed between the injury and the implementation of treatment. Stucker et al advocate primary repair of clean nonhuman bites if performed within 5 hours of injury. All human bite wounds and avulsion injuries are managed in a delayed fashion.

Rabies prevention, including hyperimmune serum and immunization, should be instituted for animal bites. For all wounds, a tetanus toxoid booster is given if the child has been immunized within the past 10 years. In unimmunized patients, tetanus immune globulin should be administered.

TRAUMATIC INJURIES TO THE TYMPANIC MEMBRANE AND OSSICLES

In a review of 57 cases of traumatic tympanic membrane rupture, Armstrong (1970) found the cotton-tipped Q-tip to be the leading offender. Tympanic membrane rupture can occur from indirect trauma as well. A shock wave in the external auditory canal from an explosion, such as a firecracker, or a blow to the ear that occludes the meatus compressing the air column, can subsequently stretch the tympanic membrane beyond its elastic limit, leading to rupture. Regardless of the mechanism, these injuries require immediate attention.

Microscopic examination of the ear after a suspected injury is recommended within the first 24 hours. Fortunately, traumatic tears of the tympanic membrane tend to heal spontaneously.

Even large perforations can heal without surgical repair.

Examination, either under local or general anesthesia, involves aspiration of blood clots, sterile irrigation, inspection of the drum and middle ear, and palpation of the ossicular chain. Medially displaced flaps can be replaced to their original position. These flaps can be held in place with a cigarette paper patch or Gelfoam.

A tympanic membrane that has healed incompletely, depending on the size, can be treated with chemical cauterization with 50% trichloroacetic acid, or 10% silver nitrate. Slightly larger perforations can be repaired utilizing the technique of fat myringoplasty.

Large perforations or those unresponsive to the above-mentioned techniques can be treated using standard myringoplasty techniques. For small posterior perforations, an underlay technique may suffice. For most other perforations of the tympanic membrane, either the lateral surface grafting technique or underlay technique may be used.

Following a traumatic rupture of the tympanic membrane, a mild conductive hearing loss, 10 to 30 dB, will be observed on audiometric testing. Small perforations are associated with very slight degrees of conductive loss.

> **PEARL...** The presence of a perforation in the posterior-superior quadrant or conductive losses exceeding 35 dB should alert the physician to the possibility of ossicular injury.

Blunt nonpenetrating trauma to the ear or temporal bone is frequently associated with ossicular injury. Longitudinal temporal bone fractures are often accompanied by ossicular subluxation or fracture.

The mechanism of ossicular injury with penetrating trauma is self-evident. However, the mechanism of injury with blunt trauma is speculative. Hough (1969) hypothesized several mechanisms acting individually or in concert: (1) the explosive effects of concussion producing temporary tissue weakening and separation, (2) the effects of inertia on the patient's head

during reaction to acceleration and deceleration, (3) the tetanic contraction of the intratympanic muscles, and (4) the torsion effect of skull fracture causing shifting of the middle ear structures.

Regardless of the mechanisms leading to injury, posttraumatic ossicular injury and subsequent conductive hearing loss are well described. The most common site of injury is the incudostapedial (IS) joint. The point of disarticulation or fracture is determined by the strength of each ossicle and its soft tissue support. The malleus is supported by its five ligaments and its attachments to the tympanic membrane at the umbo and short process. The stapes is supported by its annular ligament and the stapedius tendon. The incus is left spanning the distance between the malleus and stapes, supported only by its articulation with the malleus and its supporting ligaments in the attic and fossa incudis. The incus, therefore, is the ossicle most commonly disrupted in temporal bone trauma.

The stapes is the second most frequently injured ossicle. Because the footplate is secured in the oval window by the annular ligament, the site of stapedial injury is most often the crura.

> ## SPECIAL CONSIDERATION
>
> Subluxation of the stapes footplate, although uncommon, is an otologic emergency.

Footplate subluxation is often associated with sensorineural hearing loss, tinnitus, and vertigo with nystagmus. The exposed vestibule should be covered as soon as the patient is suitable for surgery. Early intervention may prevent deafness, resolve vertigo, and provide a barrier to infection for the inner ear and adjacent cerebrospinal fluid (CSF).

The recognition and repair of traumatic middle ear injuries were realized with the advent of the operating microscope and tympanoplastic techniques. A variety of techniques for repair have been described including ossicular repositioning, type III tympanoplasty, and incus replacement prostheses.

SPECIAL CONSIDERATION

Children with unilateral conductive hearing loss and normal contralateral hearing can be managed conservatively until the child is old enough to participate in the decision and postoperative care of ossicular reconstruction. Additionally, surgery for conductive hearing loss should not be performed on an only-hearing ear.

In general, a postauricular approach for tympanoplasty is preferred. The type of reconstruction will depend on the surgical findings. For the most common injury, IS joint dislocation, we have utilized the Applebaum hydroxylapatite IS joint prosthesis. If the incus is more severely subluxed, it is removed and continuity restored either by reshaping the incus and placing it between the malleus and stapes, by placing a hydroxylapatite incus replacement prosthesis, or by placing a prosthesis from the undersurface of the drum to the stapes [partial ossicular replacement prosthesis (PORP) or total ossicular replacement prosthesis (TORP)]. The latter technique is favored in cases with an anteriorly positioned malleus. Injuries to the incus and stapes suprastructure are reconstructed with a TORP. Autologous cartilage is placed on the platform of all partial and total ossicular reconstruction prostheses to prevent extrusion and to reinforce the tympanic membrane in this group of patients prone to eustachian tube dysfunction.

TEMPORAL BONE FRACTURES

Studies of the mechanisms and anatomic distributions of temporal bone fractures reveal that they tend to occur in specific locations and result in characteristic signs and symptoms. The petrous portion of the temporal bone forms approximately two thirds of the floor of the middle cranial fossa and one third of the floor of the posterior cranial fossa. The foramina at the base of the skull are areas of stress concentration; consequently, fractures tend to occur in their vicinity.

Temporal bone fractures have classically been described as longitudinal, transverse, and mixed. Approximately 90% of fractures are of the longitudinal type. Longitudinal fractures are associated with a temporal or parietal blow, and result in a fracture of the petrous bone extending anteromedially along the petrous ridge to the foramen lacerum and foramen ovale (Fig. 7–1). The fracture line often begins in the squamous portion, extends through the posterior and superior walls of the external canal, traverses the tegmen tympani, and extends anterior to the otic capsule on its way to the petrous apex. The facial nerve is injured in approximately 15% of cases, usually in the perigeniculate region. Longitudinal fractures are often associated with the traumatic conductive triad described by Hough (1969) as follows: (1) loss

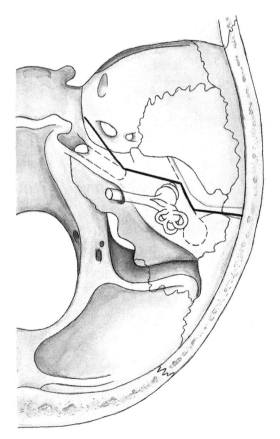

FIGURE 7–1 Schematic diagram of a longitudinal temporal bone fracture. Note the fracture line anterior and lateral to the otic capsule.

of hearing, (2) bleeding from the ear through a lacerated tympanic membrane, and (3) unconsciousness.

Transverse fractures are less frequent, constituting 10 to 15% of temporal bone fractures. Frontal or occipital blows result in a fracture that extends from the posterior cranial fossa to the middle cranial fossa at a right angle to the petrous bone (Fig. 7–2). The fracture may run from the foramen magnum or jugular foramen across the internal auditory canal to the foramen lacerum or foramen spinosum. Other fractures begin at the internal acoustic meatus and cross the vestibule to the region of the oval or round windows. Regardless of the path, most series reveal anacusis in all affected ears. These fractures are often associated with hemotympanum but not otorrhea, as the tympanic membrane is intact. The facial nerve is injured in approximately 50% of cases, usually proximal to the geniculate ganglion.

Many fractures of the temporal bone are not uniform. Tos (1971) found that approximately 50% of transverse fractures were actually mixed. In a review of 25 pediatric temporal bone fractures using three-dimensional computed tomography (CT) reconstruction, Williams et al (1992) identified oblique fractures as the most common type. These fractures are oriented in a vertical direction to the temporal bone, extending anteroinferior across the external auditory canal to the glenoid fossa. Regardless of the anatomic classification of the fracture, management depends on the injury to the contents of the temporal bone, which overlaps considerably in each of the fracture types.

Initial management of patients with head injury involves the establishment of a safe airway and adequate ventilation. Following airway, hemodynamic, and neurologic stabilization, the workup of a suspected temporal bone fracture may commence.

High-resolution axial and coronal CT scans of the temporal bone provide excellent anatomic detail. When stable, all patients suffering head injury should undergo pure-tone air, bone, and speech audiometry with appropriate masking. Finally, as discussed in subsequent sections, facial nerve testing may be indicated if decompression is contemplated.

COMPLICATIONS (TABLE 7–1)

Hearing Loss

According to Barber (1969), damage to the inner ear is the most common sequela of head injury. Several early studies revealed hearing loss in 33 to 50% of patients after head injury. Recent studies with more sophisticated audiologic data indicate between 20 and 40% of head-injured patients will suffer from hearing loss.

When longitudinal fractures are considered alone, conductive hearing loss seems to be most common. The mechanisms most frequently cited are hemotympanum, ruptured tympanic membrane, and ossicular disruption. Hemotympanum, the most frequent cause of conductive loss,

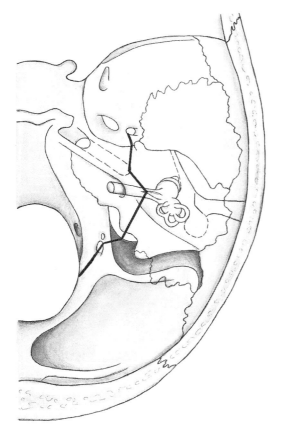

FIGURE 7–2 Schematic diagram of a transverse temporal bone fracture. Note the potential for the fracture line to cross the vestibule and enter the middle ear cleft.

TABLE 7–1 COMPLICATIONS OF TEMPORAL
BONE FRACTURE

Hearing loss
   Conductive loss
   Sensorineural loss
Vestibular injury
Facial nerve injury
Cerebrospinal fluid (CSF) fistula and meningitis

usually presents with a 30- to 45-dB loss with complete recovery within 6 weeks. The prognosis for conductive hearing loss is good. Tos (1971) revealed an 80% rate of spontaneous resolution of conductive hearing loss in his series.

PEARL••• Tos emphasized that one should be suspicious of an ossicular injury if the air–bone gap exceeds 50 dB at presentation, or 30 dB at 6-week follow-up.

The patterns of ossicular injury and techniques of repair have already been described.

High-frequency sensorineural hearing loss after head injury has been documented in 10 to 24% of patients. Transverse temporal bone fractures are almost universally followed by anacusis in the involved ear. The pathophysiology of sensorineural hearing loss in transverse fractures is self-evident.

Vestibular System Injury

Dizziness is a frequent complication of head injury. The pathogenesis of the vestibular injury is not completely understood. Most authors feel that as with injury to the auditory system, there are both peripheral and central components to the vestibular injury. Unlike the prognosis in auditory injury, however, that for posttraumatic vestibular injury is good. The majority of patients will be free of symptoms with resolution of electronystagmography (ENG) abnormalities by 6 to 12 months. Nonsurgical management with physical therapy will, in most cases, lead to resolution.

Facial Nerve Injury

The facial nerve is more often paralyzed than any other motor nerve. This fact is likely due to its long course in the bony confines of the fallopian canal. In a review of facial palsy after head injury, Potter (1964) found a 1% incidence of facial nerve injury in 2,712 cases.

The mechanisms of injury to the facial nerve are different for longitudinal and transverse fractures. Fisch (1974) found transection of the nerve in 100% of the group of transverse fractures. In contrast, the pathology in the group of longitudinal fractures revealed intraneural hematoma in 50%, bony impingement in 17%, and complete transection in 26%. He concluded that lesions of the facial nerve in temporal bone fractures, particularly longitudinal, were the result of traction on the greater superficial petrosal nerve.

CONTROVERSY

The management of facial nerve injuries associated with temporal bone fractures is controversial. The decision to proceed with surgical decompression is based on the neurologic status of the patient, the onset and severity of the paralysis, the radiographic findings, and the results of electrical testing.

Coker et al (1987) described an algorithm for the management of temporal bone fractures complicated by facial paralysis, which includes high-resolution CT (axial and coronal views) of the temporal bone, audiometric evaluation, and electrical testing with either nerve excitability (NET) or electroneuronography (ENoG) (Fig. 7–3).

In general, the prognosis for spontaneous recovery of posttraumatic facial paralysis is quite favorable. Turner (1944) reviewed 70 cases of traumatic facial paralysis, 34 of which were delayed, and found 32 of the 34 (94%) delayed onset palsies recovered spontaneously. Similarly, McKennan and Chole (1992) found 94% of their patients with delayed-onset facial

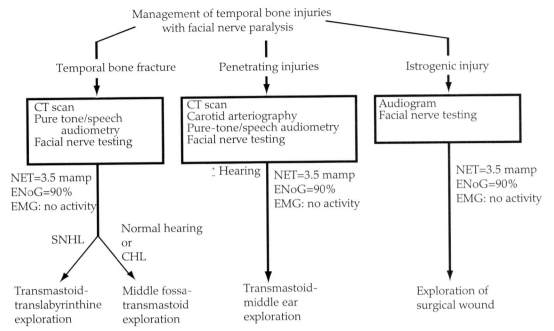

FIGURE 7–3 Recommended management scheme for temporal bone trauma with facial nerve paralysis. From Coker NJ, Kendall KA, Jenkins HA, et al. Traumatic intratemporal facial nerve injury: management rationale for preservation of function. *Otolaryngol Head Neck Surg* 1987;97:262. Reprinted by permission of the publisher.

paralysis recovered (House grade I) without surgical intervention. May advocates surgical exploration in cases of immediate-onset paralysis without response on maximal stimulation within 5 days of injury and evidence of fracture or bony impingement on high-resolution CT. Lambert and Brackmann (1984) and Coker et al (1987) recommend surgery based on the results of electrical testing. Early exploration is indicated if after a fracture, more than 90% degeneration of facial nerve fibers is demonstrated on ENoG within 6 days of the onset of the palsy. Lambert and Brackmann, like Fisch, recommend decompression in cases of delayed paralysis within 6 months if no evidence of regeneration is present on electromyography.

The approach to repair is primarily dictated by the status of the hearing. Patients with non-serviceable sensorineural loss undergo decompression via the transmastoid-translabyrinthine approach. Those patients with normal hearing or conductive loss undergo the middle cranial fossa-transmastoid approach. In cases of edema or hematoma, decompression is facilitated by

CONTROVERSY

The timing of surgery is also a controversial issue. McCabe (1972) recommended delaying repair of facial nerve paralysis in temporal bone fracture for 21 days, the amount of time necessary for the nerve cell body to push axoplasmic filaments across the nerve gap. More recent work suggests the optimum time for repair is dictated by the overall condition of the patient.

removing the bone of the fallopian canal and slitting the epineural sheath at the injured site. Partial transections greater than one-third the diameter and complete transections should be repaired either by rerouting and direct anastomosis or by interposition grafting. Moderate to severe dysfunction (House grade IV) is the likely outcome in cases requiring grafting.

The role of steroids in the management of traumatic facial nerve injury is undefined. There are no randomized prospective trials available that demonstrate efficacy. Therefore, at the present time, no specific recommendations can be made for the use of steroids in traumatic facial nerve injury.

CSF Fistula and Meningitis

CSF otorhinorrhea with resultant meningitis is a potentially lethal complication of temporal bone fracture. The diagnosis can be made by the observation of clear otorrhea or rhinorrhea, the presence of a double-ring or halo sign, or laboratory evaluation for total protein, glucose, and β_2-transferrin. High-resolution CT scans with intrathecal metrizamide are sensitive for identifying subtle leaks.

The incidence of meningitis associated with CSF leaks ranges from 15 to 24% in reported series. The most common etiologic organism is *Streptococcus pneumoniae*.

CONTROVERSY

There is much controversy in the literature regarding the use of prophylactic antibiotic therapy. Tos (1971) reported on 113 patients treated prophylactically with penicillin and 80 patients who were not. Meningitis occurred in 8% and 5% of the patients, respectively. In a placebo-controlled double-blind study evaluating the efficacy of prophylactic penicillin in 52 patients with CSF leak after head injury, Klastersky et al (1976) found no cases of meningitis in the treated group and one case in the placebo group. Jones et al found four cases of meningitis in 27 pediatric patients with posttraumatic CSF fistulas.

The treatment of CSF leaks complicating temporal bone trauma is nonsurgical in the vast majority of cases. The treatment consists of bed rest, elevation of the head, stool softeners, and avoidance of straining. Surgical therapy is recommended for leaks persisting beyond 2 to 3 weeks, large bony defects, recurrent meningitis, late-onset leaks, and brain herniation. Surgical repair can be accomplished through a transmastoid or middle cranial fossa approach. The dura can be repaired primarily or patched with fascia and reinforced with muscle or fat. If hearing has been lost, the middle ear and eustachian tube can be obliterated with muscle. This procedure can be combined with blind sac closure of the external canal for cases of persistent otorrhea.

SUGGESTED READINGS

Armstrong BW. Traumatic perforations of the tympanic membrane: observe or repair? *Laryngoscope* 1970;82:1822.

Barber HO. Head injury audiological and vestibular findings. *Ann Otol Rhinol Laryngol* 1969;78:239.

Bellucci RJ. Traumatic injuries of the middle ear. *Otol Clin North Am* 1983;16:633.

Brook I. Microbiology of human and animal bite wounds in children. *Pediatr Infect Dis J* 1987; 6:29.

Cannon CR, Jahrsdoerfer RA. Temporal bone fractures. Review of 90 cases. *Arch Otolaryngol* 1983;109:285.

Coker NJ, Kendall KA, Jenkins HA, et al. Traumatic intratemporal facial nerve injury: management rationale for preservation of function. *Otolaryngol Head Neck Surg* 1987;97:262.

Fisch U. Facial paralysis in fractures of the petrous bone. *Laryngoscope* 1974;84:2141.

Fredrickson JM, Griffith AW, Lindsay JR. Transverse fracture of the temporal bone. *Arch Otolaryngol* 1963;78:54.

Giffin CS. The wrestler's ear (acute auricular hematoma). *Arch Otolaryngol* 1985;11:161.

Griffiths MV. The incidence of auditory and vestibular concussion following minor head injury. *J Laryngol Otol* 1979;93:253.

Grove WE. Skull fractures involving the ear. A clinical study of 211 cases. *Laryngoscope* 1939;49:833.

Hough JVD. Restoration of the hearing loss after head trauma. *Ann Otol* 1969;78:210.

Kelemen G. Fractures of the temporal bone. *Arch Otolaryngol* 1944;40:333.

Klastersky J, Sadeghi M, Brihaye J. Antimicrobial prophylaxis in patients with rhinorrhea or otorrhea: a double-blind study. *Surg Neurol* 1976;6:111.

Kochhar LK, Deka RC, Kacker SK, Raman EV. Hearing loss after head injury. *Ear Nose Throat J* 1990;69:537.

Lambert PR, Brackmann De. Facial paralysis in longitudinal temporal bone fractures: a review of 26 cases. *Laryngoscope* 1984;94:1022.

McCabe BF. Injuries to the facial nerve. *Laryngoscope* 1972;82:1972.

McGuirt WF, Stool SE. Temporal bone fractures in children: a review with emphasis on long-term sequelae. *Clin Pediatr* 1992;1:12.

McKennan KX, Chole RA. Facial paralysis in temporal bone trauma. *Am J Otol* 1992;13:167.

Ohlsen L, Skoog T, Sohn SA. The pathogenesis of cauliflower ear. *Scand J Plast Reconstr Surg* 1975;9:34.

Olson JE, Shagets FW. Blunt trauma of the temporal bone. *Am Acad Otolaryngol* 1980:14.

Podoshin L, Fradis M. Hearing loss after head injury. *Arch Otolaryngol* 1975;101:15.

Potter JM. Facial palsy following head injury. *J Laryngol Otol* 1964;78:654.

Proctor B, Gurdjian ES, Webster JE. The ear in head trauma. *Laryngoscope* 1956;66:16.

Schuller DE, Dankle SD, Strauss RH. A technique to treat wrestlers' auricular hematoma without interrupting training or competition. *Arch Otolaryngol Head Neck Surg* 1989;115:202.

Sheehy JL. Surgery of Chronic Otitis Media. In: English GM, ed. *Otolaryngology.* New York: Harper and Row; 1984:1.

Silverstein H. Trauma of the tympanic membrane and ossicles. In: Nadol JD, Schuknecht HF, eds. *Surgery of the Ear and Temporal Bone.* New York: Raven Press; 1993:325.

Stucker FJ, Shaw GY, Boyd S, Shockley WW. Management of animal and human bites in the head and neck. *Arch Otolaryngol Head Neck Surg* 1990;116:789.

Tos M. Prognosis of hearing loss in temporal bone fractures. *J Laryngol Otol* 1971;85:1147.

Turner JWA. Facial palsy in closed head injuries. *Lancet* 1944;1:156.

Wiet RJ, Valvassori GE, Kotsanis CA, Parahy C. Temporal bone fractures. State of the art review. *Am J Otol* 1985;6:207.

Williams WT, Ghorayeb BY, Yeakley JW. Pediatric temporal bone fractures. *Laryngoscope* 1992;102:600.

SECTION II

NOSE AND
PARANASAL
SINUSES

Chapter 8

ANATOMY AND PHYSIOLOGY

Thomas A. Tami

EMBRYOLOGY

EXTERNAL NOSE AND NASAL CAVITY

In the 32-day embryo, the nasal cavity begins as a thickened ectodermal area of the frontal process—the *olfactory placode.* This olfactory placode becomes the *nasal fovea* and ultimately the *nasal sac,* which splits into a medial and a lateral frontonasal process.

Initially the nasal cavity communicates directly with the oral cavity. The primitive tongue lies between two *lateral palatine processes.* As the mandible develops, the tongue migrates inferiorly, and by the 8th week the palatine processes grow medially and fuse to form the primitive palate. Posteriorly they fuse with each other and anteriorly with the *premaxilla.* The premaxilla is an area of ossification in the medial part of the floor of the pyriform aperture. The septum develops superiorly, extends inferiorly, and fuses with the palatine processes.

Beginning around week 6 the bony and cartilaginous framework develops from mesenchymal elements of the medial and lateral nasal swellings. These structures are well developed by week 12.

PARANASAL SINUSES

The development and pneumatization of the paranasal sinuses occurs in two stages: *Primary*

pneumatization is the initial folding and outpouching of the primitive sinuses; however, these structures remain confined to the cartilaginous ectethmoidal unit. *Secondary pneumatization* begins when pneumatization extends outside of this primitive cartilaginous framework to involve extranasal bony structures.

Maxillary

Beginning around fetal day 60 to 75, primary pneumatization occurs. These small mucosal outpouchings from the lateral nasal wall remain confined within the cartilaginous ectoethmoid until late in the 4th fetal month.

During the 5th month, secondary pneumatization begins with lateral extension into the maxilla. At birth the maxillary sinus is quite small; however, by the 2nd year of life it has expanded laterally and inferior to the infraorbital canal. Vertical growth parallels dental and midfacial development. By 15 to 18 years, maxillary sinus development is essentially complete.

Frontal

During the 4th month of fetal development, *ethmoid furrows* are seen on the lateral nasal walls representing primary pneumatization into the frontoethmoid region. At this stage, the frontal sinus is essentially an ethmoid cell that happens to be pneumatizing the frontal area.

Although secondary pneumatization of the frontal bone begins between 6 months and 2 years, this can rarely be recognized radiographically until 6 or 7 years of age. Growth often continues well into adolescence.

Ethmoid

As for the frontal sinus, primary pneumatization begins in the 4th fetal month. The ethmoid sinuses, which develop from the middle meatus, become the anterior ethmoids, whereas those from the superior meatus become the posterior ethmoids.

Secondary pneumatization begins between birth and 2 years, and is complete by early adulthood.

Sphenoid

There is no primary pneumatization of the sphenoid sinus. Instead, constriction occurs in the sphenoethmoid recess during the 3rd fetal month. As this recess begins to deepen during the 4th month, the posterior superior part is separated from the nasal cavity by a nasal mucosal fold. A *sphenoidal cartilaginous concha* forms and encloses the sphenoidal recess and becomes attached to the body of the sphenoid by 3 to 5 years of life.

Secondary pneumatization begins around year 7 with expansion into the perisphenoid and basisphenoid regions. By 8 to 10 years a demonstrable sphenoid sinus can be recognized.

Sphenoid pneumatization is variable. Three distinct patterns are usually described:

1. *Conchal (fetal) type:* This pattern is seen when there has been minimal posterior pneumatization and extension.
2. *Presellar (juvenile) type:* Sinuses with this pattern have posterior extension to the region of the anterior sellar wall.
3. *Postsphenoidal (adult) type:* This pattern is characterized by extension posteriorly and

below the sella or, in some instances, beyond this region.

ANATOMY

EXTERNAL NOSE

Nasal Bones

These paired bones fuse with the frontal bone above and the maxilla laterally and are supported by the nasal spine of the frontal bone and the perpendicular plate of the ethmoids (septum). The pyriform aperture is bordered above the nasal bones and below and laterally by the maxilla and premaxilla (Fig. 8–1A).

Cartilaginous Framework

The paired *lower lateral nasal cartilages* are composed of the *lateral crura* and *medial crura.* These cartilages provide much of the support and structure for the nasal tip and lobule.

The paired *upper lateral cartilages* attach to the dorsum of the cartilaginous septum medially. They extend beneath the nasal bones superiorly and are overlapped inferiorly by the lower lateral cartil'ages.

Muscular Attachments

Five muscle or muscle groups attach to the external nasal framework (Fig. 8–1B):

1. *Depressor muscle of the septum:* This muscle is part of the orbicularis oris. It arises from the alveolus of the incisors and inserts on the medial crura of the lower lateral cartilages and the caudal septum. The primary action is to depress the nasal tip.
2. *Nasal muscle:* This muscle consists of two parts. The *transverse* part arises on the lateral pyriform aperture and passes superiorly and medially over the nasal dorsum. The *alar* part (alar muscle of Eisler) attaches from the pyriform aperture at the nasomaxillary suture and extends to the nasal alae. These muscles aid in dilation of the alae.

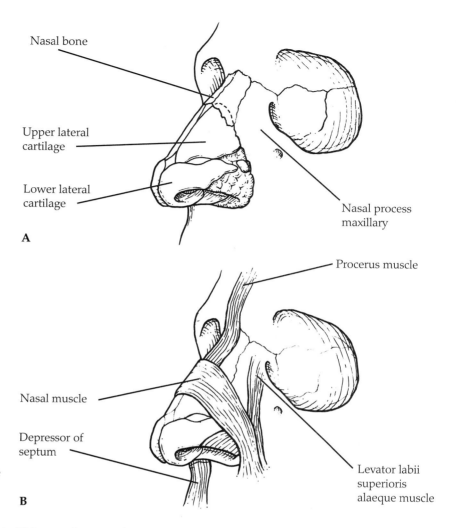

Nasal bone

Upper lateral cartilage

Lower lateral cartilage

Nasal process maxillary

A

Procerus muscle

Nasal muscle

Depressor of septum

Levator labii superioris alaeque muscle

B

FIGURE 8–1 (A). The nasal bones. (B). Muscles of the nose.

3. *Muscle of the nasal tip:* This muscle extends from the posterior inferior border of the upper lateral cartilage to the junction of the lateral and medial crura of the lower lateral cartilage. It dilates the anterior part of the nares, but can cause narrowing at the nasal valve region.

4. *Procerus muscle:* Arising from the frontal belly of the fronto-occipital muscle and inserting into the aponeurosis of the nasal dorsum, the procerus pulls the medial segment of the brow inferiorly and produces transverse folds in the glabellar region.

5. *Levator labii superioris alaeque nasi:* This muscle extends from the frontal process of the maxilla to the lateral crus of the lower lateral

cartilages. It pulls the lateral crus superiorly and is the primary nasal dilator.

CONTROVERSY

Although not universally accepted, electromyogram (EMG) studies reveal that the nasal dilators form the efferent part of a respiratory reflex arc with afferents arising from the intrathoracic mechanoreceptors, traveling via the vagus nerve to the medulla. The efferents run via the facial nerve to produce nasal dilation in response to normal respiration.

Arterial Supply

The blood supply to the external nose arises from both the external and the internal carotid systems.

The *facial artery* (external carotid a.) provides the inferior blood supply, coursing over the posterior body of the mandible and angling superiorly toward the nasolabial fold. The *nasal dorsal artery* (internal carotid) contributes superiorly as a terminal branch of the ophthalmic artery. These two system anastomose via the *angular artery* in the medial canthal region.

Venous Drainage

The veins of the face and nose do not run parallel to the arteries, but rather drain based on anatomic units. The frontomedian segment of the face is drained by the facial veins, which travel inferolaterally toward the angle of the jaw. The orbitopalpebral region is drained via the ophthalmic venous plexus.

Innervation

The skin of the nose is innervated by the ophthalmic (V1) and maxillary (V2) branches of the trigeminal nerve.

PEARL... This communication of the midfacial and nasal venous network is significant in cases of infections and inflammatory conditions because it provides a direct route for spread of infection to the orbits and cavernous sinus.

V2 supplies the lateral nose, nasal alae, and columellar area. V1 supplies the nasal root and dorsum, including the nasal tip.

SPECIAL CONSIDERATION

Recognizing that the nasal tip is included in the V1 distribution (and not V2) is important, especially in cases of herpes zoster. If the nasal tip is involved with herpetic lesions, accompanying lesions of the surface of the eye must also be considered.

NASAL CAVITY AND SEPTUM

Bony-Cartilaginous Framework

The septum consists of the cartilaginous quadrangular cartilage anteriorly and the bony septum posteriorly. This bony septum is composed of the perpendicular plate of the ethmoid superiorly and the vomer inferiorly.

The *maxillary crest* is a V-shaped bony prominence beginning just posterior to the incisive foramen and extending posteriorly beneath the cartilaginous septum and the vomer.

The *incisive foramen* is located at the region of fusion of the premaxilla and the lateral palatine processes. The *nasopalatine nerve* traverses this bony canal to provide innervation to the anterior roof of mouth.

The bony floor of the nose is formed by the maxilla anteriorly and the horizontal plates of the palatine bones posteriorly.

The nasal roof can be divided into three sections:

1. *The anterior roof (nasal)* consists of the nasal bones, nasal spine, and the frontal bones.
2. *The central (ethmoidal)* part consists of the cribriform plate of the ethmoid bone.
3. *The posterior (sphenoidal)* roof overlies the region of the sphenoethmoid recess and the superior concha.

The primary structures of the lateral nasal wall are the conchae (turbinates). The *inferior concha* attaches directly to the maxilla. The *middle concha* is part of the ethmoid bone. It attaches directly to the cribriform plate superiorly and anteriorly. Posteriorly it attaches to the laminae papyracea via the *basal lamella*. The *superior concha* forms the sphenoethmoidal region of the posterior lateral nasal wall. It forms the medial border of the posterior ethmoid labyrinth.

The anatomic regions beneath the conchae form distinct meati of the lateral nasal wall. Beneath the inferior concha is the *inferior meatus.* The nasal lacrimal duct empties into this anatomic region.

The *middle meatus* beneath the middle turbinate is an anatomically complex and important region. The anterior paranasal sinuses (frontal, maxillary, and anterior ethmoids) all have their primary ostia in this region and drain into the *semilunar hiatus.* This hiatus is bounded medially and inferiorly by the *uncinate process* of the maxilla and superiorly and laterally by the floor of the orbit and lamina papyracea.

The superior meatus opens into the region of the posterior ethmoids and posteriorly into the sphenoethmoid recess (Fig. 8–2).

Arterial Supply

The nasal cavity and septum are supplied by branches of the external carotid *(internal maxillary artery)* as well as the internal carotid *(anterior* and *posterior ethmoidal arteries)* systems.

The internal maxillary artery enters the nasal cavity through the sphenopalatine foramen. This artery then descends as the *descending palatine artery* supplying branches to the inferior lateral nasal wall. Another branch arising at the sphenopalatine foramen is the *posterior septal artery,* which courses medially across the face of the sphenoid sinus to supply the posterior nasal septum.

The superior portions of the lateral nasal wall (middle and superior turbinates) as well as the upper portions of the nasal septum is supplied by the anterior and posterior ethmoidal arteries.

The anterior nasal septum is richly vascularized in an area referred to as *Kiesselbach's plexus.* The blood supply for this vascular region of the septum is derived from the ascending branch of the anterior palatine, the posterior septal, the anterior ethmoidal, and the superior labial arteries.

Innervation

Sensory innervation for the nasal cavity and septum is provided by V1 and V2. Contributions from V1 arrive via the *anterior ethmoidal nerve,* which runs with the anterior ethmoidal artery through the *criboethmoidal foramen* to the anterior superior nasal septum and lateral nasal wall.

The *nasopalatine nerve* (Scarpa's nerve) arises from V2 in the pterygopalatine fossae and enters the nasal cavity through the sphenopalatine foramen. After passing along the face of the sphenoid to reach the posterior nasal septum, it courses anteroinferiorly toward the incisive canal. Along its course it gives off numerous branches to the nasal septum and terminates in the incisive canal innervating the gingiva of the middle and lateral incisors. The inferior lateral nasal wall receives sensory innervation from numerous branches of V2 exiting the

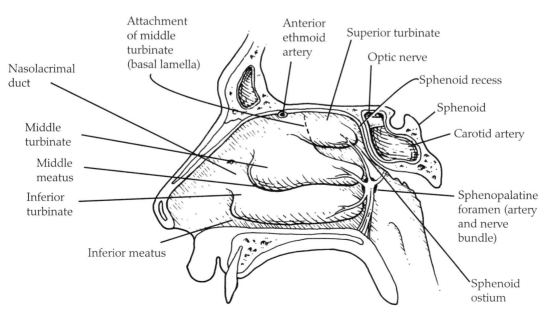

FIGURE 8–2 The nasal cavity and septum.

sphenopalatine foramen and tracking forward along the inferior and middle conchae.

Autonomic innervation consists of both sympathetic and parasympathetic fibers. The sympathetic innervation originates in the superior cervical ganglion and arrives in the nasal cavity via the carotid sympathetic plexus. These fibers leave the carotid artery in the region of foramen lacerum as the *deep petrosal nerve* and enters the *vidian (pterygoid) canal.*

Parasympathetic innervation is provided by preganglionic fibers of cranial nerve VII. Exiting the facial nerve at the geniculate ganglion, the *greater superficial petrosal nerve* courses across the floor of the middle cranial fossae and enters the vidian canal where it is joined by fibers of the deep petrosal nerve to from the *vidian nerve (nerve of the pterygoid canal).* These fibers synapse in the pterygopalatine fossae at the *pterygopalatine ganglion* and are distributed throughout the nasal cavity and paranasal sinuses.

PARANASAL SINUSES

Although the paranasal sinuses are described on an anatomic basis (e.g., sphenoid, frontal, etc.), they are more appropriately classified based on their ostia and drainage patterns. The *anterior sinuses* consist of the frontal, maxillary, and anterior ethmoids, whereas the *posterior sinuses* consist of the sphenoid and posterior ethmoids.

Maxillary Sinus

The maxillary sinus, the largest and most prominent of the paranasal sinuses, is housed entirely within the maxilla. Superiorly it is bordered by the floor of the orbit. A bony ridge runs along the roof of the sinus and contains the infraorbital nerve and artery. The sinus floor is closely approximated to the posterior molars, especially the second premolar and the first molar. The apices of the roots of these teeth often protrude into the sinus and are occasionally dehiscent. The nerve supply to these teeth often lies immediately under the mucosa of the sinus.

The ostium of the maxillary sinus is located anterosuperiorly on the medial sinus wall. It opens into the hiatus semilunaris through the ethmoid infundibulum.

The arterial supply is via middle meatal branches of the sphenopalatine artery and the ethmoid arteries.

The sensory innervation is supplied by contributions from the lateral posterior superior nasal branches of the maxillary nerve (V2) as well as by branches of the superior alveolar and infraorbital nerves.

Frontal Sinus

These sinuses extend from the most anterior part of the middle meatus (the frontal recess) into the frontal bone. Although usually paired, it is not unusual to find hypoplasia of one or both frontal sinuses. The sinus floor is bordered by the orbital portion of the frontal bone. The thin posterior wall separates the frontal sinus mucosa from the underlying frontal lobe dura. The supraorbital and supratrochlear nerves run superiorly over the anterior wall of the frontal sinuses. The ostium of this sinus is located in the posterior medial floor of the sinus and opens into the frontal recess of the middle meatus.

The arterial supply to the frontal sinus is the anterior ethmoid artery as well as middle meatal branches of the sphenopalatine artery. Venous drainage is via transosseous vascular channels into the subcutaneous system, the orbit, and intracranially.

> **PITFALL•••** This valveless venous network, which communicates intracranially, accounts for the high incidence of intracranial complications secondary to infections in this sinus.

The mucosa of the frontal sinus is innervated by nasal branches of V2 as well as by the anterior ethmoid branch of V1.

Ethmoid Sinuses

The ethmoid labyrinth is bordered laterally by the lamina papyracea of the orbit and medially by the middle turbinate (anterior ethmoids) and the superior turbinate (posterior ethmoids). The roof of the ethmoids is formed by the *fovea ethmoidalis,* which is a medial extension of the frontal bone. The medial roof, where the middle turbinate attaches at the junction of the fovea and the cribriform plate (of the ethmoid bone), is the thinnest point of the anterior skull base.

> **PITFALL...** The anterior ethmoid artery traverses the roof of the anterior ethmoids in an area just posterior to the frontal recess. At its most medial extent, this artery enters the anterior cranial vault in the suture line created by the fovea ethmoidalis and the cribriform plate. This site is a common point of entry into the anterior cranial fossae during endoscopic sinus surgery, often resulting in bleeding (due to injury to the artery) and leakage of cerebrospinal fluid.

The largest and most prominent of the anterior ethmoid cells is the *bulla ethmoidalis.* This cell lies just medial and posterior to the anterior end of the middle turbinate and is an important surgical anatomic landmark. The most anterior ethmoid cells, which pneumatize the bone around the lacrimal fossa and lie anterior and lateral to the middle turbinate, are the *agar nasi cells.* These are often important causes of obstruction of the frontal sinus in cases of frontal sinusitis. The anterior and posterior ethmoids are anatomically and functionally distinct sinuses, separated by the bony *basal (ground) lamella.* This bony plate serves as the lateral attachment of the middle turbinate to the lamina papyracea.

The ostia of the anterior ethmoid sinuses open into the region of the middle meatus, whereas the posterior ethmoid ostia drain into the sphenoethmoid recess.

The arterial supply to the ethmoid sinuses is from the middle meatal branches of the sphenopalatine artery and anterior ethmoid artery (anterior ethmoids), and via the superior conchal branch of the sphenopalatine artery and posterior ethmoid artery (posterior ethmoids). Sensory innervation is provided by the posterior superior nasal branches of V2 and the anterior ethmoid branch of V1.

> **PEARL...** Haller cells are ethmoid cells that pneumatize laterally into the floor of the orbit. These can be clinically significant when they produce narrowing of the ethmoid infundibulum and obstruction of the ostium of the maxillary sinus.
>
> Frontal cells are derived from the agar nasi region and pneumatize superiorly into the frontal bone. These cells often cause narrowing and occasionally obstruction of the frontal sinus resulting in frontal sinus infection.
>
> The Onodi cell is a posterior ethmoid cell that pneumatizes posteriorly above or laterally to the sphenoid sinus. When these cells are present, the optic nerve usually traverses the lateral superior portion of this cell, and can be dehiscent in up to 5% of cases.

Sphenoid Sinus

This sinus is located in the sphenoid bone and is surrounded by several important structures. Superior to the sinus is the pituitary fossa, the olfactory tracts, and frontal lobes, as well as the optic chiasm.

Inferiorly is the nasopharynx and the vessels and nerve (vidian nerve) of the pterygoid canal. The pterygoid canal is often located directly beneath the mucosa of the floor of the sphenoid sinus.

Posteriorly a thick bony wall separates the sinus from the basilar artery and the pons.

Laterally, a thin bony wall, which is occasionally dehiscent, covers the cavernous portion of the internal carotid artery. Other lateral structures include the cavernous sinus, the abducens nerve, and the maxillary division (V2) of the trigeminal.

The ostium of the sphenoid is located anterior and medially near the roof of the sinus. This ostium is often located just posterior to the posterior end of the superior turbinate.

The arterial supply to the sphenoid sinus is via branches of the nasopalatine and sphenopalatine arteries. Branches from the artery of the pterygoid canal can also provide a vascular supply to this sinus.

Sensory innervation is provided by the posterior superior nasal branches of V2 as well as the posterior ethmoid branch of V1.

SUGGESTED READINGS

Blitzer A, Lawson W, Friedman WH, ed. *Surgery of the Paranasal Sinuses.* Philadelphia: WB Saunders; 1985.

Lang J. *Clinical Anatomy of the Nose, Nasal Cavity and Paranasal Sinuses.* New York: Thieme; 1989.

Chapter 9

CLINICAL TESTS

Thomas A. Tami

PHYSICAL EXAMINATION

VISUAL EXAM

The anterior nasal cavity and in many instances the posterior nasal cavity can be easily examined using a head light and nasal speculum. The examination should be performed both before as well as after nasal decongestion to assess reversible edema and inflammatory changes. Septal deviations of both the cartilaginous and the bony septum and hypertrophy of the middle and inferior turbinates can be easily assessed. If present, gross nasal polyposis can usually be seen emanating from the regions of the middle and superior nasal meatus. Following decongestion, a clear view to the nasopharynx can usually be obtained and nasopharyngeal masses detected.

NASAL ENDOSCOPY

Nasal endoscopy is a natural extension of the anterior nasal examination. To perform this technique, the nasal cavity is decongested and topically anesthetized with either lidocaine or tetracaine and with phenylephrine or oxymetazoline. A 30-degree nasal telescope (either 2.7 or 4.0 mm) provides the best visualization. The scope is first passed along the floor of the nose. By angling the scope superiorly, pathology in

the sphenoethmoid recess can usually be identified. The telescope is then passed into the middle meatus area. When direct visualization into a tight middle meatus is necessary, further local anesthetic application is often required. Nasal endoscopy facilitates the early identification of inflammatory and anatomic changes contributing to sinusitis. This technique also facilitates the performance of directed cultures of the middle meatus. When used as an initial screening tool, nasal endoscopy can often eliminate the need for radiographic studies to establish the diagnosis of sinusitis.

> **PEARL...** Nasal endoscopy is an ideal technique to provide visualization and access to middle meatus secretions for obtaining cultures. Both aspiration and swabs can be directed at this infectious source to enable organism-specific antibiotic therapy.

RADIOGRAPHIC EXAMINATION

PLAIN SINUS X-RAYS

For many years, the plain sinus X-ray series was the mainstay of radiographic examination of the paranasal sinuses. Four anatomic views are usually included in this examination. The *Caldwell* view is a direct posterior-anterior view and is used to evaluate the frontal and ethmoid sinuses. The maxillary sinuses are obscured by the petrous portion of the temporal bone in the standard Caldwell view. The anterior ethmoids, posterior ethmoids, and the sphenoid sinus are all superimposed on each other, making it difficult to specifically assess these individual sinuses. The *Waters* view is a 45-degree off-axis view that throws the petrous temporal bone away from the maxillary sinus. This is the classic view for evaluating the maxillary sinuses. The ethmoids cannot be examined in this view and the frontal sinuses are viewed at an oblique angle. The *lateral* view is used to detect air-fluid levels in the sphenoid and frontal sinuses. Owing to variations in pneumatization of the sphenoid sinus, this view has poor sensitivity and specificity. The *submental vertex* view examines the sinuses in a cephalorostral orientation. In this view the ethmoids and sphenoid sinuses can be compared from left to right; however, the superimposition of the inferior and middle turbinates on the ethmoids makes this evaluation very difficult.

Although plain sinus X-rays are still often used to assist in the evaluation of patients with paranasal sinus problems, their use is accompanied by poor diagnostic sensitivity and specificity, particularly when evaluating the ethmoid and/or sphenoid sinuses. The use of plain sinus radiography has been largely supplanted by computed tomography (CT) scanning.

COMPUTED TOMOGRAPHY SCANNING

CT scanning has replaced plain sinus radiography as the gold standard for radiographic evaluation of the paranasal sinuses. Bone windows are usually used to evaluate the sinuses; the most popular orientation of scanning is in the direct coronal view. This coronal orientation is particularly helpful when surgery is contemplated. Direct coronal CT scanning requires full extension of the neck, which is occasionally difficult. In these cases, off-axis scanning or axial scans with coronal reconstructions are performed. With CT scanning, major anatomic structures such as the turbinates, the ethmoid

and sphenoid sinuses, frontal recess anatomy, and the osteomeatal complex can all be easily visualized. Evidence of bony erosion or extra-sinus complications of sinusitis are also usually easily detected (Fig. 9–1).

Recently, CT scan images have been coupled to computer localization equipment to provide image-guided intraoperative surgical localization. These systems are ideal for the safe and efficient performance of complex surgical procedures of the anterior skull base and are particularly helpful for anatomically difficult or revision endoscopic sinus surgery.

MAGNETIC RESONANCE IMAGING (MRI)

MRI is a superior imaging technique when soft tissue detail is required. Images can be produced in any anatomic plane without repositioning the patient. MRI scanning provides poor definition of bony structures, thus limiting its usefulness in most cases of sinusitis. However, it can be very helpful when soft tissue masses ac-

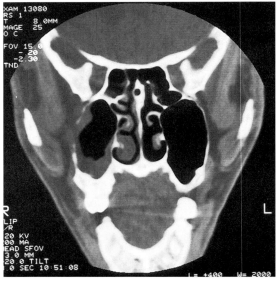

FIGURE 9–1 Computed tomography (CT) scanning is ideal for the clinical anatomic evaluation of the paranasal sinuses. Erosion of the lateral wall of the maxillary sinus can be easily appreciated on this coronal CT image.

company infectious processes or when intracranial and intraorbital extension of sinusitis is present. MRI is also an ideal technique to differentiate among mucoceles, tumors, and nasal polyposis.

SPECIAL CONSIDERATION

MRI has also been found useful for detecting fungal infections within the paranasal sinuses. A marked decrease in signal intensity can be noted on T2-weighted images, whereas routine inflammatory changes tend to be enhanced.

RHINOMANOMETRY

The evaluation of nasal obstruction has traditionally been fraught with the problem of patient and physician subjectivity. Most patients with nasal obstruction have obvious clinical abnormalities; however, because symptoms are subjective, the degree of mechanical abnormality needed to produce significant symptoms has never been established. Rhinomanometry is a clinical test that is used as an objective measure to document nasal obstruction. During this test, a tight-fitting face mask is attached to a resistance flowmeter. Nasal pressure and flow are plotted for each nasal passage to determine the presence of increased resistance (nasal obstruction). Standard reporting of flow and resistance is done at the pressure of 150 Pa (1.5 cm H_2O). Turbulence can be measured by comparing flow rates at three different pressures (75, 100, and 300 Pa) and by calculating the increase in flow between the lower and upper pressure levels (Fig. 9–2).

PITFALL••• Anterior rhinomanometry is inherently flawed by changes in nasal valve anatomy secondary to equipment application. Posterior rhinomanometry obviates this problem, but is much more difficult to perform.

ACOUSTIC RHINOMETRY

Acoustic rhinometry is a technique that examines the geometry of the nasal cavity as determined by reflected acoustic signals. When correlated with CT scans and cadaver sections, this technique has been fairly reproducible and accurate in determining actual nasal cross-sectional anatomy.

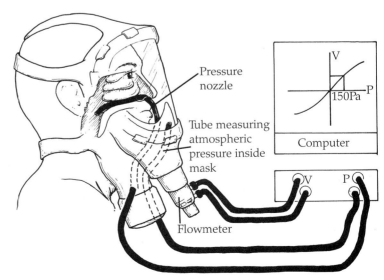

FIGURE 9–2 Rhinomanometry can be used to measure nasal airway resistance. In the anterior technique, placing the pressure transducer at the anterior nares can result in deformity of the nasal alae and factitious pressure determinations. Although the posterior technique results in a more accurate assessment of airway resistance, it is somewhat more difficult to perform.

Pressure nozzle

Tube measuring atmospheric pressure inside mask

Flowmeter

Computer

SPECIAL CONSIDERATION

Because patient cooperation is not needed, acoustic rhinometry can be used even in the pediatric population. The role of this examination in the clinical assessment and management of patients with nasal problems is still somewhat obscure.

CILIARY FLOW MEASUREMENTS

Several techniques can be used to evaluate mucociliary activity in the nasal cavity. *Mucous transport velocity* is a complex test that utilizes technetium 99–labeled albumin. This radioactive tracer is introduced onto the anterior nasal mucosal surface. By using a gamma camera, the velocity of posterior transport can be measured in millimeters per minute.

The *saccharin transport time* is clinically easier to perform but is a less accurate test. This test is performed by placing a 1-mm saccharin particle on the anterior floor of the nasal cavity, just behind the anteriormost segment of the inferior turbinate. The time that elapses for the patient to report a sweet taste in the mouth is then noted. The normal time range is fairly wide (3–20 minutes). Values greater than 30 minutes are considered pathologic and indicate altered mucus flow.

The determination of *ciliary beat frequency* is a complex test that is now performed in many laboratories throughout the United States. In this test, ciliated mucosa is obtained from the nasal surface and placed in a culture medium. By using a phase-contrast microscope coupled to a photoelectric detector, the cilia are visualized and real-time measurement of ciliary beating frequency made. Normal beat rate is from 10 to 12 per second. Reduced beat frequencies are seen in diseases associated with poor ciliary motility such as Kartagener's syndrome.

NASAL CYTOLOGY

The nasal smear is an effective test to quickly and simply determine the etiology of rhinitis. To perform this test, mucus is obtained from the surface of the inferior turbinate, smeared on a slide, and then stained and examined microscopically. A preponderance of eosinophils suggests an allergic etiology, whereas a preponderance of neutrophils suggests an infectious etiology.

ALLERGY TESTING

Allergy testing is indicated for patients with signs and symptoms consistent with seasonal or perennial allergic rhinitis and who have not responded to first-line medical therapy. These tests are all designed to demonstrate antigen-specific immunoglobulin E (IgE).

SKIN TESTING

To perform *prick skin tests,* a drop of antigenic extract is placed on the skin of the back or arm and specially designed needles are employed to introduce the extract into the subcutaneous tissue. A wheal-and-flare response is typically observed and reported as 0 to 4+ reactivity. Because multiple tests can be performed during a single sitting, this is a popular screening test.

The prick test is occasionally not sensitive enough to demonstrate low levels of allergy. *Intradermal testing* is more sensitive, although slightly more painful and much more time-consuming. To administer intradermal testing, antigens must be individually injected. By measuring the subsequent skin reaction, a more quantitative result can be reported.

Skin end-point titration (SET) is a technique used to determine the concentration of a known allergen that should be used to begin immunotherapy. Progressively decreasing concentrations of a known antigen are injected intradermally until a negative result is obtained. The end point is then that dilution at which progressive positive skin responses occur. This indicates the concentration that should be used to begin desensitization.

IN VITRO ALLERGY TESTS

Direct measures of allergen-specific IgE in patient serum are also available. The most common of these is the radioallergosorbent

CONTROVERSY

Although SET is advocated by most otolaryngic allergists in the United States, this technique is not used by most medical allergists or by the European community. Those who have abandoned this technique cite its poor sensitivity, specificity, and reproducibility.

test (RAST). These in vitro tests are more specific but less sensitive then skin tests and, although often used for screening, are generally considered inadequate for beginning desensitization.

OLFACTORY TESTING

Olfactory testing is commonly performed in patients complaining of disordered smell or taste. There are two types of tests: *threshold testing,* which determines the threshold concentration of an odorant that can be perceived, and *identification testing,* which measures the patient's ability to correctly identify a number of common odorants. The most commonly used and easily administered olfactory test is the University of Pennsylvania Smell Identification Test (UPSIT). This self-administered and easily scored test of odor identification is ideally suited to screening for olfactory dysfunction. It has built-in controls to detect functional olfactory disorders or malingering. Forty odorants are tested. Table 9–1 displays the scoring used on the UPSIT to categorize olfactory function, the score being based on the number correct.

TABLE 9–1 UNIVERSITY OF PENNSYLVANIA SMELL IDENTIFICATION TEST (UPSIT) DIAGNOSTIC SCORES

	Male	*Female*
Normal	34–40	35–40
Hyposmia	20–33	20–34
Anosmia	6–19	6–19
Malingering	<5	<5

MISCELLANEOUS TESTS

Although there are no specific laboratory tests of nasal function, many systemic disorders can present as problems in the nasal cavity. When these are suspected, appropriate laboratory testing should be performed, including fluorescent treponemal antibody absorption/Venereal Disease Research Laboratory tests (FTA-Abs/VDRL) when syphilitic infection is a consideration; antinuclear cytoplasmic antibody (c-ANCA), a fairly sensitive test for Wegener's granulomatosis; angiotensin-converting enzyme (ACE) levels, a test that is often elevated in patients with sarcoidosis; cultures and sensitivities (fungal, mycobacterial, and routine) to detect an unusual organism that may be responsible for infectious symptoms; and erythrocyte sedimentation rate (ESR), rheumatoid factor, and antinuclear antibody (ANA) when rheumatologic diseases are suspected as the cause of nasal symptoms.

SUGGESTED READINGS

Doty RL. Practical approaches to clinical olfactory testing. In: Seiden AM, ed. *Taste and Smell Disorders.* New York: Thieme; 1997:38–51.

Endoscopic radiologic diagnosis. In: Stamberger H, Hawke M, eds. *Essentials of Functional Endoscopic Sinus Surgery.* St. Louis: CV Mosby; 1993:chap 4.

Mabry RL. Skin endpoint titration. In: Mabry RL, ed. *American Academy of Otolaryngic Allergy.* 2nd ed. New York: Thieme; 1994:1–98.

Marais J, Murray JA, Marshall, Douglas N, Martin S. Minimal cross-sectional areas, nasal peak flow and patient satisfaction in septoplasty and inferior turbinectomy. *Rhinology* 1994;32:145–147.

Petersson G. Allergy practice and the otolaryngologist. *Curr Opin Otolaryngol Head Neck Surg* 1995;3:218–223.

Riechelmann H, Hinni ML, Klimek L, Mann WJ. Objective measures of nasal function. *Curr Opin Otolaryngol Head Neck Surg* 1995;3:207–212.

Chapter 10

CONGENITAL DISORDERS

Thomas A. Tami

EXTERNAL NASAL DEFORMITIES

Deformities of the external nasal structures can vary from subtle cosmetic deformities to complete absence of the external nose. A discussion of several of these congenital deformities follows.

Congenital absence of the nose (arhinia) has been reported by several authors. Although often associated with other developmental disorders, including central nervous system anomalies, it has also been described with no other associated anomalies. This condition is usually associated with both anterior and posterior atretic plates that enclose a single hypoplastic nasal cavity. Surgical management is usually recommended during the early days or weeks of life because of the severe associated feeding difficulties.

Bifid nose is a common nasal abnormality when mild; however, a complete bifid nose is uncommon. This defect is usually associated with other midfacial anomalies, such as clefting of the lip and palate and occasionally anterior skull base anomalies. Because there is no standard surgical management for these severe deformities, each patient must be individually evaluated and managed.

Lateral nasal clefts are very unusual deformities that involve the lateral nasal alae and nasal wall. The clefting defects can involve only the nasal alar region, or can extend into the medial canthal and lacrimal duct region. Surgical repair is usually delayed as long as possible to allow maximum normal facial and nasal development.

A fairly unusual anomaly for which no established cause has been found is *proboscis lateralis*. Proboscis lateralis is a rare craniofacial malformation and is commonly associated with deformities of the ipsilateral half of the nose, the eye, and its adnexa. This condition has also been seen in association with severe cranial base deformities such as holoprosencephaly as well as anterior encephaloceles. Usually, a complete absence of half of the nose is replaced by a lateral trunk or proboscis, usually occurring in the region of the inner canthus. Surgical correction is usually required.

A fairly common external congenital deformity encountered in otolaryngologic practice is the *cleft lip nasal deformity*. The major characteristics of this deformity include retrodisplacement of the lower lateral cartilage on the side of involvement. This produces a lateral and inferior displacement of the alar base with blunting of the alar-facial angle. The caudal end of the septum as well as the collumella is dislocated toward the normal side. The dome of the lower lateral cartilage is depressed, with resultant loss of tip projection on the involved side (Fig. 10–1). In cases of bilateral cleft lip nasal deformities, the nasal deformity is usually much more severe, with underdevelopment of the premaxilla, shortened collumella, and caudal septum. Sur-

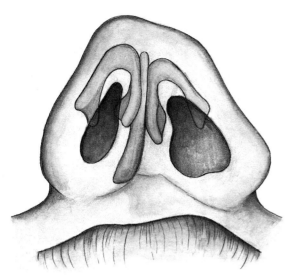

FIGURE 10-1 Cleft lip nasal deformity.

gical correction is usually best accomplished through an open approach.

The goal of surgery is to rotate the depressed lower lateral cartilage into a position more symmetrical with the opposite side. In the case of unilateral deformity, the caudal septal deviation must also be carefully addressed to attain a symmetrical final result. Onlay grafting techniques are often used in cases of pronounced deformity.

SPECIAL CONSIDERATION

Children with clefts also frequently have severe nasal septal deformities. Although best delayed until the teenage years, surgery on the septum is occasionally unavoidable at a much earlier age. Surgery should be extremely conservative due to the unknown effects of nasal septal surgery (specifically in the region of the septal nasovomerine angle) on the subsequent growth of the nose and midface. Also, in patients with severe nasal obstruction, the establishment of an improved nasal airway can often produce velopharyngeal insufficiency, which was not evident prior to surgery.

For bilateral deformities, the addition of a collumellar lengthening procedure is needed to release and project the nasal tip.

INTRANASAL CONGENITAL DEFORMITIES

Congenital septal deviation is often discovered in the newborn. This problem is generally thought to be caused either in utero secondary to abnormal head presentation, or during vaginal delivery through the birth canal. Interestingly, the incidence of this abnormality in infants delivered by cesarean section is dramatically less than for vaginal deliveries. If repaired within the first several days of birth, this deformity can usually be easily managed in the nursery using a blunt elevator to return the septum to the maxillary crest.

Posterior choanal atresia is one of the most common serious nasal congenital deformities. The almost complete dependency of neonates upon nasal breathing is highlighted by the near-life-threatening clinical presentation of bilateral posterior choanal atresia. The incidence of this abnormality is approximately 1 in 5000 live births. The presentation can range from unilateral to bilateral, complete or incomplete, membranous or bony. The diagnosis is usually identified in the immediate neonatal period by the failure to transnasally pass a soft catheter. In cases of unilateral atresia, the diagnosis is occasionally missed in the neonatal period. These patients are often picked up at a later time due primarily to the symptom of unilateral chronic mucus drainage from the nose. Choanal atresia is often associated with other abnormalities. The acronym CHARGE is often used to describe the following association: coloboma, heart disease, atresia choanae, retarded development of central nervous system, genital hypoplasia, and ear abnormalities or deafness.

The diagnosis and characterization of choanal atresia are best performed using axial computed tomography (CT) scanning. Using this technique, the precise characteristics of the atretic plate can be delineated and the appropriate surgical approach planned.

Embryologically, the choanal atretic plate is classically thought to be secondary to failure of resorption of the buccopharyngeal membrane during fetal development.

Initial management of infants with choanal atresia centers on airway and feeding. The McGovern nipple, which is a nipple modified by having its end cut off, is place into the infant's mouth and secured by ties around the back of the occiput. This basically serves as an oropharyngeal airway. During feeding, these children tend to swallow more air than usual, so frequent rests for breathing and belching are necessary. These children usually learn mouth-breathing, at which time the emergent nature of this clinical situation is lessened.

Surgical management has traditionally been the *transpalatal* approach. This approach usually affords the best visualization and preserves nasal mucosa; however, it may produce a restricting effect on lateral maxillary growth due to the scars from the palatal incision. Most surgeons tend to wait until the child is between 1 and 1½ years of age prior to recommending this approach. The *transnasal* approach has become much more popular recently, particularly since the advent of endoscopic endonasal surgery, and it is often now preferred by many surgeons. Cases of membranous atresia are particularly well suited to this approach; however, even bony atretic plates can be addressed using lasers, drills, or other aggressive surgical instru-

---

CONTROVERSY

Although the transpalatal approach has been considered by many surgeons as the gold standard for repairing posterior choanal atresias, the advent of advanced endoscopic techniques has challenged this position. Newer instrumentation, including lasers, drills, and power-driven shavers, has made the transnasal approach much more feasible and acceptable. Furthermore, in cases of difficult or unusual bony anatomic abnormalities, computer image–guided surgical techniques may also play an increasing role.

---

ments. Prolonged stenting is usually recommended in these cases, however, cases using minimal or no nasal stents have been described.

A much less commonly described congenital cause of nasal obstruction is *congenital nasal pyriform aperture stenosis.* In this recently described cause of nasal airway obstruction in the newborn, the nasal pyriform aperture is narrowed owing to bony overgrowth of the nasal process of the maxilla. This abnormality is often found in association with a single prominent central maxillary incisor and can also be associated with pituitary hypofunction and central nervous system (CNS) and ophthalmologic anomalies. CT confirms the diagnosis and delineates the anomaly. Surgical enlargement of the nasal pyriform aperture can be performed through either a sublabial or a transnasal approach.

Nasal encephaloceles and *gliomas* are congenital nasal masses with similar presentations and embryogenesis. Both of these congenital masses consist of CNS glial tissue. Gliomas have lost their CNS/subarachnoid attachments, whereas encephaloceles have a persistent cerebrospinal fluid (CSF) connection to the subarachnoid space. Encephaloceles are generally divided into sincipital and basal types. Sincipital encephaloceles generally present in the nasal dorsum, forehead, or orbital region and are associated with an external mass. Basal types are less common and appear in the nasal cavity and nasopharynx. There is generally no associated external mass.

PITFALL... Unilateral nasal masses must be approached with extreme caution and close scrutiny. Office biopsy of these lesions is unwise, because most offices are ill-equipped to deal with a sudden iatrogenic CSF leak!

Most nasal encephaloceles are formed by a failure of closure of the embryologic foramen cecum during the 3rd week of fetal development. The degree of separation of the glial element from the CNS by ingrowth of mesoderm determines whether the resultant deformity will be an encephalocele or a glioma. Approximately 15% of gliomas retain a fibrous connection with the CNS.

Gliomas are most commonly extranasal and present as a noncompressible mass at the root of the nose. Less commonly, they can present as an intranasal mass.

Sincipital encephaloceles occur between the frontal and ethmoid bones anterior to the crista galli (foramen cecum). Although the osseous defect is constant (foramen cecum), the presenting location can vary. Sincipital encephaloceles almost always present as an externally detectable mass. Three common presentations for sincipital encephaloceles are *nasofrontal* (protruding between the frontal and nasal bones); *nasoethmoidal* (protruding through the foramen cecum into the space between the nasal bones and the nasal cartilages); and *nasoorbital* (protruding laterally through a defect in the frontal process of the maxilla into the medial orbit, just anterior to the lacrimal bone).

Basal encephaloceles are less common than the sincipital type. The skull base defect is in the anterior cranial fossa, behind the anterior border of the cribriform. These encephaloceles therefore produce herniation into the nose, nasopharynx, or orbit. The common presentations are *transethmoidal* (intranasal mass emerging from a defect in the cribriform plate); *sphenoethmoidal* (defect at the posterior cribriform); *transsphenoidal* (large defect from posterior cribriform to posterior clinoid with mass protrusion into the nasopharynx); and *sphenorbital* (mass extending through the superior orbital fissure into the posterior orbit).

In evaluating patients with unilateral nasal masses, or with masses in the nasal root area, the possibility of a neurogenic etiology must be considered. Encephaloceles generally feel soft, appear bluish, and are compressible. A positive Furstenburg sign can often be elicited (expansion of the mass when the jugular vein is compressed). Ultimately, the evaluation of patients with possible encephaloceles or gliomas should consist of high-resolution CT scanning to evaluate the extent of the bony defect, followed by a magnetic resonance imaging (MRI) scan to determine if there is a connection with the intracranial subarachnoid space (Fig. 10–2).

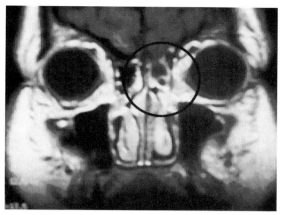

FIGURE 10–2 Magnetic resonance imaging (MRI) in a patient with a nasal mass.

PEARL... A thorough evaluation of the bony skull base while assessing the CT scan of a patient with unilateral nasal pathology will often reveal findings suggestive of an encephalocele. This should be part of the routine preoperative examination of coronal sinus CT scans.

Surgical management consists of removal of the mass, and in cases of encephaloceles, identification of the skull base defect and repair of the dural defect. The standard frontal craniotomy approach has been the traditional technique for managing these patients; however, recent success has been described with the endoscopic approach, especially for those lesions with intranasal extension.

SUGGESTED READINGS

Batsakis JG, ed. *Tumors of the Head and Neck.* 2nd ed. Baltimore: Williams & Wilkins, 1979:chap 17.

Brown OE, Myer CM 3d, Manning SC. Congenital nasal pyriform aperture stenosis. *Laryngoscope* 1989;99(1):86–91.

Harris J, Robert E, Kallen B. Epidemiology of choanal atresia with special reference to the CHARGE association. *Pediatrics* 1997;99(3):363–367.

Hengerer AS, Newburg JA. Congenital malformations of the nose and paranasal sinuses.

In: Bluestone CD, Stool SE, Scheetz MD, eds. *Pediatric Otolaryngology.* 2nd ed. Philadelphia: WB Saunders; 1990:chap 36.

Josephson GD, Vickery CL, Giles WC, Gross CW. Transnasal endoscopic repair of congenital choanal atresia: long-term results. *Arch Otolaryngol Head Neck Surg* 1998;124(5):537–540.

Khoo BC. The proboscis lateralis—a 14-year follow-up. *Plast Reconstr Surg* 1985;75(4):569–577.

Shewmake KB, Kawamoto HK Jr. Congenital clefts of the nose: principles of surgical management. *Cleft Palate Craniofac J* 1992;29(6):531–539.

Chapter 11

FUNCTIONAL DISORDERS

Thomas A. Tami

Other than for breathing, nasal function is rarely given more than passing attention until it is disordered or lost. This chapter discusses the functional nasal conditions obstruction and olfaction, as well as the vomeronasal organ, a possible receptor organ for pheromone stimulation.

NASAL OBSTRUCTION

The primary function of the nose is respiration, and the most common nasal condition managed by otolaryngologists is nasal obstruction. This problem can have numerous etiologies, and each should be considered systematically prior to recommending a therapeutic strategy. Mechanical blockage is the most common and usually the most obvious etiology of nasal blockage. Physical examination can usually pinpoint the precise structural problem. Common possibilities include the following:

▼ *Nasal septal deviation* occurs often on a traumatic basis, although congenital deviation is probably much more common. Deviation can be produced in the caudal septum, bony septum, or a combination of these two (S-shaped deformity). Septoplasty is usually very successful if the precise deformity is identified and addressed during surgery.

▼ *Inferior turbinate hypertrophy* is usually associated with an inflammatory condition within the nose and often responds readily to medical management. In some cases where obstruction persists despite medical management, surgical reduction should be considered. Various techniques have been advocated including partial anterior resection, bipolar cautery, laser reduction, and radiofrequency reduction.

CONTROVERSY

Some surgeons advocate total inferior turbinectomy; however, most rhinologists recommend against this technique due to the severe drying effects that this can have on the nasal mucosa.

▼ *Nasal valve collapse* is a common, yet quite difficult problem to manage surgically. This condition can occasionally occur following aggressive rhinoplasty surgery with narrowing of the nasal dorsum or disruption of the attachment of the upper lateral cartilage. Because the nasal valve region (lower margin of the upper lateral cartilage and septum) is the narrowest part of the nasal airway, dorsal narrowing can further compromise this

95

anatomic region. With inhalation, the negative pressure created in this region, as well as the mobile (floppy) nature of the upper lateral cartilage, allows it to collapse onto the septum. Various treatment options include onlay nasal dilator strips, internal nasal dilators, and surgical spreader grafts (cartilage implanted between the septum and attachment of the upper lateral cartilage).

▼ *"Tunnel nose" syndrome* is a condition in which the patient feels an obstruction to nasal flow; however, upon inspection, the nasal cavity is quite patent. In fact, it usually has the appearance of a wide open "tunnel." Because of a loss of intranasal sensory ability, either due to prior surgery or due to atrophic inflammatory changes, the patient may have good airflow, but because it can't be perceived by the intranasal sensory receptors, the nose always feels obstructed.

▼ *Nasal polyps* are usually quite obvious upon direct anterior rhinoscopic examination, although posterior nasal polyps can occasionally be somewhat obscure. A classic, yet often misdiagnosed etiology of nasal obstruction is the antrochoanal polyp. This nasal polyp arises from the maxillary sinus and extends directly into the nasopharynx, often producing unilateral or bilateral obstruction. Careful endoscopic examination of the nasal cavity and nasopharynx is necessary to establish this diagnosis.

PITFALL••• Except for the antrochoanal polyp, nasal polyps are usually bilateral. Always consider an alternative diagnosis in cases of unilateral polyposis.

CONTROVERSY

Although the traditional treatment for antrochoanal polyp was Caldwell Luc surgery, recent success has been demonstrated using the endoscopic approach.

▼ *Choanal atresia* is usually a life-threatening condition when it is bilateral and presenting in the neonate, but unilateral choanal atresia occasionally goes undiagnosed until adulthood. These patients often present with chronic unilateral rhinorrhea and obstruction. Endoscopy and computed tomography imaging can definitely establish this diagnosis.

▼ *Adenoidal hypertrophy* in children is an especially common cause of nasal obstruction. Even in adults, the adenoids can occasionally enlarge to obstructing dimensions; however, in these cases other possible causes must be considered, such as a primary nasopharyngeal neoplasm, infection (e.g., mononucleosis), or infection with the human immunodeficiency virus (HIV).

▼ *Nasal cavity neoplasm* is covered in more depth in Chapter 13.

SPECIAL CONSIDERATION

A neoplasm should always be considered when the diagnosis of nasal polyp is being entertained. Various possibilities include inverting papilloma, squamous cell carcinoma, undifferentiated sinonasal carcinoma, esthesioneuroblastoma.

OLFACTION

Smell is one of the most primal senses for animals. In the animal world, the sense of smell facilitates the identification of food, mates, and predators; provides sensual pleasures; and warns of danger. It has always been an extremely important means of communication with the environment.

Odorants are chemical compounds carried by inhaled air into the olfactory region on the roof of the nose. In the human, this region consists of an approximately 2.5-cm^2 region containing about 50 million olfactory receptor cells. This olfactory region consists of cilia projecting from the olfactory epithelium into a layer of mucus 60 μm thick. Bowman's glands residing within the olfactory epithelium produce this lipid-rich mucus layer, which bathes the surface of the receptors. This lipid-rich mucus facilitates the transportation of odorants to the olfactory receptors to produce neural signals, which are interpreted centrally as odors. Each olfactory neuron has from 8 to 20 cilia, each extending up to 200 μm in length. It is at the surface of these cilia that the molecular sensory transduction of smell begins.

OLFACTORY EPITHELIUM

The olfactory epithelium contains the following structures and cells (Figs. 11–1 and 11–2):

▼ *Primary olfactory neurons:* These cells rest near the basement membrane of the epithelium as a densely packed layer of cell bodies. The dendritic cilia project onto the surface, whereas the unmyelinated axons form into fascicles of 50 to 100 axons, which then project through the cribriform plate to synapse with second-order olfactory neurons within the olfactory bulb. The olfactory neurons are unique in that they are capable of regeneration.

▼ *Bowman's glands:* These glands produce the lipid-rich mucus that bathes the surface of the receptors.

▼ *Supporting cells:* These cells, also known as sustentacular cells, are tall slender cells with an apically located nucleus. Microvilli, which project from their surface, entangle with olfactory cilia. These cells probably function by increasing the overall surface area of the respiratory epithelium via their microvilli. They may also possess metabolic and phagocytotic functions to remove odorant molecules following stimulation.

▼ *Basal cells:* These cells are the source of new receptor neurons and supporting cells when lost following injury or due to normal cell turnover.

▼ *Microvillar cells:* These are flask-shaped cells the function of which is as yet unknown.

THEORIES OF OLFACTION

Although it is still not clear how the olfactory mechanism functions at a receptor/molecular level, several theories have been offered:

▼ *Molecular-shape theory:* This original "lock and key" theory was modeled after the kinetic properties of enzymes. In this theory there are several primary odors (camphor, musk,

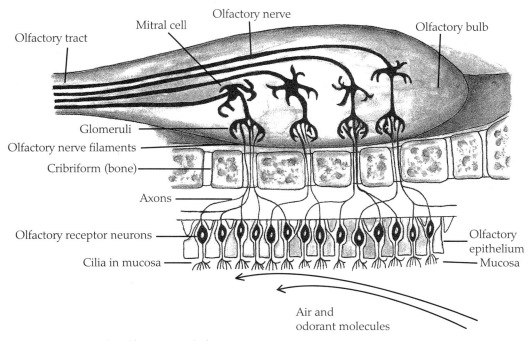

FIGURE 11-1 The olfactory epithelium.

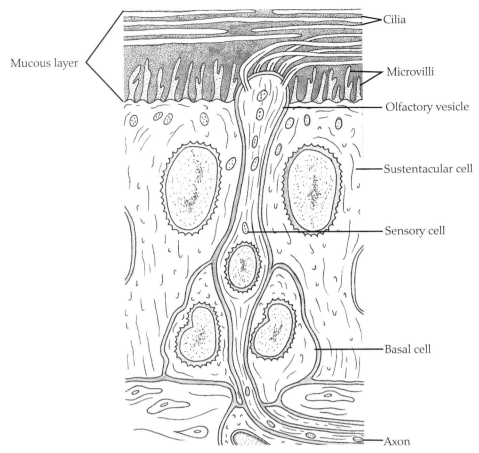

FIGURE 11-2 The olfactory mucosa.

floral, peppermint, ether, pungent, and putrid). Recent evidence of odorant-binding proteins has revived interest in this theory. There appear in fact to be many odorant-binding proteins as well as hundreds of odorant receptors. Many of these have been recently cloned, and messenger RNA (mRNA) encoding these proteins has been identified.

▼ *Diffusion pore theory:* This theory held that olfactory molecules diffuse across the receptor membrane forming an ion pore in its wake. Although this theory could account for some of the qualities of smell, such as threshold, it offered little to explain differential smell qualities.

▼ *Piezo effect theory:* This theory proposed that the odorant molecules combined with carotenoids in the pigment of olfactory cells to give rise to a semiconductor current. This theory has been largely discounted.

▼ *Molecular resonance theory:* Because many odorants have natural vibratory frequencies in the infrared spectrum, it was felt that frequency coding was somehow responsible for smell perception.

OLFACTORY DYSFUNCTION

A disordered sense of smell can present in a variety of ways. The following terms are generally used to describe each of the more common presentations of olfactory dysfunction:

▼ *Anosmia:* a complete loss of smell perception
▼ *Hyposmia:* a decreased, yet still present sense of smell

▼ *Hyperosmia:* an increased or enhanced odor sensitivity

▼ *Dysosmia:* a distorted or abnormal smell response

▼ *Phantosmia:* an abnormal smell perception in the absence of an external stimulus

▼ *Parosmia:* an abnormal response to an environmental stimulus

There are a number of common, and some not so common, etiologies of smell dysfunction. Some are treatable, and others are difficult or impossible to manage effectively. One of the most common etiologies is *head trauma*. This diagnosis is based on a history of trauma immediately preceding the onset of the loss. It is generally thought that the mechanism of this loss is from shearing of the olfactory neurons at the cribriform plate region. Occasionally, posttraumatic olfactory loss is secondary to obstruction of airflow into the olfactory groove. In these cases, relief of the obstruction can result in improved olfaction. Unfortunately, most cases of traumatic loss are secondary to neural disruption, and the prognosis for recovery in these cases is usually poor.

Postviral olfactory loss is another common presentation of anosmia. Although this is a well-known cause of anosmia, the precise mechanism is not known. Viral infection can produce direct injury to the olfactory epithelium or might produce an immunologic response, which injures these cell. There is also some evidence of damage to central olfactory pathways secondary to viral injury. Although recovery from virally induced injury does usually occur, it may be delayed, may occur very slowly, and may be incomplete. There is no evidence that steroids, vitamins, zinc, or any other medications are beneficial.

> **PEARL...** Always consider the possibility of an obstructive etiology for anosmia in the setting of viral infection. The diagnosis of postviral anosmia should only be assigned after the possibility of obstruction from inflammation has been excluded.

Primary nasal and paranasal sinus conditions can also produce alterations in olfaction. *Nasal obstruction* is an obvious etiology. If air can't pass into the olfactory sensory region of the nose, odorants will not be detected. Symptomatic nasal obstruction does not have to be present before smell is significantly affected. Although nasal septal deviation is often an etiologic consideration, there are no studies clearly demonstrating such a relationship. *Tumors* or *nasal polyposis* causing obstruction to airflow into the olfactory region can also produce dysfunction on the basis of nasal obstruction. *Chronic sinusitis,* with or without nasal polyposis, can also be associated with olfactory disorders. Even in the absence of gross polyposis, edemia of the middle and superior turbinates can produce intranasal obstruction to the olfactory region and result in hyposmia or anosmia. Functional endoscopic sinus surgery can often be curative in these cases.

Toxic exposure has long been known to be associated with some cases of olfactory pathology. It is generally agreed that high levels of toxins are necessary to induce pathologic changes. Usually this results from a sudden excessive exposure rather than a prolonged, low-level chronic exposure. Agents that have been shown to affect olfactory function include metallic compounds (cadmium, nickel); nonmetallic inorganic compounds (ammonia, carbon disulfide, carbon monoxide, chlorine); organic compounds (acetone, benzene, ethyl acetate); dusts (cement, hardwoods, lime, printing); and manufacturing processes (acids, asphalt, lead paints, spices). In addition to trying to remove the suspected causative agent, topical steroids have shown some efficacy in promoting olfactory recovery.

Kallmann's syndrome is a congenital cause of anosmia. Also associated with this syndrome is primary hypogonadotrophic hypogonadism. Anosmia results from a failure in formation of connections between nerve fibers from the nose and the brain, whereas the gonadal dysfunction results from insufficient secretion of a key peptide, gonadotropin-releasing hormone (GnRH), from the hypothalamus.

The Vomeronasal Organ (Jacobson's Organ)

The vomeronasal organ (VNO), or Jacobson's organ, is an intranasal chemoreceptor organ present in most vertebrate species. This organ is separate from the main olfactory system and is thought to be important in species-specific chemical (pheromone) communication. In most species this organ is located within a capsule at the juncture of the vomer and bone or vomer and cartilage. The epithelium of the VNO contains bipolar receptor neurons with microvilli on their exposed surface. Most of the work on vomeronasal function has been in rodents and snakes and has demonstrated dramatic effects on reproductive behavior as well as some aggressive behavior. In these species, vomeronasal input may be critical for reliable preprogrammed behavior (e.g., mating).

The VNO has long been known to be present in human fetuses and has been reported sporadically in adults; however, recent studies have demonstrated the presence of vomeronasal duct openings in most human adults. There are cells in the human VNO that have the appearance of bipolar neurons; however, connections between these neurons and the brain have not been demonstrated in humans. Although an actual role for the VNO has yet to be established for humans, commercial enterprises have begun to market fragrances with purported pheromonic activity. The precise role and existence of these compounds are yet to be determined. As nasal septal surgical procedures may result in dysfunction or ablation of this organ, its existence should be a consideration during conservative intranasal surgical procedures.

Suggested Readings

Gaafar HA, Tantawy AA, Melis AA, Hennawy DM, Shehata HM. The vomeronasal (Jacobson's) organ in adult humans: frequency of occurrence and enzymatic study. *Acta Otolaryngol (Stockh)* 1998;118(3):409–412.

Garcia-Velasco J, Garcia-Casas S. Nose surgery and the vomeronasal organ. *Aesthetic Plast Surg* 1995;19(5):451–454.

Jones N, Rog D. Olfaction: a review. *J Laryngol Otol* 1998;112(1):11–24.

Monti-Bloch L, Jennings-White C, Berliner DL. The human vomeronasal system. A review. *Ann NY Acad Sci* 1998;855:373–389.

Seiden AM, ed. *Taste and Smell Disorders.* New York: Thieme; 1997.

Settipane GA, ed. *Rhinitis.* Providence, RI: OceanSide; 1991.

Chapter 12

INFECTIOUS AND INFLAMMATORY DISORDERS

Thomas A. Tami

ALLERGIC RHINITIS

PATHOPHYSIOLOGY

Allergic rhinitis is an inflammatory disorder characterized by an immunoglobulin E (IgE)-mediated hypersensitivity to foreign allergens. The concentration of allergen in the ambient air correlates directly with rhinitis symptoms. When these antigens contact the respiratory mucosa, specific IgE antibody is produced in susceptible hosts. This results in the classic clinical picture of nasal congestion, itching eyes and nose, rhinorrhea, and sneezing.

At a cellular level, several different cells and molecules participate in the pathophysiology of allergic rhinitis. Among these, T cells and their secreted products play an important role. The initial presentation of an allergen to the immune system usually produces no symptoms but prepares the host to respond to future exposures. Macrophages initially degrade the allergen and present antigen fragments to the CD4+ T lymphocytes. These activated T cells deliver signals to B cells, which are then stimulated to produce IgE antibodies in response to this T-cell interaction. Other components that also participate in this process include the major histocompatability complex and interleukin-4.

Following their production, IgE antibodies attach to receptors on mast cells and circulating basophils. In subsequent contact with the allergen, antigen molecules bind to these mast cell IgE surface molecules. The bridging of two IgE antibodies on the cell surface activates a cascade reaction resulting in mast cell degranulation. The release of histamine and other mediators produces the immediate allergic symptoms of nasal congestion, mucosal edema, increased granular secretion, nasal itching, and sneezing. This cascade also induces the synthesis of other inflammatory mediators including the leukotrienes C_4, D_4, and E_4, prostaglandins, and extracellularly derived kinins.

SPECIAL CONSIDERATION

Approximately 4 to 24 hours after mast-cell activation, the late-phase reaction in the nose continues to produce allergic symptoms.

This late-phase reaction is associated with infiltration of inflammatory cells, the reappearance of inflammatory mediators, as increased responsiveness to allergens, and hyperresponsiveness to irritants. Neural mechanisms also contribute to nasal symptoms because inflammatory mediators cause activation of the nonadrenergic, neural C-fiber system.

DIAGNOSIS

The most important component in establishing the diagnosis is the history. It is important to obtain a detailed account describing when and where the symptoms occur. The usual symptoms, including sneezing, nasal congestion, watery nasal discharge, and itching, may be seasonal (typically in the spring or late summer) or perennial (with or without seasonal exacerbations). Seasonal allergens include trees, grasses, weed pollens, and airborne molds, and symptoms are highly correlated with the timing of pollen release according to geographic location. Perennial allergens, such as dust mites, pet danders, and mold spores, often cause chronic symptoms and rarely have a seasonal relationship.

Typical physical eye findings include injected conjunctiva with a watery discharge and eyelid puffiness. In chronic cases, a transverse crease is often seen across the bridge of the nose (allergic crease), which results from rubbing the nose to relieve nasal obstruction and itching (the allergic salute). Darkening of the infraorbital skin ("allergic shiners") may also be present.

Nasal examination may be normal or may reveal watery mucus on the epithelial surface. The mucosa is usually edematous and may have a bluish-gray appearance in cases of severe mucosal edema. This mucosal appearance is not specific to allergic rhinitis, because nonallergic rhinitis often presents with similar findings. Swollen inferior turbinates often appear polypoid due to edema.

Allergy skin testing and the radioallergosorbent test (RAST) are the most useful diagnostic tests for determining the presence of IgE directed against specific allergens. RAST tends to be used generically, whereas most in vitro testing methods today utilize enzyme and not radioactive labeling. Nasal cytology in patients with allergic rhinitis usually reveals an abundance of eosinophils, and serum IgE levels may be elevated.

TREATMENT

Patients with allergic rhinitis require a customized approach to management. Patient education regarding avoidance of specific allergens, pharmacotherapy, and immunotherapy are the cornerstones of treatment.

Patient Education

Patient education is particularly important because of the recurrent and chronic nature of allergic rhinitis. Patients who have seasonal symptoms due to molds or pollen should keep their home and work environments closed if possible. Air conditioning and filters can reduce the amount of pollen exposure. Dust mites are a major source of perennial allergen. Dust mites live in carpets, mattresses, and bedding, and thrive on human dander. They excrete enzymatic proteins in their feces, which are the primary source of antigen. Encasing the mattress and pillows in plastic minimizes conditions for mite growth. Patients with mold allergy eliminate sources of mold growth in their homes, such as old mattresses and furniture and damp areas. Cat and dog allergens are also quite common perennial triggers for allergic rhinitis. Cat allergens in particular are easily airborne and allergic patients often experience symptoms immediately upon entering a room with a cat. Pets should be removed from homes of the pet-allergic patients; however, this is often a difficult and emotional process.

Pharmacotherapy

Pharmacotherapy for allergic rhinitis includes antihistamines, decongestants, and topical nasal sprays.

Antihistamines

Antihistamines have always been an important component of therapy for allergic rhinitis and are easily obtained in over-the-counter preparations. These H_1-receptor antagonists work best if taken before allergen exposure. First-generation antihistamines, such as diphenhydramine and chlorpheniramine, are effective in producing symptomatic relief from sneezing and itching of the eyes, nose, and palate. However, these first-generation antihistamines often produce significant sedation and anticholinergic effects. Because the newer second-generation antihistamines (e.g., terfenadine, astemizole, loratadine, cetirizine) do not cross the blood–brain barrier, they are relatively nonsedating in most patients. These agents are also quite effective in producing symptom relief.

Antihistamines are relatively safe drugs for most patients. Certain antihistamines have been reported to produce cardiac arrhythmias, particularly torsades de pointes. This rare cardiac arrhythmia has been reported to occur with both terfenadine and astemizole when hepatic metabolism of these drugs is impaired.

Antihistamines are useful for the relief of itching of the eyes, nose, and throat and for sneezing and watery rhinorrhea when used on a short- or long-term basis, but are less effective for nasal congestion. Treatment of nasal congestion usually requires the use of a topical nasal glucocorticoid spray or an oral decongestant.

Decongestants

Managing nasal congestion usually requires the use of a topical or oral decongestant. Both topical and systemic decongestants produce vasoconstriction of the nasal mucosa in allergic rhinitis patients. Topical decongestants (e.g., oxymetazoline) are very effective for the acute relief of nasal congestion; however, prolonged use can be associated with the development of rhinitis medicamentosa with severe rebound nasal congestion. They should be used only for short-term relief (several days) so as to minimize these risks.

Oral decongestants (e.g., pseudoephedrine and phenylpropanolamine) are also very effective at reducing nasal congestion and are frequently used in combination with antihistamines. Unlike topical nasal decongestants, oral agents are not associated with rhinitis medicamentosa and can therefore be safely used for longer periods of time. Common side effects of these agents include insomnia, headache, irritability, and palpitations. These drugs should also be used with caution in patients with uncontrolled hypertension, coronary artery disease, or concomitant therapy with monoamine oxidase inhibitors.

Topical Nasal Sprays

NASAL STEROIDS Nasal steroid sprays have been important agents in the treatment of almost all types of rhinitis. Preparations that are currently available include both aqueous as well as nonaqueous forms of beclomethasone, flunisolide, budesonide, triamcinolone, and fluticasone. These drugs can sometimes improve symptoms of nasal obstruction due to nasal polyps and may also help prevent recurrence following surgery.

The primary clinical benefits of topical nasal steroid preparations are produced by reducing nasal mucosal inflammation. This effect is obtained by reducing the cell-mediated inflammatory response (basophils, mast cells, eosinophils, and neutrophils), in addition to decreasing inflammatory mediator levels in the nasal mucosa and nasal secretions. These actions inhibit both the early as well as the late allergic responses.

> **PEARL...** A major cause of treatment failure using nasal steroids is poor patient education regarding the correct use of these agents. Patients should be informed that 7 to 14 days are often necessary for the medication to achieve clinical effectiveness. Regular use is necessary to obtain continued symptom relief, and an as-needed dosing regimen is usually ineffective.

Side effects from the use of these agents are unusual. The most common is nasal irritation and occasionally epistaxis. These problems are usually avoidable if the patient is instructed in the proper delivery of the medication. If there is a severe nasal septal deviation, constant spraying into this portion of the septum can produce mucosal irritation and crusting.

Long-term use of these agents does not produce suppression of the hypothalamic-pituitary-adrenal axis. Biopsy studies evaluating nasal mucosa have also shown that intranasal beclomethasone produces no mucosal atrophy.

NASAL DISODIUM CROMOGLYCATE Disodium cromoglycate acts by preventing chemical mediator release from mast cells in response to an-

CONTROVERSY

The use of the nonaqueous preparations seems to be particularly prone to local nasal irritative symptoms. Frank septal perforation has been rarely reported as a result of the use of these agents. Although the use of topical steroids in patients with glaucoma has been somewhat controversial, nasal steroid preparations have not been shown to have any significant effect on intraocular pressure measurements.

tigen stimulation. Disodium cromoglycate works best if used before exposure to antigen and prior to onset of allergic symptoms. Because this agent must be used prior to exposure and requires multiple daily dosing, it has become less popular in the management of allergic rhinitis.

TOPICAL NASAL ANTIHISTAMINE Levocabastine is currently the only available H_1 antagonist available as a topical spray for allergic rhinitis. When applied intranasally, it can also modulate the nasal symptoms of itching, sneezing, and rhinorrhea. This agent requires multiple daily dosing to achieve maximum clinical effectiveness.

NASAL IPRATROPIUM BROMIDE Ipratropium bromide is a topical anticholinergic agent that can decrease watery rhinorrhea in patients with vasomotor rhinitis; however, it has little or no effect on nasal congestion. It can be very helpful if used prophylactically to reduce watery rhinorrhea associated with specific inciting situations (e.g., cold air exposure, the rhinitis associated with eating spicy foods). This topical anticholinergic has no significant effects on intraocular pressure or urinary retention.

ORAL STEROIDS For patients with severe allergic symptoms that cannot be controlled with other agents, oral prednisone or long-acting intramuscular steroids can often provide dramatic symptomatic relief.

IMMUNOTHERAPY Immunotherapy is the repeated administration of specific allergens to patients with IgE-mediated disease. This process appears to provide protection against allergic symptoms caused by the inflammatory reaction that follows exposure to these allergens. The precise mechanisms responsible for this clinical response is unclear. Possible mechanisms include decreased postexposure cellular responsiveness; the production of blocking antibodies, induction of B- or T-cell tolerance, the production of antiidiotypic antibodies, or possibly the activation of a T-cell suppressor mechanism.

Studies have clearly shown that immunotherapy is very effective for the management of allergic rhinitis. Patients should demonstrate specific IgE antibodies to clinically relevant allergens. For maximal clinical benefit, there should be a good correlation between the history of the patient's symptoms and positive skin tests to the allergens with which the patient will be hyposensitized. Patients should not be immunized with allergens that do not cause clinical symptoms.

The direct measurement of serum IgE levels in patients with suspected allergic rhinitis can also be helpful, but is considered by many to be an insensitive test. Although total serum IgE is frequently elevated an allergic rhinitis, it may occasionally be normal.

RASTs and other serologic techniques can provide in vitro measures of antigen-specific IgE. RASTs are generally considered less sensitive than skin tests. However, they may be useful for some patients.

> **PITFALL...** Indiscriminate and inappropriate use of immunotherapy for nonallergic rhinitis has contributed to the erroneous view held by some practitioners that it is a generally ineffective form of treatment.

The need for immunotherapy depends on the degree of symptom reduction obtained by pharmacotherapy. The local and regional prevalence of pollens, fungi, and dust mites should drive the selection of specific allergens used for testing.

The major risk associated with immunotherapy is anaphylaxis. For this reason, immunotherapy should be administered under the supervision of a physician who can recognize and manage this life-threatening condition.

PEARL... Patients who are receiving β-adrenergic–blocking agents generally should not receive allergen immunotherapy.

The duration of immunotherapy after obtaining maximal clinical response is unknown. Many clinicians advise the continuation of therapy for 4 to 5 years, whereas others recommend treatment indefinitely, fearing a clinical exacerbation if therapy is withdrawn. If symptoms have been controlled and there has been no change after 12 to 18 months of treatment, immunotherapy should probably be discontinued.

VASOMOTOR RHINITIS

PATHOPHYSIOLOGY

Vasomotor rhinitis consists of a complex of symptoms including sneezing and watery rhinorrhea and may occasionally be associated with nasal congestion. These symptoms frequently occur in response to environmental triggers such as cold air, bright lights, specific odors or chemicals, exercise, emotional upset, and eating certain foods. Many patients with these symptoms, but who have no obvious allergic or infectious etiology, are often lumped into the category nonallergic vasomotor rhinitis, even though this classification often contains a heterogeneous group of disorders. The exact pathophysiologic mechanism is unknown; however, it is clear that IgE-mediated mechanisms do not play a role. Cholinergic hyperactivity within the nasal cavity is generally felt to be responsible for the rhinorrhea that these patients experience, and treatment is usually directed toward addressing this hyperactive cholinergic system.

TREATMENT

Pharmacotherapy

Because cholinergic hyperreactivity has been hypothesized in these patients, most treatments tend to address this issue. Ipratropium bromide is a muscarinic receptor antagonist that is poorly absorbed across mucous membranes (less than 20% of an 84-μg dose is absorbed from nasal mucosa). It affects the nasal mucosa by causing a reduction in cholinergic activity and thereby a reduction of nasal secretory activity. It has little or no effect on nasal congestion.

The most common adverse effect from ipratropium is mild, transient episodes of epistaxis and nasal dryness. The usual dose of the 0.03% preparation is two sprays per nostril two to three times daily.

PEARL... Rhinorrhea associated with the common cold is due in part to parasympathetic stimulation. Treatment with an anticholinergic agent such as ipratropium bromide (Atrovent nasal 0.06%) provides some relief of rhinorrhea associated with the common cold.

Topical nasal steroid sprays have also been used in vasomotor rhinitis. Although success has been reported with these agents, the precise mechanism for their efficacy is unclear. Some reports have also discussed a possible role for capsaicin spray as a substance-P–depleting agent. Long-term usage of this agent has not been evaluated.

Surgical Therapy

If the rhinitis symptoms do not respond to medical therapy, one of several surgical procedures can be considered. Cryosurgery produces damage with subsequent healing of the intranasal mucosa and submucosa. This is generally a successful procedure for congestion; however, it is less effective for chronic rhinorrhea.

Vidian neurectomy is a procedure classically described for this condition but with inconsistent results. By disrupting parasympathetic fibers to the nasal mucosa, rhinorrhea can be reduced. Several approaches have been described including the classic transantral procedure as well as the more recent endoscopic technique. Because the nasal parasympathetics are also part of the parasympathetic system to the lacrimal gland, chronic xerophthalmia is a well-described complication of this procedure.

Laser therapy has also been advocated for this disorder. The most popular has been the use of a laser to burn a grid onto the mucosa of the middle and inferior turbinates. Subsequent scarring produces symptomatic improvement by eliminating much of the secretory activity of the nasal mucosa.

NONALLERGIC RHINITIS WITH EOSINOPHILIA (NARE)

This syndrome is characterized by nasal itching, sneezing, and watery rhinorrhea. These symptoms are usually perennial, but tend to have paroxysmal exacerbations. Polypoid changes may occur in the nasal mucosa. The nasal secretions contain abundant eosinophils; however, there is no obvious IgE-mediated hypersensitivity. The pathophysiologic mechanisms of this syndrome are unknown.

> **PEARL•••** The etiology of the syndrome is obscure; however, it may represent an early stage of aspirin sensitivity.

The treatment of this condition includes decongestants, occasionally antihistamines, and topical nasal steroid sprays. These patients usually have a dramatic response to steroid therapy.

NASAL POLYPS

Nasal polyposis may be associated with several different conditions: nonallergic asthma; Samter's triad (asthma, aspirin intolerance, nasal polyps); cystic fibrosis; Kartagener's syndrome; Churg-Strauss syndrome; and chronic

sinusitis. Polyps are usually bilateral and most often emanate from the middle meatus and ethmoid region.

> **PITFALL•••** Unilateral nasal polyposis should always raise clinical suspicions of a noninflammatory process such as encephaloceles or nasal tumors.

Antrochoanal polyps, arising from the maxillary sinus and extending into the nasopharynx, are often unilateral; however, they can produce bilateral nasal obstruction by expanding into the entire nasopharynx (Fig. 12–1).

The histopathologic appearance of inflammatory nasal polyps consists of a pseudostratified columnar epithelium with extensive thickening of the basement membrane overlying an edematous, vascular stroma often containing numerous eosinophils, lymphocytes, and plasma cells. The glandular components of the mucosa are few, and these glands are usually denervated.

Numerous chemical mediators have been identified in nasal polyp tissue. These include the leukotrienes, histamine, serotonin,

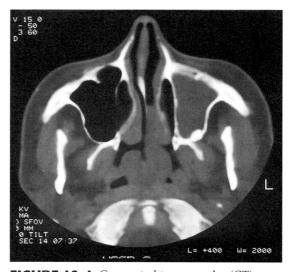

FIGURE 12–1 Computed tomography (CT) scan of a typical antrochoanal polyp, which originates in the maxillary sinus; however, it extends into and fills the nasopharynx, thereby causing bilateral nasal obstruction.

prostaglandins, and kinins. Up to 70% of patients with nasal polyps also have reactive airway disease and asthma; however, the majority of these patients do not have evidence of atopic disease. Samter's triad is associated with severe asthma that is often steroid dependent. Aspirin and other nonsteroidal antiinflammatory drugs (NSAIDs) inhibit the enzyme cyclooxygenase, thereby increasing the production of leukotrienes and other arachidonic acid metabolites.

> **PITFALL•••** Patients with Samter's triad must be cautioned against the use of any NSAID because all have similar effects on cyclooxygenase.

These patients do not usually have allergic disease as determined by skin or serologic testing. Surgical management is associated with an extremely high recurrence rate in these patients.

> ## CONTROVERSY
>
> Although polypectomy in these patients has been traditionally thought to be associated with an increased risk of perioperative bronchospasm, studies have confirmed that there is essentially no change in bronchial reactivity following polypectomy.

> ## SPECIAL CONSIDERATION
>
> Nasal polyps are unusual in children and teenagers. When present, the possibility of another concurrent disease such as cystic fibrosis or Kartagener's syndrome should be entertained.

VIRAL INFECTIONS

By far, the most common infectious cause of nasal inflammation is viral infection. A host of viruses can produce acute infection; however, those most commonly isolated include rhinovirus, parainfluenza virus, and influenza virus. Respiratory syncytial virus and coronavirus also probably play an important role in these infections; however, they are hard to grow and isolate in culture, making the investigation of these agents difficult.

Rhinovirus exerts its clinical effect by stimulating the release of inflammatory mediators rather than by causing direct mucosal damage and destruction. On the other hand, influenza virus is often isolated from sinus aspirates of patients with acute sinusitis and seems to cause a fairly destructive infection of the respiratory mucosa.

During typical rhinovirus infections symptoms usually progress from the nasopharyngeal region anteriorly into the nose. Symptoms subside dramatically by day 4 or 5 and have usually ended by 1 week. On average, viral shedding continues for up to 3 weeks.

> **PITFALL•••** Bacterial infections can usually be distinguished from viral infections by the time course. If symptoms continue beyond 10 to 14 days, secondary bacterial rhinosinusitis is probably present. Recent studies have demonstrated a higher incidence of computed tomography (CT) abnormalities during simple rhinovirus infections. Because these changes can easily be interpreted as bacterial sinusitis, timing of CT scans when evaluating patients with recurrent or chronic sinusitis is important to avoid confusion in interpretation.

BACTERIAL INFECTIONS

ACUTE SINUSITIS

Acute bacterial infection of the paranasal sinuses is most often the result of a prolonged viral upper respiratory infection. The pathophysiology of sinusitis is now generally accepted as being due to obstruction of the ostia of the sinuses. The most common sinuses involved are the anterior sinuses (anterior ethmoid, maxillary, and frontal) due to their common outflow tract through the middle meatus. The most common bacteriologic organisms isolated in acute sinusitis are *Streptococcus pneumoniae, Haemophilus influenzae,* and *Moraxella catarrhalis.* Recent resistance data confirm that the incidence of antibiotic resistance among these three organisms is steadily increasing. Currently, nearly 100% of *M. catarrhalis* are β-lactamase producers, 30 to 40% of *H. influenzae* produce β-lactamase, and up to 35% of *S. pneumoniae* are penicillin resistant.

SPECIAL CONSIDERATION

Penicillin-resistant *S. pneumoniae* (PRSP) is due to an alteration of surface penicillin binding proteins and is not secondary to β-lactamase production. As these resistant strains become increasingly more common, many of the standard therapies for sinusitis are becoming less effective. PRSP is also frequently resistant to macrolides and sulfonamides.

Duration of treatment for acute sinusitis remains controversial. Although recent cost-containment trends in medicine have argued for shorter durations of therapy, it is generally held that at least 2 weeks of antibiotic treatment is necessary to ensure resolution of acute sinusitis.

Adjuvant therapeutic options include systemic decongestants (pseudoephedrine or phenylpropanolamine), topical decongestants (such as oxymetazoline), mucoevacuants (guaifenesin), and antipyretic/analgesics (acetaminophen).

Although maxillary antral irrigation is still occasionally recommended, little data is available to confirm its effectiveness in facilitating resolution of infection or shortening the duration of symptoms. Antral tap can be useful if cultures are required to direct antibiotic therapy; however, endoscopically directed middle meatal cultures can probably provide similar clinical information.

CHRONIC SINUSITIS

The difficulties encountered in actually defining chronic sinusitis have impeded the systematic study of this problem. Although definitions vary, sinusitis is generally considered chronic when symptoms have been present, usually despite medical therapy, for greater than 8 to 12 weeks. Although the same bacterial organisms associated with acute sinusitis may also be isolated in these patients, *Staphylococcus aureus* and various anaerobic bacteria also become important pathogens. Culture-directed antibiotic therapy is often a useful management tool.

Besides antimicrobials, other adjuvant therapy is often recommended. Nasal saline irrigation can improve mucociliary clearance and is frequently recommended for these patients. Decongestants can also be helpful; however, topical agents are best avoided in this situation. For patients with underlying allergic rhinitis, appropriate allergy management, including antihistamines, can be beneficial. Topical nasal steroids have been shown not only to help improve patient symptoms, but also to decrease the inflammatory cell infiltrate within the mucosal tissues. Systemic corticosteroids have been gaining increasing popularity in patients with chronic sinusitis, especially when nasal polyposis complicates chronic sinusitis. Systemic steroids can produce dramatic antiinflammatory effects; however, these changes are not always long-lasting.

PEARL... Care should always be exercised when steroids are used in patients with diabetes. Glucose intolerance associated with high-dose steroids can be associated with devastating invasive infections in these patients.

Surgical therapy is recommended when symptoms persist despite maximal medical therapy. Functional endoscopic sinus surgery (FESS) as popularized by Kennedy has become the mainstay of surgical management. Although this technique addresses the pathophysiology of sinusitis by improving drainage and facilitating normal mucociliary flow, standard open techniques such as Caldwell Luc, external frontoethmoidectomy, and frontal sinus obliteration are still occasionally necessary for recalcitrant cases.

FUNGAL SINUSITIS

Fungal infections of the paranasal sinuses are not uncommon. There are three primary types of fungal involvement.

Mycetoma

Noninvasive fungal sinusitis (mycetoma) is a relatively benign process. Symptoms often consist of localized pain (usually the maxillary region), postnasal drainage, and nasal congestion. The fungal mass (mycetoma or fungal ball) is contained within the sinus (usually the maxillary) and does not produce invasion of surrounding bony or soft tissues. By causing intermittent obstruction of the ostium of the sinus, it can predispose to recurrent bacterial infections. The most common cause is *Aspergillus* species. Radiographically the mass appears as a soft tissue density, often with calcifications, confined to one sinus. Treatment is quite effective either by endoscopic or open techniques to completely evacuate the fungal elements from the sinus.

> **PEARL...** Tissue biopsies should be obtained and closely evaluated by the histopathologist to exclude an invasive component.

Allergic Fungal Sinusitis (AFS)

This entity is not a true infection, but represents an immunologic (allergic) response to fungal growth within the sinuses. These patients typically present with chronic symptoms and have often undergone numerous previous surgical procedures. The accumulation of allergic mucin within the sinus cavity contributes to expansion and bony erosion of the sinus walls. Although this can be a process involving all of the sinuses, it is not unusual to see unilateral disease.

The diagnosis is made by observing bony expansion of the paranasal sinuses on CT scanning (often producing proptosis if involving the ethmoids). Histopathologic examination of allergic mucin reveals sheets of eosinophils, Charcot-Leyden crystals, and occasional fungal hyphae in the mucin. The pathophysiology is thought to be related to a hypersensitivity to fungi colonizing the paranasal sinus cavities. Eosinophils gather in the region and secrete inflammatory mediators that damage cilia and contribute to polyp formation. These mediators further obstruct mucus flow from sinus ostia. Treatment begins with surgical evacuation of all sinus contents.

> **PEARL...** Bony erosion, especially at the skull base and orbit region, must be carefully evaluated (Fig. 12–2). Although complete removal of sinus contents is important, attention to anatomic detail and avoiding penetration through dehiscent bony landmarks is essential. Computer image—guided surgery is often ideal for these cases.

Most authors agree that medical treatment with systemic and topical steroids is the cornerstone of long-term management of this disease. Because the primary problem is an inflammatory one, antiinflammatory treatment is used. Controversy exists regarding the duration of therapy as well as the role of immunotherapy for this disorder. Although data are limited supporting fungal desensitization, its popularity appears to be increasing.

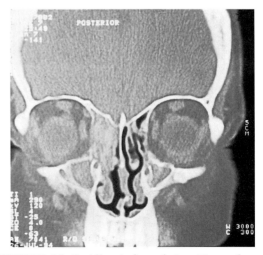

FIGURE 12–2 Allergic fungal sinusitis can be unilateral as shown on CT in this case. Note the expansion of the right ethmoid labyrinth with bony erosion of the orbital lamina.

Systemic antifungal therapy has traditionally played no role in the management of AFS. Recent experience with oral itraconazole, the only oral agent active against dematiaceous fungi, has provided encouraging, yet inconclusive support for its use.

Invasive Fungal Sinusitis

There are two forms of invasive fungal disease. In *chronic invasive fungal sinusitis,* the symptoms have usually been present and progressive for a long period of time (months or years). The infection is invasive and usually erodes through bony anatomic barriers into adjacent structures such as the orbit, infratemporal fossa, anterior cranial fossa, or premaxillary region. When present within the sphenoid sinus, the consequences can be particularly grave due to extension into the cavernous sinus or optic nerve. The dematiaceous fungi, including bipolaris and aspergillus, are the most common pathogens isolated in this disease.

SPECIAL CONSIDERATION

Although often associated with an alteration of host defenses (e.g., HIV disease, immunoglobulin deficiency), chronic invasive fungal sinusitis has also been reported in otherwise healthy individuals.

Treatment consists of complete surgical debridement, if possible, followed by systemic antifungal chemotherapy. Initial medical treatment usually consists of intravenous amphotericin B; however, long-term treatment using oral itraconazole has been gaining popularity.

Fulminant invasive fungal sinusitis is a devastating, often life-threatening condition. There are two primary conditions that predispose to this overwhelming infection. The first is diabetes mellitus. Patients with diabetes have poorly functioning neutrophils to begin with. In the presence of acidosis and elevated glucose levels that accompany diabetic ketoacidosis, the *Rhizopus* family of fungi thrive. As the fungus spreads, it invades vascular and neural structures, producing thrombosis and necrosis. Unless underlying metabolic abnormalities are corrected, the infection will continue to rapidly and aggressively spread into adjoining tissues, such as the orbit and central nervous system.

Treatment is highly dependent on early identification and recognition. Understanding the pathophysiology of this disorder should help in identifying patients at risk. Careful examination intranasally (looking for areas of avascular tissue necrosis) as well as a careful neurologic evaluation (V2 hypesthesia is a common early finding) can help identify this process before it has caused extensive irreparable damage. The underlying metabolic problem must be corrected as quickly as possible. Surgical debridement of all devitalized tissue followed by systemic amphotericin B can often be lifesaving. However, delay in diagnosis guarantees a poor clinical result with substantial morbidity, and often mortality.

Another clinical scenario associated with invasive fungal sinusitis is neutropenia. Bone marrow transplant patients are a typical group developing neutropenia following bone marrow ablation. Although the neutrophil count usually increases as the transplant begins to function, prolonged neutropenia can be associated with fulminant fungal infection, usually caused by *Aspergillus* species. As with diabetes mellitus, successful treatment depends on early diagnosis, correction of the underlying immunologic deficit, and aggressive surgical debridement, followed by intravenous amphotericin B therapy.

GRANULOMATOUS RHINOSINUSITIS

WEGENER'S GRANULOMATOSIS

This is a fairly unusual form of vasculitis that often affects the sinopulmonary tract. This disease has a peak incidence in the third and fourth decades of life and has a slight predilection for women. Classic Wegener's consists of the triad of necrotizing granulomas of the upper and lower respiratory tract, glomerulitis, and disseminated vasculitis. When the kidneys are not involved, it is usually referred to as limited

Wegener's. Nasal symptoms often include nasal congestion, nasal crusting, and epistaxis. As the destructive process progresses, nasal saddling and chronic nasal crusting are common.

When entertaining this diagnosis, a search for possible systemic involvement is mandatory. Chest radiographs (often including CT scans) and urine analysis for protein should be undertaken. An elevated sedimentation rate is common. Serologic studies often reveal an elevated antinuclear cytoplasmic antibody (c-ANCA). Although not diagnostic, this test is highly suggestive for Wegener's. Histopathologic examination of involved tissue will often reveal necrotic granulomas with typical vasculitis. Treatment consists of aggressive antiinflammatory therapy using high-dose steroids, cyclophosphamide, and occasionally methotrexate. For limited Wegener's trimethoprimsulfamethoxazole may play a role. Frequent intranasal debridements and irrigations can help provide good nasal hygiene until the active inflammatory process is controlled.

SARCOIDOSIS

Sarcoidosis is a chronic granulomatous process of unknown etiology. This condition often occurs in the third or fourth decades of life and seems to predominate in African Americans. Although it most often affects the lower respiratory tract, it is not unusual to find sarcoidosis occurring in the nose and paranasal sinuses. Other areas often involved include the skin, lymph nodes, salivary glands, lacrimal glands, neurologic structures, heart, and joints. Heerfordt's syndrome consists of parotid gland involvement, uveitis, and facial nerve paralysis.

Diagnostic evaluation should include a chest radiograph, serum calcium level (often elevated), serum angiotensin-converting enzyme (ACE) level, and ultimately a biopsy. Transbronchial biopsy is often necessary to confirm this diagnosis; however, when the sinonasal tract is involved, nasal biopsy can often be diagnostic. The classic histopathologic finding is a noncaseating granuloma with no evidence of acid-fast organisms on either staining or culture.

Treatment is usually dictated by the extent and severity of the pulmonary involvement.

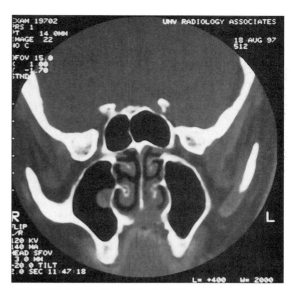

FIGURE 12–3 Sarcoidosis of the nose can present as an aggressive invasive process as shown on CT, often imitating an invasive tumor. This patient had an ulcerating lesion extending through the floor of the nose into the oral cavity.

High-dose steroids are often needed to stem the inflammatory process. Recent therapy has also included methotrexate, which seems to decrease steroid requirements. Sinonasal disease can present as an extremely aggressive and erosive condition, occasionally mimicking neoplasia (Fig. 12–3).

UNUSUAL CAUSES OF RHINOSINUSITIS

RHINOSCLEROMA

This fairly unusual condition is rarely seen in the United States, but is much more common in Central America and Eastern Europe. This disease is caused by the gram-negative bacteria *Klebsiella rhinoscleromatis.* There are three classic stages described: catarrhal (prolonged chronic rhinorrhea); granulomatous (characterized by granuloma formation); and cicatricial or sclerotic (dense fibrous scarring within the involved anatomic region). Although the nose is considered the classic area of involvement, other regions where scleroma can present include the nasopharynx, oropharynx, larynx, and subglottic region. Histopathologically, the classic finding in this disease is the vacuolated or "foamy histiocytes" (Mikulicz cells), often with intracytoplasmic gram-negative organisms. Treatment consists of streptomycin or tetracycline. Medical management is best if the diagnosis can be made prior to the cicatricial stage.

MYCOBACTERIAL INFECTIONS

These infections of the nose are fairly uncommon. *Mycobacterium tuberculosis, M. avium-intracellulare,* and *M. leprae* (leprosy) have all been described in the nasal cavity and paranasal sinuses. Treatment is primarily medical and is dictated by the sensitivity patterns of the particular organisms.

RHINOSPORIDIOSIS

This nasal infectious condition is endemic in India and Sri Lanka. It is caused by *Rhinosporidium seeberi,* which inoculates the nasal epithelium through public bathing in contaminated waters. The presentation consists of tumor-like lesions within the nose and nasopharynx producing epistaxis and nasal obstruction. Treatment consists of surgical debridement and occasional steroid injections for recurrences.

ATROPHIC RHINITIS

Primary atrophic rhinitis usually occurs in elderly patients. They often report nasal congestion and a foul smell (ozena) in the nose. This is accompanied by progressive atrophy of the nasal mucosa and underlying turbinates. Thick crusts form on the septum, floor of the nose, and turbinates. The nasal cavities become cavernous, and squamous metaplasia occurs on the surface epithelium. This syndrome can also be a secondary condition usually in response to radical nasal surgery or irradiation. Although the incidence of primary atrophic rhinitis has declined, it is still prevalent in Eastern Europe, Greece, Egypt, India, and China. The etiology of primary atrophic rhinitis is thought to be an infection with *Klebsiella ozaenae* or some other bacteria. Treatment consists of nasal irrigation, debridement, humidification, antibiotic therapy, and occasionally surgery. Nasal vault closure (Young's procedure) has been advocated for this condition and is purported to reverse the process.

SUGGESTED READINGS

Donald P, Gluckman J, Rice D. *The Sinuses.* New York: Raven Press; 1995.

Druce HM, ed. *Sinuisitis: Pathophysiology and Treatment.* New York: Marcel Dekker; 1994.

Report of the Rhinosinusitis Task Force Committee Meeting. *Otolaryngol Head Neck Surg* 1997;117(2, suppl):S1–S68.

Settipane G, ed. *Rhinitis.* Providence, RI: Oceanside; 1991.

Chapter 13

NEOPLASMS AND CYSTS

Thomas A. Tami

Although fairly unusual, tumors of the nose and paranasal sinuses can produce devastating outcomes if unrecognized and untreated. These tumors, both benign and malignant, often remain undetected for prolonged time periods due to their location, only to be recognized when adjacent structures are affected. Common presenting symptoms include the following:

▼ Nasal symptoms: epistaxis, nasal discharge, nasal obstruction, recurrent sinusitis, external nasal deformity
▼ Orbital symptoms: epiphora, diplopia, visual loss, proptosis, telecanthus
▼ Oral symptoms: velopharyngeal insufficiency, palatal hypesthesia, palatal ulceration, oronasal fistula, dental pain, or infection
▼ Central nervous system symptoms: meningitis, stroke, seizures, hydrocephalus, mental status changes
▼ Skull base symptoms: cranial nerve deficits
▼ Facial symptoms: facial cellulitis, facial swelling, pain, anesthesia

BENIGN NASAL AND PARANASAL SINUS TUMORS

EPITHELIAL TUMORS

Papilloma of the nasal cavity is fairly common. Fungiform papillomas generally occur on the anterior nasal septum and are easily managed with simple excision. They have no predisposition to malignant transformation and rarely recur if totally excised.

Inverting papillomas are potentially more important than the fungiform variety. These tend to arise from the lateral nasal wall, often in the region of the middle turbinate. Although the etiology of these tumors is unknown, some evidence suggests an association with human papilloma virus. Inverting papillomas usually present as unilateral nasal masses and are often mistaken for unilateral nasal polyps. As they increase in size they can expand, cause bone erosion, and often extend into the paranasal sinuses causing obstruction, infection, and occasionally mucocele formation. Malignant transformation into squamous cell carcinoma has been reported in approximately 15% of cases.

CONTROVERSY

Controversy exists as to whether squamos cell carcinoma arises synchronously or due to malignant degeneration.

Complete excision and submission for serial histopathologic evaluation is important to identify carcinomatous changes within the tumor.

The traditional surgical approach to inverting papillomas has been the lateral rhinotomy and medial maxillectomy. Since the introduction of this approach, the previously reported high rate of local recurrence has been reduced to less than 5%. This approach has now become the standard against which other surgical approaches are measured. Recent experience with endoscopic endonasal surgery has created enthusiasm for using this approach to manage these tumors. Postoperative endoscopic evaluation for possible tumor recurrence lends itself ideally to long-term monitoring and surveillance of these patients.

CONTROVERSY

Although initially controversial, endoscopic removal is becoming much more common and in some arenas is being heralded as the ideal technique for surgical management.

Tumors of the minor salivary glands can also present in the nose or paranasal sinuses. Of the nonmalignant varieties, the benign mixed tumor (pleomorphic adenoma) is by the far the most common. Oncocytomas and basal cell adenomas have also been described in these areas. Although often becoming quite large prior to detection, these tumors can usually be removed safely and effectively via wide local excision.

ANGIOMATOUS TUMORS

As in other anatomic locations, tumors of angiogenic origin occasionally occur in the nasal and paranasal sinus regions. The most common of these is the *juvenile nasopharyngeal angiofibroma (JNA)*. This tumor usually arises at the juncture of the posterior nasal cavity and nasopharynx, in the region of the sphenopalatine foramen. JNA occurs almost exclusively in teenage boys. This very vascular tumor usually presents clinically as recurrent epistaxis following relatively minimal head trauma. As the tumor enlarges, nasal obstruction often becomes a more prominent symptom. Although this is considered a benign process, local expansion can occasionally produce symptoms of proptosis, facial swelling, cra-

nial nerve palsies, or central nervous system findings secondary to intracranial extension.

The diagnosis of JNA can be confirmed using computed tomography (CT) or magnetic resonance imaging (MRI) scanning.

PEARL••• Due to its location, a typical finding is anterior bowing of the posterior wall of the maxillary sinus.

MR angiography can also be helpful in determining the vascularity of these tumors.

PITFALL••• Although it is often tempting to obtain a transnasal biopsy of these lesions, this procedure can be accompanied by tremendous blood loss. If this diagnosis is entertained, even remotely, then imaging should be used as the diagnostic procedure of choice.

Surgery remains the mainstay of treatment. Preoperative embolization is usually recommended to reduce the bleeding, which is otherwise attendant to the procedure. Recently, the endoscopic approach has been advocated by some to surgically approach these masses.

CONTROVERSY

The role of radiotherapy for JNA is somewhat controversial. While in some centers, particularly the group at Princess Margaret Hospital in Toronto, excellent results have been reported, most centers tend to avoid radiation. The primary objection raised to this treatment mode revolves around potential long-term effects of high-dose radiation therapy in this young population group.

Other angiogenic tumors occasionally encountered in this anatomic locale include the hemangiopericytoma, hemangioma, and lymphangioma.

MESENCHYMAL TUMORS

Fibrous dysplasia is a fibro-osseous disorder of the facial skeleton. There are two forms of this disorder: the monostotic form (accounting for up to 80% of cases) represented by a solitary lesion, and the polyostotic form, in which multiple sites of involvement are identified. Albright's syndrome consists of the triad of polyostotic fibrous dysplasia, cutaneous pigmentation, and sexual precocity.

Facial lesions of fibrous dysplasia usually appear during the first two decades of life. Although facial deformity is the most common presentation, pain can also be a component. The frontal bone is the most common area of involvement. Radiographic appearance is the classic ground-glass presentation with a thin shell of cortical bone. The ground-glass appearance is due to a mixture of fibrous and osseous histopathologic changes.

Treatment is indicated in cases of sinus dysfunction, gross facial deformity, cranial foramina narrowing (such as the optic foramen), or severe pain. Treatment is aimed primarily at symptomatic improvement because this process is basically benign and usually stops progressing by early adulthood. Surgical resection is the treatment of choice. However, in cases of extensive disease, complete resection without significant skeletal deformity is often impossible. Conservative surgical management in these cases is advised.

Osteomas are very common benign tumors of the sinuses. Although the etiology of these tumors is unknown, they occur most commonly in the frontoethmoid region. They tend to grow very slowly and rarely cause symptoms. Occasionally the tumors can enlarge and cause pain or produce obstruction to sinus outflow. In these cases, surgical removal is curative.

Other less common mesenchymal tumors include the giant cell tumor, fibroma, and fibromyxoma.

> **PITFALL...** Most osteomas are asymptomatic. The presence of an osteoma alone should not be used as an indication for surgery, because more often than not it is an incidental finding.

ODONTOGENIC TUMORS

Odontogenic tumors are occasionally encountered in the maxillary sinuses and nasal cavity due to the close proximity of the maxillary dentition. The most aggressive of these benign tumors is the *ameloblastoma,* which tends to be more of a problem when occurring in the maxilla than when occurring in the mandible, and usually requires aggressive surgical management.

Other even more uncommon tumors of odontogenic origin include the cementifying fibroma, adenoblastoma, Pinborg tumor, and odontogenic fibroma.

NEUROGENIC TUMORS

Benign neurogenic tumors, which can occur in this region, include the *schwannoma* and the *neurofibroma*. Both can be found throughout the sinonasal tract, but are fairly unusual. Neurofibromas can occasionally be associated with von Recklinghausen's disease and may be multiple. These are also occasionally associated with malignant degeneration into neurofibrosarcoma.

MALIGNANT NASAL AND PARANASAL SINUS TUMORS

EPITHELIAL TUMORS

Squamous cell carcinoma is by far the most common malignant tumor encountered in the nose and paranasal sinuses. When occurring in the nasal cavity, it usually arises from the turbinates or the nasal septum. These tumors are often detected at an early stage because they tend to produce symptoms of nasal obstruction or epistaxis, which brings this problem to the early attention of the patient and physician. On the other hand, when occurring in the paranasal sinuses, they usually become quite large before symptoms are appreciated.

The staging system for maxillary sinus tumors is shown in Table 13–1. Staging for tumors of the nasal cavity or of the other paranasal sinuses is not currently available through the American Joint Committee on Cancer. Maxillary sinus staging is based on Ohngren's line dividing the maxillary sinus; it is drawn from the

TABLE 13–1 MAXILLARY SINUS TUMOR STAGING

TX	Primary tumor cannot be assessed
T0	No evidence of primary tumor
Tis	Carcinoma in situ
T1	Tumor limited to the antral mucosa with no erosion or destruction of bone
T2	Tumor with erosion or destruction of the infrastructure, including the hard palate and/or the middle nasal meatus
T3	Tumor invades any of the following: skin of cheek, posterior wall of maxillary sinus, floor or medial wall of orbit, anterior ethmoid sinus
T4	Tumor invades orbital contents and/or any of the following: cribriform plate, posterior ethmoid or sphenoid sinuses, nasopharynx, soft palate, pterygomaxillary or temporal fossae, or base of skull

medial canthus of the eye to the angle of the mandible. Tumors situated posterior/superior tend to have a poorer prognosis because they invade the orbit and pterygopalatine fossae at a much earlier stage in their growth.

Some data suggest that squamous cell cancers of the sinonasal tract may be associated with specific industrial exposures. Workers in the boot and shoe industry, nickel workers, chromate workers, isopropyl alcohol workers, workers exposed to flour dust, and textile workers have all been suggested as having increased risks of sinonasal carcinoma. Interestingly, little data supports any connection between tobacco use and sinonasal carcinoma.

Sinonasal undifferentiated carcinoma (SNUC) is a fairly uncommon malignancy, which has only recently been recognized as a distinct clinical entity. It is a highly aggressive tumor that often must be differentiated from other poorly differentiated tumors. This can usually be accomplished using both histopathologic criteria as well as by applying various tumor specific stains. Although the clinical outcomes are often quite poor following treatment, aggressive management, often utilizing surgery, radiation therapy, and adjuvant chemotherapy, is usually recommended.

Adenoid cystic carcinoma of the sinonasal tract arises from the glandular elements within the mucosa. Although these tumors can occur throughout the sinonasal tract, they are most

common in the lower nasal regions and the paranasal sinuses. As with adenoid cystic carcinomas elsewhere, there is a tendency to progress slowly and relentlessly with perineural spread. Hematogenous spread is also common, with distant metastatic rates of up to 40%, often occurring 10 to 15 years after initial diagnosis. Combined therapy using surgery and radiation is usually recommended for these patients.

SPECIAL CONSIDERATION

Even when these tumors seem to be small and unimportant, the perineural spread can be considerable. The histopathologist should give special attention to this aspect of the pathologic evaluation.

Esthesioneuroblastoma, or olfactory neuroblastoma, is a fairly uncommon tumor that arises in the olfactory epithelium. This tumor is generally thought to be a neoplasm of bipolar olfactory neurons. Histologically, this tumor is classified into grades I through IV (Table 13–2). Staging follows the Kadish staging system (Table 13–3). These tumors are locally aggressive and often invade structures such as orbit and cranium. Metastatic spread occurs most frequently to lymphatics, bone, and lungs, and occurs in up to 40% of cases.

Malignant melanoma of the sinonasal tract composes 1 to 2% of all melanomas. Most occur

TABLE 13–2 ESTHESIONEUROBLASTOMA HISTOLOGIC CLASSIFICATION

Grade I	Lobular architecture, uniform round neuroblasts, well-defined neurofibrillary component, frequent pseudorosettes (Homer-Wright rosettes), variable calcification
Grade II	Less defined neurofibrillary component, scattered mitoses
Grade III	Increased cellularity, individual cell pleomorphism, increased mitoses, necrosis
Grade IV	Necrosis is common, nuclei are hyperchromatic and anaplastic, cytoplasm indistinct, calcification uncommon

TABLE 13–3 ESTHESIONEUROBLASTOMA STAGING (KADISH) SYSTEM

Stage A	Tumor confined to nasal cavity
Stage B	Tumor involves nasal cavity and one or more paranasal sinuses
Stage C	Tumor extends beyond sinonasal tract

in the nasal cavity (usually on the turbinates and septum). Up to 30% of these melanomas can be amelanotic, requiring immunohistochemical staining to confirm the diagnosis. Nasal melanoma has a worse prognosis than cutaneous melanomas. Five-year survival ranges from 10 to 30%. Treatment usually consists of combined surgery and radiation.

LYMPHORETICULAR TUMORS

Lymphoma of the nose and paranasal sinuses is usually of the non-Hodgkin's variety. Although these occur most often in the maxillary sinus, they can occur anywhere in the sinonasal region. Non-Hodgkin's lymphomas, in particular the B-cell variety, are much more common in patients infected with the human immunodeficiency virus (HIV). Following the appropriate staging workup, treatment is usually instituted using chemotherapy and/or radiation therapy.

Polymorphic reticulosis (lethal midline granuloma) is a rare progressively destructive lesion that usually originates in the nasal septum or palate. Although the etiology of this condition was once in question, it is now generally accepted that it represents poorly differentiated T-cell lymphomas. Radiotherapy is usually recommended for treatment.

> **PEARL...** The differential diagnosis must include a search for nasal granulomatous processes such as Wegener's granulomatosis, mycobacterial disease, and sarcoidosis.

The sinonasal tract is the most common site in the upper respiratory system for *extramedullary plasmacytoma,* which must be differentiated from multiple myeloma; some cases have been associated with a delayed onset of multiple myeloma. Treatment can often be accomplished using radiation therapy alone, although surgery can occasionally be useful.

MESENCHYMAL TUMORS

Osteogenic sarcoma occurs much more commonly in the maxilla than in the mandible. A previous history of Paget's disease or prior local radiotherapy seems to predispose to this tumor. The 5-year survival for maxillary osteosarcoma is only 25%. Failures are characterized by both distant as well as local recurrence.

Rhabdomyosarcoma is a highly malignant tumor, which often presents in the sino-orbital region. Usually occurring before the age of 15, this is the most common sarcoma of the head and neck. Histologically, it can be separated into embryonal, alveolar, and pleomorphic types. Combination therapy using surgery, radiation, and chemotherapy has dramatically improved the survival of this malignancy.

Other fairly unusual mesenchymal tumors also encountered include fibrosarcoma and chondrosarcoma. Both of these are exceedingly rare in the nose and paranasal sinuses, and are usually managed using combination surgery and radiation therapy.

SUGGESTED READINGS

Batsaakis J. *Tumors of the Head and Neck.* 2nd ed. Baltimore: Williams & Wilkins; 1982.

Donald P, Gluckman J, Rice D. *The Sinuses.* New York: Raven Press; 1995.

Hyams V, Batsakis J, Michaels L. *Tumors of the Upper Respiratory Tract and Ear.* Washington, DC: Armed Forces Institute of Pathology; 1988.

Chapter 14 ———————————————

SPECIAL CONSIDERATIONS

EPISTAXIS

Approximately 10% of the American population has had at least one episode of epistaxis. Most never come to medical attention, and fewer than 10% require the attention of an otolaryngologist. Although most episodes of epistaxis are minor, potentially serious consequences can result, including aspiration hypotension, or hypoxia with resultant myocardial infarction.

VASCULAR ANATOMY

The nasal mucosa has a rich blood supply derived from both the internal and external carotid systems, with extensive anastomoses. The external carotid is the main contributor to this blood supply. Of its branches, the facial and internal maxillary arteries are the primary sources of blood to the nose. The facial artery gives rise to the superior labial artery, which enters the nose just lateral to the nasal spine. The third part of the internal maxillary artery enters the pterygopalatine fossa, giving off the sphenopalatine and greater palatine arteries. The sphenopalatine artery enters the nasal cavity through the sphenopalatine foramen at the posterior attachment of the middle turbinate. It gives off the posterior septal branch, which courses over the face of the sphenoid to supply the septum pos-

teriorly. The posterior lateral nasal branch supplies the turbinates and middle meatus region as well as the ethmoid and maxillary sinuses. The greater palatine artery originates from the internal maxillary and descends through the pterygopalatine canal, to emerge from the greater palatine foramen as the greater palatine artery. It then courses anteriorly and passes through the incisive foramen to supply the anterior nasal septum.

The internal carotid supplies the nasal cavity via its first intracranial branch, the ophthalmic artery, which enters the superior orbital fissure and gives rise to the posterior and anterior ethmoid arteries. The posterior ethmoid artery branches from the ophthalmic artery shortly after it enters the orbit. The posterior ethmoid is located 3 to 7 mm anterior to the optic nerve. It travels through the posterior ethmoid air cells, enters the anterior and cranial fossa, and penetrates the cribriform plate to reach the nose. The anterior ethmoid artery branches from the opthalmic artery anteriorly and exits the orbit through the anterior ethmoid foramen usually about 10 mm anterior to the posterior ethmoid foramen. It travels through the anterior ethmoid air cells, enters the anterior cranial fossa, and enters the nose to supply the anterior third of the lateral and medial nasal walls.

Kiesselbach's plexus (Little's area) is located along the caudal nasal septum where the sphenopalatine, greater palatine, anterior ethmoid, and superior labial arteries anastomose. Most episodes of epistaxis occur in this area, especially in children and young adults. Woodruff's plexus is an area on the lateral nasal wall, below the inferior turbinate where the sphenopalatine artery enters the nasal cavity. Although most episodes of posterior epistaxis have been traditionally described as occurring in this region, some recent evidence suggests that posterior epistaxis may also be a primarily septal phenomenon. Posterior epistaxis occurs primarily in older adults.

Anterior epistaxis is more likely in children and young adults, whereas posterior epistaxis is more common in older adults, especially men with hypertension and arteriosclerosis. Epistaxis is more common during the winter months due to increased upper respiratory infections and dryer air. Nosebleeds are very unusual in infants. The causes of epistaxis can be attributed to either local or systemic problems. Probably the most common cause of epistaxis is direct trauma to the nose, with or without fracture. Habitual nose picking, especially in children, is an extremely common reason for anterior septal nosebleeds. Chronic irritation produces crusting and granulation tissue that bleeds easily on further nose picking. Other less common reasons for the anterior epistasis include surgical procedures of the nose and sinuses; barotrauma from flying or diving; nasal septal deviations interrupting the normal airflow pattern and producing turbulent flow inside the nasal cavity; septal perforations; foreign bodies; and tumors, both benign and malignant.

SPECIAL CONSIDERATION

Juvenile nasopharyngeal angiofibroma should be considered when a male adolescent presents with nasal obstruction, epistaxis, and a nasal or nasopharyngeal mass.

Aneurysms of the extradural or cavernous sinus portion of the internal carotid artery can cause life-threatening epistaxis. Systemic conditions that can predispose to epistaxis include hypertension/arteriosclerosis and blood dyscrasias or any condition that impairs or decreases clotting factors and/or platelet function.

MANAGEMENT

Initial rapid evaluation and stabilization of the patient is mandatory. Patients with significant acute blood loss can present with acute hypovolemia, which must be recognized and managed. Once stabilized, a good history and physical examination should be undertaken. Specific areas of importance include a history of hypertension, diabetes mellitus, liver disease, cardiopulmonary disease, or alcoholism; a personal or family history of prolonged bleeding or easy bruisability; and a medication history, with special attention to aspirin-containing compounds, coumadin, and nonsteroidal antiinflammatory agents. A thorough exam of the nasal cavity should then be undertaken to identify the bleeding site if possible, as well as to assess any other structural abnormalities. Adequate vasoconstriction and topical anesthesia are necessary for a good evaluation. Nasal telescopes can also be extremely helpful. Laboratory studies, including a complete blood count, clotting profile, and liver function tests, should be considered.

Most nosebleeds will either stop spontaneously or can be easily controlled with simple measures including having the patient sit quietly, applying direct squeeze pressure over the anterior nose, or applying topical decongestants such as oxymetazoline. The subsequent use of humidification and saline nasal sprays can provide further relief and prevent recurrent bleeding.

If an active bleeding site can be identified, chemical or electrical cautery can be used to stop the bleeding. A petroleum-based antibiotic ointment should be used on the cauterized area for 7 to 10 days to promote healing of the site. Even posterior bleeding sites can occasionally be treated with chemical or electrical cautery after visualization with rigid nasal endoscope.

If these measures fail, anterior nasal packing can be considered. The nose should be adequately anesthetized prior to packing, especially

PITFALL... Beware of performing overly aggressive cautery on both sides of the septum as cartilage exposure or septal perforation can occur.

if the classical ½-inch petrolatum gauze is used. Merocel nasal tampons provide a more recent alternative, and often require little topical anesthesia. Anterior packs are usually left in place for 2 to 5 days. Prophylactic antibiotics should be considered to manage sinusitis from blockage of the sinus ostia as well as to potentially prevent toxic shock syndrome secondary to toxin producing *Staphylococcus aureus.* Porcine adipose strips (salt-pork) also appear to be useful in patients with profound thrombocytopenia or in pediatric populations with blood dyscrasias.

Posterior packs are usually considered when nosebleeds are refractory to conservative measures or when they continue despite anterior packing. A standard posterior pack made of rolled gauze tied to umbilical tape or 0-silk ties or an inflatable balloon pack such as a Foley catheter or commercially available balloon tampons can be used.

SPECIAL CONSIDERATION

All patients with posterior packs should be admitted for close observation. Potentially serious hypoventilation, hypoxemia, and cardiac arryhthmias may occur and are occasionally attended by cardiac arrest.

PEARL... Nasal hemorrhage involving the distribution of the sphenopalatine artery can be controlled by injecting Xylocaine with epinephrine into the pterygopalatine fossa through the greater palatine foramen. This technique provides good nasal anesthesia and temporary control of epistaxis (about 3 hours).

Surgery is usually employed for epistaxis refractory to packing, but some advocate surgery for immediate control of severe epistaxis to avoid the morbidity of packing and to shorten hospital stay. In general, ligation as close as possible to the bleeding site is preferable due to failure to control collateral circulation with more proximal ligations. Transantral ligation of the internal maxillary artery (IMA) is usually performed through a Caldwell-Luc approach to gain access to the internal maxillary artery through the posterior wall of the maxillary sinus. Through an operating microscope the distal branches of the IMA are clipped. An intraoral approach to ligation of this artery has also been described. It provides access to the first and second parts of the IMA between the ramus of the mandible and temporalis muscle. The site of ligation is more proximal than with the transantral approach and has a theoretically greater chance of failure due to collateral circulation. Trismus is also a frequent postoperative complaint secondary to trauma to the temporalis muscle. Recently, the transnasal endoscopic approach has gained increasing popularity. The distal branches of the IMA can usually be easily approached at the lateral attachment of the middle turbinate and ligated or bipolar cauterized. The morbidity associated with this approach is minimal. Ligation of ethmoidal arteries can be performed in patients who have superior nasal cavity epistaxis. This procedure is also often performed in conjunction with IMA ligation when the bleeding site is ill-defined.

SPECIAL CONSIDERATION

Care must be taken in this area because the optic nerve is only 5 mm posterior to the posterior ethmoid artery.

Selective angiography and embolization of the IMA can be used as a diagnostic or therapeutic tool to control epistaxis. This procedure is most effective in patients with epistaxis refractory to arterial ligation, with bleeding sites difficult to reach surgically, or in patients who are poor surgical candidates. Recent studies have suggested that embolization may be more cost-effective than surgical ligation. Although the complication rates are similar for these two alternatives, the serious complications that can attend embolization (stroke, carotid injury) are often deterrents to its routine application.

Hereditary hemorrhagic telangiectasia (HHT) or Osler-Weber-Rendu is an autosomal-dominant disorder affecting precapillary arterioles. These patients have multiple mucosal and cutaneous telangiectasias. When located on the anterior nasal mucosa, recurrent brisk epistaxis can result. Approximately 15% of patients with HHT also have arteriovenous malformations of the lungs or central nervous system. As part of their routine workup, imaging of the chest and brain should be performed. Treatment consists of multiple cautery (which is usually unsuccessful), repeated laser treatment of telangiectasia using the neodymium:yttrium-aluminum-garnet (Nd:YAG) or potassium tytanil phosphate (KTP) laser, or septodermoplasty.

IMAGE-GUIDED SINUS SURGERY

Computer image guidance first gained recognition as a valuable surgical adjunct through its introduction into the neurosurgical arena. As its use became more widespread, the anterior skull base and paranasal sinuses became an ideal setting for image-guided surgery (IGS). The initial devices consisted of articulated digitized mechanical arms, which were used to correlate three-dimensional anatomic landmarks with corresponding computed tomography (CT) images. Although these early systems were useful, they depended on the placement of fiducials on the patient's head and required that the head be immobilized throughout the procedure. Currently available systems dispense with the need for both the articulating arm as well as the necessity for head

immobilization. Current technology employs one of two types of sensoring mechanisms: infrared sensors and electromagnetic sensors.

The basic technology for IGS involves several general steps. First, the patient must undergo an axial CT scan. This scan is performed using protocols that will allow the thin-cut images to be uploaded to a computer workstation in the operating room. For the electromagnetic systems, the patient must wear a headset during the scanning, which is subsequently used for intraoperative image calibration. The infrared systems do not require the use of a device during the scan. When the patient is brought into the operating room, the computer images are calibrated with anatomic landmarks on the patient. This might entail the use of surface fiducial markers, surface anatomic points, or, in the case of the electromagnetic system, the fiducial headset. Following calibration of the instrument, the system is verified visually to ensure that known intranasal landmarks correctly correlate with the reconstructed CT image.

SPECIAL CONSIDERATION

Verification sites should give assurance that the anterior/posterior, superior/inferior, and medial/lateral correlations are correct. Favorite sites for verification include the floor of nose, face of sphenoid, nasal septum, and middle turbinate.

Table 14–1 reviews inherent differences between the infrared and electromagnetic IGS systems. Current-generation systems provide

TABLE 14–1 CHARACTERISTICS OF THE ELECTROMAGNETIC AND INFRARED IMAGE-GUIDED SURGERY SYSTEMS

Electromagnetic	Infrared
Radiofrequency transmitter in headset	Optical sensors in three infrared cameras on a movable base
Receiver in handpiece	Light-emitting diodes (LEDs) on instruments
Nonferous instruments	LEDs on headset
Scan with headset on	Scan without headset
Instatrak (VTI)	LandmarX (Xomed)

TABLE 14–2 INDICATIONS FOR THE USE OF IMAGE-GUIDED SURGERY

Revision surgery

Scarring, obscure or absent landmarks

Gross nasal polyposis

Unusual anatomy

Bony dehiscences

the ability to attach numerous operative instrumentations to the localizers, such as suction devices, cutting or biting instruments, probes, seekers, and powered shavers.

PITFALL••• The use of IGS systems must not be a substitute for a thorough understanding of paranasal sinus surgical anatomy. Powered instrumentation in a bloody field attached to an IGS device could be a sure formula for disaster if the surgeon uses the IGS alone to guide the surgical procedure.

Although IGS systems are not needed for routine sinus surgical procedures, they do offer definite advantages during difficult cases, especially for revision sinus surgery. Surgical training can also benefit tremendously by the immediate anatomic feedback offered by these systems. Table 14–2 lists the common indications for the use of IGS in paranasal sinus surgery.

SUGGESTED READINGS

Anon JB, Klimek L, Mosges R, Zinreich SJ. Computer-assisted endoscopic sinus surgery. *Otolaryngol Clin North Am* 1997;30(3):389–401.

Cullen MM, Tami TA. Comparison of internal maxillary artery ligation versus embolization for refractory posterior epistaxis. *Otolaryngol Head Neck Surg* 1998;118(5):636–642.

DeFilipp GJ, Steffey D, Rubinstein M, et al. The role of angiography and embolization in the management of recurrent epistaxis. *Otolaryngol Head Neck Surg* 1988;99(6):597–600.

Josephson GD, Godley FA, Stierna P. Practical management of epistaxis. *Med Clin North Am* 1991;75(6):1311–1320.

McGarry GW. Nasal endoscope in posterior epistaxis: a preliminary evaluation. *J Laryngol Otol* 1991;105(6):428–431.

Padgham N. Epistaxis: anatomical and clinical correlates. *J Laryngol Otol* 1990;104(4):308–311.

SECTION III

ORAL
CAVITY

Chapter 15

ANATOMY AND PHYSIOLOGY

Judith Czaja McCaffrey

EMBRYOLOGY

The primitive digestive tract is primarily composed of endoderm; however, contributions from the embryonic ectodermal layer occur early in aerodigestive tract development. The digestive tract is initially divided into three separate segments including the mouth, the pharynx, and the digestive tube. Caudal to the developing branchial arches, the primitive foregut develops into the oral cavity, the oro- and hypopharynx, as well as the alimentary tract to the level just distal to the proximal duodenum. The stomodeum or primitive oral cavity develops as a depression in the ectodermal foregut. The depression is surrounded superiorly by the projecting forebrain and laterally by the maxillary processes that are developing into the midface. Separating the stomodeum from the foregut, which subsequently develops into the oropharynx, is the buccopharyngeal membrane (Fig. 15–1). The buccopharyngeal membrane is covered by both ectodermal and endodermal layers and is well developed in the 2.5-mm embryo. At approximately 3 to 4 weeks of gestation, the buccopharyngeal membrane should disintegrate and the stomodeum becomes contiguous with the portion of the foregut developing into the oropharynx. The upper and lower lips are formed from the developing mandibular and maxillary processes, respectively. Fusion of the primary and secondary palates also occurs within this time period.

Development of the tongue occurs in two parts (Fig. 15–2). The anterior portion of the tongue develops from the tuberculum impar growing in a cephalad direction from lateral swellings that form symmetrically on either side of the primitive foregut. Medial portions of the first mandibular arch develop simultaneously and merge with the tuberculum impar, thus developing the anterior two-thirds of the tongue. The base of the tongue posterior to the circumvallate papillae develops from the primitive copula and from the second, third, and fourth arch mesoderm. At approximately 12 weeks' gestation, the thyroid gland develops as an endodermal outgrowth at the foramen cecum, which is the point separating the anterior from the posterior portions of the tongue. Normal thyroid development is covered in Chapter 80.

> **PITFALL•••** Although the complicated embryology of the tongue would imply that this is a branchial arch derivative, it is not. Striated lingual muscles are derived from the ventral migration of occipital myotomes and are innervated by the hypoglossal nerve.

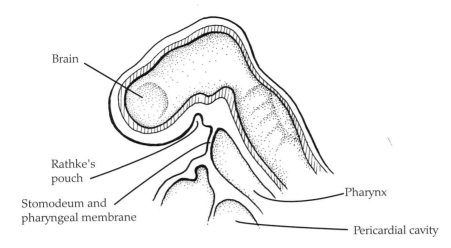

FIGURE 15–1 The brain, pharynx, and pericardial cavity as they appear in a 2.5-mm embryo.

ANATOMY OF THE ORAL CAVITY

The oral cavity is divided into two sections: (1) the vestibule is the space between the mucosa covering the inner surface of the lips and buccal cavities and the lateral aspect of the mandibular and maxillary alveoli, and (2) the oral cavity proper is the space bounded by the medial surfaces of the maxillary and mandibular alveoli.

The main musculature associated with the vestibule includes the orbicularis oris and the buccinator muscles. The orbicularis oris is a muscle of facial expression that is oriented circumorally around the opening of the mouth. The origin and insertion of this muscle is entirely into the skin and mucosa of the lips and surrounding skin of the face. The levator anguli oris, levator labii superioris alaeque nasi, and levator labii superioris muscles also contribute to the musculature of the oral cavity superiorly. The depressor anguli oris, the depressor labii inferioris, and strips of the risorius and platysma muscles contribute to the musculature of the oral cavity inferiorly.

The buccinator muscle arises from the maxilla and mandible medially and the pterygomandibular raphe posteriorly. The muscle inserts into the skin and mucosa of the lips and buccal cavity.

The blood supply to the oral cavity musculature is via the perforating branches of the superior and inferior labial arteries that are terminal branches of the external facial artery. The motor innervation is from the facial nerve, as all of these muscles are muscles of facial expression. General sensation to the buccal mucosa and mucosa covering the inner surface of the lips arises from the maxillary division of the trigeminal nerve.

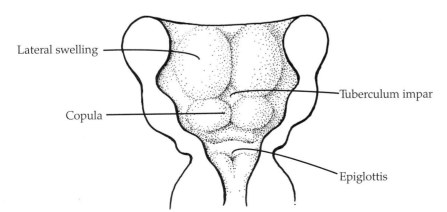

FIGURE 15–2 Development of the tongue (9-mm embryo).

ORAL CAVITY PROPER

The hard palate separates the nasal and oral cavities. Fusion of the symmetric palatine processes of the two developing maxillae occurs in the midline. The incisive fossa is a persistent foramina positioned anteriorly between the primary and secondary hard palates and allows for passage of the nasopalatine artery and nerves. Posteriorly the greater and lesser palatine foramina are present laterally in the hard palate and allow for passage of the greater and lesser palatine arteries and nerves (Fig. 15–3).

FLOOR OF THE MOUTH

The frenulum connects the anterior two-thirds of tongue to the floor of the mouth. The openings of Wharton's ducts are located on either side of the frenulum. These are the openings of the submandibular ducts into the floor of the mouth. Adjacent to the openings of the submandibular ducts are the sublingual glands that give a cobblestoned appearance to the mucosa in the floor of the mouth. Multiple minor sublingual ducts open into the mucosa of the floor of the mouth and, although difficult to visualize, produce large amounts of saliva.

TONGUE

As previously mentioned, the tongue is divided into two portions: (1) the anterior two-thirds or oral tongue, which is the mobile portion; and (2) the posterior one-third or base of tongue, which is nonmobile but contributes signifi-

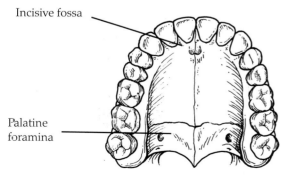

Incisive fossa

Palatine foramina

FIGURE 15–3 The bony palate.

cantly to swallowing. The latter portion of the tongue is present in the oropharynx and therefore will not be covered in detail here. A thick, stratified squamous epithelium covers the entire dorsal oral tongue. The dorsal surface of the oral tongue is covered by multiple fungiform, filiform, and foliate papillae. At the junction of the anterior and posterior portions of the tongue are the circumvallate papillae. These are arranged in a V-shaped row just anterior to the foramen cecum. Taste buds or receptors are present in all but the filiform papillae.

The tongue musculature is divided into both intrinsic and extrinsic muscles. Intrinsic muscles of the tongue are arranged with vertical, transverse, and longitudinal muscle fibers, and it is this arrangement that determines the shape of the tongue.

SPECIAL CONSIDERATION

There is a true septation dividing the intrinsic musculature into a discrete left and right side; however, this septation does not prevent the free spread of hematoma, abscess, or cancer throughout the tongue.

The extrinsic muscles of the tongue include the genioglossus, hyoglossus, and styloglossus muscles. The intrinsic and extrinsic muscles of the tongue are innervated by the hypoglossal nerve. Two major sensory nerves innervate the tongue. These include the lingual nerve and glossopharyngeal nerve. The lingual nerve gives sensation to the anterior two-thirds of the oral tongue and carries with it the chorda tympani nerve that provides the preganglionic parasympathetic fibers to the submandibular ganglion as well as taste reception to the anterior two-thirds of the tongue.

The glossopharyngeal nerve approaches the tongue on the lateral surface of the stylopharyngeus muscle and enters the posterior one-third of the tongue deep to the extrinsic muscles. This nerve supplies both taste and general sensation. Blood supply to the tongue is primarily from the lingual artery that gives off

PEARL... The lingual nerve crosses the submandibular duct twice in the submandibular triangle. Just posterior to the submandibular gland, the nerve runs inferiorly and crosses the lateral surface of the duct. The nerve then loops upward below and rises superiorly on the medial side of the duct to reach the anterior two-thirds of the tongue.

multiple branches including the dorsal lingual, the sublingual, and the deep lingual arteries.

LYMPHATICS

The cheeks, upper lip, and lateral parts of the lower lip drain into submandibular nodes. The central portion of the lower lip drains into submental lymph nodes. Lymphatics from the vestibular mucosa drain into the facial and submandibular nodes. The anterior two-thirds of the tongue drains into the upper deep jugular digastric nodes (Fig. 15–4).

TEETH

In the adult mouth, there are 32 teeth, numbered consecutively beginning in the right upper maxilla with number 1 and ending in the right lower mandible with number 32.

PEARL... All teeth have a single root except the molars. Molars of the maxilla have three roots; mandibular molars have two roots.

The child has 20 deciduous teeth.

The nerve supply to the teeth of the maxilla arises from the maxillary division of the trigeminal nerve. The anterior, middle, and posterior superior alveolar nerves provide sensation to the maxillary teeth. The anterior-superior alveolar nerve arises as a branch of the infraorbital nerve, descending on the anterior wall of the maxillary sinus before exiting the infraorbital foramen, to innervate the canine and incisor teeth. The vascular supply to the maxillary den-

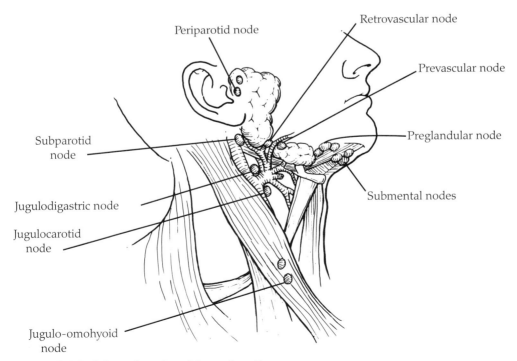

FIGURE 15–4 Lymph nodes of the oral cavity.

tition arises from the internal maxillary artery. The posterior superior alveolar artery provides blood supply to the posterior molars, whereas the infraorbital artery gives rise to the anterior and middle superior alveolar arteries that anastomose anteriorly to provide blood supply to the remaining portion of the upper teeth. The mucosa over the maxillary alveolus shares similar blood and nerve supply. The dentition of the mandible is innervated by the inferior alveolar nerve, a branch of the mandibular division of the trigeminal nerve.

> **PEARL...** The inferior alveolar nerve as well as the artery of the same name enters the mandibular foramen just posterior to the lingula on the internal surface of the mandible. The inferior alveolar nerve and artery are completely encased in bone and travel in the canal, exiting distally at the mental foramen. Intraoral mandibular block with anesthetic can be performed by injecting the nerve as it enters the mandibular foramen. This provides excellent anesthesia for the entire hemimandible and skin over the chin.

The blood supply to the lower teeth and body of the mandible is from the inferior alveolar branch of the internal maxillary artery.

PHYSIOLOGY OF THE ORAL CAVITY

The functions of the oral cavity are (1) swallowing, (2) speech and voice production, (3) taste sensation, and (4) accessory respiratory function.

SWALLOWING

Swallowing is divided into two active and two passive phases of a normal swallowing cycle. The oral preparatory phase or masticator phase begins with salivation at the site and smell of food, continuing when a food bolus is placed into the oral cavity. Salivary flow is critical for effective swallowing function; 1500 cc of saliva are made per day, composed of 99% water and 1% inorganic and organic protein, enzymes,

and salts. The pH of saliva is 6.2 to 7.4. Electrolyte composition includes Na^+, 10 mEq/L; K^+, 26 mEq/L; Cl^-, 10 mEq/L; and $HCO_3^=$, 30 mEq/L.

The second or oral phase of swallowing consists of chewing as well as propulsion of the food bolus posteriorly into the pharynx. Both of these initial phases are active. The third and fourth involuntary phases are pharyngeal and esophageal phases and are portions of a reflex arc that are initiated by appropriate sensory stimuli through cranial nerves IX and X. Involuntary peristalsis then occurs in conjunction with reflex laryngeal protective mechanisms to complete the swallow cycle.

SPEECH AND ARTICULATION

Normal speech and language development require a competent oral cavity without significant congenital anomalies that may prevent the formation of normal speech patterns. Speech occurs when respiration, phonation, and articulation act in concert to produce spoken words for communication. Air expelled from the lungs vibrates the vocal folds to produce sound that resonates in the upper pharynx or nose. Articulation is used to shape the bolus of sound waves into an understandable spoken word. The movement of the mouth, tongue, lips, and teeth shapes the bolus to modify the speech sounds.

TASTE SENSATION

The tongue tastes only salt, sweet, sour, and bitter through the action of taste buds. The flavor of food is a combination of gustatory transduction through the taste buds in combination with olfactory sensation through the nose. There are three cranial nerves (CNs) responsible for the sensation of taste in the oral cavity and oropharynx. The facial nerve (CN VII) carries the special visceral efferents for taste to the anterior two-thirds of the tongue via the chorda tympani nerve. The posterior one-third of the tongue is innervated by taste fibers from the glossopharyngeal nerve (CN IX). In addition, the vagus nerve (CN X) innervates several taste buds around the base of the epiglottis.

SPECIAL CONSIDERATION

The sensation of taste may decrease or be absent in many endocrine as well as metabolic disorders. Patients with hypothyroidism as well as diabetes may have decreased taste sensation. In addition, chronic cigarette smoking decreases taste sensitivity. Elderly patients may also complain that taste sensitivity has diminished over the years. Multiple objective tests for the evaluation of smell and taste are available and can be used to assess taste sensitivity. Patients with complaints regarding taste disturbance should be assessed for olfactory disturbance as well.

ACCESSORY RESPIRATORY FUNCTION

During normal quiet breathing, the nose and its internal resistors provide a comfortable environment for respiration. During times of increased stress, however, or when demands of the cardiovascular system require that the respiratory rate be increased, oral respiration begins. "Mouth breathing" also occurs during times of nasal congestion, as in an upper respiratory tract infection.

SPECIAL CONSIDERATION

Air respired through the mouth is not humidified, filtered, or warmed, as it would be when respiring through the nose, therefore making mouth respiration less satisfying as well as less physiologic.

SUGGESTED READINGS

Crafts RC. *Textbook of Human Anatomy.* 2nd ed. New York: Wiley; 1975.

Gartner LP. Oral anatomy and tissue types. *Semin Dermatol* 1994;13(2):68–73.

Hillel AD, Robinson LR, Waugh P. Laryngeal electromyography for the diagnosis and management of swallowing disorders. *Otolaryngol Head Neck Surg* 1997;116(3):344–348.

Hollinshead WN, Rosse C. *Textbook of Anatomy.* 4th ed. Philadelphia: Harper and Row; 1985.

Koch WM. Swallowing disorders. Diagnosis and therapy. *Med Clin North Am* 1993;77(3):571–582.

Laine FJ, Smoker WR. Oral cavity: anatomy and pathology. *Semin Ultrasound CT MRI* 1995;16(6):527–545.

Lazarus CL, Logemann JA, Pauloski BR, et al. Swallowing disorders in head and neck cancer patients treated with radiotherapy and adjuvant chemotherapy. *Laryngoscope* 1996;106(9 pt 1):1157–1166.

Logemann JA. Rehabilitation of oropharyngeal swallowing disorders. *Acta Otorhinolaryngol Belg* 1994;48(2):207–215.

Logemann JA. Role of the modified barium swallow in management of patients with dysphagia. *Otolaryngol Head Neck Surg* 1997;116(3):335–338.

Whetzel TP, Saunders CJ. Arterial anatomy of the oral cavity: an analysis of vascular territories. *Plast Reconstr Surg* 1997;100(3):582–587.

Chapter 16

CONGENITAL DISORDERS

Judith Czaja McCaffrey

There are multiple congenital disorders of the oral cavity and oropharynx that are not related to cleft pathology. For these conditions to be appropriately treated, adequate assessment of the anomaly must be performed. This should include an extensive history and physical examination as well as a complete family history and appropriate clinical tests. In cases of severe congenital syndromes, multiple anomalies may occur in one patient; therefore, a complete physical examination should be performed. Assistance of a pediatrician as well as a geneticist is often necessary as well. Skull and facial X-rays should be taken, and swallowing function should be assessed with either videofluorography and/or a modified barium swallow. In many cases, full skeletal surveys are needed to explore for bony anomalies. Certain patients who are old enough to undergo examination of speech and articulation should be examined by a speech pathologist. Consideration must be given to upper airway obstruction and its subsequent sequelae in patients with severe noncleft craniofacial anomalies. Tracheotomy or other means to temporarily secure the airway may be

necessary. In addition, nutritional status of the patient must be assessed as augmentation of feedings may be necessary. The temporary placement of a nasogastric tube or a gastrostomy may be required. Assessment of hearing function is critical in patients with craniofacial anomalies. Any portion of the oral cavity may be affected by non-cleft congenital anomalies (Table 16–1).

WHITE SPONGY NEVUS

This nevus is characterized by the formation of white spongy asymptomatic plaques in the oral mucosa. There is no malignant potential to these lesions and treatment is expectant.

FORDYCE SPOTS (FORDYCE GRANULES)

These granules are small, elevated, flat, yellowish-brown spots either occurring singly or in clusters on the mucous membranes in the oral cavity. They are reported to be ectopic sebaceous glands, and they occur in other mucocutaneous sites. No treatment is needed.

TABLE 16-1 OTHER CONGENITAL SYNDROMES AFFECTING THE ORAL CAVITY

Syndrome	Systemic Findings	Oral Signs/Symptoms
Achondroplasia	Dwarfism	Malocclusion, overbite
Ascher's syndrome	Nontoxic thyromegaly	Duplication of the upper lip
Ataxia-telangiectasia	Ataxia	Mucosal telangiectasias
Beckwith-Wiedemann syndrome	Omphalocele	Macroglossia, malocclusion, airway obstruction
Cleidocranial dysostosis	Large cranium, clavicular aplasia	High arched or cleft palate, mandibular nonunion, maxillary hypoplasia
deLange syndrome	Genitourinary, musculoskeletal anomalies	Migrognathia, cleft palate, oral self-mutilation
Marfan's syndrome	Tall stature, aortic aneurysm	High arched or cleft palate, prognathic mandible
McCune-Albright syndrome	Endocrine and bone anomalies	Large distorted mandible and maxilla, maxillary mass obstructing oral cavity
Peutz-Jeghers syndrome	Gastrointestinal polyposis	Brown maculae on lips and buccal mucosa

CONGENITAL EPULIS

This nontender mass typically forms on the free edge of the gingiva covering the maxillary or mandibular alveolus. On histopathologic examination, an epulis resembles a granular cell myoblastoma. Treatment is excision.

ANOMALIES OF THE DENTAL ORGAN

These are anomalies of the enamel as well as dentin, with poorly calcified and immature defects of the dental lamina that cause erosion and breakage of the teeth. Caries form readily and assistance of a dentist is required to manage these patients.

ORAL CAVITY COMMISSURE PITS

These depressions form in the commissure of the mouth, measuring approximately 2 to 3 mm deep and wide. They are transmitted as an autosomal-dominant trait and have no clinical significance. They may be associated with cleft lip and cleft palate. The pits that produce saliva or become repeatedly infected may be excised.

TORUS PALATINUS

This bony exostosis forms on the surface of the hard palate. It appears as a well-mucosalized firm bony, occasionally lobulated, mass. Treatment of torus palatinus may be required in cases where the tori are large and make the fitting of an upper denture difficult.

TORUS MANDIBULARIS

This bony exostosis forms on the lingual surface of the mandible either unilaterally or bilaterally. Treatment of torus mandibularis may be required if difficulty with fitting a lower denture is encountered.

HYPOPLASTIC MANDIBLE

This finding typically occurs with first arch syndromes, each of which will be described in brief.

Pierre-Robin Anomaly

This anomaly is a triad of cleft palate, micrognathy, and glossoptosis. This triad typically occurs secondary to an arrest in normal first arch development.

SPECIAL CONSIDERATION

Because of mandibular micrognathy and relative glossoptosis, airway obstruction in neonates and young children with Pierre-Robin syndrome may occur and become life-threatening. In these cases, adequate respiration is secured through tracheotomy.

Mild cases of airway obstruction may be treated expectantly by placing the child in the prone position. Glossepexy has also been used for expectant management of these children. Mandibular growth may reach a normal state by approximately 6 years; however, this is not always the case. Parents should be counseled accordingly. Decannulation of these children should be delayed until adequate support for the tongue is present.

Treacher-Collins Syndrome

This mandibulofacial dysostosis is manifested as abnormal fusion of the zygomatic arches and malar complex, abnormal orbital bony rims and low set ears with congenital aural atresia, hypoplastic mandible, and cleft palate.

Crouzon Syndrome

This craniofacial dysostosis occurs secondary to premature synostosis of multiple skull suture lines. Maxillary hypoplasia occurs commonly in this syndrome, resulting in an abnormal dental arch. Other common findings include mild mental retardation, congenital aural atresia, hypertelorism, and a prognathic mandible.

Apert's Syndrome

This syndrome, also known as acrocephalosyndactyly, often occurs in an autosomal-dominant pattern; however, it can occur sporadically as well. This syndrome is associated with occasional mental retardation and a cleft palate. Early fusion of cranial suture lines causes a brachycephalic appearance to the head. Syndactyly of the hands and feet occurs with fusion of the digits. Dental eruption may be delayed.

Goldenhar Syndrome

This oculoauriculovertebral dysplasia results in multiple vertebral anomalies as well as abnormalities of the first and second branchial arches.

ANKYLOGLOSSIA

Ankyloglossia, commonly known as tongue-tie, occurs in a small percentage of patients; however it can result in significant symptoms if left untreated. The presence of an elongated lingual frenulum tethering the entire oral tongue to the floor of mouth alters the mobility of the tongue (Fig. 16–1). In symptomatic cases, patients may have difficulty with eating as well as difficulty with linguodental speech. On physical examination, there is often a forked tongue, secondary to the tongue tethering.

> **PEARL...** Early surgical intervention is best and can be done at a young age, allowing for adequate growth and development without delays in speech and trouble with eating.

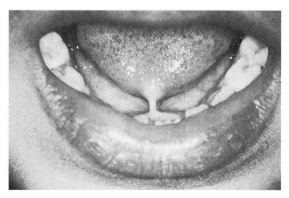

FIGURE 16–1 Tongue-tie.

Simple division of the frenulum may be all that is needed in the presence of a thin frenulum. In cases with a thick frenulum, a formal Z-plasty may need to be performed. A V-Y plasty is also effective.

MEDIAN RHOMBOID GLOSSITIS

When the lateral halves of the tongue fail to fuse prior to interposition of the tuberculum impar during embryonic development of the tongue, median rhomboid glossitis occurs. Another speculated etiology for this condition is chronic candidal infection. Many studies have reported that cultures of these areas on the tongue have grown *Candida albicans.* Patients with positive cultures should be treated with topical antifungal therapy. Patients with recurrent lesions may be suspected of having immunodeficiency, most commonly HIV infection. The area of median rhomboid glossitis is a histologically benign portion of mucosa, devoid of papillae. The lesion typically appears anterior to the circumvallate papillae.

FISSURED TONGUE

The presence of a fissured tongue is of no clinical significance except when occurring in a patient with recurrent episodes of facial nerve paralysis and facial edema.

PEARL••• When the latter triad is described, Melkersson-Rosenthal syndrome should be suspected.

LINGUAL THYROID

Normal thyroid development occurs between the 7th and 12th weeks of embryogenesis. Thyroid tissue is derived from the base of the foramen cecum in the tongue base and descends to its normal anatomic position anterior to the second and third tracheal rings by 12 weeks. The normal pathway of thyroid descent is typically obliterated; however, it may persist in the neck as a thyroglossal duct cyst. In cases when there is failure of thyroid descent, a lingual thyroid may persist. Patients typically present with complaints of dysphagia, dyspnea, and changes in voice. Patients may also be hypothyroid. Physical examination of the oral cavity demonstrates the presence of a well-mucosalized red mass in the posterior aspect of the tongue.

PEARL••• When lingual thyroid is suspected, a search for normal functioning thyroid tissue should be undertaken. Workup includes thyroid function tests as well as cervical ultrasound to determine the presence of any thyroid tissue in the normal anatomic position. Thyroid scanning should be done to assess the function of the lingual mass as well as any cervical thyroid tissue.

Management of symptomatic patients with lingual thyroid may include suppression with thyroid hormone. This decreases the size of the lingual thyroid and improves the patient's symptoms. Radioactive iodine ablation may also be used; however, lifetime thyroid hormone replacement is necessary. Surgical excision may be performed either transorally or through a midline glossotomy. Thyroid hormone replacement is needed with the latter form of treatment.

SUGGESTED READINGS

Baughman RA. Lingual thyroid and lingual thyroglossal tract remnants: a clinical and histopathologic study with review of the literature. *Oral Surg Med Pathol* 1972;34:781.

Catlin FI, DeHaas V. Tongue-tie. *Arch Otolaryngol* 1971;94:548.

Cohen MM Jr, Kreiborg S. A clinical study of the craniofacial features in Apert syndrome. *Int J Oral Maxillofac Surg* 1996;25(1):45–53.

Fuhr AH, Krogh PH. Congenital epulis of the newborn: centennial review of the literature and a report of cases. *J Oral Surg* 1972;30:30.

Gorlin RJ, Pindborg JJ, Cohen MM Jr. *Syndromes of the Head and Neck.* 2nd ed. New York: McGraw-Hill; 1976.

Moore MH. Upper airway obstruction in the syndromal craniosynostoses. *Br J Plast Surg* 1993;46(5):355–362.

Perkins JA, Sie KC, Milczuk H, Richardson MA. Airway management in children with craniofacial anomalies. *Cleft Palate Craniofac J* 1997; 34(2):135–140.

Peterson SJ, Pruzansky S. Palatal anomalies in the syndromes Apert and Crouzon. *Cleft Palate J* 1974;11:394.

Posnick JC. Treacher Collins syndrome: perspectives in evaluation and treatment. *J Oral Maxillofac Surg* 1997;55(10):1120–1133.

Rogers BO. Treacher-Collins syndrome: a review of 200 cases (mandibulo-facial dysostosis, Franceshetti-Zwahlen-Klein syndromes). *Br J Plast Surg* 1964;17:109.

Routledge RT. The Pierre-Robin syndrome: a surgical emergency in the neonatal period. *Br J Plast Surg* 1960;13:204.

Sirotnak J, Brodsky L, Pizzuto M. Airway obstruction in the Crouzon syndrome: case report and review of the literature. *Int J Pediatr Otorhinolaryngol* 1995;31(2–3):235–246.

Chapter 17

INFECTIOUS AND INFLAMMATORY DISORDERS

Judith Czaja McCaffrey

Oral mucosa provides an effective protective barrier to the spread of infectious and inflammatory diseases of the oral cavity. The protective covering of stratified squamous epithelium composing the oral cavity mucosa provides a physical as well as a biochemical barrier for resistance to diseases. The latter functional barrier is provided by saliva and its components, including salivary immunoglobulins.

In the normal state, oral mucosa is moist, smooth, and pink. There is keratinized masticatory mucosa on the gingiva, hard palate, and periodontium that is firmly adherent to underlying structures. The lining mucosa of the buccal cavities, soft palate, floor of mouth, retromolar trigone, and tongue is nonkeratinized and easily deformed by excessive movement of the oral cavity during speech and mastication.

Inflammatory and infectious diseases originate commonly in the gingiva as well as the surrounding loose mucosa. Multiple etiologies for infection include bacteria, viruses, and fungi as well as chemical irritants, systemic diseases, and neoplasms. Predisposing factors to the development of inflammatory and infectious diseases of the oral cavity include poor dental hygiene, dietary deficiencies, vitamin deficiencies (e.g., vitamin C deficiency leads to scurvy), mineral deficiencies (zinc and iron), radiation therapy, autoimmune diseases, leukemia, pernicious anemia, thalessemia, mononucleosis, polycythemia vera, and diabetes mellitus.

GINGIVITIS

Traumatic, chemical, thermal, and bacterial factors have been implicated in the development of gingivitis. Poor dental hygiene causes an overgrowth of pathogenic bacteria and appears to be essential for the development of gingivitis. There are multiple types of gingivitis, and the diagnosis is made by physical examination.

CHRONIC GINGIVITIS

This is the most common form of gingivitis, occurring in approximately 70% of young adults and up to 90% of patients by middle age. Irritation of the gingiva is caused by bacteria and food particles in the presence of poor dental hygiene. Proliferation of commensal bacteria of the oral cavity within the uncleaned plaque (calculus) present on the tooth enamel causes chronic gingivitis. Therapy requires appropriate dental hygiene and correction of any carious lesions.

CHRONIC DESQUAMATIVE GINGIVITIS

A painless diffuse erythema of the gingiva as well as adjacent oral mucosa occurs and may be severe. This is a rare condition more commonly found in women. Hormonal imbalance has been implicated; however, it has not been proven to be the exact etiology. It is speculated that local irritation with repeated trauma as well as thermal and chemical injury may be the source of the problem. Treatment is avoidance of irritants that aggravate the gingivitis. Systemic oral steroids have been used in severe cases.

ACUTE GINGIVITIS

This is another rare form of gingivitis that is caused by β-hemolytic streptococci. Gingivae are inflamed and erythematous, bleeding easily with trauma. There is no loss of gingival tissue. Treatment is management of the acute bacterial infection with oral antibiotics and oral hygiene.

ACUTE NECROTIZING ULCERATIVE GINGIVITIS (VINCENT'S STOMATITIS, TRENCH MOUTH)

This form of gingivitis occurs as an acute inflammation of the gingival margin. The surface of the gingiva is necrosed and sloughed. A pseudomembrane covering necrotic epithelium occurs on the previously intact gingival margin. Fusiform bacteria are the causative organism. Lesions appear punched-out and crater-like along the entire gingivae and alveolar margin. The condition is painful and there is an associated characteristic fetid halitosis. Gingival bleeding occurs readily. In severe cases, there may be associated lymphadenitis and development of gangrenous stomatitis and toxemia. Treatment of this condition is aggressive dental hygiene directed against the fusiform bacteria.

HYPERTROPHIC GINGIVITIS

In this chronic condition there is an overgrowth of gingiva surrounding the base of the teeth. In extreme cases, gingival hyperplasia may cover the teeth completely. This is seen in patients with chronic systemic conditions including certain vitamin deficiencies and hematopoietic diseases and rarely in pregnancy. Noninflammatory gingival hyperplasia occurs in patients receiving Dilantin therapy for epilepsy. Treatment requires careful dental hygiene and correction or removal of the causative factor.

PERIODONTITIS

Chronic infection in the periodontal membrane leads to a destructive process with secondary ulceration and separation of the surrounding gingiva. Teeth become loose and often painful; periodontal abscesses may develop in the surrounding periodontal membrane. Therapy is directed at appropriate oral hygiene as well as removal of affected teeth in severe cases.

ODONTOGENIC INFECTIONS

Pulp necrosis secondary to dental caries allows for proliferation of bacteria and bacterial invasion through the enamel organ and into the periodontal space. Subsequent necrosis of bone surrounding the tooth root and periodontal membrane then occurs. It is at this point that patients will undergo tooth extraction and drainage of the tooth root abscess, and resolution of the symptoms occurs. If the tooth root abscess goes unchecked, the infection can erode through the surrounding bone and spread freely into the soft tissue fascial compartments of the neck.

Odontogenic infection is more common in mandibular teeth; however it does occur in maxillary teeth as well. The relationship between muscular attachments and landmarks of the mandible allows for direction of spread of odontogenic infection into the deep neck spaces (Fig. 17–1).

Although uncommon, spread to deeper neck spaces does occur, once infection has spread either to the submandibular space or pterygomandibular spaces of the cheek. Some of the more common spaces that can be involved with life-threatening infection include the parapharyngeal space as well as the retropharyngeal space. The prevertebral space may also be significantly involved after retropharyngeal space involvement.

Multiple life-threatening complications may follow deep neck infections. Most disconcerting of these is upper airway obstruction.

When maxillary teeth are affected by odontogenic abscesses, the masseteric space as well as the temporal space can be affected. In addition, the parotid gland can be involved in cases of extensive infection. Cavernous sinus thrombosis has been reported to occur, not only with a maxillary, but also with a mandibular odontogenic infection. This typically occurs by a hematogenous spread rather than a direct route.

When all three of the primary mandibular spaces are involved with the spread of infection (this includes bilateral submandibular spaces and the sublingual space), this is known as Ludwig's angina. Patients typically present with a history of recent dental work and poor oral hygiene. The most common symptoms with which patients present include fever, pain in the floor of mouth, trismus, drooling, and dyspnea. On physical examination, there is brawny edema beneath the chin spreading down onto the skin of the anterior neck. The skin has an erythematous appearance and this cellulitis can descend rapidly onto the chest wall.

The characteristic findings in patients with infections in other deep neck spaces secondary to odontogenic infections are similar to those found in patients with Ludwig's angina. Patients with these infections generally have poor dentition, trismus, pain, fever, dysphagia, and dyspnea. Patients with involvement of deep lateral neck spaces may also have torticollis.

Workup of patients with complications of odontogenic infections includes establishment

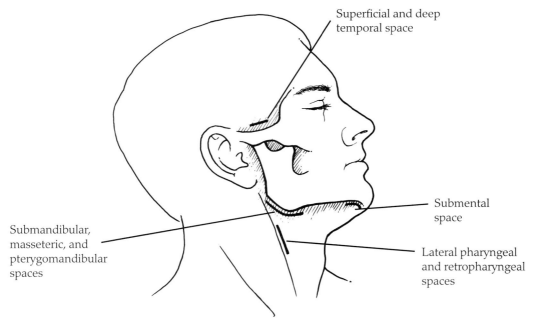

FIGURE 17–1 Deep neck spaces that may be infected by the spread of odontogenic infections. Lines mark approximate sites for incision to drain spaces.

of intravenous lines and resuscitation with fluids. Complete blood count as well as bacterial blood cultures should be obtained. Empiric antibiotic therapy should be started prior to definitive bacterial culture. The initiation of immediate antibiotic therapy may prevent the patient from progressing to a more life-threatening problem. The appropriate diagnosis of deep neck space abscess may be made by computed tomography (CT) scanning of the head and neck with contrast. Often, the CT scan of the head and neck will demonstrate evidence of nonspecific or diffuse cellulitis within the deep neck spaces, without definite abscess formation. In these cases, patients may respond to aggressive management with intravenous antibiotics and appropriate resuscitation. However, in the presence of obvious abscess formation demonstrated on CT scan, surgical intervention is required in order to treat the patient appropriately and eliminate the life-threatening condition. Other absolute indications for surgical exploration include the presence of gas within the soft tissues of the face or neck, indicating the presence of an aggressive anaerobic fasciitis. When choosing the more conservative approach in the management of patients with deep neck cellulitis, the general rule is that patients not responding to maximal intravenous antibiotic therapy and resuscitative measures within 18 to 24 hours should be surgically explored to rule out the presence of an occult abscess.

When the decision has been made to bring the patient with a deep neck space abscess to the operating room, coordination between the otolaryngologist and the anesthesiologist is critical. Life-threatening airway obstruction may occur; therefore, the surgeons must be in communication with the anesthesiologist regarding the plans for securing the airway. Most patients are able to undergo either blind nasotracheal or fiberoptic-guided naso- or orotracheal intubation. An experienced bronchoscopist should be able to secure the airway with fiberoptic guidance. A planned elective tracheostomy may also be performed in patients who have obvious contraindications to a nasal or oral endotracheal tube airway.

Careful planning of incisions is necessary to access all loculations of abscess within these

CONTROVERSY

Some authors believe that a tracheotomy in the face of active deep neck space infection is contraindicated secondary to the possible development of mediastinitis. If this is a major concern, patients may be initially intubated, the abscess drained, and if repeated debridements in the operating room are necessary, a tracheotomy may be performed at a later time, once the abscess cavity shows no progression of infection.

spaces. Typically, horizontal incisions either in the temporal area or below the angle of the mandible will adequately access the temporal, buccal, masseteric, pterygomandibular, submandibular, and sublingual spaces. The submental space is opened through a horizontal incision paralleling the mandible anteriorly over the mylohyoid muscle (Fig. 17–1). Access to the retropharyngeal and parapharyngeal spaces is gained through a curvilinear incision paralleling the relaxed skin tension lines of the neck approximately midway up the sternocleidomastoid muscle. This allows for exposure of the anterior border of the sternocleidomastoid muscle and the carotid sheath. Blunt dissection is then carried superiorly into the parapharyngeal space. This may require division of the stylomandibular ligament and styloid process. Similarly, the retropharyngeal space may be entered by dissecting medial to the carotid sheath and posterior to the laryngopharynx where the abscess cavity is encountered.

Upon opening of the abscess cavity in the neck, aerobic and anaerobic bacterial cultures should be obtained. Culture and sensitivity should be performed on all aspirates and, in questionable cases where tenacious purulent material is not encountered but is replaced by a thin, dishwater brawny edema, the surrounding muscles or fascia may be biopsied for culture. After all loculated areas of the abscess have been opened and drained, copious saline irrigation is used to clean the neck spaces. The wounds are left open. A Penrose drain may be used to provide adequate drainage of the deep neck spaces. The drain is passed into the cavity and brought out onto the patient's skin. Over the course of several postoperative days, the drain is advanced with subsequent collapse of the healing abscess cavities. An alternative treatment option is packing the wound with clean ½- or 1-inch gauze strips changed three to four times daily.

A persistently elevated fever and white blood cell count may indicate the persistence of a loculated abscess cavity. In these cases, a repeat CT scan should be performed with contrast to visualize the area of previous drainage and examine for residual abscess. Cases that show residual abscess or reformation of abscess require further surgical drainage.

> **PEARL...** A parotid abscess is drained through a standard parotidectomy incision. After the skin flap is elevated over the parotid, the fascia is incised in a direction parallel to the branches of the facial nerve. A drain is left in place for several days.

Antibiotic management is dictated based on the most common offending organisms as well as those organisms that are cultured. The most common bacteria are anaerobes, mainly streptococcus and peptostreptococcus as well as bacteroides, fusobacterium, and *Bacteroides melaninogenicus*. Common aerobic bacteria include α- and β-hemolytic streptococcus, gram-negative cocci and bacilli, and gram-positive bacilli. Patients with life-threatening deep neck space infections require parenterally administered antibiotics. The antibiotics that are effective against the anaerobic or mixed odontogenic infection include penicillin and clindamycin.

Mucosal Stomatitis

Herpetic Gingival Stomatitis

This painful erythema of the gingiva and the oral mucosa occurs with a characteristic low-grade fever, malaise, and lymphadenitis. In the anterior portion of the oral cavity, small gray vesicular lesions of herpes appear and rupture within 24 hours.

> **PEARL...** Within the oral cavity, herpetic lesions generally appear only on mucosa that is bound to bone, that is, the alveolus and hard palate.

Small ulcers with an elevated margin subsequently develop. The disease process is self-limited and often does not recur; however, certain patients are predisposed to recurrent infections. Therapy may include antiviral medications to decrease the viral load.

Moniliasis (Mucosal Candidiasis)

Often chronically debilitated patients, as well as those who are immunocompromised (organ transplant recipients, HIV infection, AIDS), and those who have received radiation therapy, may develop candidiasis. In addition, patients admitting to recent antibiotic use may also be predisposed to developing candidal infections of the oral cavity.

On physical examination, lesions are generally red, flat, and irregular. In the pseudomembranous form, there is a painful white plaque with a red halo. The plaque may be wiped or scraped with a tongue blade, revealing friable, freely bleeding mucosa beneath. In the erythematous form the plaques have largely disappeared. Treatment in uncomplicated cases requires topical swish and swallow liquid antifungal medications or troches. In complicated cases, systemic antifungal medications (e.g., amphotericin B) may be necessary.

Herpes Zoster

Dormant varicella zoster virus may be reactivated and affect those areas innervated by the second and third division of the trigeminal nerves. Vesicular lesions similar to chicken pox virus arise in a dermatomal distribution, often found in the buccal cavity, gingival surfaces over the alveolus, palate, and lips. Antiviral medications such as acyclovir can be used to decrease the intensity of the infection.

HERPANGINA (COXSACKIE A VIRUS)

This is a self-limited process in which small, 2- to 3-mm vesicles form on the soft palate and uvula. These are surrounded by a circumferential red halo. The lesions ultimately rupture and heal quickly. Coxsackie A virus may be accompanied by a prodromal systemic illness characterized by malaise, fever, a headache, and emesis. Vesicles occur later.

APHTHOUS STOMATITIS

The etiology of aphthous ulcers is unknown; however, it has been suggested that this is a chronic inflammatory condition with heavy infiltration of lymphocytes in the submucosa of the ulcers. Multiple spherical depressed craters form in the buccal spaces and mobile mucosa of the oral cavity. There is some speculation that these occur more commonly in times of stress; however, the true etiology of this disease process is unknown. A condition known as giant aphthous stomatitis may occur in young adult males. Lesions have been reported to grow up to 10 cm, involving the entire oral cavity and oropharynx. Treatment of this condition is rather difficult and the natural course of the disease is that of unrelenting recrudescences.

BEHÇET'S SYNDROME

This syndrome of aphthous ulcers, genital ulcers, and uveitis occurs most often in men.

VESICULOBULLOUS DISORDERS

These are a group of autoimmune diseases with antibodies targeted against the epithelial basement membrane or suprabasilar layer of the epithelium, leading to bullous desquamation. Several different varieties occur, usually in women of varying ages. Table 17–1 compares the clinical features of the four most common of these diseases.

Immunofluorescence is used for diagnosis after biopsy of a suspicious bullous lesion. Both direct and indirect techniques can be used to detect autoantibodies against the epithelium in bullous conditions.

SYPHILIS

Primary, secondary, and tertiary syphilis may all have manifestations in the oral cavity. In primary syphilis, a solitary painless chancre may occur either on the lips or intraorally. In secondary syphilis, mucous patches ("snail tracks") may occur on the lips and oral mucosa. The secondary manifestations of syphilis are more common than the primary chancre. Because of inflammation accompanying secondary mucous patches, these lesions are often painful. Gumma develops in tertiary syphilis. Gumma are dense infiltrations of inflammatory cells that eventu-

TABLE 17–1 MUCOCUTANEOUS BULLOUS LESIONS

	Erythema Multiforme	Bullous Pemphigoid	Cicatricial Pemphigoid	Pemphigus Vulgaris
Oral manifestations	Vesicles, papules	Rare	Ruptured blisters	Blisters
Skin manifestations	Macules, vesicles	Blisters, scar formation	Rare	Skin blisters
Histology	Subepithelial split	Subepithelial split	Subepithelial split	Supraepithelial split, Tzanck cells
Treatment	Topical or systemic steroids	Self-limited, systemic steroids	Topical steroids	Systemic steroids

ally heal, resulting in scar formation, typically over the gingiva (Table 17–2).

ACTINOMYCOSIS

The commensal bacteria in the oral cavity known as actinomycetes cause actinomycosis.

> **PITFALL•••** Actinomycosis is a bacterial infection, not a fungal infection. Therefore, it is treated with appropriate antibacterial agents rather than antifungals.

Actinomycosis infection typically starts as a painless nodule that slowly grows in the mucosa and submucosal tissues of the oral cavity. Its burrowing and invasive nature causes infected sinus tracts to erupt, either into the oral cavity through the mucosa or, in deeper infections, onto the surface of the skin. Eruption through the skin typically occurs if the parotid or submandibular glands are infected. Chronic draining sinuses persist, and treatment requires appropriate identification of actinomycoses and penicillin therapy.

LICHEN PLANUS

Multiple varieties of lichen planus have been described. The most common form in the oral cavity is the reticular form, located on the buccal mucosa. A lace-like reticular pattern of white lines forms and may be self-limited or require the use of topical steroids to prevent the seque-

TABLE 17–2 ORAL CAVITY MANIFESTATIONS OF SYPHILIS

Stage	Signs
Primary	Painless chancre at inoculation site
Secondary	Papules on oral mucosa, mucous membrane patches of "snail tracks" especially on lips
Tertiary	Hard palate ulceration secondary to granulomatous (gumma) infiltration, gumma on the alveoli

lae of mucosal and submucosal scarring. Erosive lichen planus, another variety of this autoimmune condition, may ulcerate, occurring commonly on the lateral tongue and buccal mucosa. Oral cavity squamous cell carcinoma has been reported to occur in erosive lichen planus.

WEGENER'S GRANULOMATOSIS

This condition is characterized by necrotizing vasculitis of the upper and lower respiratory tracts as well as the renal system. Persistent hyperplastic or ulcerated gingival lesions may occur in the oral cavity. Biopsy is diagnostic, demonstrating necrotizing vasculitis with surrounding palisading histiocytes on histopathologic examination. Antineutrophil cytoplasmic antibody (C-ANCA) titers are often elevated in the acute phase of Wegener's granulomatosis. Therapy includes trimethoprim/sulfamethoxazole in mild cases and cyclophosphamide, methotrexate, and oral corticosteroids in more severe cases.

LYMPHOMATOID GRANULOMATOSIS

Polymorphic reticulosis, lymphomatoid granulomatosis, and lethal midline granuloma are all synonyms for what is now known to be a mucocutaneous T-cell lymphoma. The common finding is ulceration of mucosal surfaces, most commonly the nose and sinuses; however, erosions of the hard palate have been reported. This disease is associated with a high mortality rate, approximately 50 to 70% over a 5-year period. Treatment for localized disease is low-dose radiation therapy. In disseminated disease, the treatment is systemic chemotherapy.

NECROTIZING SIALOMETAPLASIA

This is a lesion characteristically found on the hard palate, typically at the junction between the hard and soft palates. The lesion appears as a painful, necrotic ulcer that has the appearance of carcinoma. On histopathology, there is a characteristic metaplastic change to epithelial cells lining small salivary gland ducts. There is preservation of the lobular architecture of the salivary tissue in necrotizing sialometaplasia, in contrast to squamous cell carcinoma and salivary gland malignancies, which also show mitotic figures and pleomorphism. Treatment is expectant with topical viscous lidocaine. Spontaneous resolution should occur. Biopsy is necessary for appropriate diagnosis.

SJÖGREN'S SYNDROME

Sjögren's syndrome represents a systemic autoimmune disorder that destroys the exocrine glands, most commonly the lacrimal and salivary glands in middle-aged women. Primary Sjögren's disease or the sicca syndrome isolates the symptoms to the eye and oral cavity. Xerophthalmia is demonstrated on ocular examination. Patients often present with an extremely dry mouth with the inability to salivate appropriately to moisten dry food when eating. Speech may also be affected. Secondary Sjögren's syndrome is the sicca syndrome (lacrimal and salivary gland destruction) accompanied by another connective tissue disorder, most commonly rheumatoid arthritis. Patients with Sjögren's syndrome have an increased incidence in the development of lymphoma.

SPECIAL CONSIDERATION

Lymphoma should be suspected in patients with known Sjögren's or other autoimmune diseases who develop the sudden onset of uni- or bilateral painless parotid enlargement.

Severe dental caries can develop in patients with Sjögren's syndrome secondary to poor salivary flow. Careful dental management is essential.

HAIRY LEUKOPLAKIA

This lesion is exclusively found in patients with severe immunocompromised conditions, most commonly HIV infection. A shaggy appearance to the mucosal surface of the tongue is apparent and may vary in color from a white or gray to black. It is present on the lateral surfaces of the tongue and is infrequently found over the dorsal surface. It is speculated that the etiology of this condition is infection of the tongue mucosa with Epstein-Barr virus. This condition, when present in patients with HIV infection, heralds the onset of full-blown acquired immunodeficiency syndrome (AIDS). There is no treatment other than symptomatic care.

SUGGESTED READINGS

Albandar JM, Brown LJ, Genco RJ, Loe H. Clinical classification of periodontitis in adolescents and young adults. *J Periodont* 1997; 68(6):545–555.

Albandar JM, Brown LJ, Loe H. Clinical features of early-onset periodontitis. *J Am Dent Assoc* 1997;128(10):1393–1399.

Bokor M. Immunoglobulin A levels in the saliva in patients with periodontal disease. *Med Pregl* 1997;50(1–2):9–11.

Gidley PW, Ghorayeb BY, Stiernberg CM. Contemporary management of deep neck space infections. *Otolaryngol Head Neck Surg* 1997; 116(1):16–22.

Johnson JT. Abscesses and deep space infections of the head and neck. *Infect Dis Clin North Am* 1992;6(3):705–717.

McDonald TJ, DeRemee RA. Head and neck involvement in Wegener's granulomatosis (WG). *Adv Exp Med Biol* 1993;336:309–313.

Nisengard RJ, Neiders M. Desquamative lesions of the gingiva. *J Periodont* 1981;52(9):500–510.

Pacini N, Zanchi R, Ferrara A, Canzi E, Ferrari A. Antimicrobial susceptibility tests on anaerobic oral mixed cultures in periodontal diseases. *J Clin Periodont* 1997;24(6):401–409.

Rao JK, Allen NB, Feussner JR, Weinberger M. A prospective study of antineutrophil cytoplasmic antibody (c-ANCA) and clinical criteria in diagnosing Wegener's granulomatosis. *Lancet* 1995;346(8980):926–931. [Published erratum appears in *Lancet* 1995;346(8985): 1308.]

Rogers RS 3d, Sheridan PJ, Nightingale SH. Desquamative gingivitis: clinical, histopathologic, immunopathologic, and therapeutic observations. *J Am Acad Dermatol* 1982;7(6): 729–735.

Sewon LA, Parvinen TH, Sinisalo TV, Larmas MA, Alanen PJ. Dental status of adults with and without periodontitis. *J Periodont* 1988; 59(9):595–598.

Stiernberg CM. Deep-neck space infections. Diagnosis and management. *Arch Otolaryngol Head Neck Surg* 1986;112(12):1274–1279.

Yumoto E, Saeki K, Kadota Y. Subglottic stenosis in Wegener's granulomatosis limited to the head and neck region. *Ear Nose Throat J* 1997; 76(8):571–574.

Chapter 18

NEOPLASMS AND CYSTS

Judith Czaja McCaffrey

Cysts that develop in the oral cavity are primarily of odontogenic origin. These cysts are either inflammatory or developmental. Some of the more common odontogenic cysts have little to no malignant potential; however, some of the rare cysts have shown a tendency for malignant degeneration. There is a large amount of diversity within the group of odontogenic cysts secondary to the complexity of the dental organ and the numerous stem cells from which the cysts can arise. Developing tooth buds consist of three separate parts including the enamel organ, derived from oral ectoderm, the dental papilla, derived from ectomesenchyme, and the dental sac, also derived from the ectomesenchyme.

Benign and malignant neoplasms arise in the oral cavity. Although some characteristics of the primary tumor may suggest the benign or malignant nature of the tumor, a biopsy is necessary to confirm the diagnosis. Tumors that are entirely submucosal and that have been present for prolonged periods of time without change may be benign; however, a slow-growing salivary gland malignancy cannot be ruled out without appropriate histopathologic examination. Changes to the overlying mucosa including ulceration, violaceous appearance to the mucosa, pain, bleeding, or friability of the mucosa may suggest malignancy; however, erosive infectious or inflammatory diseases may be in the differential diagnosis; therefore, definitive biopsy is needed.

ODONTOGENIC CYSTS

These cysts are inflammatory or developmental.

INFLAMMATORY CYSTS

Radicular cysts or periapical cysts are the most common type of inflammatory cysts, accounting for greater than 50% of all odontogenic cysts. Often lesions are asymptomatic and found on routine screening with dental X-rays. Occasionally, however these lesions may become acutely inflamed and symptomatic, with pain on mastication. Teeth associated with these cysts are nonvital. Extraction of the tooth in question is necessary in the treatment of symptomatic periapical radicular cysts.

DEVELOPMENTAL CYSTS

Dentigerous Cyst

This cyst is the second most common odontogenic cyst and is associated with an unerupted tooth, most commonly the impacted third mandibular or maxillary molars. Characteristic radiographic findings include a radiolucency on plain film, surrounding a well-formed crown of an unerupted or impacted tooth. Although most dentigerous cysts are asymptomatic and found on routine dental X-ray, often these may grow large and produce infection or pathologic fracture of the mandible or maxilla.

SPECIAL CONSIDERATION

It has been speculated that ameloblastoma as well as squamous cell carcinoma may arise in the wall of a dentigerous cyst.

Odontogenic Keratocyst (OKC)

Although the cystic neoplasm is benign, its propensity for local destruction secondary to continued lobular growth causes bony destruction of the mandible and maxilla. Often, multiloculated lesions may affect the entire hemimandible, as two-thirds of the cases of OKC occur in the mandible. The angle and body are most commonly affected, showing cortical destruction as the OKC grows freely through the cancellous bone. The most common presenting symptom in patients with OKC is a painless facial swelling.

Odontogenic keratocysts have a characteristic pattern on histopathology (Fig. 18–1). A stratified squamous lining of the cyst wall is present with a polarized basal layer of epithelial cells with hyperchromatic nuclei. Often there is a corrugated appearance to the surface epithelium and within the cyst cavity are numerous whorls of keratinous debris. Multiple satellite cysts or daughter cysts may be present in the subepithelial layers of the main cyst. A common treatment for this condition is simple curettage of the cyst cavity. With curettage, recurrence rates have been reported to be as high as 50 to 60% and may occur late after the treatment of the primary lesion. Secondary to the propensity for recurrence with further destruction of the hemimandible, definitive initial procedures have been advocated by many authors. Treatment recommendations include resection of the affected bony segment with an appropriate margin and reconstruction.

A condition known as basal cell nevus syndrome is associated with odontogenic keratocysts. Patients present with multiple basal cell carcinomas of the face, neck, back, and trunk as well as multiple mandibular radiolucencies consistent with OKC. Skeletal abnormalities in these patients include bifid ribs, frontal bossing, and a hypoplastic midface.

ANEURYSMAL BONE CYST

This is a uniloculated or multiloculated radiolucency that is composed of multiple blood vessels with multinucleated giant cells in the peripheral cyst wall. The tumor is highly vascular and bleeds profusely with curettage. Curettage may lead to multiple recurrences of the tumor that then require definitive resection. These lesions can be pulsatile, and a bruit may be auscultated over the mandible in certain cases.

NONODONTOGENIC CYSTS

NASOPALATINE DUCT CYST

Embryologic remnants of the nasopalatine duct persist in the area between the primary and secondary palates, leading to the formation of a ductal cyst. This often is found in the area of the incisive canal and may extend into the floor of the nose and be evident as a well-mucosalized or skin covered firm mass. Treatment is enucleation of the cyst.

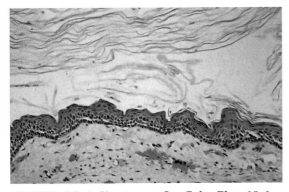

FIGURE 18–1 Keratocyst. See Color Plate 18–1.

MEDIAN PALATAL CYST

This cyst represents one of the only true fissural cysts that form during the embryonic development of the palatal shelves. Epithelial rests are trapped during fusion of the palatal shelves and a midline cysts forms. These lesions may become large and symptomatic. Treatment is enucleation of the cyst.

ODONTOGENIC TUMORS

Odontogenic tumors are epithelial, mesenchymal, or mixed in origin. These tumors are derived from cells arising from the enamel organ and can demonstrate varying degrees of differentiation.

EPITHELIAL

Ameloblastoma

This tumor is the most common of the epithelial odontogenic tumors. Although ameloblastoma is histopathologically benign, its biology is aggressive and it becomes extensively invasive, often through the entire posterior hemimandible, causing significant facial deformity (Fig. 18–2). The common presentation is that of a painless facial swelling demonstrating on radiography the typical "soap-bubble lucency" of the mandible. As with odontogenic keratocyst, ameloblastoma may grow and expand within the body of the mandible, causing cortical bone thinning and possible pathologic fracture as well as

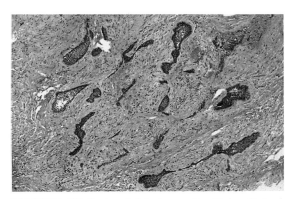

FIGURE 18–2 Ameloblastoma. See Color Plate 18–2.

penetration into the soft tissues of the floor of mouth or anterior face. Appropriate treatment of ameloblastoma is definitive resection rather than curettage. Resection may include partial or complete hemimandibulectomy, often with a vascularized free tissue transfer for reconstruction.

Calcifying Epithelial Odontogenic Tumor (CEOT; Pindborg Tumor)

This benign infiltrating tumor affects the mandible most commonly, often in the later decades of life. The tumor is histologically different from ameloblastoma, with islands of squamous cells infiltrating bony trabeculae. The treatment of CEOT is similar to that of ameloblastoma; however, the propensity for recurrence of this tumor is significantly lower.

Calcifying Odontogenic Cyst (Gorlin's Cyst)

A painless swelling in the mandible or maxilla is the typical presentation of this tumor. These tumors are well encapsulated, and although they can grow to considerable size, they behave in a benign manner. Multiple reactive processes occur in the tissue surrounding the tumor. Cell death occurs readily within the tumor wall and local inflammatory responses and calcification occur readily. Treatment includes either curettage or resection.

MESENCHYMAL

Odontogenic Myxoma

This tumor similarly behaves like an ameloblastoma, but differs histologically. Often the tumor is filled with a soft gelatinous material demonstrating numerous fibroblasts and myxomatous ground substance. Secondary to the infiltrative nature of this tumor, recurrence is common. Segmental bony resection is needed for complete removal.

Cementoblastoma

This tumor represents a true benign neoplasm of the cementum. Cementoblastoma occurs in young people and its characteristic symptom is an asymptomatic swelling. A radiolucent rim surrounds the periphery of the tumor as seen on radiography.

Mixed

Odontoma

This tumor is a hamartoma of the enamel organ. Enamel, cementum, and pulp are found mixed with dentin material in the tumor. Multiple odontomas have been described, including the complex as well as the compound odontoma. The latter is considered to be the most differentiated of the odontogenic tumors. Multiple small teeth may be found within the compound variety. Odontomas occur more commonly in the anterior maxilla. Treatment is simple enucleation.

Evaluation of Odontogenic Cysts and Tumors

The most common symptom of odontogenic cysts and tumors is a gradual painless swelling over the lower jaw.

> **PEARL•••** The presence of dysesthesias, pain, or loose dentition may suggest a malignancy within the jaw.

The use of Panorex X-ray to evaluate the maxilla and mandible is critical to the diagnosis and management of odontogenic cysts and tumors. Although there may be classic findings on X-ray, the definitive diagnosis is made by histopathologic examination of the tumor mass. Fine-needle aspiration (FNA) in the evaluation of these tumors may be performed; however, the mass is often completely surrounded by bone and therefore FNA is impossible. In such cases, a transoral or external incisional biopsy of the tumor is necessary in the operating room. Curettage can also be performed and sent for pathologic examination. Definitive resection, if necessary, is best done at a separate sitting, in order to preoperatively counsel the patient re-

garding the operative defect and options for reconstruction.

Benign Neoplasms of the Oral Cavity

There are multiple structures within the oral cavity from which benign tumors develop. These include tumors of the epithelium, the mesenchyme, and ectodermal elements, including nerves within the oral cavity.

Epidermoid Cysts

Epidermoid, as well as dermoid, cysts have been reported to appear in the buccal space, lips, and floor of the mouth. These present as firm, well-encapsulated masses. Upon histopathologic examination, the tumors do not differ from epidermoids and dermoids in other regions of the body. A simple stratified squamous epithelial lining without adnexal structures is present in the case of an epidermoid. If adnexal structures are found (e.g., hair follicles, sebaceous glands), a dermoid cyst is diagnosed. Treatment is excision and recurrence is uncommon.

Mucocele

A mucocele is common, typically found in areas of repeated trauma on the inner surface of the lip mucosa. These appear as well-circumscribed, 2- to 5-mm soft lesions in the submucosa. They tend to have a bluish hue below the thin mucosa. Mucoceles form as inspissated secretions of mucus accumulate under the mucosa secondary to injured minor salivary glands. Treatment is excision if the tumors are bothersome to the patient or are frequently traumatized by repeated biting during mastication.

Fibroma

Chronic irritation on surfaces of the oral cavity lead to the development of a fibroma. Fibromas typically have a smooth overlying mucosa and are frequently pedunculated. Often, they are asymptomatic, but can be bothersome to the patient during mastication. Excision is the treatment of choice, and on histopathologic examination, a fibrous stroma is present within a collagenous matrix surrounded by multiple inflammatory cells.

GRANULAR CELL MYOBLASTOMA

The most common location for a granular cell tumor is the oral cavity. The majority of cases that occur in the oral cavity are on the tongue. The tumor appears as a firm submucosal nodule; however, the overlying epithelium may rarely ulcerate. For this reason, it may have the appearance of keratinizing squamous cell carcinoma. Definitive diagnosis is based on biopsy and histopathologic examination. A large number of cases demonstrate pseudoepitheliomatous hyperplasia. Management after making the correct diagnosis is conservative surgical removal.

HEMANGIOMA

Hemangioma represents a tumor composed of multiple proliferating capillaries (capillary hemangioma) or large dilated mature blood sinuses (cavernous hemangioma). These present at birth or shortly thereafter. The tumors can become extensive and are apparent on examination of the oral cavity.

> **PEARL••• To adequately assess the size of a hemangioma, it is helpful to have the patient lie down on an exam table or recline in an exam chair. The blood sinuses will expand, showing the true, and often underestimated, extent of the tumor.**

The tumors appear as enlarged blood-filled sinuses just under the mucosa of the floor of mouth, buccal space, or lips. Often the intraoral portion of the tumor is contiguous with an external facial hemangioma and the entire tumor presents a significant cosmetic and functional abnormality. Hemangiomas frequently involve the tongue. In many cases with tongue invasion, airway obstruction may be a problem and a prophylactic tracheotomy may be needed to secure the airway. The natural history of hemangioma is that of spontaneous regression over the course of several years. This does not occur in all cases.

> ## CONTROVERSY
>
> Some authors advocate the surgical management of hemangioma in patients at an early age, prior to spontaneous regression. However, the general opinion regarding the management of hemangiomas is that in asymptomatic cases, spontaneous regression should be allowed to occur. Cases that may require earlier intervention include hemangiomas affecting the periorbital area or upper aerodigestive tract.

LEIOMYOMA

This benign neoplasm is composed of smooth muscle cells derived from mesenchymal origin. The tumor is extremely rare in the oral cavity and is more commonly found in the esophagus.

LYMPHANGIOMA (CYSTIC HYGROMA)

This neoplasm is composed of multiple dilated lymphatic ducts that proliferate in any region of the head and neck. These tumors typically present at or shortly after birth. Unlike the vascular counterpart, hemangioma, spontaneous regression of lymphangioma does not occur. These neoplasms can grow to become significant in size, involving the entire floor of mouth and tongue and descending deeply into the neck. The tumors are intimately associated with many vital structures in the neck, making removal difficult (Fig. 18–3). The natural history of the disease is that of unrelenting recurrences of the tumor after excision. Patients and parents of patients with lymphangioma should be counseled regarding the inevitable recurrence of this tumor. Attempts at complete removal should be performed at the initial operation. Repeated surgical procedures are fraught with increased risk of damage to surrounding vital structures.

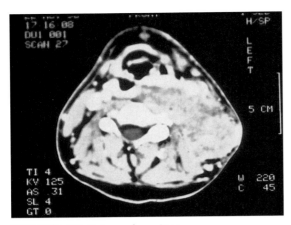

FIGURE 18-3 Lymphangioma.

RANULA

Ranula is a mucocele of the sublingual glands. This tumor is apparent as a bluish mass with a well-mucosalized covering in the floor of the mouth, just lateral to the sublingual frenulum. When confined above the mylohyoid muscle in the floor of mouth, these tumors remain within the oral cavity and are best removed through a transoral approach.

Plunging ranulas require both transoral and external approaches for excision. The sublingual gland should be removed completely for the operation to be adequate and to prevent recurrence.

PAPILLOMA

Papilloma represents a benign proliferative epithelial overgrowth. On histopathology, multiple fingerlike fungiform projections of proliferating squamous epithelium are present over a benign subepithelial fibrous stroma. Treatment is surgical excision.

NEUROFIBROMA

Isolated neurofibromas may occur in the oral cavity and represent tumors of the peripheral nerve sheath. More commonly, however, multiple neurofibromas occur in the oral cavity. When this occurs, it is often associated with von Recklinghausen's disease. Another condition in which multiple mucosal neuromas occurs is the multiple endocrine neoplasia (MEN) syndrome type IIb. This includes mucosal neuromas, pheochromocytoma of the adrenal glands, and medullary thyroid carcinoma. Patients with multiple mucosal neuromas should be screened for the MEN IIb syndrome. When neurofibromas occur singly, simple excision is all that is required if the tumor is bothersome to the patient. Tumors that are demonstrating malignant potential (e.g., sudden increase in size, pain, neurologic dysfunction) should be excised. Patients with massive clusters of neurofibromas pose a difficult problem. Extensive surgery is required to remove the tumors, and significant morbidity may result; therefore, conservative expectant management may be the best option.

TRAUMATIC NEUROMA

Patients sustaining trauma to the oral cavity may have injury to a motor or sensory nerve, thereby setting up a nidus for traumatic neuroma formation. These tumors may cause considerable pain. Conservative management includes simple excision.

Leukoplakia

Leukoplakia is a benign overgrowth of hyper-keratotic epithelium of the oral mucosa. Within the oral cavity, leukoplakia may occur on any surface. Leukoplakia is more often seen in smokers and patients who wear dentures. Hyperkeratosis is often an indicator of repeated trauma and eliminating the offending agent (stopping smoking, adjustments to denture plates) may resolve the leukoplakia. Areas of leukoplakia with surrounding erythema (i.e., erythroplakia) should be suspected of having malignant potential. These areas should be biopsied to rule out malignancy, especially in smokers and alcohol users.

Malignant Neoplasms of the Oral Cavity and Lip

Despite the different biologic behaviors of squamous malignancies at various sites in the oral cavity, all primary sites are similarly staged. The current staging system for oral cavity carcinomas is found in Table 18–1.

Epidemiology of Oral Cavity Carcinoma

Greater than 95% of cancers in the oral cavity are squamous cell carcinomas. There is a direct relationship between duration and amount of cigarette smoking and alcohol abuse and the development of oral cavity squamous cell carcinoma. Squamous cell carcinoma is more common in males; however, the incidence in women has increased, secondary to the increase in smoking in the female population. It is well known that in patients with oral cavity cancer who continue to smoke after treatment of an initial squamous cell carcinoma, there is a 40% incidence in development of a second primary malignancy. Alcohol and tobacco carcinogens act synergistically to increase the incidence of oral cavity carcinoma. Alcohol causes a chemical irritation to the mucosal epithelium of the oral cavity. Damage to the protective mucosal barrier

allows tobacco carcinogens to exert local toxic effects on the epithelial lining. Chewing tobacco has also been shown to be a direct mucosal epithelial carcinogen. The use of snuff in the buccogingival sulcus has increased not only the incidence of leukoplakia and erythroplakia, but also the incidence of invasive carcinoma.

Assessment and Tumor Management

Although there is little doubt that erythroplakia is a premalignant lesion, with a reported malignant tranformation rate of 30 to 40%, there is some debate regarding the malignant potential of leukoplakia. Some authors report a leukoplakic malignant transformation rate of up to 10%. Careful screening of patients with leukoplakia is therefore mandatory in this high-risk group. Erythroplakia, in contrast to leukoplakia, has a roughened red appearance with occasional superficial ulceration and may be friable.

> **PEARL...** It is difficult to differentiate the noninvasive, nonmalignant erythroplakia from carcinoma in situ or early stage invasive carcinoma. For this reason, the physician examining patients with erythroplakia must maintain a high index of suspicion and a low threshold for the frequent biopsy of questionable lesions.

Careful surveillance and early management will cure most patients with small invasive lesions.

The typical presentation of squamous cell carcinoma of the oral cavity is a persistent mouth sore. The patient complains of pain upon eating and drinking, especially citrus fruits and juices. A freely bleeding area aggravated by toothbrushing may be noted by the patient. A careful head and neck evaluation in patients with these complaints, especially in smokers or alcohol abusers, is essential to discover lesions at an early stage. Many lesions remain asymptomatic and are only found on careful examination of the oral cavity, many times by a dentist during routine dental care. Unfortunately, many patients with oral cavity carcinoma do not undergo

TABLE 18–1 STAGING OF LIP AND ORAL CAVITY CARCINOMA

TX: Primary tumor cannot be assessed

T0:   No evidence of primary tumor

Tis: Carcinoma in situ

T1:   Tumor 2 cm or less in greatest dimension

T2:   Tumor between 2 and 4 cm in greatest dimension

T3:   Tumor greater than 4 cm in greatest dimension

T4:   Tumor invades adjacent structures (through cortical bone, into deep extrinsic tongue muscles, skin, etc.)

NX: Regional nodes cannot be assessed

N0:   No regional nodal metastases

N1:   Metastasis to single lymph node measuring less than or equal to 3 cm

N2a: Metastasis in a single ipsilateral lymph node between 3 and 6 cm in greatest dimension

N2b: Metastasis in multiple ipsilateral lymph nodes all less than 6 cm in greatest dimension

N2c: Metastasis in bilateral or contralateral lymph nodes, none greater than 6 cm in greatest dimension

N3:   Metastasis in a lymph node more than 6 cm in greatest dimension

MX: Presence of distant metastasis cannot be assessed

M0:   No distant metastasis

M1:   Distant metastasis

Stage 0	Tis	N0	M0	
Stage I	T1	N0	M0	
Stage II	T2	N0	M0	
Stage III	T3	N0	M0	
		T1	N1	M0
		T2	N1	M0
		T3	N1	M0
Stage IV	T4	N0	M0	
		T4	N1	M0
		any T	N2	M0
		any T	N3	M0
		any T	any N	M1

routine dental care and have poor dental hygiene; thus, tumors may become quite large before patients are aware of the symptoms.

Patients with advanced-stage disease (T3 and T4) have involvement of surrounding oral cavity structures, especially the mandible and tongue. Mandibular involvement with oral cavity carcinoma may be difficult to assess. Physical findings of inferior alveolar or mental nerve anesthesia indicate mandibular invasion. In addition, loose dentition surrounding the area of tumor involvement may indicate spread of tumor into the marrow space.

PITFALL... Palpation of a large oral cavity tumor can suggest mandibular invasion; however, this may be inaccurate. The best radiographic test to determine gross mandibular invasion is the computed tomography (CT) scan. Bone windows to evaluate the mandibular cortex is helpful in questionable cases. When done preoperatively, the CT scan assists in surgical planning.

The ultimate assessment of mandibular invasion comes at the time of surgical resection. Direct inspection of the mandibular periosteum and cortical bone reveals the extent of mandibular involvement.

Full preoperative head and neck evaluation in patients with oral cavity carcinoma must be performed. Once assessment of the primary tumor and examination for regional metastases have been completed, a biopsy to confirm malignancy is necessary. The biopsy may be done either under local anesthesia in the office at the time of initial consultation or may be included at the time of panendoscopic evaluation under general anesthesia in the operating room. Panendoscopy should be completed either after or at the time of biopsy of the tumor and includes nasopharyngoscopy, direct laryngoscopy, bronchoscopy, and rigid esophagoscopy. Panendoscopy and exam under anesthesia allow the surgeon to evaluate the extent of the primary tumor, regional metastases, and the possible presence of a second primary tumor. Distant metastatic evaluation should include a chest X-ray and a chemistry panel that includes liver function tests and serum Ca^{2+}. Patients with advanced stage tumors who have complaints of localized bone pain should undergo bone scan to rule out distant bony metastases. Elevated liver function enzymes or lesions on screening chest X-ray should be evaluated with CT scan of the abdomen and chest, respectively.

> **PEARL...** Extensive evaluation for distant metastases is critical in advanced-stage oral cavity carcinoma to avoid morbid and deforming surgery in patients with poor overall prognosis.

LIP CARCINOMA

The most common carcinoma of the lip is squamous cell on the lower lip of men. There is some speculation that lip carcinoma is increased in cigar smokers. There is little debate that patients with prolonged exposure to sunlight have a significantly higher risk for development of lip carcinoma than the general population. Lip carcinoma is easily identified; therefore, the patient seeks attention sooner than for lesions of the oral cavity proper. However, if left unchecked by the patient or undiagnosed by an unwary physician, lip carcinoma may grow extensively and involve adjacent structures during the progression of disease. For early-stage lip cancers (T1), surgical excision has local control and disease-free survival rates equal to those of radiotherapy. The curability of T1 lip cancer is high, and most surgeons treating this disease will use excision with negative margins as the treatment modality of choice. Patients unable to undergo surgical removal of tumors can undergo radiotherapy. The results with primary radiotherapy for tumors greater than T1 (T2–T4) is poor; therefore, combined modality therapy is recommended in advanced cases. Patients with clinical adenopathy should undergo therapeutic modified or radical neck dissection.

> ## CONTROVERSY
>
> Some authors advocate the use of functional or selective neck dissection in patients with clinically positive adenopathy. This debate is beyond the scope of this chapter.

Patients with high-risk lesions (T2–T4 and recurrent tumors) without evidence of clinical adenopathy (N0) may undergo elective staging supraomohyoid neck dissection. In such cases, those patients found to have obviously involved cervical lymph nodes should undergo either completion modified or radical neck dissection. An alternative to neck dissection for patients with the N0 neck is postoperative radiotherapy for treatment of the cervical nodes.

Lip Reconstruction

Multiple algorithms of cheiloplasty reconstructive techniques have been described for upper and lower lip defects. Defects involving less than half of the width of the lip may be closed primarily without difficulty. Defects involving between one-half and two-thirds of the lip may be reconstructed using techniques that borrow

CONTROVERSY

There is a debate between head and neck surgical oncologists and radiotherapists regarding the management of the N0 neck. There is little debate that the N0 neck in patients with advanced head and neck tumors should be treated with some modality. Although surgery and radiation may be comparable in N0 neck management, radiotherapists argue that unnecessary surgery is avoided, and surgeons argue that surgical salvage after radiation failure has disastrous results.

tissue from the opposite intact lip, such as the Abbe-Estlander flap, or the Karapandzic flap.

The Karapandzic flap was first described in 1974. This flap uses local surrounding facial skin after careful placement of multiple circumoral releasing incisions and extensive undermining to bring remaining lip segments together under minimal tension (Fig. 18–4).

The Abbe flap is a transposition flap from the opposite lip. Tumors involving the oral commissure may be reconstructed with a variation of the Abbe flap known as the Abbe-Estlander flap (Fig. 18–5). This reconstructive technique borrows tissue from the opposite lip at the area of the oral commissure. Although the Abbe flap requires a secondary procedure to divide the pedicle of the donor lip flap, the Estlander variation does not. The Karapandzic technique maintains adequate blood supply as well as normal sensation to the reconstructed lip; however, the Abbe and Abbe-Estlander flaps denervate the donor tissue, and if the pedicle to the donor tissue is damaged, the flap may fail. The use of insensate reconstruction flaps may yield higher rates of oral incompetence. Careful apposition of the lip vermillion borders is necessary for good cosmetic closure.

In cases where the entire lip has been removed, total lip reconstruction is an option. Local facial advancement flaps have been used and are a good technique for reconstruction. Regional myocutaneous as well as free tissue transfers have also been used to reconstruct lip defects.

Both cosmesis and function must be considered in the reconstruction of lip defects. The goals of lip reconstruction are to provide the patient with a cosmetically acceptable oral stoma as well as a competent sphincter that prevents drooling and provides for adequate mastication and speech.

BASAL CELL CARCINOMA OF THE LIP

Sun exposure predisposes to basal cell as well as squamous cell carcinoma. Basal cell carcinoma typically appears on the upper lip, most commonly in men. A rodent-ulcer lesion with pearly raised edges suggests a basal cell tumor. Treatment is excision with primary closure for small lesions. Mohs' excision of lip basal cell carcinomas is an effective management strategy. Occasionally, neglect of a small basal cell carcinoma allows the tumor to grow to significant size, involving local structures. Resection and cure are

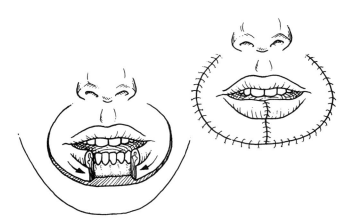

FIGURE 18–4 Karapandzic flap.

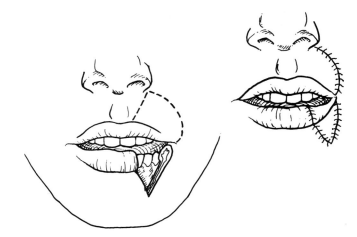

FIGURE 18–5 Abbe-Estlander flap.

possible in these advanced-stage tumors; however, the challenges of lip reconstruction make these cases difficult. Nodal metastases are rare in basal cell carcinoma.

BUCCAL MUCOSAL CARCINOMA

Buccal mucosal carcinoma, although rare, can be aggressive and presents late in the course of the disease. Tumors arising deep in the buccogingival sulcus may be difficult for the patient to appreciate until local structures are involved. These tumors grow laterally to involve the buccinator space and can involve the parotid gland as well. If the tumor is allowed to grow superiorly, it may enter the maxillary sinus through the anterior sinus wall. In patients with infraorbital nerve hypesthesia and a buccal space lesion, an advanced-stage tumor should be suspected. Tumors may grow medially to involve the bony alveolus or posteriorly to involve the ascending ramus of the mandible. Early-stage lesions may be locally excised, and the defect is either closed primarily or covered with a skin graft to prevent scar contracture.

> ## SPECIAL CONSIDERATION
>
> Tumors greater than T1 have a high incidence of regional metastases; therefore, staging elective neck dissection is advocated in the management of patients with large tumors and N0 necks.

Radiotherapy may also be used to treat the cervical region in patients with an N0 neck. Patients with clinically positive nodes at the time of diagnosis should undergo modified or radical neck dissection. Adjuvant postoperative radiotherapy is recommended in advanced disease to improve local control and disease-free survival.

FLOOR-OF-MOUTH CARCINOMA

Secondary to delay in symptoms with floor-of-mouth carcinoma, many patients present with advanced disease. Pain and a mass typically present later in the course of disease; therefore, careful surveillance of patients with smoking and alcohol history is necessary to detect early-stage disease. Early T1 and T2 tumors are readily treated either with primary radiotherapy or surgical removal. Because of the high morbidity associated with full-course radiotherapy to the oral cavity and surrounding structures (mandible), recommended treatment for early stage tumors is transoral excision. Small floor-of-mouth tumors removed transorally can be reconstructed with either primary closure or a skin graft to prevent contracture. Advanced-stage floor-of-mouth carcinoma may grow unchecked for a protracted period of time and involve surrounding structures. Mandibular and oral tongue invasion occur readily. The full extent of the floor-of-mouth lesion is appreciated at physical examination. Deep bimanual palpation of the oral cavity mass allows the surgeon to fully evaluate the extent of the neoplasm.

Deeply invasive tumors have a very high incidence of regional metastases relatively early in the course of floor-of-mouth malignancy. As many as 50% of patients with floor-of-mouth carcinomas (all T stages) present with palpable cervical adenopathy at the time of diagnosis. In patients with a clinically N0 neck, there is a high likelihood of occult metastases. Therefore, in cases greater than T1 with a clinically N0 neck, an elective staging neck dissection is advocated. Many authors will use depth of tumor invasion in the floor of mouth (as well as tongue) as a prognostic indicator and as an indicator for occult regional metastases. Patients with tumors having depth of invasion between 3 and 4 mm should undergo staging neck dissection. Advanced-stage, floor-of-mouth tumors often involve the mandible or tongue, necessitating a wider resection including partial mandibulectomy, hemimandibulectomy, and/or partial or near-total glossectomy for adequate tumor removal. Adjuvant radiotherapy is necessary to improve local control and disease-free survival rates. En-bloc resection including floor-of-mouth primary, mandible, portions of the tongue, and neck dissection should be done to remove the intervening lymphatics that may have tumor seeding. Primary radiotherapy as single-modality therapy for advanced floor-of-mouth carcinoma has poor results and is typically used alone only for palliation.

ALVEOLAR CARCINOMA

Gingival squamous cell carcinoma is relatively uncommon.

SPECIAL CONSIDERATION

One of the main considerations in this neoplasm is the presence or absence of teeth. In patients with dentition, alveolar and gingival neoplasms may grow into the tooth socket, invade the periodontal membrane, and extend freely into the mandibular or maxillary bone. Edentulous patients may be somewhat resistant to free bone invasion of alveolar tumors.

Because of the free pathway for tumor spread along tooth roots, even small alveolar lesions may be advanced stage (i.e., T4: maxilla or mandible invasion) at the time of diagnosis. Early-stage alveolar and gingival lesions require transoral excision with exploration of the periosteum surrounding the bone. If gross tumor invasion is found through the periosteum and into the mandibular bone, then a segmental mandibulectomy or superior mandibular shave (see Chapter 20) can be performed to adequately resect the tumor. Marrow margins may be assessed for spread of malignancy. Tumors arising on the maxillary alveolus may require partial alveolectomy of maxillectomy for complete removal. Defects in the maxilla may be closed in this area with surgical obturator.

As with most advanced oral cavity carcinomas, patients with advanced alveolar tumors should be treated with adjuvant postoperative radiotherapy. Patients with clinically positive lymphadenopathy should undergo modified or radical neck dissection. Patients with small T1 alveolar lesions have a low incidence of occult metastases in the N0 neck; therefore, staging neck dissection is not recommended. However, patients with T2–T4 lesions with an N0 neck should undergo prophylactic staging neck dissection or radiotherapy.

TONGUE CARCINOMA

In general, there are two forms of tongue carcinoma: exophytic and infiltrative. In the exophytic form, a thickened plaque-like tumor grows off the surface of the tonque mucosa. There is little deep infiltration of squamous cell cancer in exophytic carcinoma. Infiltrative tumors typically have a large submucosal extension deep into the tongue and demonstrate ulceration of the mucosal surface late in the course of disease.

The most common site for oral tongue carcinoma is the lateral surface. Pain or a sore on the tongue brings the patient for evaluation. Tumor size is often underestimated at initial examination and it is with deep palpation of the tongue that the true size of the tumor is appreciated. Adjacent oral cavity structures may be involved with tongue carcinoma; therefore, a thorough evaluation to assess the extent of tumor is necessary prior to resection.

There is a high rate of cure in patients with early-stage oral tongue cancers. T1 and T2 lesions are effectively treated with either surgery or radiotherapy alone. Although external beam radiotherapy may be administered for oral tongue carcinoma, this is technically difficult to deliver. The use of brachytherapy with insertion of implant catheters into the tumor had become a widely accepted form of therapy for many tongue lesions. Both external beam therapy and brachytherapy are associated with complications and many surgeons favor simple transoral excision for early-stage tumors. This management strategy is similar to that for floor-of-mouth carcinoma. Most T1 and T2 tongue carcinomas can be resected with an adequate margin and either closed primarily or with a split-thickness skin graft to prevent contracture.

Advanced-stage carcinomas of the oral tongue (T3 and T4) are best treated with combined modality therapy including surgery and postoperative radiotherapy. Reconstruction in cases of advanced-stage tongue carcinoma include regional myocutaneous flaps and free tissue transfers.

CONTROVERSY

T4 oral tongue carcinomas that involve the base of tongue and vallecula extensively require total glossectomy with total laryngectomy for complete removal and to prevent chronic aspiration. The total laryngoglossectomy, in the opinion of some head and neck surgeons, results in an overall poor quality of life for patients and therefore is not justifiable as a surgical option. Patients treated by physicians with this philosophy undergo combined chemotherapy and radiotherapy for palliation. However, many head and neck surgeons have the opposite opinion and perform total laryngoglossectomy with fair functional results.

Rehabilitation of speech and swallowing are the most difficult challenges in these patients. Many of these patients never regain understandable speech and are gastrostomy-dependent.

If the vallecula of the tongue base is free in advanced oral tongue carcinomas, a total glossectomy may be performed without total laryngectomy. Some of the patients undergoing this procedure function well with respect to speech and articulation, especially when reconstructed adequately; however, many are rendered gastrostomy-dependent. The exceptionally rehabilitated patient, in addition to gaining communicable speech, will also swallow without aspiration after total glossectomy. Careful preoperative patient and family counseling regarding the functional outcome for these patients is required, and the physician should be honest about the expectations.

As with most oral cavity carcinomas, there is controversy regarding the management of the N0 neck. Most surgeons favor elective supraomohyoid neck dissection in patients with tongue tumors that show greater than 3 to 4 mm depth of invasion. Few advanced-stage tongue cancers (T3 and T4) present with N0 necks; therefore, controversy regarding management in these cases is moot. Modified or radical neck dissection should be performed in all patients with clinically positive nodes at the time of diagnosis. An acceptable form of treatment in patients with the N0 neck is postoperative radiotherapy to the neck in cases that are suspicious for occult malignancy.

HARD PALATE CARCINOMA

Patients presenting with hard-palate carcinoma often complain of a lump on the roof of the mouth or an ill-fitting denture plate. When seeing a patient with a lump on the roof of the mouth, the surgeon must be cognizant of the "tip of the iceberg" phenomenon. Careful history regarding the nose and paranasal sinuses should be obtained to rule out a paranasal sinus malignancy that has directly extended into the oral cavity. Appropriate workup in these cases includes a direct coronal CT scan of the sinuses to rule out paranasal sinus involvement. (A CT scan will also show the extent of palatal bone invasion.)

> **PEARL...** It may be difficult to determine whether the tumor is a hard-palate primary with sinus extension or a paranasal sinus malignancy with extension into the oral cavity. The history should assist in differentiating the two. Patients with a long history of nasal congestion, epistaxis, hyposmia, anosmia, vision changes, or numbness over the cheek have symptoms suggesting paranasal sinus malignancy.

Management of hard-palate squamous cell carcinoma for early-stage tumors includes either external beam radiotherapy or transoral excision. Treatment for advanced-stage tumors should include combined modality therapy with surgical resection followed by postoperative radiotherapy. Surgery for advanced-stage lesions includes a partial maxillectomy and reconstruction with surgical obturator. Other considerations in the management of advanced-stage hard-palate carcinomas include the extent of involvement of the maxillary sinus, ethmoid sinus, sphenoid sinus, and orbit. The surgical procedure of choice in the management of these tumors is dictated by the extent of the primary. Craniofacial resection may be necessary for tumors that extend superiorly to the cribriform plate. Gross extension into the sphenoid sinus is a sign of unresectable and incurable disease.

Management of the neck in hard-palate neoplasms is seldom necessary. The incidence of clinically positive neck metastasis remains low, even in advanced-stage tumors; however, the incidence of occult metastasis in T3 and T4 tumors is high enough to warrant treatment of the neck with either surgery (supraomohyoid staging neck dissection) or radiotherapy.

Secondary to the large amount of salivary gland tissue in the hard-palate mucosa, there is a high incidence of non–squamous cell malignancies. These salivary gland malignancies account for 50% of hard-palate neoplasms. The most common form is the low-grade polymorphous adenocarcinoma, followed by the other minor salivary gland malignancies including mucoepidermoid, adenoid cystic, and acinic cell carcinomas.

RETROMOLAR TRIGONE CARCINOMA

Retromolar trigone carcinomas may grow to be extensive prior to appropriate diagnosis.

> **PITFALL...** This area of the oral cavity is often inadequately examined, thereby allowing tumors to grow to large size before diagnosis. Because of the intimate relationship between the retromolar trigone and surrounding structures, tumors progress to advanced stages, involving mandible or tongue, early in the course of disease.

The thin mucosal covering over the ascending ramus and angle of the mandible with little intervening submucosal tissues is an ineffective barrier to tumor spread. Although the periosteum of the mandible may provide a barrier, in advanced cases, the bony cortex is readily invaded and the tumor spreads into the mandibular marrow space. Spread of tumor along the inferior alveolar nerve may also occur with marrow invasion. Complete tumor removal in such cases requires en-bloc tumor resection with hemimandibulectomy.

Similarly, extension into the floor of mouth and tongue may occur, and the true extent of the retromolar trigone tumor may be underestimated on clinical examination. For this reason, all oral cavity carcinomas should be thoroughly assessed in the operating room under general anesthesia. This allows the surgeon to stage the primary tumor and counsel the patient regarding surgical resection and options for reconstruction.

As with other oral cavity primaries, management of early-stage tumors of the retromolar trigone with either external beam radiotherapy or transoral excision may be performed. However, secondary to complications arising from high-dose radiotherapy to the oral cavity, surgery is favored for early-stage tumors. Advanced-stage tumors should be treated with combined modality therapy. Advanced-stage lesions require mandibulectomy for adequate resection. Cervical metastases occur readily with retromolar trigone tumors, and clinically positive nodal metastases should be resected with modified or radical neck dissection. Clinically N0 necks may be treated either with staging supraomohyoid neck dissection or radiotherapy.

Verrucous Carcinoma

Verrucous carcinoma occurs commonly in the oral cavity and differs from invasive keratinizing squamous cell carcinoma. Verrucous carcinoma or Ackerman's tumor clinically has a papillomatous, shaggy appearance and spreads like a carpet in a benign manner over large surfaces in the oral cavity. Common on the buccal and palatal mucosa, verrucous tumors have a characteristically benign appearance on histopathology. They typically do not invade through the basement membrane of the involved epithelium but have pushing borders of squamous cells that extend deeply into the subepithelial layers of the affected tissue. Pathologists may often call the tumor benign based on the hematoxylin and eosin (H&E) preparation without any information from the surgeon about the tumor's clinical appearance. Treatment is wide excision. Regional metastases are rare; therefore, neck treatment is unnecessary. When nodes are present, this portends a poorer prognosis.

SPECIAL CONSIDERATION

Frankly invasive squamous cell carcinoma may develop in a verrucous carcinoma.

Nonsquamous Carcinomas of the Oral Cavity

The most common non–squamous cell carcinoma of the oral cavity is of minor salivary gland origin. Ulceration of minor salivary gland malignancies in the oral cavity is uncommon, and these tumors typically present as firm submucosal masses most frequently located on the hard and soft palates. The adenoid cystic carci-noma is the most common minor salivary gland malignancy in the oral cavity; however, low-grade polymorphous adenocarcinoma is most common on the hard palate. The natural history of adenoid cystic carcinoma is frequent local recurrence as the patient is followed for prolonged periods of time. A patient will remain disease-free up to 10 to 15 years after surgical resection of adenoid cystic carcinoma, and then present with either a local recurrence or a distant metastasis.

Another common scenario in adenoid cystic carcinoma is a patient who remains disease-free at the primary site but has evidence of distant metastasis that rarely cause any symptoms. Management of adenoid cystic carcinoma consists of wide surgical resection with attempt at negative margins. There is inevitable perineural invasion that makes complete excision of these tumors in the oral cavity difficult. Postoperative radiotherapy is used by many surgeons in patients with both negative and positive margins.

PEARL... In patients with negative margins, there may be some justification for saving radiotherapy for management of the eventual recurrence. When local recurrence occurs, cranial nerve involvement may be present and the tumor may be unresectable. In these cases, radiotherapy can be used to palliate the patient.

Chemotherapy has been used in certain clinical protocols; however, it has not been shown to improve either local control or survival. Regional neck dissection is not advocated for clinically N0 necks; however, in patients with positive regional metastasis at the time of diagnosis, a neck dissection should be performed.

Adenocarcinoma may be either high or low grade. The low-grade polymorphous type typically has a good prognosis and requires excision with adequate margins for cure. The high-grade adenocarcinomas are aggressive, demonstrating local destruction, and resection is more difficult. The prognosis in the latter form of tumor is poor.

Mucoepidermoid carcinoma also will occur on the hard or soft palate. These tumors are graded in a similar manner to the mucoepidermoid carcinomas of the major salivary glands. The determination of grade is based on histopathologic examination of mucous and epidermoid components of the tumor. Low-grade tumors characteristically have a larger number of mucous cells; therefore, they behave in a more indolent manner. The high-grade tumors have a large number of epithelial cells, accounting for their aggressive behavior, which is similar to squamous cell carcinomas. Oral mucoepidermoid carcinomas are treated most effectively with primary surgical excision or combined modality therapy including surgery and radiotherapy. Neck dissection should be performed in patients with high-grade mucoepidermoid carcinomas. These patients will often present with clinically positive adenopathy. In cases with a clinically N0 neck, there is high likelihood of occult cervical metastases, and most surgeons favor prophylactic neck dissection in the management of these patients. Local recurrence is common in high-grade tumors, and those recurrences that are amenable to resection should be excised.

MELANOMA

Melanoma of the oral cavity is rare, representing less than 1% of all melanomas. However, the oral cavity is the most common location for mucosal melanoma. Appropriate diagnosis relies on assessment of pigmented oral cavity lesions and biopsy in suspicious cases. Treatment of mucosal melanoma is wide excision and neck dissection in patients with clinically positive adenopathy. The overall prognosis in patients with mucosal melanoma remains poor, despite attempts at adjuvant chemotherapy and radiotherapy.

SUGGESTED READINGS

Browne RM. The odontogenic keratocyst. Histological features and their correlation with clinical behaviour. *Br Dent J* 1971;131(6):249–259.

Fang FM, Leung SW, Huang CC, et al. Combined-modality therapy for squamous carcinoma of the buccal mucosa: treatment results and prognostic factors. *Head Neck* 1997;19(6):506–512.

Fitzpatrick PJ. Cancer of the lip. *J Otolaryngol* 1984;13(1):32–36.

Fukano H, Matsuura H, Hasegawa Y, Nakamura S. Depth of invasion as a predictive factor for cervical lymph node metastasis in tongue carcinoma. *Head Neck* 1997;19(3):205–210.

Ichimura K, Ohta Y, Tayama N. Surgical management of the plunging ranula: a review of seven cases. *J Laryngol Otol* 1996;110(6):554–556.

Jovanovic A, Schulten EA, Kostense PJ, Snow GB, van der Waal I. Squamous cell carcinoma of the lip and oral cavity in the Netherlands: an epidemiological study of 740 patients. *J Craniomaxillofac Surg* 1993;21(4):149–152.

Keszler A, Cabrini RL. Histometric study of leukoplakia, lichen planus and carcinoma in situ of oral mucosa. *J Oral Pathol* 1983;12(5):330–335.

Kirita T, Okabe S, Izumo T, Sugimura M. Risk factors for the postoperative local recurrence of tongue carcinoma. *J Oral Maxillofac Surg* 1994;52(2):149–154.

Lee SP, Shimizu KT, Tran LM, Juillard G, Calcaterra TC. Mucosal melanoma of the head and neck: the impact of local control on survival. *Laryngoscope* 1994;104(2):121–126.

Maceri DR, Saxton KG. Neurofibromatosis of the head and neck. *Head Neck Surg* 1984;6:842–846.

Maiorano E, Altini M, Favia G. Clear cell tumors of the salivary glands, jaws, and oral mucosa. *Semin Diagn Pathol* 1997;14(3):203–212.

Manolidis S, Donald PJ. Malignant mucosal melanoma of the head and neck: review of the literature and report of 14 patients. *Cancer* 1997;80(8):1373–1386.

Nuutinen J, Karja J. Local and distant metastases in patients with surgically treated squamous cell carcinoma of the lip. *Clin Otolaryngol* 1981;6(6):415–419.

Pindborg JJ. *Atlas of Diseases of the Oral Mucosa.* 4th ed. Copenhagen: Munksgaard, 1985.

Sankaranarayanan R, Mathew B, Varghese C, et al. Chemoprevention of oral leukoplakia with vitamin A and beta carotene: an assessment. *Oral Oncol* 1997;33(4):231–236.

Shear M. Cysts of the jaws: recent advances. *J Oral Pathol* 1985;14:43–48.

Wald RM Jr, Calcaterra TC. Lower alveolar carcinoma. Segmental v. marginal resection. *Arch Otolaryngol* 1983;109(9):578–582.

Weissman BW, Wetli C. Ameloblastoma of the maxilla. *South Med J* 1977;70(2):251–253.

Wetmore SJ, Billie JD, Howe A, Wetzel W. Odontogenic keratocyst: diagnosis and treatment. *Otolaryngol Head Neck Surg* 1983;91(2): 167–172.

Yuen AP, Wei WI, Wong YM, Tang KC. Elective neck dissection versus observation in the treatment of early oral tongue carcinoma. *Head Neck* 1997;19(7):583–588.

Zitsch RP 3d. Carcinoma of the lip. *Otolaryngol Clin North Am* 1993;26(2):265–277.

Chapter 19

TRAUMA
Judith Czaja McCaffrey

The mandible is the second most commonly fractured facial bone after the nasal bones. Fractures of the mandible often occur secondary to motor vehicle accidents or in physical confrontations. Muscles attached to the mandible tend to draw broken fragments toward one another in a *favorable* fracture. *Unfavorable* fractures occur when the muscular attachments to the mandible distract broken fragments away from one another. Unfavorable fractures need definitive open reduction more commonly than favorable fractures. Fractures may also be defined as *horizontal* or *vertical* (Fig. 19–1). Horizontal fractures exhibit either displacement or stabilization in a vertical direction secondary to action of the temporalis, masseter, and pterygoid muscles. Vertical fractures exhibit displacement or stabilization in a horizontal direction secondary to action of the mylohyoid muscle.

Angle's classification of dental occlusion (Fig. 19–2) is based on the relationship of the maxillary first molar to the mandibular first molar. Class I occlusion occurs when the mesiobuccal cusp of the maxillary first molar sits directly in the buccal groove of the mandibular first molar. Class II occlusion occurs when the mesiobuccal cusp lies posterior to the buccal groove of the mandibular first molar (underbite). Class III occlusion occurs when the mesiobuccal cusp lies anterior to the buccal groove of the mandibular first molar (overbite). Understanding the classes of occlusion is important in es-

tablishing premorbid occlusion in patients with mandibular fractures. In addition to understanding the appropriate relationship between the maxillary and mandibular molars, making note of wear facets and cuspal interdigitation is important for reestablishment of the patient's premorbid occlusion, which is often *not* class I.

Patients with mandibular fractures typically present with complaints of unilateral or bilateral mandibular pain, a history of trauma, loose dentition, and malocclusion. Careful physical examination includes measurement of interincisal distance. The normal interincisal distance is 40 mm or greater. Secondary to splinting, patients with mandibular fractures often have interincisal distances less than 35 mm. Careful intraoral inspection reveals concurrent tooth fractures and intraoral hematoma.

The most common site of mandibular fracture is the condyle followed by the angle and body. Parasymphyseal fractures may also occur.

PITFALL... In evaluation of patients with mandibular fractures, a second fracture should be sought when a first fracture is discovered. A common injury that is unrecognized in poorly evaluated patents is a contralateral displaced subcondylar fracture in the presence of a body or angle fracture.

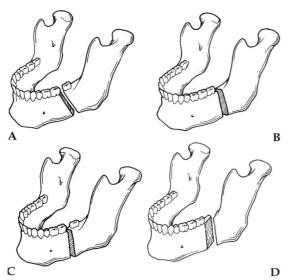

FIGURE 19–1 Fractures of the jaw. (A) horizontally unfavorable. (B) Horizontally favorable. (C) Vertically unfavorable. (D) Vertically favorable.

Appropriate evaluation includes a Panorex plain radiograph that shows the entire mandible from condyle to condyle. Special condylar tomograms may also be obtained to thoroughly evaluate subcondylar or condylar fractures.

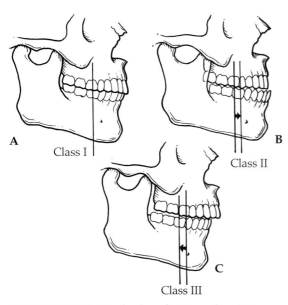

Class I

Class II

Class III

FIGURE 19–2 Angle classification of occlusion.

MANAGEMENT OF MANDIBULAR FRACTURES

All mandible fractures should be considered compound; therefore, antibiotic prophylaxis should be started immediately after identification of a mandible fracture. In general, however, mandible fractures do not need immediate closure, but should be reduced within 24 hours after injury for best healing results. Delay may result in an increased rate of infection and subsequently poor union or nonunion of bony fragments.

There are two forms of reduction for mandibular fractures: closed and open. Most favorable fractures can be treated with closed reduction. The muscles of the mandible pull fragments together; therefore plating is usually unnecessary. Arch bars with mandibulomaxillary fixation (MMF) for 6 weeks should be adequate treatment for closed reduction of most favorable fractures. Minimally displaced condylar fractures can be treated with MMF for periods shorter than 6 weeks to prevent joint ankylosis. Subcondylar fractures that are either minimally displaced or in edentulous patients can be treated with soft diet alone, especially in patients who would not tolerate MMF.

When bony fractures lie in unfavorable positions, where attached muscles distract fragments, open reduction is typically necessary to reapproximate fragments and hold them in rigid fixation. Rigid fixation using plates and screws from an intraoral approach is most commonly used today for management of displaced mandibular fractures. Miniplates can be used over the fracture site, typically with three screws on either side of the plate spanning the defect. A second plate or an arch bar on mandibular teeth is commonly used as a tension band to prevent distraction at the upper end of the fracture.

> **PITFALL...** One must take care not to damage tooth roots in the placement of the plates. Monocortical screws are used to prevent tooth root damage. Body or angle fractures that are amenable to lag screw fixation can be treated with this technique.

CONTROVERSY

Open reduction of mandibular condyle fractures is somewhat controversial. There are absolute indications for this technique, including displacement of the condyle into the middle cranial fossa with dural injury and cerebrospinal fluid (CSF) leak, and bilateral subcondylar fractures in edentulous patients where splinting is difficult or impossible. Another relative indication for open reduction is bilateral condylar fractures in the presence of multiple midface fractures where it is impossible to determine the premorbid occlusion and height of the facial skeleton.

There are special situations that arise in the care of mandibular fractures, including mandibular fractures in the pediatric population, the management of vital dentition in the line of fracture, the complications of mandibular fractures, and emergencies arising in the care of patients with these fractures.

Most authors agree that open rigid fixation in the management of pediatric mandibular fractures is unnecessary and puts undue risk on the developing tooth buds. Most pediatric mandibular fractures can be treated with 2 to 3 weeks of closed reduction with MMF.

SPECIAL CONSIDERATION

Shorter closed reduction time is necessary because the complications resulting from long-term reduction in children can be disastrous.

Complications include temporomandibular joint ankylosis and severe alterations in mandibular growth leading to jaw deformities. Ankylosis is best avoided by allowing for mandibular movement on a regular basis during the period of MMF.

Uninjured stable teeth in the line of mandibular fracture should be left intact and reduction performed without extraction. Careful dental hygiene is required to maintain integrity of the tooth. Any unstable teeth or broken teeth in the line of a fracture should be extracted and reduction subsequently performed.

There are multiple complications related to mandibular fractures including infection, malocclusion, malunion, temporomandibular ankylosis and dysfunction, and inferior alveolar nerve injury.

PITFALL... Uncontrolled infection secondary to delay in reduction or inadequate reduction may lead to osteomyelitis and subsequent nonunion of bony fragments. Management of the mandible in such instances is difficult and requires extensive debridement, antibiotic therapy, and bone grafts to reestablish bone continuity.

Emergencies related to mandibular fractures include airway obstruction secondary to posterior displacement of the mandibular arch as well as expansion of floor-of-mouth hematoma with posterior tongue displacement. Acute intervention with tracheotomy may be required. The condyle may be driven into the middle cranial fossa with resultant dural tear, CSF leak, and brain injury. In such cases, neurosurgery is required. Finally, in patients sustaining comminuted ascending ramus and condylar fractures secondary to a penetrating gunshot wound or blast injury, concomitant injury to the adjacent carotid artery may be present. Expanding hematoma in the presence of an ascending ramus fracture requires urgent operative intervention and possible interventional angiography for vascular control.

PEARL... Penetrating injury in this zone of the neck, in the absence of expanding hematoma or hemodynamic instability, should be evaluated with angiography to determine the integrity of the carotid artery.

THERMAL INJURY

The most common thermal injury of the oral cavity is electrical burns in children. Chewing on exposed electrical appliance cords causes burn injury to the oral commissures of the mouth orifice.

CONTROVERSY

There is controversy regarding the management of patients sustaining such injuries. It is generally accepted that the injury appears deceptively small early after electrocution and time is required in order for the wound to completely demarcate.

Oral commissure splints are commonly used typically 2 to 3 weeks after injury to prevent severe oral stoma contracture. Surgery for reconstruction may not be necessary when splints are used in a timely fashion.

SPECIAL CONSIDERATION

The long-term complication of thermal injury is severe microstomia secondary to profuse scarring. Once heavy scarring has occurred, surgery is required to enlarge the microstomia. Complete lip reconstruction is difficult after thermal injury and requires the use of local and regional flaps as well as skin grafts.

Caustic ingestions can also yield oral cavity burns. Severe mucositis develops, especially after the oral cavity is exposed to alkali substances. The effect may be delayed, with deeper burns occurring later after initial exposure. Blisters and sloughed mucosa may appear. Caustic burns of the lips and oral cavity are the sentinel for severe chemical burns of the hypopharynx and esophagus. The severity of the hypopharyngeal and esophageal burns, with their subsequent morbidities, far outweighs the seriousness of the oral cavity burns. Treatment of oral cavity caustic burns includes mild oral rinses, dental hygiene, and a bland soft diet, advancing as tolerated, in cases where patients are permitted to eat.

LACERATIONS

Lacerations of the oral cavity occur secondary to penetrating trauma from foreign bodies or from dental trauma. Most oral cavity lacerations do not require definitive closure and heal readily by secondary intention. Careful inspection of the lacerations is necessary, however, as a retained foreign body can delay healing and induce infection. Intraoral wounds or through-and-through cheek wounds may sever the parotid duct. Probing of the duct is necessary. Stenting is required in through-and-through lacerations that extend into the parotid bed. There is a high risk for facial nerve injury with such lacerations.

Penetrating tongue trauma may be accompanied by hematoma within the tongue musculature. This should be sought when evaluating patients with tongue lacerations to prevent subsequent complications related to airway obstruction.

SUGGESTED READINGS

Bruce R, Fonseca RJ. Mandibular fractures. In: Fonseca RJ, Walker RV, eds. *Oral and Maxillofacial Trauma.* Philadelphia: WB Saunders; 1991:359–417.

Dierks EJ. Management of associated dental injuries in maxillofacial trauma. *Otolaryngol Clin North Am* 1991;24:165–180.

Helfrick JF. Early assessment and treatment planning of the maxillofacial trauma patient. In: Fonseca RJ, Walker RV, eds. *Oral and Maxillofacial Trauma.* Philadelphia: WB Saunders; 1991:279–300.

Kellman RM, Marentette LJ. *Atlas of Craniomaxillofacial Fixation.* New York: Raven Press; 1995.

Powers MP. Diagnosis and management of dentoalveolar injuries. In: Fonseca RJ, Walker RV, eds. *Oral and Maxillofacial Trauma.* Philadelphia: WB Saunders; 1991:323–358.

Shumrick KA. Facial trauma: soft-tissue lacerations and burns. In: Cummings CW, Fredrickson JM, Harker LA, Krause CJ, Schuller DE, eds. *Otolaryngology Head and Neck Surgery.* 3rd ed. St. Louis: CV Mosby; 1998:1388–1406.

Chapter 20

SPECIAL CONSIDERATIONS

Judith Czaja McCaffrey

ORAL CAVITY RECONSTRUCTION

Most superficial defects in all parts of the oral cavity can be either left open to heal by secondary intention or closed at the time of initial resection. Secondary healing is adequate for superficial wounds where scar contraction and subsequent limitation in function are not a concern. Primary closure of defects can be used in lieu of healing by secondary intention. This technique is excellent for superficial floor-of-mouth defects as well as defects of the oral tongue. There is little loss of function with primary closure of most tongue defects. As much as one-half of the tongue can be removed and closed primarily without significant morbidity to the patient.

In areas where significant scar contracture would lead to tethering of the tongue and subsequent decrease in function or limitations in oral cavity opening, split-thickness skin grafts can be used. When placed adequately in the wound bed and secured with bolster dressings, healing is excellent and contracture is prevented.

The three techniques discussed are excellent options for the closure of small to moderately sized defects of the floor of mouth, buccal mucosa, and tongue. Many lesions of the hard palate that are excised without underlying bone can be left open to heal by secondary intention.

This technique works best and most wounds heal without problems. In patients unable to tolerate an open hard-palate mucosal defect, having problems with either irritation from oral intake or repeated tongue trauma, coverage can be provided with either a small bolster dressing, Silastic sheeting, or a prefabricated surgical obturator.

The next category of defects in the oral cavity represent the through-and-through floor-of-mouth defects (Fig. 20–1). These defects typically remain after resection of large floor-of-mouth tumors and may be contiguous with mandibular as well as tongue defects. Through-and-through defects are best closed with regional myocutaneous flaps or free tissue transfers. These reconstruction options can be performed with or without consideration for reconstruction of the mandible.

The pectoralis major regional myocutaneous flap provides excellent bulk and a large skin paddle for reconstruction of floor-of-mouth and tongue defects. This flap is based on the thoracoacromial and lateral thoracic arteries (see Chap. 87). When preparing the flap for elevation, one must take care to consider the insertion of the pectoralis major muscle inferiorly on the ribs. Skin flaps that are only partially supported by the underlying elevated muscle are considered partially random and at risk for loss in the reconstruction. The skin paddle should be

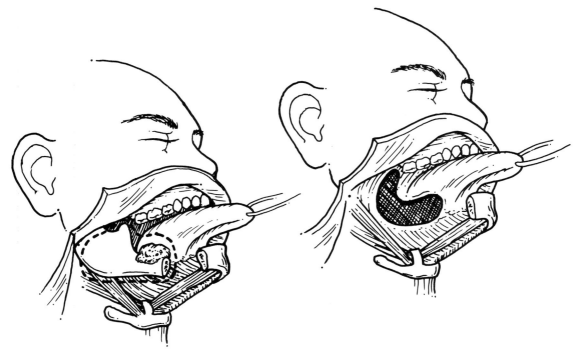

FIGURE 20–1 Full-thickness resection of the jaw for cancer invading the depths of the mandible.

designed to lie within the boundaries of the pectoralis major insertion at the sixth rib inferiorly. Care should be taken to prevent avulsion of the attached skin paddle.

> **PITFALL...** Consideration must also be given to preservation of the deltopectoral regional skin flap when designing the pectoralis major flap defect. The deltopectoral skin flap is excellent and can be used in cases of primary reconstruction failure; therefore it should not be violated in the planning of primary reconstructive regional flaps.

Once the pectoralis flap has been completely elevated and muscle has been trimmed down to the pedicle, the skin paddle can be rotated into the surgical defect. Sizing the skin paddle is done prior to elevation of the myocutaneous flap. Paddles as large as 8 × 8 cm can be reliably raised with the pectoralis major flap. Near-total reconstruction of the oral cavity including the floor of mouth and tongue may be completed with the pectoralis major flap. The flap is also versatile in

reconstructing lateral pharyngeal and tonsillar fossa/soft palate defects.

> **PEARL...** An inframammary incision in the crease of the female breast should be used in creating the pectoralis major myocutaneous defect in women. This provides adequate exposure to the muscle, and allows one to fashion a large skin paddle that does not leave the patient with an unsightly scar over the chest wall, which is not tolerated in many female patients.

Superiorly and inferiorly based myocutaneous trapezius flaps can also be used to reconstruct the oral cavity. The superiorly based trapezius flap blood supply is from the occipital artery as well as perforators from the paraspinal arteries (see Chap. 87). The inferiorly based flap receives its blood supply from the transverse cervical artery (Figs. 20–2 and 20–3). In the presence of a radical neck dissection, the blood supply to both the superiorly and inferiorly based flaps may be tenuous or may have been sacrificed. In this case, the trapezius flaps are not viable options for oral cavity reconstruction. The limitations to these flaps are the size of the skin paddle and the distance that the flap can be transposed to fill a defect.

The latissimus dorsi myocutaneous flap is based on the thoracodorsal artery (see Chap. 87). The main limitation to this flap in reconstruction of oral cavity defects is the need for repositioning of patients from the supine to the decubitus position during reconstruction. This is a minor inconvenience and one that may be overcome if the necessity for the flap arises. The muscle and skin paddle are elevated and the flap is tunneled through the axilla. The main advantage to the flap is its length and it may be used for defects as high as the nasopharynx and skull base.

CONTROVERSY

Many surgeons believe that the use of myocutaneous flaps when the mandible is present provides a bulky reconstruction that may inhibit normal function. This is not the opinion of all authors.

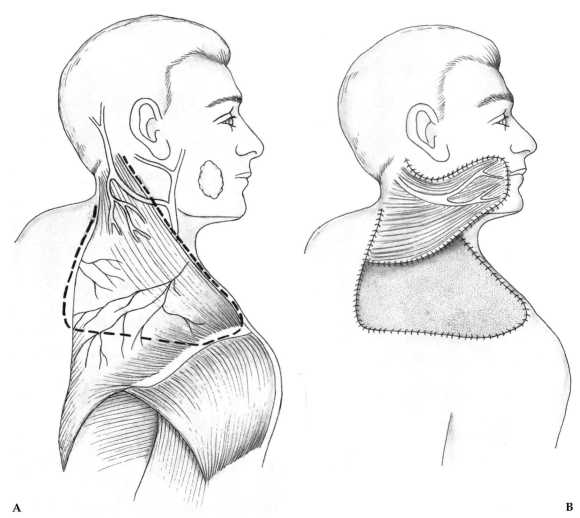

A   B

FIGURE 20–2 Superiorly based trapezius myocutaneous flaps. (A). Flap formed. (B). Flap covers defect.

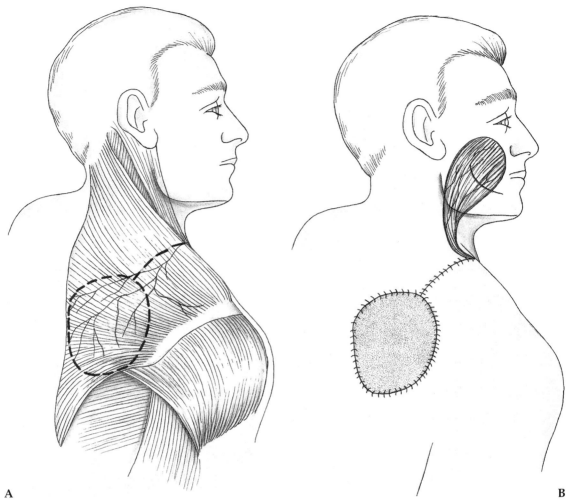

A   B

FIGURE 20–3 Inferiorly based trapezius myocutaneous flap. (A). Flap formed. (B). Flap rotated and sutured into oral cavity buccal defect.

The deltopectoral (DP) regional skin flap is an excellent flap for reconstruction of floor-of-mouth defects (see Chap. 86). This flap is based on the first four perforators of the internal mammary artery (Fig. 20–4). The distalmost portion of the flap over the deltoid may be random. The DP flap's limitation in floor-of-mouth reconstruction is its pliability and lack of bulk. For this reason, the flap is probably best used as a material for coverage of raw surfaces to prevent contractures. Buccal as well as superficial floor-of-mouth defects are readily closed with the deltopectoral flap. The defect of the deltopectoral region is most often closed with a split-thickness skin graft.

MANDIBULAR RESECTION

The extent of bony mandibular resection required in the management of oral cavity carcinoma is determined by the depth of invasion of the tumor. At the time of initial resection, intraoral mucosal incisions are made and the extent of mandibular invasion is evaluated by careful dissection of the tumor away from the mandible. When assessing bony involvement in this manner, the surgeon typically encounters one of three possible patterns of invasion. In the first scenario, the deeply invasive tumor has extended to, but not through, the mandibular periosteum. In these cases, the periosteum lifts

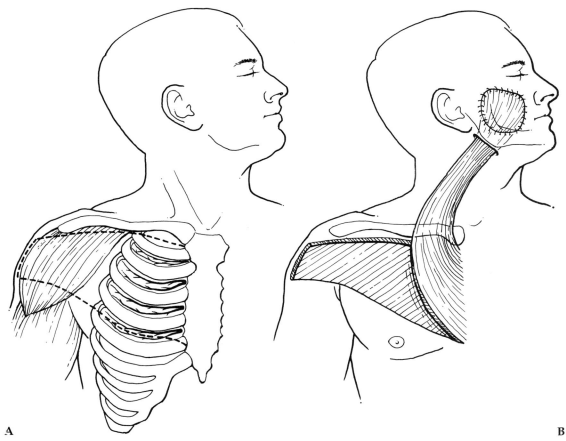

FIGURE 20–4 Deltopectoral flap. (A). Skin flap outlined. (B). Flap rotated superiorly to form tube.

cleanly from the underlying bone in continuity with the resected specimen and no further bony resection is necessary.

In the second scenario, tumor has extended through the bony periosteum and is adjacent to, but not eroding into, the mandibular cortex. In these cases, to obtain an adequate surgical margin, a mandibular shave excision must be performed. Shaving removes a split thickness of cortical bone in continuity with the tumor specimen. Shaving can only be performed in certain regions of the mandible where bone is thickest, including the mentum and body. The thin bone at the angle and ascending ramus is difficult to shave, and segmental mandibulectomy is usually required for adequate resection in cases where periosteum is violated. Occasionally, shaving can also be performed when the tumor approximates the periosteum, but does not invade through, as in the first scenario presented.

In the third scenario, tumor has invaded deeply through periosteum and cortical bone. When this occurs, the surgeon must assume that cancer has spread throughout the marrow space of the hemimandible. Tumor entering the marrow space freely invades the inferior alveolar nerve; therefore, in such cases, the hemimandible is resected to include the entire course of the inferior alveolar nerve from the lingula to the mental foramen (Fig. 20–1).

Alveolar malignancy that has grown to involve the mandible in the edentulous patient may be treated with shave excision. In this manner, the superior margin of the mandibular alveolus is resected with the primary tumor. The technique works well in the edentulous mandible that has lost little bony height, thereby allowing the surgeon to preserve a continuous inferior bony strip and not disturb mandibular continuity. In cases where an edentulous mandible has lost considerable height secondary to bony resorption, the superior mandibular shave may leave the patient with a thin inferior strip, and pathologic fracture may occur. In such cases, a segmental mandibulectomy is a better option. Alveolar tumors that deeply invade bone of the dentulous mandible are best treated with segmental mandibulectomy, as the marrow space may be involved with tumor.

MANDIBULAR RECONSTRUCTION

Many techniques of mandibular reconstruction have been described in the literature.

SPECIAL CONSIDERATION

Regardless of the technique chosen, the two most important considerations in reconstruction are function and cosmesis. It is difficult to have hard-and-fast rules regarding mandibular reconstruction as all cases presenting to the surgeon have different surrounding circumstances. In general, however, the location of the defect, the prognosis of the disease process, and the patient's comorbidities are essential to consider in the management of mandibular defects.

The first option in mandibular reconstruction is no bony replacement. This is best chosen for the lateral segmental mandibular body, angle, or ascending ramus defect. In such cases, soft tissue coverage alone with a myocutaneous flap (pectoralis major) is adequate. Patients function normally with adequate masticatory compensation from the opposite side. Speech is unaffected if enough tongue remains to provide adequate articulation. The main disadvantage in not providing bony reconstruction is the cosmetic deformity that results.

The second option in mandibular reconstruction is to replace bone with foreign material. Although in the past, trays filled with cancellous bone and marrow have been used, this

technique has fallen out of favor. The placement of prefabricated titanium plates to approximate proximal and distal bony remnants is more commonly used. A variety of different plate styles are commercially available and include those with artificial condyles that can sit in the glenoid fossa.

PITFALL... The artificial condyle may erode into the middle cranial fossa, and several authors have abandoned this plate style, believing there is significant risk of morbidity with little improvement in function.

In patients who may be concerned about facial appearance after segmental body, angle, or ramus mandibulectomy, a plate covered by a myocutaneous flap can be placed to stabilize the bony fragments and improve mandibular contour. Some disadvantages to the use of reconstructive plates include the potential development of mandibular osteomyelitis, intraoral or external plate exposure, plate fracture, and pathologic bone fracture of remaining remnants. Both pathologic fracture and osteomyelitis are difficult to treat and, at a minimum, require plate removal.

The third option in mandibular reconstruction is to replace bone with bone. In the past, a popular technique for replacing bone was to harvest the fifth or sixth rib with a pectoralis major myocutaneous flap. This is no longer used as the rib was found to be nonviable. Since the development of microvascular techniques allowing for the harvest and reimplantation of vascularized free tissue, "free flaps" are now almost exclusively used for the replacement of bone with bone in mandibular reconstruction (see Chap. 88). Iliac crest from the contralateral hip provides bone with excellent mandibular contour for body and angle reconstruction. Donor-site morbidity includes significant pain in the hip with exercise.

One of the more favored free tissue transfers for mandibular defects is the fibula. This tissue may be elevated as an osseous flap alone or as an osseocutaneous free tissue transfer with a portion of the lateral calf skin for reconstruction of soft tissue defects. The fibular bone is easily contoured and has enough length to reconstruct the mandible from condyle to condyle in most cases. Split-thickness skin graft is often required to close the donor site defect on the leg. Delayed wound healing of the donor site in poorly vascularized lower extremities may occur. Immobilization of the lower extremity is often necessary in the postoperative period.

The scapular flap including the spine of the scapula as well as two separate skin islands is also excellent for mandibular reconstruction. This flap provides bone that is less stable than the fibula; however, it does yield large skin paddles that may be used to reconstruct massive soft tissue defects.

There is little doubt that free tissue transfer is an excellent method of mandibular reconstruction, yielding adequate results in function and cosmesis. However, there are disadvantages to the technique as well, including prolonged operating time, the need for a second surgical team, the degree of technical difficulty in performing the vascular anastomosis, arterial and venous insufficiency leading to flap failure and reoperation, and donor-site morbidity.

SPECIAL CONSIDERATION

Many consider anterior segmental mandibulectomy to be an absolute indication for reconstruction of the mandibular defect using free tissue transfer. These patients lose support of the anterior tongue and floor of mouth. The resulting "Andy Gump" deformity leads to oral incompetence and airway compromise.

SUGGESTED READINGS

Ariyan S, Cuono CB. Myocutaneous flaps for head and neck reconstruction. *Head Neck Surg* 1980;2(4):321–345.

Ariyan S, Ross DA, Sasaki CT. Reconstruction of the head and neck. *Surg Oncol Clin North Am* 1997;6(1):1–43.

Biller HF, Baek SM, Lawson W, Krespi YP, Blaugrund SM. Pectoralis major myocutaneous island flap in head and neck surgery: analysis of complications in 42 cases. *Arch Otolaryngol* 1981;107(1):23–26.

Davis JP, Nield DV, Garth RJ, Breach NM. The latissimus dorsi flap in head and neck reconstructive surgery: a review of 121 procedures. *Clin Otolaryngol* 1992;17(6):487–490.

Gilas T, Sako K, Razack MS, Bakamjian VY, Shedd DP, Calamel PM. Major head and neck reconstruction using the deltopectoral flap. A 20 year experience. *Am J Surg* 1986; 152(4):430–434.

Guillamondegui OM, Larson DL. The lateral trapezius musculocutaneous flap: its use in head and neck reconstruction. *Plast Reconstr Surg* 1981;67(2):143–150.

Haughey BH. The jejunal free flap in oral cavity and pharyngeal reconstruction. *Otolaryngol Clin North Am* 1994;27(6):1159–1170.

Komisar A, Lawson W. A compendium of intraoral flaps. *Head Neck Surg* 1985;8(2):91–99.

Moscoso JF, Urken ML. Radial forearm flaps. *Otolaryngol Clin North Am* 1994;27(6):1119–1140.

Urken ML. Composite free flaps in oromandibular reconstruction. Review of the literature. *Arch Otolaryngol Head Neck Surg* 1991;117(7): 724–732.

Wurster CF, Ossoff RH. Reconstructive techniques after ablative head and neck surgery. *Otolaryngol Clin North Am* 1985;18(3):551–572.

SECTION IV

PHARYNX

Chapter 21

ANATOMY AND PHYSIOLOGY

Lyon L. Gleich

EMBRYOLOGY

The pharynx forms from the elongation and growth of the primitive foregut. The foregut also develops into the esophagus, stomach, and proximal small intestine. Outgrowths from the ventral wall of the caudal pharynx develop into the lower respiratory tract. The pharyngeal arches indent against the foregut during development. Mesodermal migrations from the branchial arches lead to development of the larynx within the caudal portion of the pharynx. The endoderm of the foregut and pharyngeal pouches forms the internal lining of the pharynx.

ANATOMY

The pharynx is a musculomembranous tube that extends from the base of the skull to the level of the sixth cervical vertebra, where it is contiguous with the esophagus. The pharynx is subdivided into the nasopharynx, the oropharynx, and the hypopharynx. The nasopharynx is that part of the pharynx above the soft palate (see Section V). The oropharynx extends from the soft palate superiorly to the level of the hyoid inferiorly. Anteriorly it extends to the circumvallate papilla of the tongue. Major structures of the oropharynx are the palatine tonsils, soft palate, and tongue base. The hypopharynx includes that portion of the pharynx below the level of the hyoid. The regions of the hypopharynx are the pyriform sinus, posterior pharyngeal wall, and postcricoid region.

The pharyngeal walls consist of mucosa, muscle, and intervening fascia. The mucosal lining of the oropharynx and hypopharynx is a nonkeratinizing stratified squamous epithelium that is tightly adherent to an underlying layer of fascia called the pharyngobasilar fascia. The pharynx is surrounded by three constrictor muscles—the superior, middle, and inferior constrictors (Fig. 21–1). The constrictor muscles each insert on the posterior midline raphe, and the inferior muscles overlap the more superior muscles. The palatopharyngeus, salpingopharyngeus, and stylopharyngeus muscles each provide additional support to the pharynx. The pharyngeal muscles are enclosed by the buccopharyngeal or visceral fascia. Areas of loose connective tissue surround the visceral fascia of the pharynx and are potential spaces for infection. The retropharyngeal space is posterior to the buccopharyngeal fascia, and the lateral pharyngeal spaces are lateral.

The pharyngeal submucosa contains numerous mucous and serous glands. Lymphatics are plentiful and drain throughout the neck, but most specifically to the upper and middle deep cervical nodes and to the retropharyngeal nodes.

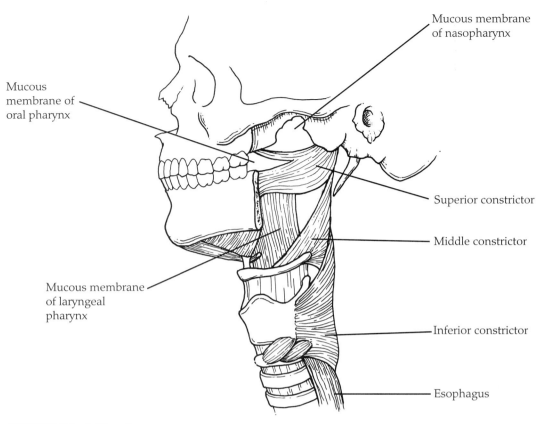

Mucous membrane of nasopharynx

Mucous membrane of oral pharynx

Superior constrictor

Middle constrictor

Mucous membrane of laryngeal pharynx

Inferior constrictor

Esophagus

FIGURE 21-1 The pharynx.

Despite the overlap between the constrictor muscles, these regions are potential areas of weakness. The gap between the superior and middle constrictor muscles is filled by the stylopharyngeus muscle along with the ninth cranial nerve and the lingual artery and nerve. The gap between the middle and inferior constrictor muscles is filled by the thyrohyoid membrane. The thyrohyoid membrane is pierced by the superior laryngeal vessels and the internal branch of the superior laryngeal nerve. The anatomy of the upper esophageal sphincter region is discussed in Section VIII.

THE TONSILS

Waldeyer's ring is a continuous band of lymphoid tissue that surrounds the upper pharynx. The superior portion of the ring is located in the nasopharynx and is composed of the adenoids. Laterally the palatine tonsils and anteriorly the lingual tonsils complete the ring. Lymphoid tissue is present in the soft tissues surrounding and connecting these structures.

The palatine tonsils represent the largest accumulation of lymphoid tissue in Waldeyer's ring. The palatine tonsils are remnants of the second branchial groove. The supporting soft tissues of the tonsillar fossa are derived from the second and third branchial arches. The tonsillar fossa is formed by the palatopharyngeus muscle, which contributes to the posterior pillar, and by the palatoglossus muscle, which contributes to the anterior pillar. The palatine tonsil is composed of lymphoid cells and connective tissue. Tonsillar crypts extend deeply into the body of the tonsil and are surrounded by lymphoid nodules. Debris and foreign particles collect within the crypts.

A specialized portion of the pharyngobasilar fascia envelops the deep portion of the tonsil. This tonsillar capsule permits the tonsil to be removed from the surrounding tissue in the peritonsillar space. After infection, this space may become increasingly fibrotic, causing increasing difficulty during tonsillectomy.

The palatine tonsil has a rich blood supply from the external carotid artery branches. The lower pole of the tonsil receives branches from the following arteries: the dorsal lingual artery, the ascending palatine artery from the facial artery, and the tonsillar branch of the facial artery. The upper pole of the tonsil receives branches from the ascending pharyngeal artery and the lesser palatine artery. The tonsillar branch of the facial artery is the largest vessel. The venous drainage is via a pericapsular plexus of veins into the lingual vein or the pharyngeal plexus.

> **PEARL...** The internal carotid artery lies approximately 2 cm from the palatine tonsils, but contributes no branches.

The lymphatic drainage of the tonsils is primarily to the superior deep cervical nodes and deep jugular nodes. Sensory innervation is via the lesser palatine nerve and tonsillar branches of the glossopharyngeal nerve.

> **SPECIAL CONSIDERATION**
>
> Tonsillar tumors or infections may result in ear pain due to referred pain conducted by cranial nerve IX.

TONGUE BASE

The sulcus terminalis, just posterior to the circumvallate papillae, divides the anterior two-thirds of the tongue from the posterior oropharyngeal portion. The hypobranchial eminence from the third and fourth arches forms the posterior third of the tongue. The posterior tongue has no papillae, but is covered with the lymphoid tissue of the lingual tonsils. The hypoglossal nerve provides motor innervation. Taste from the posterior tongue is mediated by the glossopharyngeal nerve. The lingual artery provides an abundant arterial supply.

The tongue base develops embryologically as a single structure and therefore has a rich lymphatic communication across the midline. The lymphatic drainage is primarily to the upper deep cervical nodes and retropharyngeal nodes. The tongue lymphatics are plentiful, and tumors therefore present with early metastases.

> **SPECIAL CONSIDERATIONS**
>
> The tongue base arises embryologically as a single midline structure and therefore has significant vascular and lymphatic anastomoses. The oral tongue, however, arises as separate structures that fuse. Tongue base tumors, therefore, have a higher risk of contralateral spread than oral tongue tumors that are not at the midline.

HYPOPHARYNX ANATOMY

The hypopharynx is a mucosa-lined tube bounded by muscles posteriorly and laterally and by the larynx anteriorly. For classification purposes, it is subdivided into the pyriform sinus, posterior pharyngeal wall, and postcricoid region; however, these areas are all histologically similar to each other and to the oropharynx. The pyriform sinus is an inverted pyramid that is open superiorly where it is contiguous with the glossopharyngeal sulcus of the oropharynx and inferiorly ends in an apex. The pyriform sinus is limited medially by the larynx, anteriorly by soft tissue, and laterally by the thyroid cartilage. The posterior pharyngeal wall is contiguous with the lateral wall of the pyriform sinus. The constrictor muscles are deep to this region. The postcricoid region extends from the posterior surface of the arytenoids and covers the posterior aspect of the cricoid cartilage.

The glossopharyngeal and vagus nerves form a flexus that provides the motor and sensory innervation to the hypopharynx. The lymphatic supply is rich and drains to the upper, middle, and lower deep cervical nodes as well as to the retropharyngeal nodes. Nodal metastases therefore occur early in hypopharyngeal tumors. Additionally, the vagal innervation to the pyriform sinus frequently results in referred pain to the ear mediated via Arnold's nerve.

PHYSIOLOGY

The tongue forces the food bolus through the oropharyngeal isthmus into the oropharynx. The palatoglossus muscle then contracts to prevent reflux into the oral cavity. The larynx then elevates, and through a combination of tongue thrusts and pharyngeal muscular contractions the food is propelled through the hypopharynx and into the esophagus. Any lack of muscular coordination or sensation can significantly impair swallowing, resulting in aspiration.

SUGGESTED READING

Hollinshead WH. The pharynx. In: Hollinshead WH, ed. *Anatomy for Surgeons: The Head and Neck.* 3rd ed. Philadelphia: JB Lippincott; 1982:389–410.

Chapter 22

CLINICAL TESTS

Lyon L. Gleich

The most important clinical test for evaluating pharyngeal disorders, after a thorough history, is visual inspection and palpation. The oropharynx can be well visualized with good lighting, and the tongue base can be palpated to detect subtle changes. Cranial nerve function should be evaluated. Any abnormal lesions seen or palpated that may be neoplastic generally warrant biopsy.

SPECIAL CONSIDERATION

In performing the head and neck examination, it is crucial to palpate the oral cavity and oropharynx, as tumors can be palpable with only subtle surface abnormalities.

RADIOLOGY

Radiologic evaluations have a role in specific disease entities of the oropharynx. For a suspected retropharyngeal abscess, a lateral neck film can reveal thickening anterior to the vertebrae. Computed tomography (CT) scans are useful in further delineating the extent of pharyngeal tumors and masses. For small tumors a CT scan is less valuable, as the endoscopic exam may permit complete tumor visualization. However, for larger tumors a CT scan may demon-

strate unsuspected involvement of the infratemporal fossa and skull base or of the prevertebral space. In general, CT is preferable to magnetic resonance imaging (MRI) for its ability to better distinguish the tumor's relationship to osseous structures. MRI is particularly useful in evaluating tongue base lesions, where its ability to distinguish soft tissue interfaces is valuable.

PEARL... The barium swallow can be useful in evaluating dysphagia of unclear etiology. The barium swallow can also be modified as needed to test for particular swallowing difficulties. This will often be accomplished by having the patient swallow not only liquid barium but also barium mixed in pudding and cookies to determine what difficulties occur with different substances. A modified swallow of this type can delineate abnormalities of pharyngeal contraction and enable the therapist to find positions or exercises that may permit the patient to overcome the region where there is an inability to propel the food bolus.

THROAT CULTURES

A common question that arises is the need for throat cultures in cases of tonsillitis. At the initial presentation of tonsillitis, empiric antibiotic therapy is sufficient and cultures are not cost-effective. If the patient fails to respond to the antibiotic or the infection recurs soon after, a culture may be useful in directing future therapy.

CONTROVERSY

When cultures are obtained to evaluate tonsillitis, usually only aerobic cultures are performed. In studies that have collected specimens appropriately for both aerobic and anaerobic culture, anaerobes have been frequently detected. The clinical significance of these anaerobic cultures is undefined and, because anaerobic cultures require rapid processing and special handling, their clinical application is unclear in the routine management of tonsillitis.

POLYSOMNOGRAPHY

Polysomnography is the most reliable method to evaluate for obstructive sleep apnea. Patients who are being evaluated for snoring should be evaluated for obstructive sleep apnea because, whereas benign snoring may be bothersome, obstructive sleep apnea can be dangerous. A polysomnogram includes monitoring of an electroencephalogram, airflow, rib cage and abdominal effort, esophageal pressure, oxygen saturation, and EKG.

PEARL... To reduce costs, portions of the testing are frequently omitted, or the study is performed for shorter periods, or it is performed in the home. These limited tests are assumed to be less sensitive.

From the polysomnography, the apnea index is defined as the average number of apneas per hour. The respiratory disturbance index is the number of apneas or hypopneas divided by the total sleep time. A respiratory disturbance index of 6 to 20 is reported as mild obstructive sleep apnea, an index of 21 to 40 as moderate, and an index of greater than 40 as severe.

SUGGESTED READINGS

Brook I, Yocum P, Foote PA Jr. Changes in the core tonsillar bacteriology of recurrent tonsillitis. *Clin Infect Dis* 1995;21:171–176.

Tami TA, Duncan HJ, Pfleger M. Identification of obstructive sleep apnea in patients who snore. *Laryngoscope* 1998;108:508–513.

Chapter 23

CONGENITAL DISORDERS

Lyon L. Gleich

Congenital disorders affecting only the pharynx are uncommon. Most often a congenital disorder that involves the pharynx also involves other regions as well, especially the oral cavity. An example would be Treacher-Collins syndrome, in which the mandibulofacial dysostosis affects structures that arise from the first branchial arch, groove, and pouch. In this syndrome the mandibular hypoplasia results in a relative glossoptosis that can cause pharyngeal obstruction leading to respiratory embarrassment. The congenital abnormalities in this syndrome are therefore in the oral cavity, but the pharynx is directly impacted upon by the disorder. The changes that occur in congenital disorders of regions that abut the pharynx, such as the oral cavity or midface, can therefore result in significant pharyngeal compromise or malformation. Maldevelopment can occur in the tongue as part of a syndrome, such as macroglossia in Down syndrome, or as an isolated occurrence.

LINGUAL THYROID

The most common congenital disorder that affects the base of the tongue is lingual thyroid. The thyroid gland embryologically descends from the foramen cecum, immediately posterior to the circumvallate papillae. If there is a failure of either all or part of the thyroid to descend, a mass will persist at the tongue base. This occurs clinically in 1 in 10,000 individuals.

With time the lingual thyroid mass can increase in size due to thyroid-stimulating hormone affecting this marginally functional tissue. This may cause dysphagia, dyspnea, or dysphonia. On examination the mass is smooth and mucosally covered. Thyroid function tests should be performed.

> **PEARL•••** Treatment with thyroid hormone usually results in regression and the relief of symptoms. If the mass is symptomatic and fails to respond to thyroid hormone, or begins to hemorrhage, surgical excision is indicated.

SPECIAL CONSIDERATION

The cervical thyroid is absent in approximately 70% of patients with a lingual thyroid.

SOFT PALATE

Abnormal development of the soft palate can have significant consequences. The soft palate forms from a posterior extension of the mesoderm of the fused palatine processes. The soft palate can be short, resulting in velopharyngeal incompetence. This may be seen in patients with Down syndrome or may occur as an isolated abnormality.

PEARL... Adenoidectomy should be avoided in patients with a short palate because the adenoid mass may aid in preventing velopharyngeal incompetence.

A bifid uvula is associated with a submucus cleft palate. Adenoidectomy should be approached cautiously in these patients as well. If there is also palatal insufficiency, there may be hypernasal speech. In a cleft of the secondary palate, the numerous muscles involved in the function of the soft palate are hypoplastic and insert into the posterior edge of the remnant hard palate instead of the midline raphae. This results in severe velopharyngeal incompetence with hypernasal speech and nasal regurgitation when swallowing.

Clefts limited to the soft palate are frequently closed at 6 to 18 months. Surgical repair is generally preferable to prosthetic rehabilitation because children under 3 years of age rarely tolerate the prostheses. If a patient is already successfully using an obturator, surgery may not be indicated. Surgical methods of soft palate cleft repair include (1) the Von Langenbeck's palatoplasty, which utilizes bipedicled mucoperiosteal flaps that are advanced medially to close the cleft, and (2) the V-Y pushback, which involves creating two posteriorly based unipedicled flaps to lengthen the palate.

PEARL... The most common complication of soft palate cleft repair is persistent hypernasal speech. Speech therapy can aid the child in overcoming this. If further palatal lengthening cannot be performed, a pharyngoplasty may aid in further reducing the velopharyngeal inlet.

OTHER DISORDERS

Branchial cleft cysts may extend into the pharynx. A second branchial cleft cyst can extend to the tonsillar fossa, and a third branchial cleft cyst can extend to the hypopharynx. Congenital tumors that may present in the pharynx include teratomas, chordomas, craniopharyngiomas, cystic hygromas, and hemangiomas.

Chapter 24

INFECTIOUS AND INFLAMMATORY DISORDERS

David L. Walner and Sally R. Shott

INFECTIOUS DISORDERS

Pharyngitis is prevalent during the cold weather season. It is more common in children than in adults. In children, pharyngitis is most common after the age of 6 months. As maternal immunity fades, children become more susceptible to upper respiratory infections. An increased rate of infection should be expected if the child attends a day-care center. Children may experience up to six or eight upper respiratory infections per year, with approximately 50% of them associated with pharyngitis.

BACTERIAL

Adenotonsillitis

The onset of acute adenotonsillitis is often abrupt and manifested by chills, low-grade fever, malaise, thirst, odynophagia, dysphagia, nasal speech, and swollen and tender cervical lymph nodes. On examination, the tonsils are red and swollen, often contacting each other in the midline with yellowish or white spots or vesicles formed on them. Malodorous breath can also accompany this disorder.

Staphylococcus aureus, group A β-hemolytic streptococcus, and *Haemophilus influenzae* are the most common bacterial causes of acute pharyngitis/tonsillitis. However, other potential etiologic agents include anaerobic bacteria, actinomyces, viruses (especially adenovirus), Epstein-Barr virus (EBV) gonococci, and cornibacterium diphtheria. The normal adult flora also contains both gram-positive and gram-negative organisms as well as anaerobic bacteria, although gram-positive bacteria usually predominate and include lactobacilli, actinomyces, and leptothix.

The treatment of acute adenotonsillitis includes increased oral intake, bed rest, analgesics, and antipyretic medications. In the majority of cases, the symptoms are self-limited, and recovery occurs regardless of whether antibiotics are given. Antibiotics are indicated, however, in cases where the offending organism is group A β-hemolytic streptococcus. The purpose of antibiotic treatment in these cases is prevention of potential renal and cardiac sequelae. In addition, treatment of strep tonsillitis shortens the length of the illness, eradicates the streptococcus from the pharynx so the infection cannot be transmitted to others, and prevents possible suppurative complications. The drug of choice is penicillin (if the patient is not penicillin allergic) for a 10-day course. Erythromycin can be used as a second-line agent. Clindamycin can also be utilized in patients who are allergic to penicillin.

Another treatment option would be a first-generation cephalosporin. Pichichero (1993) found that the first-generation cephalosporins have a lower clinical failure rate compared to penicillin, and treatment success was achieved in only 5 days of treatment, compared to the 10 days needed with penicillin. Overall however, it is generally accepted that if the community failure rate with penicillin is low, less than 10%, penicillin should be the first-line treatment. In addition, one may want to consider the use of the cephalosporin in cases where posttreatment reculturing is not planned.

Although acute bacterial tonsillitis is generally self-limited, it can be complicated by peritonsillar edema and airway obstruction leading to a peritonsillar abscess, deep neck infection, septicemia, rheumatic fever, and even glomerulonephritis, if neglected. This disorder must be differentiated from diphtheria, scarlet fever, Vincent's angina or trench mouth, and various viral disorders.

Chronic Tonsillitis

Chronic tonsillitis represents persistent inflammation of the tonsils as a result of recurrent acute or subclinical infections. Enlargement of the tonsils can occur due to hyperplasia of the parenchymal structures or fibrinoid degeneration with obstruction of the tonsil crypts. This condition is more commonly seen in adults but can occur at any age.

The organisms responsible for chronic tonsillitis are similar to those involved in acute infections, generally due to gram-positive bacteria. These patients usually have complaints of recurrent sore throats that may be associated with viral illness, malaise, and joint pain. Cervical adenopathy is also commonly present, as is halitosis from obstructed tonsillar crypts.

On examination, the tonsils are usually covered by some degree of debris or purulent material within tonsillar crypts. The tonsillar pillars may show signs of scarring or chronic inflammation.

Treatment generally consists of increased oral intake, adequate rest, analgesics, and antibiotics when indicated. In cases of chronic or recurrent tonsillitis/pharyngitis, the use of an antibiotic with β-lactamase coverage (e.g., cephalosporins),

or anaerobic coverage (e.g., clindamycin) may be helpful prior to moving onto more definitive surgical treatment. Definitive therapy would involve tonsillectomy, generally suggested if the patient has more than five to seven infections in 1 year, four to five infections each year for 2 successive years, or 3 infections each year for 3 successive years. These guidelines must be taken into consideration with regard to the patient's lifestyle changes due to the chronic condition such as inability to attend school or work.

DIPHTHERIA

Diphtheria is generally suspected if a dirty-gray membrane covers the tonsils, tonsillar pillars, soft palate, and uvula.

> **PEARL...** Contact with these lesions generally causes bleeding.

The symptoms of this condition are generally mild but can progress to upper airway obstruction or cardiac toxicity. Cultures of the plaques need to be studied with fluorescent antibodies. The presence of Klebs-Löffler bacillus in the membrane is diagnosed by Gram stain and culture.

> **SPECIAL CONSIDERATION**
>
> The treatment for diphtheria is generally considered an emergency, and antitoxins should be given within the first 48 hours of onset to be effective.

Penicillin in high doses should be administered. Patients need to be evaluated for airway obstruction. If present, a tracheostomy may be required for the most severe infections.

Vincent's Angina

Vincent's angina is due to *Spirochaeta denticulata*. This condition generally appears when living conditions are overcrowded, and it tends to have a slow, sometimes insidious onset. Patients present with jugular-digastric lymph node enlargement, sore throat, headache, and malaise. Often a membrane is found on the tonsil that sloughs and goes on to form an ulcer. Treatment is with penicillin.

VIRAL AND FUNGAL

Infections of the oropharynx and nasopharynx can also be caused by viruses. Most of these conditions are self-limited and resolve within 48 hours. Positive agents that have been identified include adenoviridae and enteroviridae. The treatment for these infections is generally nonspecific and symptomatic.

> **PITFALL...** Antibiotics should not be used unless a secondary bacterial infection has evolved.

Infectious Mononucleosis

Infectious mononucleosis often resembles a severe attack of acute tonsillitis. The patient may present with fever, pharyngitis, cervical adenopathy, and splenomegaly. Other symptoms include malaise, sore throat, dysphagia, and odynophagia. Examination will reveal enlarged tonsils, often with a dirty-gray exudate. The soft palate may be edematous with petechiae.

> **PITFALL...** It has been estimated that one-third of these patients will have β-hemolytic streptococcus cultured from the throat. Therefore, it is appropriate to cover these patients for a bacterial tonsillitis. The Epstein-Barr virus, which is a ubiquitous member of the human herpes virus group, is the causative agent. This heterophile antibody positive disease is also known as "glandular fever." Tonsillar hypertrophy may be significant enough to cause airway obstruction. On the other hand, fleeting scarlatiniform rashes may develop in association with ampicillin, and less often with other antibiotic use.

In mononucleosis, the white blood cell count is elevated to 10,000 to 15,000 with 50% or more lymphocytes, which are atypical in structure. The EBV-specific heterophile antibody serologic test is positive. Monospot tests for infectious mononucleosis are directed against heterophile antibodies and are the tests most frequently employed in the diagnosis.

In most cases the disease resolves completely in 1 to 3 weeks but occasionally it persists longer. Treatment is supportive, including bed rest, until the fever has resolved, with a gradual return to physical activity. Care must be taken in patients with splenomegaly to avoid physical activity. Rarely, hospital admission is required due to tonsillar hypertrophy and airway obstruction. In these cases monitoring for potential airway obstruction is appropriate, and corticosteroids may be of use. If the severity of airway obstruction is significant and/or the airway obstruction fails to resolve with supportive care and corticosteroids, tonsillectomy and/or adenoidectomy may be warranted.

Varicella

This condition generally has an incubation period of 13 to 17 days and presents with a rash followed by vesicular lesions that start on the trunk and spread to the extremities. These vesicular lesions can also be found on any mucous membrane and thus may be seen in the pharynx. The most common complication of varicella is a secondary bacterial infection usually due to staphylococcal or streptococcal species. In addition, progression can lead to myocarditis, pericarditis, endocarditis, hepatitis, and glomerulonephritis. If the condition spreads to the central nervous system, it can cause encephalitis, cerebellar ataxia, transverse myelitis, or an ascending paralysis (Guillain-Barré syndrome). However, if uncomplicated, treatment for the majority of patients is symptomatic for relief of severe itching of the skin lesions.

Measles (Rubeola)

Measles may be characterized by conjunctivitis and a generalized maculopapular rash with Koplik spots in the mouth. The Koplik spots are most commonly found opposite the lower molars but can involve the pharynx. In the immunocompromised patient this condition can be life threatening.

Candida Albicans

Infections involving the pharynx caused by *Candida albicans* are called "thrush." Thrush can be a common finding in children up to 6 months of age or occurs after a course of antimicrobial therapy. Thrush has also been associated with other conditions such as hyperparathyroidism, diabetes, adrenal insufficiency, leukemia, or acquired immunodeficiency syndrome (AIDS). In the pseudomembranous form, yellow-white plaques are present that have an appearance resembling "milk curds" (Fig. 24–1). In the erythematous form, such plaques have disappeared (Fig. 24–2). Treatment is with oral nystatin.

Human Immunodeficiency Virus (HIV)

Patients with HIV infection can present with a multitude of lesions in the pharynx. These can include fungal infections such as candida or numerous viral infections including herpes simplex, herpes zoster, or others.

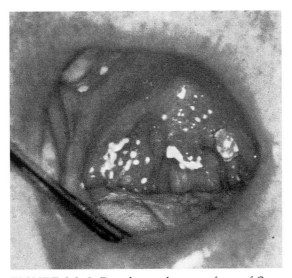

FIGURE 24–1 Pseudomembranous form of *Candida albicans* showing yellow-white plaques. See Color Plate 24–1.

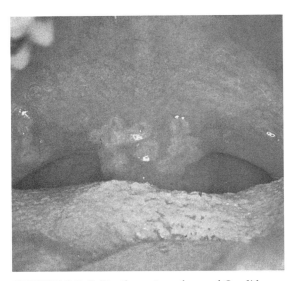

FIGURE 24–2 Erythematous form of *Candida albicans*. Yellow-white plaques visible in the pseudomembranous form have disappeared. See Color Plate 24–2.

COMPLICATIONS OF OROPHARYNGEAL INFECTIONS

Peritonsillar Abscess (Quinsy)

Peritonsillar abscesses usually occur in patients with recurrent tonsillitis or those with chronic tonsillitis that has been inadequately treated. However, the absence of any history of tonsillitis is not uncommon. This disease process is more common in young adults. Usually the process begins with a peritonsillar cellulitis that progresses into an abscess that extends beyond the tonsillar capsule. The abscess forms in the potential space between the buccopharyngeal fascia and the capsule itself. Abscess within the body of the tonsil itself is actually rare. The swelling usually causes edema of the soft palate and displaces the tonsil medially forward and downward. This generally causes deviation of the uvula to the normal side. It is unusual for this process to be bilateral.

Patients generally complain of extreme unilateral soreness of the throat with odynophagia, drooling, and trismus. Otalgia on the side of the infection is not uncommon. If the process has been present for a period of time, the patients are often dehydrated. Airway obstruction can occur due to the swelling caused by the infection and inability to handle one's secretions.

CONTROVERSY

Treatment of this condition has become a source of great debate. Intravenous antibiotics, needle aspiration, incision and drainage and tonsillectomy are all commonly practiced. Treatment for children and adults may vary. Recognition of the process and initiation of some form of therapy are essential.

Because it can be difficult at times to differentiate a peritonsillar cellulitis from a true abscess, some opt to initially treat with 24 hours of intravenous antibiotics and hydration. If the patient improves during this time, the infection is most likely a cellulitis that will probably continue to improve with parental antibiotics. Others perform needle aspiration followed by intravenous antibiotics. Many advocate incision and drainage of all peritonsillar abscesses. Because of the lack of cooperation in the pediatric population for an incision procedure in the office, many choose to perform a tonsillectomy as the definitive treatment, often after a trial of parenteral antibiotics and hydration. Cultures of the pus obtained generally show mixed bacteria, both aerobic and anaerobic. Treatment with intravenous antibiotics is generally with penicillin or clindamycin.

Retropharyngeal Space Infection

The retropharyngeal space lies behind the pharynx and esophagus, just anterior to the prevertebral fascia. It extends superiorly to the base of the skull and inferiorly to the bifurcation of the trachea. A midline raphe, formed from the attachment of the superior constrictor muscle to the alar layer of the deep cervical fascia, separates two chains of lymph nodes that lie in this potential space.

Patients generally present with trismus, drooling, dyspnea, dysphagia, and a mass, often fluctuant, on one side of the posterior pharyngeal wall.

PEARL... In children, in whom examination of the oropharynx is difficult and sometimes quite brief, use of the nasopharyngoscope will provide better visualization of the posterior pharyngeal wall.

Lateral radiographs of the neck are also helpful in diagnosis. It is important, however, to have proper positioning of the patient at the time of X-ray; otherwise the results may be misleading. The patient should have the neck extended in a true lateral position for the X-ray.

PEARL... If widening of the soft tissue shadow at the level of C2 is more than 7 mm in width or wider than the vertebral body, it is considered abnormal. At the level of C6 widening of the retrotracheal tissue is abnormal in children under 5 years if it is more than 14 mm and in adults if it is more than 22 mm.

A more sensitive evaluation is through a computed tomography (CT) scan of the retropharynx. A ring-enhanced lesion in this area is suggestive of an abscess. The presence of air within the lesion confirms that an abscess is present.

Once an abscess is diagnosed or suspected, either by air within the area of swelling, by CT scan evaluation, or by failure to improve on antibiotics, a drainage procedure in the operating room is required. This is performed under general anesthesia. A vertical incision followed by blunt dissection is made just off the midline in the posterior pharyngeal wall. A CT scan is helpful in localizing the level of the abscess.

Parapharyngeal Space Abscess

The parapharyngeal space is cone shaped. Superiorly it starts at the base of the skull and inferiorly its margin ends at the hyoid bone. The superior constrictor muscle is the medial boundary, and the parotid gland, the mandible, and the pterygoid muscle are its lateral margins.

Posteriorly, the prevertebral fascia is present. This space is divided into an anterior and posterior division by the styloid process, and is intimately involved with the great vessels in the neck.

A parapharyngeal space abscess can develop when infection or pus from the tonsillar region goes through the superior constrictor muscle. The abscess then forms between the superior constrictor muscle and deep cervical fascia. Patients can present with toxemia and pain in the throat and neck, with tender swelling of the neck in the region of the angle of the mandible. Examination may reveal tonsillitis and/or medial displacement of the tonsil. Trismus may also be present due to inflammation and edema around the pterygoid musculature. If only the posterior compartment is involved, there may be no trismus, but rather swelling of the lateral pharyngeal wall and perhaps of the posterior tonsillar pillar. This condition is best diagnosed by CT scan.

Once a parapharyngeal abscess is identified it needs to be surgically drained.

PEARL... The safest approach to the parapharyngeal space is through a lateral cervical approach identifying the great vessels. Following incision and drainage the wound is packed open for residual drainage for a period of 24 to 72 hours.

INFLAMMATORY PROCESSES

The pharynx is frequently involved in systemic inflammatory or vascular processes.

KAWASAKI DISEASE

Kawasaki disease is also known as mucocutaneous lymph node syndrome. It is an acute, multisystem disease that predominantly affects children. The clinical guidelines that establish the diagnosis have been set by the Centers for Disease Control. Many of the symptoms that make up this disease can first present as complaints to an otolaryngologist. The diagnostic criteria include fever for at least 5 days and four of the following signs:

1. Bilateral conjunctivitis (nonpurulent)
2. Oral cavity changes such as fissured lips, strawberry tongue, pharyngitis
3. Red palms or soles of the feet, edema of the hands or feet, and/or desquamation of the fingers and toes
4. Rash—polymorphous on trunk or face
5. Cervical lymphadenopathy

Early treatment can prevent potential complications of coronary artery aneurysm and thrombosis. Treatment consists of high-dose intravenous gammaglobulin and oral aspirin.

SYSTEMIC LUPUS ERYTHEMATOSUS

This condition most often affects adolescents and women. The oral cavity and oropharynx is involved in 25% of patients. The initial symptoms include fatigue, weakness, fever, and weight loss. Also seen is a butterfly rash over the malar region, arthritis, vasculitis, and photosensitivity. Cardiac involvement can also be present as can renal involvement. Lesions can be identified on the tongue, hard palate, and mucosa of the lips and cheek and are typically white plaques with dark reddish-purple margins. Superficial ulcerations are not infrequent and xerostomia is often present.

Diagnosis is made by positive antinuclear antibody screening as well as positive lupus erythematosus preparations and antibodies to double-stranded DNA. These patients can be anemic, have decreased platelet count with complement disorders, and a positive Coombs' test.

Treatment can begin with salicylates, but corticosteroids are often required, and if the disease is extensive cyclophosphamide may be necessary.

SJÖGREN'S SYNDROME

This syndrome includes keratoconjunctivitis and xerostomia with progressive infiltration of the salivary and lacrimal glands. These patients can have dry mouth and thus complain of pharyngeal cracking. An elevated sedimentation rate is often present as are positive tests for antinuclear antibody (ANA) and rheumatoid factor. The treatment is symptomatic, with corticosteroids used for more severe systemic involvement.

CONCLUSION

Overall, infectious processes of the pharynx are much more common than inflammatory processes. Practitioners must take a thorough history and perform a complete physical examination in addition to formulating a complete differential diagnosis. Due to concerns about the emergence of bacterial resistance, antibiotic treatment for uncomplicated infections should be guided by culture documentation. Inflammation of the pharynx as a component of a systemic process should not be overlooked.

SUGGESTED READINGS

Ballenger JJ. Diseases of the oropharynx. In: Ballenger JJ, Snow JB, eds. *Otorhinolaryngology*. 15th ed. Baltimore: Williams & Wilkins; 1996: 236–244.

Holt GR, Tinsley PP Jr. Peritonsillar abscess in children. *Laryngoscope* 1981;91:1226.

Kornblut AD. Non-neoplastic diseases of the pharynx and adenoids. In: Paparella MM, Shumrick DA, Gluckman JL, Meyerhoff WL, ed. *Otolaryngology*. 3rd ed. Philadelphia: WB Saunders; 1991:2129–2165.

Pichichero ME. Cephalosporins are superior to penicillin for treatment of streptococcal tonsillopharyngitis: is the difference worth it? *Pediatr Infect Dis J* 1993;12:268–274.

Pichichero ME, Margolis PA. A comparison of cephalosporins and penicillins in the treatment of group A beta-hemolytic streptococcal pharyngitis: a meta-analysis supporting the concept of microbial copathogenicity. *Pediatr Infect Dis J* 1991;10:275–281.

Seid AB, Dunbar JS, Cotton RT. Retropharyngeal abscesses in children revisited. *Laryngoscope* 1979;89:1717–1724.

Sinai LN, Schwartz MW. Oropharyngeal manifestations of systemic disease. In: Bluestone CD, Stool SE, Kenna MA, eds. *Pediatric Otolaryngology*. 3rd ed. Philadelphia: WB Saunders; 1996:1077–1083.

Zalzal GH, Cotton RT. Pharyngitis and adenotonsillar disease. In: Cumming CW, Fredrickson JM, Harker LA, Krause CJ, Schuller DE, eds. *Otolaryngology—Head and Neck Surgery*. St. Louis: Mosby Year Book; 1993:1180–1198.

Chapter 25

NEOPLASMS AND CYSTS

Lyon L. Gleich

The vast majority of pharyngeal neoplasms are squamous cell carcinomas. Other malignant histologies include lymphoma, minor salivary cancers, sarcoma, and metastatic lesions. Benign lesions include necrotizing sialometaplasia, ectopic thyroid tissue, benign minor salivary neoplasms, Crohn's disease, and papilloma.

> **PEARL...** Necrotizing sialometaplasia can occur anywhere salivary tissue is present. The oral form most commonly arises spontaneously at the junction of the hard and soft palate. It typically appears as a deep-seated ulcer and may therefore be mistaken for carcinoma. Microscopic features include squamous metaplasia, lobular necrosis of the acini, and sialoadenitis. Necrotizing sialometaplasia resolves spontaneously without any treatment.

When the tumor does not have the typical appearance of a squamous cell carcinoma, either lymphoma or minor salivary neoplasm is most likely.

Minor salivary neoplasms are the third most common tumor type of the pharynx. Approximately 50% of these are carcinomas, with muco-epidermoid carcinoma and adenoid cystic carcinoma being the most common cell type. Treatment is primarily wide surgical excision often followed by radiation therapy when malignancy is confirmed.

> ## SPECIAL CONSIDERATION
>
> The lymphomas occur most commonly in the tonsil where they represent 16% of all neoplasms. Lymphomas can occur anywhere in Waldeyer's ring, and are almost always non-Hodgkin's lymphomas. Treatment is primarily nonsurgical.

This chapter concentrates on pharyngeal squamous cell carcinoma. These cancers are strongly associated with tobacco and alcohol use. There are weak associations with poor oral hygiene, syphilis, human papilloma virus, and Epstein-Barr virus. Patients with Plummer-Vinson syndrome have an increased risk of postcricoid carcinoma. Plummer-Vinson syndrome is composed of glossitis, splenomegaly, esophageal stenosis, achlorhydria, and iron-deficiency anemia.

PHARYNGEAL CARCINOMA

SYMPTOMS

A sore throat is the most common symptom of pharyngeal cancer. Dysphagia, trismus, a globus sensation, a neck mass, and ear pain are also commonly seen. Advanced tumors may have bleeding, airway obstruction, and weight loss. These patients can have significantly advanced cancers, however, with a paucity of symptoms.

> **PEARL•••** A persistent sore throat in a tobacco user must prompt a thorough search of the pharynx, at times including examination under anesthesia and/or radiologic scanning.

EXAMINATION

Once a mass is detected and a complete history obtained, the head and neck region should be thoroughly examined to detect any additional lesions, to detect any nodal spread, and to document the tumor. Documentation of pharyngeal tumors should include the tumor's multidimensional size, location in the regions of the pharynx, mobility of the lesion, and relationship to the prevertebral fascia, relationship to the larynx, vocal fold mobility, and invasion of surrounding structures. Computed tomography (CT) scanning or magnetic resonance imaging (MRI) can aid in evaluating the deep extent of the tumor and the tumor's relationship to surrounding structures and in detecting small lymph nodes. Endoscopy in the operating room will add to the evaluation of the primary tumor and permit biopsies to be obtained. This will also aid in detecting second primary tumors. Following full examination, the tumor should then be staged as shown below. It is important to recall that oropharyngeal primary tumors are staged mainly by size, while for hypopharyngeal tumors the location and relation to the larynx are also important.

STAGING

Oropharynx

T1 Tumor 2 cm or less in greatest dimension
T2 Tumor more than 2 cm but not more than 4 cm in greatest dimension
T3 Tumor more than 4 cm in greatest dimension

T4 Tumor invades adjacent structures (e.g., pterygoid muscles, mandible, hard palate, deep muscle of tongue, larynx)

Hypopharynx

T1 Tumor limited to one subsite of the hypopharynx and 2 cm or less in greatest dimension
T2 Tumor involves more than one subsite of the hypopharynx or an adjacent site, or measures more than 2 cm but not more than 4 cm in greatest diameter without fixation of hemilarynx
T3 Tumor measures more than 4 cm in greatest dimension or with fixation of hemilarynx
T4 Tumor invades adjacent structures (e.g., thyroid/cricoid cartilage, carotid artery, soft tissues of neck, prevertebral fascia/muscles, thyroid and/or esophagus)

Regional Lymph Nodes

NX Regional lymph nodes cannot be assessed
N0 No regional lymph hode metastases
N1 Metastasis in a single ipsilateral lymph node, 3 cm or less in greatest dimension
N2a Metastasis in a single ipsilateral lymph node more than 3 cm but not more than 6 cm in greatest dimension
N2b Metastasis in multiple ipsilateral lymph nodes, none more than 6 cm in greatest dimension
N2c Metastasis in bilateral or contralateral lymph nodes, none more than 6 cm in greatest dimension
N3 Metastasis in a lymph node more than 6 cm in greatest dimension

Once the tumor is staged, the metastatic evaluation should be reviewed. In patients with distant metastases the chance of cure is minimal, and this must be discussed with the patient and family. If no metastases are present, the approach to treatment is dictated by the tumor's location and the patient's choices. Patients with pharyngeal tumors are often nutritionally depleted due to tumor bulk and dysphagia. Nasogastric tubes or gastrostomy tubes should be considered early to improve patients' nutritional and general health so that they can survive their therapy.

TREATMENT

Tonsil Carcinoma

The tonsil is the most common site of squamous cell carcinoma of the oropharynx. Tumors frequently present at advanced stages, and approximately 70% of patients present with lymph node metastases. T1 and T2 tonsil cancers can be treated with external beam radiation to the primary site and neck with approximately 80% 5-year survival. If significant neck disease is present, this is often combined with a planned neck dissection.

SPECIAL CONSIDERATION

Tumors of the tonsillar fossa respond better to radiation than cancers of the tonsillar pillar.

Surgery can be used as the primary treatment modality for T1 or T2 tonsil cancers in select cases. Some tumors can be approached intraorally, but many will require complex approaches with significant potential morbidity.

PEARL... An important concern when treating tonsil cancers surgically is the need to assess or resect the retropharyngeal lymph nodes, as these nodes are at risk for metastases and can be overlooked.

Advanced tonsil cancers can be treated with radiation alone, and more recently attempts have been made to treat these tumors with chemo-radiation protocols. Most would agree, however, that for these tumors the best cure rates can be obtained with combined therapy consisting of surgery followed by radiation therapy. Prior to embarking on surgery the tumor's

resectability must be assessed. Important areas or structures to evaluate for invasion by cancer are the prevertebral fascia, carotid artery, and skull base. If these areas are involved, the tumor would be judged by most surgeons to be unresectable, and the patient should be treated with radiation therapy. The role of chemotherapy for these patients remains unclear.

For resectable advanced tumors of the tonsil, the mandible should be evaluated. Evaluation of the mandible includes physically examining the tumor's relation to the mandible to determine if it is fixed. The tumor may also invade the mandible through tooth roots, and these should be inspected.

PEARL... Anesthesia in the distribution of the mental nerve would also suggest mandibular involvement.

Panorex radiographs and CT scans can assist in evaluating the mandible, but physical examination is paramount. If the mandible is invaded, the best approach is a composite resection with a neck dissection.

If the tumor is free of the mandible, the most common approach to the tumor is via a parasymphyseal mandibulotomy, permitting the mandible to swing laterally. The tumor is then approached through the floor of the mouth and resected in continuity with the neck dissection specimen. Reconstructive options for the tonsil include (1) a split-thickness skin graft, (2) a myocutaneous flap—most often a pectoralis major flap, or (3) a microvascular flap—most often a radial forearm flap. Combined surgery and radiation for stage III and IV tonsil cancers can produce 5-year survival rates of approximately 40%.

Tongue Base Carcinoma

Tongue base cancers are particularly difficult to manage due to their frequently late presentation, early nodal metastases, and the important function of the tongue base. At presentation 80% of patients with tongue base cancer have nodal metastases. The tongue base can be approached surgically by a mandibulotomy, a transhyoid approach, or a lateral pharyngotomy. Regardless of the approach used, vital tissue, which is important in propelling the food bolus for swallowing and protecting the larynx from aspiration, is removed. If resection would require removal of large portions of the tongue base, a laryngectomy must be considered to prevent aspiration.

CONTROVERSY

The tongue base is important to propel food over the larynx and provide sensation and bulk to protect the larynx. The removal of the tongue base, even without any removal of the supraglottis can therefore cause severe aspiration. Procedures other than total laryngectomy have been described to protect the larynx when the tongue base is removed and include (1) suspending the hyoid to the mandible to move the larynx anteriorly and superiorly and thereby reduce aspiration and (2) laterally sewing the epiglottis together to create an overlying funnel to divert swallowed materials from the glottic inlet.

Due to these concerns, attempts have been made to treat tongue base cancers primarily with radiation. For small tongue base cancers, which are the minority, either surgery or radiation can be used to treat the primary site. In select early tumors, a radical approach may not be required for complete resection, and therefore should be offered to the patient. Approaches to the tongue base for partial resection include (1) the mandibular swing as described above in the approach to the tonsil; (2) the transhyoid approach to the central tongue base, which provides access, but with limited visibility laterally and orally; and (3) the lateral pharyngotomy approach through the pyriform sinus, which permits resection of small lateral tongue base lesions.

For advanced tongue base cancer, surgery will often necessitate a near total glossectomy with a possible laryngectomy. If this is the case, the patient should be offered both a surgical and a nonsurgical approach. Nonsurgical approaches that are advocated include (1) external beam radiation alone, (2) external beam radiation combined with brachytherapy with looping implants to maximize the radiation dose to the tumor, and (3) radiation combined with either induction or concomitant chemotherapy.

Cancers of the soft palate or pharyngeal walls are treated analogously to tonsil and tongue base tumors. Smaller tumors can be treated with surgery or radiation therapy, but for the majority of lesions combined therapy will offer the best chance of cure.

Many physicians advocate treating oropharyngeal tumors primarily with radiation. When this is done, the necks are also irradiated. For patients presenting with N2 or N3 neck disease in which the primary tumor did respond to radiation therapy, many would advocate following the radiation therapy with a planned neck dissection.

Hypopharynx Carcinoma

Greater than 95% of cancers in the hypopharynx are squamous cell carcinomas. Verrucous carcinoma can occur in the hypopharynx and, similar to its laryngeal counterpart, can be treated by wide local excision. Hypopharynx squamous cell carcinomas are typically highly infiltrative with significant submucosal spread complicating surgical treatment. Due to the high incidence of nodal disease and aggressive behavior at the primary site, the cure rates for hypopharyngeal tumors are poor. The majority of hypopharyngeal carcinomas occur in the pyriform sinus.

There are many considerations in evaluating a patient with hypopharyngeal cancer, including the patient's general health. The typical patient with a hypopharyngeal cancer presents with an advanced-stage tumor and a history of significant tobacco and alcohol abuse, weight loss, and malnourishment. These factors may influence the patient's tolerance of any surgical therapies that need to be considered.

SPECIAL CONSIDERATION

Many patients will be inappropriate for aggressive surgical procedures needed to completely excise their tumor due to either the extensive primary tumor, extensive nodal disease, distant metastasis, or poor medical condition. These patients are best treated with primary radiation therapy with or without chemotherapy for palliation. In rare instances this therapy may result in cure.

During the evaluation of a hypopharynx tumor, the tumor's relationship to the esophagus and larynx must be thoroughly evaluated. Particular attention should be paid to the upper and lower extent of the tumor. At the upper extent significant oropharyngeal involvement of the tonsil and tongue base may be detected. At the lower extent involvement of the esophagus may complicate resection, and involvement of the pyriform apex may suggest paraglottic space involvement. Vocal fold mobility must be assessed to detect subtle laryngeal involvement. Fixation against the prevertebral fascia is common and suggests unresectability.

The patient's tumor characteristics, general health, and treatment preferences must then be considered in formulating a plan. In the rare early tumor, therapy can be planned that preserves the larynx. Tumors limited to the lateral wall of the pyriform sinus without extension to the pyriform apex can be treated surgically via a lateral pharyngotomy with a neck dissection. Radiation can be used postoperatively if there are close margins or extensive nodal disease. Radiation alone is a consideration in these patients, but given that this surgical procedure is organ preserving and reliable, it is usually the treatment of choice.

Early tumors of the medial wall of the pyriform sinus can be removed in conjunction with a supraglottic laryngectomy, but this often results in severe aspiration. Early tumors of the posterior pharyngeal wall can be approached by a mandibular swing, a lateral pharyngotomy, or a transhyoid approach, similar to oropharyngeal lesions. For all these early lesions, radiation alone is an option.

Unfortunately, small tumors are rare and surgical treatment of hypopharyngeal carcinoma usually necessitates total laryngectomy. Neck dissections and postoperative radiation therapy should be used in all cases. Depending on the location and size of the primary tumor resection may require a partial or complete resection of the hypopharyngeal mucosa. The exact margin necessary is unclear, but given the infiltrative nature of these cancers at least 2-cm margins should be obtained.

Following total laryngectomy with partial pharyngectomy the defect can be closed primarily if the contralateral pyriform sinus was not involved and sufficient mucosa remains. When only a thin strip of mucosa remains, primary closure is not recommended due to the high incidence of stenosis. When there is insufficient mucosa for primary closure, a flap should be used to close the defect. Either a myocutaneous flap, such as the pectoralis major flap, or a free flap, such as the radial forearm flap, can be used and sewn to the surrounding mucosal remnants.

When the tumor bulk necessitates circumferential removal of the hypopharyngeal mucosa, primary closure and patch grafts are insufficient for repair. A tubed pectoralis flap is a consideration but will have a tendency to unfurl, creating a fistula. Free flaps are frequently employed in this setting, particularly the jejunal free flaps. Tubed fascia-cutaneous flaps, such as the radial forearm flap, have been gaining in favor for this reconstruction. The radial forearm flap requires an additional suture line to create a tube but eliminates the need for a laparotomy.

When the hypopharyngeal tumor extends significantly into the esophagus and is inferior to the thoracic inlet, surgical resection requires removal of not only the larynx and pharynx but also the esophagus. Laryngopharyngoesophagectomy permits oncologic resection of these cancers but requires entry into the cervical region, thorax, and abdomen. There is a high rate of morbidity from this procedure and long-term survival is poor due to the advanced stage of the tumor.

Surgical therapy for advanced hypopharyngeal cancer should only be employed with the patient's complete understanding of what these morbid procedures involve. In all advanced cases postoperative radiation should be employed. In patients who do not wish to undergo surgical therapy, radiation for cure should be employed. Recent randomized studies comparing induction chemotherapy and radiation to surgery and radiation for advanced hypopharyngeal carcinoma have shown similar poor cure rates in both arms.

SUGGESTED READINGS

Harrison LB, Zelefsky MJ, Sessions RB, et al. Base of tongue cancer treated with external beam radiation plus brachytherapy: oncologic and functional outcome. *Radiology* 1992;184:267–270.

Ho CM, Lam KH, Wei WI, et al. Squamous cell carcinoma of the hypopharynx—analysis of treatment results. *Head Neck* 1993;15:405–412.

Lefebvre JL, Chevalier D, Luboinski B, et al. Larynx preservation in pyriform sinus cancer: preliminary results of a European Organization for Research and Treatment of Cancer phase III trial. *J Natl Cancer Inst* 1996;88:890–899.

Ruhl CM, Gleich LL, Gluckman JL. Survival, function, and quality of life after total glossectomy. *Laryngoscope* 1997;107:1316–1321.

Spector JG, Sessions DG, Emami B, et al. Squamous cell carcinoma of the pyriform sinus: a nonrandomized comparison of therapeutic modalities and long-term results. *Laryngoscope* 1995;105:397–406.

Spiro JD, Spiro RH. Carcinoma of the tonsilar fossa. *Arch Otolaryngol Head Neck Surg* 1989; 115:1186–1189.

Chapter 26

SPECIAL CONSIDERATIONS

Thomas A. Tami

OBSTRUCTIVE SLEEP APNEA

Surgical management of patients with severe obstructive sleep apnea (OSA) traditionally consisted of tracheotomy, which often produced an unsatisfactory solution, but nevertheless gave universally successful results. It was following Fujita's classic description of the uvulopalatopharyngoplasty in 1981 that otolaryngologists became interested in this medical problem. Since then, both the medical and the surgical approaches of OSA have undergone several evolutions. Although the current treatment options for patients with sleep-disordered breathing are numerous, debate continues on the appropriate management for this condition.

DEFINITION

Sleep apnea syndromes are defined as alterations in the respiratory patterns normally expected during the sleep cycle. Normal sleep can be divided into REM (rapid eye movement) and NREM (nonrapid eye movement) stages. The NREM stage can be further divided into stages I through IV based on changes in the electroencephalogram (EEG). Following the onset of sleep in normal subjects, sleep descends through the four NREM sleep stages, entering the REM stage after approximately 90 minutes of sleep. As the night progresses, more and more time is spent in REM sleep with less and less in NREM stages III and IV. Although muscle tone is usually decreased in all states of sleep, muscle tone is essentially absent during REM sleep (except for extraocular muscle movements).

In normal subjects, ventilation continues with normal or near-normal respiratory flow volumes even during periods of maximal muscle relaxation. The introduction of formal polysomnography in the mid-1970s enabled investigators to clearly describe sleep stages and record respiratory events during sleep.

SPECIAL CONSIDERATION

Based on polysomnographic evaluations, sleep apnea syndromes can be divided into one of three basic types: central apnea, which occurs when both airflow as well as thoracic and abdominal respiratory efforts are absent; obstructive apnea, which is defined as the cessation of measurable airflow without a concurrent cessation of respiratory efforts; and mixed apnea, which has both central and obstructive characteristics.

Formal polysomnography is usually considered the "gold standard" for making this diagnosis, but it is hardly a standard procedure using standard diagnostic criteria. The polysomnographic definition of obstructive sleep apnea syndrome (OSAS) is based on the number of abnormal respiratory events occurring during each hour of sleep. In large normative populations, it has been widely accepted that five or less apneic events per hour (defined as the apnea index, AI) is normal. Studies looking at specific segments of the population, however, have revealed a wide variance of normal. For example, in the pediatric populations as few as one episode per hour is considered abnormal. In the elderly, an AI in excess of five is commonly encountered, yet doesn't appear to be associated with significant physiologic changes or daytime dysfunction. The normal AI should therefore be age weighted, but many laboratories continue to consider a value of five or greater to be abnormal.

INCIDENCE AND EPIDEMIOLOGY

The incidence of OSA in the general population has been evaluated by a number of centers during the past two decades. The most widely quoted study examining this question was published by Young et al in 1993. In that study, a random sample of 602 state employees in Wisconsin underwent formal overnight polysomnography. If an apnea/hypopnea index (AHI) of 5 was used as the upper limit of normal, the incidence of sleep-disordered breathing was 9% for women and 24% for men. If an AHI of 15 was defined as the upper limit, then the incidence of OSA was 12% for men and 5% for women. This study demonstrates that, using the AHI alone in a middle-aged working population, the prevalence of undiagnosed obstructive sleep apnea is surprisingly high.

PATHOPHYSIOLOGY

The pathophysiology of OSA relates simply to the cessation of breathing secondary to periods of upper airway collapse during sleep. Airway narrowing and collapse can occur at various regions of the upper airway; however, the areas most commonly implicated include the nasal airway, velum and nasopharynx, oropharynx and tongue-base, or the hypopharynx and larynx. In many instances, measurable narrowing of these critical anatomic sites can be appreciated even during wakefulness.

> **PEARL•••** Studies evaluating the anatomic relationships of the soft tissue and skeletal structures of the head and neck describe a high association of OSA with large tongue and soft palate volumes, a retrognathic mandible, an anteroposterior discrepancy between the maxilla and mandible, and an open bite tendency between the incisors.

Inheritance may also play a role in OSA because the rate of OSA (47%) in the offspring of patients with OSA is much higher than would be expected in the general population.

Other more obvious anatomic factors can also contribute to this condition. In children as well as in some adults, hypertrophy of the tissues of Waldeyer's ring is frequently an associated finding. Macroglossia, retro- or micrognathia, and primary or secondary tumors of the tongue, pharynx, or larynx can also predispose to OSA.

> ## CONTROVERSY
>
> Nasal obstruction is often grouped with other traditional causes of OSA, and nasal surgery is often recommended as part of the treatment for patients who snore or who suffer from OSA. The evidence to implicate nasal obstruction in the pathophysiology of this condition is minimal. One recent study that evaluated the effects of surgical correction of nasal obstruction failed to demonstrate any meaningful postoperative reduction in sleep-disordered breathing in patients with OSA.

The two primary risk factors usually associated with OSA are age and weight. The incidence of clinically significant OSA appears to peak between the ages of 40 and 50 years, but OSA can be diagnosed at any age. Although increasing age is often considered a risk factor for OSA, the Wisconsin study failed to find any significant increase in prevalence between 30 and 60 years, suggesting that age is at least not a strong risk factor for OSA. On the other hand, obesity appears to be a substantial risk factor for developing OSA. Approximately two-thirds of patients with OSA are at least 20% over ideal body weight.

Decreased neuromuscular tone is probably the most important factor leading to a loss of support and structural integrity with subsequent airway collapse. Although all sleep stages are associated with decreased muscle tone, it is during REM sleep that oropharyngeal muscles become nearly flaccid. Not surprisingly, most of the severe episodes of obstructed breathing tend to occur during REM sleep.

> **PITFALL•••** Agents that increase muscle relaxation during sleep will induce or worsen OSA. Ethanol and sedatives such as the benzodiazepines and barbiturates have all been shown to depress hypoglossal nerve activity and genioglossal muscle tone, thereby causing increased upper airway resistance.

The signs and symptoms of OSA result from respiratory events occurring during sleep. Patients with OSA experience periods of asphyxia associated with hypoxemia, progressive hypercapnia, acidemia, and progressive increasing efforts to inspire against a closed airway. These events often lead to an arousal from sleep, and during these brief periods of wakefulness, muscle tone is regained and the upper airway reestablished. Driven by hypoxemia and acidemia, ventilations characterized by high tidal volumes are followed once again by return to sleep. This cycle (sleep–obstruction–arousal–return to sleep) is repeated throughout the night in patients with OSA. This abnormal sleep cycle causes alterations in the normal REM/NREM sleep cycle, often causing relative sleep deprivation that results in daytime sleepiness. Physiologic changes caused by hypoxemia, hy-

percapnia, and acidemia produce surges in catecholamine production with potential long-term cardiopulmonary sequelae.

IMPLICATIONS AND SEQUELAE

Obstructive sleep apnea can be associated with significant medical morbidity. The cycle of frequent nighttime arousals is rarely reported by patients; however, excessive daytime sleepiness is the most common symptom reported in patients with OSA. Hypersomnolence probably results from constant sleep fragmentation and a deficit of stages III and IV NREM sleep. Daytime somnolence causes impaired performance on cognitive tasks and can interfere with the safe performance of routine activities, such as driving or operating heavy construction equipment.

> ## SPECIAL CONSIDERATION
>
> The prevalence of sleep-related disorders is now being recognized as a serious problem in the workplace. Regulatory agencies have also recognized the danger of hypersomnolence in the workplace and on the highways, and guidelines are being developed to restrict the activities of severely affected individuals.

> ## CONTROVERSY
>
> There may be a group of patients who do not have OSA but still suffer from daytime hypersomnolence. The upper airway resistance syndrome has recently been offered to account for some of these cases. These patients have multiple short arousals (measured by EEG) directly related to abnormal increases in respiratory efforts, but with no definite apnea or hypopnea. In these cases, a therapeutic trial of nasal continuous positive airway pressure (nasal CPAP) usually reverses the hypersomnia.

Severe cardiovascular disease often develops in patients with OSA. Systemic hypertension, left ventricular dysfunction, cardiac arrhythmias, myocardial infarction, pulmonary hypertension with cor pulmonale, and sudden death are all more common in OSA patients. These conditions appear to be mediated by physiologic changes during periods of obstruction. The hypoxia and hypercapnia produced by repetitive episodes of airway closure during sleep are accompanied by increased sympathetic tone. Over time, this contributes to diurnal hypertension as well as many of these other cardiovascular consequences.

> **PEARL...** Systemic hypertension has been reported in up to 50% of patients with OSA. An observation of even greater concern was a report that implicated undiagnosed OSA in as many as 40% of patients with essential systemic hypertension.

Transient and eventually persistent elevations in pulmonary arterial pressures often occur during periods of hypoxia, and in extreme and long-standing cases cor pulmonale may result. In an often-quoted study by He et al in 1988, a large cohort of patients with OSA were evaluated at the Henry Ford Hospital Sleep Disorders Center and followed for up to 9 years. Untreated subjects with AHIs greater than 20 had significantly increased mortality compared to those with less severe AHI scores, and aggressive treatment with nasal CPAP seemed to completely reverse this trend, clearly implicating OSA for this increased mortality.

MAKING THE DIAGNOSIS

Patient history is the most simple and cost-effective way to determine the likelihood of clinically significant OSA. Typical signs and symptoms of OSA such as obesity, systemic hypertension, daytime somnolence, morning headache, and loud sonorous snoring with observed interrupted breathing are easily assessed during the patient interview and would intuitively seem to be factors able to differentiate simple snorers from those with apnea. When the effectiveness of these simple measures has been tested in clinical situations, the results have been mixed at best. Because daytime somnolence is often a prominent feature of OSA, the Epworth Sleepiness Scale was developed as a predictor of increased daytime sleepiness and used as a screen for OSA. This test shows a correlation with the degree of respiratory disturbance as measured by polysomnography but is accompanied by a high false-negative rate when applied to clinical situations.

Although formal polysomnography continues to represent the industry standard for diagnosing OSA, portable computerized systems have recently been introduced to perform home sleep apnea monitoring in a potentially more cost-effective manner. The American Sleep Disorders Association has developed a system to classify polysomnographic testing equipment:

Level I

This level represents the standard attended polysomnography, often used as the gold standard. These formal studies generally include several physiologic measures:

1. EEG (electroencephalogram) evaluates the various stages of sleep, confirms the presence of sleep during the study, and determines sleep latency (time it takes to fall asleep).
2. EOG (electrooculogram) confirms REM sleep by detecting eye movement activity.
3. EMG (electromyography), usually obtained from the submental musculature, evaluates muscle tone during sleep.
4. EKG (electrocardiogram) provides important information about cardiac rhythm abnormalities during sleep.
5. Air flow measurement, either a nasal or an oral airflow detector, establishes and quantifies airflow during respiration.
6. Thoracic and abdominal respiratory effort detectors monitor, detect, and quantify thoracic and abdominal respiratory movement, which should correlate with air flow during the normal respiratory cycle.

7. Blood oxygen saturation detector, usually a pulse oximeter, monitors oxygen saturation during respiratory events.

Level II

This comprehensive portable polysomnograph measures both respiratory and sleep variables. Sleep measurements are made in essentially the same manner as with level I studies, except that there is an absence of both trained personnel to ensure continuous recording quality and of on-line paper or monitor display. As with level I studies, level II polysomnography allows the determination and quantification of sleep stages, total sleep time, arousal identification, and leg movements.

Level III

Portable testing at this level measures cardiorespiratory variables, but does not evaluate sleep parameters. These devices typically measure respiratory flow, chest and/or abdominal movements, pulse rate, and oxygen desaturation. Level III devices are currently the most commonly selected systems for diagnosing obstructive apnea in the ambulatory setting. They are most often used as portable low-cost alternatives to the formal laboratory polysomnography. Although these devices do not measure physiologic sleep parameters, studies have demonstrated their usefulness, especially for diagnosing OSA. Most level III systems include the measurement of oximetry, pulse, airflow, abdominal and chest wall sensors, and position detectors, and can provide valuable information with acceptable sensitivity and specificity if carefully used to evaluate patients with potential OSA.

Level IV

Testing with this group of devices employs a continuous single or dual-bioparameter recording. Examples of level IV devices include tracheal sound recordings, continuous pulse oximetry, continuous Holter type cardiac monitoring, continuous blood pressure measurements, and body movement detectors. In general, while these are often used to screen for OSA, their inherent diagnostic limitations make them poor choices for diagnosing OSA.

THERAPY

As the field of sleep medicine has expanded over the past two decades, the list of management options for patients with OSA has grown. This list spans a wide spectrum of therapeutic options from very conservative, noninvasive alternatives on the one hand to extensive, quite invasive surgical options on the other.

The initial step in the medical management of OSA is to eliminate associated risk factors. Patients who regularly take sedatives or who use alcohol should be encouraged to stop since these have a clear association with OSA. Overweight patients should try to lose weight since a positive correlation between obesity and OSA has been clearly described.

> **PITFALL...** Although weight reduction alone may benefit some patients, the success of weight loss in OSA has been limited at best. Even when initially successful, sustained dietary compliance is difficult to achieve.

Other noninvasive therapeutic measures, such as the use of a nasopharyngeal airway and operant conditioning to help patients avoid sleep positions that exacerbate the breathing problem, have also been attempted with variable, but generally dismal success.

The use of pharmacologic agents to treat this syndrome has been examined in several studies; however, results have been disappointing. The tricyclic antidepressant protriptyline was the most widely studied agent; however, its use is usually limited by severe anticholinergic side effects.

Orthodontic devices have also been developed to alter the upper airway by changing the tongue-jaw relationship. These are usually quite effective for snoring; however, there are little controlled data that support the efficacy of these various devices for the treatment of OSA, yet their use has become fairly widespread.

Nasal CPAP was first introduced in 1981 as a nonsurgical treatment and since then has become widely used for this condition. Nasal CPAP delivers positive airway pressure through a tightly sealed and tightly fitting nasal mask. When the pressure delivered to the patient is titrated appropriately, a constant pneumatic pressure is maintained in the upper airway, and collapse during nocturnal respiration is prevented. Excessive daytime somnolence and other neuropsychologic symptoms associated with OSA are usually quickly reversed using nasal CPAP and the cardiovascular sequelae and mortality associated with this disorder can be dramatically reduced.

The clinical effectiveness of nasal CPAP for OSA is often overshadowed by poor patient acceptance and low compliance. Several recent studies evaluating patient compliance with nasal CPAP suggest that the compliance rate is usually less than 50%. When implemented appropriately, however, nasal CPAP remains the treatment of choice for OSA.

Prior to the development of nasal CPAP, the primary modality for managing severely affected patients was formal tracheotomy. This technique provided an absolute solution to the problem but was generally associated with both patient and physician resistance. For this reason, only the most severely affected patients with severe daytime somnolence or cardiovascular sequelae were offered this option.

The introduction of uvulopalatopharyngoplasty (UPPP) by Fujita et al in 1981 represented the first specialized surgical procedure, other than tracheotomy, for the management of OSA. Although the area of upper airway obstruction is often the region of the oropharynx and velum, anatomic narrowing in the hypopharynx, larynx, and tongue base can also contribute to OSA. Predictably, the success of UPPP alone in all patients with OSA is in the range of only 50%. If patients are grouped according to site of narrowing, UPPP would theoretically be more successful if applied only to those patients with narrowing or collapse in the region of the oropharynx and velum. It has been difficult to clearly demonstrate this relationship in a scientifically acceptable manner. The literature regarding UPPP and other surgical measures for OSA is filled with inconsistencies. Differences in technique, patient selection, definitions of OSA, and surgical success make it next to impossible to perform any meaningful review of this literature.

Patients who fail UPPP may be candidates for other surgical procedures. The most common adjunctive procedure for obstruction in the hypopharynx and tongue base is the mandibular osteotomy/genioglossus advancement with hyoid myotomy/suspension (GAHM). This procedure expands the hypopharyngeal region at the tongue base by advancing the genial tubercle and hyoid bone. The group at Stanford University uses extensive preoperative data analysis including physical examination, fiberoptic nasopharyngoscopy with the Mueller's maneuver, and lateral cephalometric analysis to determine the anatomic site of obstruction. Based on these studies, recommendations are made for surgery including UPPP, GAHM, or a combination UPPP/GAHM. The group reports a high success rate using these extensive evaluation criteria. Because these adjuvant procedures can be associated with greater patient morbidity, they should be considered carefully before being recommended.

The introduction of laser assisted uvulopalatoplasty (LAUP) was initially met with excitement and optimism regarding its potential effectiveness for OSA. Unfortunately, while it has been shown to be a reasonably effective option for snoring (albeit fairly painful), it has only shown minimal effectiveness for mild OSA.

Radiofrequency ablation of the soft palate and tongue base has also been recently introduced as an option for OSA. Specifically, tongue base reduction has appeal because tongue base obstruction seems to play a role in those patients who fail treatment using UPPP. Preliminary reports using this technique have been encouraging and clinical trials looking at the effectiveness of this treatment modality are currently underway.

SUGGESTED READINGS

Fujita S, Conway W, Zorick F, et al. Surgical correction of anatomic abnormalities in obstructive sleep apnea syndrome: uvulopalato-pharyngoplasty. *Otolaryngol Head Neck Surg* 1981;89:923–934.

He J, Kryger MH, Zorick FJ, et al. Mortality and apnea index in obstructive sleep apnea. *Chest* 1988;94:9–14.

Riley RW, Powell NB, Guilleminault C. Obstructive sleep apnea syndrome: a review of 306 consecutively treated surgical patients. *Otolaryngol Head Neck Surg* 1993;108:117–125.

Tami TA, Duncan HJ, Pfleger M. Identification of obstructive sleep apnea in patients who snore. *Laryngoscope* 1998;108:508–513.

Young T, Palta M, Dempsey J, et al. The occurrence of sleep-disordered breathing among middle-aged adults. *N Engl J Med* 1993;328:1230–1235.

SECTION V

NASOPHARYNX

Chapter 27

ANATOMY AND PHYSIOLOGY

Benjamin E. J. Hartley

ANATOMY OF THE NASOPHARYNX

The nasopharynx lies behind the nose and above the level of the soft palate (Fig. 27–1). With the exception of the floor, its walls are immobile and, unlike the other parts of the pharynx, it is not collapsible. It is lined with ciliated respiratory columnar epithelium above Passavant's ridge, and below this ridge, with stratified squamous epithelium. In these respects it shows more similarities to the nasal cavity than to the pharynx.

ANTERIOR BOUNDARY

This boundary is formed by two openings known as the posterior choanae through which the nasopharynx communicates with the nasal cavity. These are separated by the posterior edge of the nasal septum formed by the underlying vomer and the perpendicular plate of the ethmoid bone.

POSTEROSUPERIOR WALLS

These walls form a continuous sloping surface that inclines downward and backward. The posterosuperior wall is supported by the basilar part of the occipital bone and the posterior part of the body of the sphenoid with the anterior arch of the atlas below. The pharyngeal tonsil (adenoid) appears as a prominence of the posterior pharyngeal wall in the late months of fetal life and

increases in size to age 6 or 7 years, after which it tends to progressively atrophy. The adenoid prominence contains a number of mucosal folds. It consists principally of lymphoid tissue but also contains some deep mucous glands.

LATERAL WALLS

The lateral walls of the nasopharynx contain on each side the pharyngeal opening of the eustachian tube. This lies 10 to 12 mm behind and a little below the posterior end of the inferior concha (inferior turbinate). The opening is bounded above and behind by the tubal elevation. This is a firm prominence formed by the underlying cartilage of the eustachian tube, which forms the shape of an inverted J. The long limb is continuous in a downward direction as the salpingopharyngeal fold produced by the underlying salpingopharyngeus muscle. Behind the tubal elevation lies the pharyngeal recess (fossa of Rosenmüller).

SPECIAL CONSIDERATION

The pharyngeal recess is filled by the levator palati muscle and overlies the internal carotid artery, which courses at this point against the wall of the pharynx.

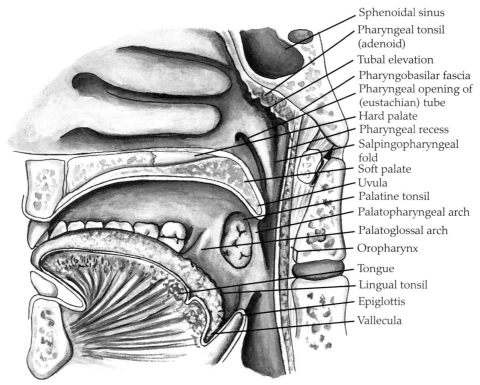

Sphenoidal sinus
Pharyngeal tonsil (adenoid)
Tubal elevation
Pharyngobasilar fascia
Pharyngeal opening of (eustachian) tube
Hard palate
Pharyngeal recess
Salpingopharyngeal fold
Soft palate
Uvula
Palatine tonsil
Palatopharyngeal arch
Palatoglossal arch
Oropharynx
Tongue
Lingual tonsil
Epiglottis
Vallecula

FIGURE 27–1 Sagittal section through the head demonstrating anatomy and relations of the nasopharynx.

The term *tubal tonsil* is given to the prominence at the lips of the eustachian orifice, where the cartilage is covered with lymphoid tissue.

INFERIOR WALL

The inferior wall of the nasopharynx is formed by the soft palate. When the soft palate is elevated, it contacts an area posteriorly known as Passavant's ridge.

BLOOD SUPPLY AND LYMPHATIC DRAINAGE

The nasopharynx derives its blood supply from the branches of the external carotid artery, including the ascending pharyngeal and facial arteries. Venous drainage is into the pterygoid venous plexus superiorly and the pharyngeal plexus inferiorly. Lymphatic drainage is via the retropharyngeal nodes and the deep cervical lymph node chain.

NERVE SUPPLY

The nasopharynx is supplied by the trigeminal nerve via the pharyngeal branch of the sphenopalatine ganglion. Below Passavant's ridge the nerve supply is the same as for the rest of the pharynx—by the glossopharyngeal and vagus nerves.

PHYSIOLOGY OF THE NASOPHARYNX

AIRFLOW

The nasopharynx is part of the upper airway. Like the nose, it is a noncollapsible structure. It may be obstructed by enlargement of the adenoids or congenital and acquired diseases as discussed below. Usually nasopharyngeal obstruction results in reflex use of the oral airway. The exception is in neonates, who are regarded as obligate nasal breathers. Congenital obstruction in bilateral choanal atresia becomes a respiratory emergency (see Chapter 29).

BACTERIAL COLONIZATION

Bacteria colonizing the nasopharynx are of little clinical significance locally but are important because they may spread via the eustachian tube and play an important role in the pathogenesis of acute otitis media.

EUSTACHIAN TUBE FUNCTION AND EFFECTS ON THE MIDDLE EAR

The eustachian tube orifice opens into the nasopharynx. The tube functions to allow secretions to exit and air to enter the middle ear space. Sade and Lundtz (1989) demonstrated that the normal middle ear loses gas by diffusion and this is constantly replaced by the eustachian tube. When this system fails, the result is a negative middle ear pressure. The pneumatized mastoid system acts as a buffer to protect against this, and hence poor mastoid pneumatization correlates with chronic middle ear disease.

CONTROVERSY

Which came first is a subject of controversy. Do congenitally small mastoid air systems cause chronic middle ear disease or does chronic infection lead to sclerosis of the mastoid air cells?

There is increasing evidence that altering the nasopharyngeal environment by performing adenoidectomy has an effect on the natural history of otitis media with effusion.

SPEECH AND SWALLOWING

Airtight closure of the oropharyngeal isthmus is important in the production of certain sounds. Failure of closure will result in air escape and hypernasal speech. Effective closure of the oropharyngeal isthmus during swallowing is essential to prevent nasal regurgitation. Mechanisms of palatal closure and the assessment and management of velopharyngeal incompetence are discussed in Chapter 30.

SUGGESTED READINGS

Baden H, Waz MJ, Bernstein JM, Brodsky L, Stanievich J, Ogra PL. Nasopharyngeal flora in the first three years of life in normal and otitis prone children. *Ann Otol Rhinol Laryngol* 1991;100:612–615.

Dempster JH, Browning GG, Gatehouse SG. A randomized study of surgical management of children with persistent otitis media with effusion associated with a hearing impairment. *J Laryngol Otol* 1993;107:284–289.

Gates GA, Avery CA, Prihoda TJ, Cooper JC. Effectiveness of adenoidectomy and tympanostomy tubes on chronic otitis media with effusion. *N Engl J Med* 1987;317:1444–1451.

Maw AR, Bawden R. Spontaneous resolution of severe chronic glue ear in children and the effect of adenoidectomy, tonsillectomy and the insertion of ventilation tubes (grommets). *Br Med J* 1993;306:756–760.

Paradise JL, Bluestone CD, Rogers KD, et al. Efficacy of adenoidectomy for recurrent otitis media in children previously treated with tympanostomy tubes. Results of parallel randomized and non-randomized trials. *JAMA* 1990;263:2066–2073.

Sade J, Lundtz M. Gaseous pathways in atelectatic ears. *Ann Otol Rhinol Laryngol* 1989; 99:335–338.

Chapter 28

CLINICAL TESTS

Benjamin E. J. Hartley

Patients present with a wide variety of signs and symptoms. In addition to understanding these symptoms, the clinician must conduct a thorough physical examination and order appropriate tests.

SYMPTOMS

Nasal obstruction may result from any space-occupying lesion whether congenital or acquired. The patient's age may indicate the likely cause; for example, severe nasal obstruction at birth suggests bilateral choanal atresia, and onset at age 2 to 3 years is suggestive of adenoidal hypertrophy, although rhinitis is another possibility in this age group.

Rhinorrhea may be secondary to an upper respiratory infection or less commonly chronic inflammation in the adenoids. Increasing awareness of allergic rhinitis has meant that chronic rhinorrhea in children is now less commonly attributed to the adenoids.

> **PEARL...** Unilateral rhinorrhea in children may suggest an intranasal foreign body or a unilateral choanal atresia. The rhinorrhea from a foreign body is usually offensive in nature and often has a shorter history than rhinorrhea due to unilateral choanal atresia.

Mouth breathing and snoring may be associated with adenoidal hypertrophy. Posterior epistaxis may be a presenting feature of nasopharyngeal disease. Conductive hearing loss may be the first indicator of nasopharyngeal disease, for example, a nasopharyngeal carcinoma causing obstruction of the eustachian tube orifice. Spread of nasopharyngeal carcinoma superiorly across the skull base may cause cranial neuropathy. A neck mass is another initial presentation of nasopharyngeal carcinoma. Hypernasal speech or regurgitation indicates velopharyngeal incompetence.

PHYSICAL EXAMINATION

The patient with adenoid facies classically presents with open mouth, flat midface, and dark under the eyes, together with a dull appearance. These appearances, however, are nonspecific and may be associated with nasal obstruction, whatever the etiology. They are rarely seen today in their classic form. A postnasal mirror placed in the oropharynx directed upward allows visualization of the nasopharynx. An adequate view of the nasopharyngeal structures, the posterior choanae, and the posterior end of the inferior and sometimes middle turbinate can be obtained in most adults and some children.

PEARL... A simple assessment of nasal airflow is to look for two mist patches on a cold metal instrument or mirror held in front of the nose on exhalation. The presence of misting in children can quickly rule out choanal atresia and may avoid the need for more invasive techniques or imaging.

SPECIAL INVESTIGATIONS

Modern fiberoptic or rigid endoscopes provide excellent visualization of the anatomy of the nasopharynx. Local anesthetic sprays may be administered to the nose first. The endoscope is passed along the floor of the nose through the inferior meatus. The optical quality of the rigid endoscopes are superior, but they are less maneuverable within the nasopharynx. The 0-degree 4-mm endoscope is standard; however, an angled 30-degree rigid endoscope can be rotated to clearly view the lateral walls and eustachian orifices. In compliant children, a 2.7-mm rigid endoscope or a fiberoptic flexible endoscope usually enables visualization of the adenoids (Fig. 28–1). The 120-degree endoscope can be used intraoperatively with the palate retracted to provide an excellent view of the nasopharynx (Fig. 28–2).

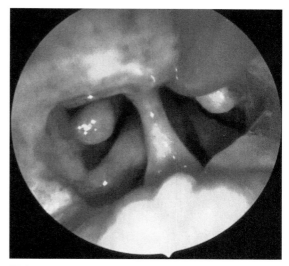

FIGURE 28–2 A 120-degree endoscopic view of the nasopharynx and posterior choanae. A red rubber catheter is seen on the left and is used to elevate the palate. See Color Plate 28–2.

Fiberoptic flexible endoscopy during speech and swallowing maneuvers gives functional information about velopharyngeal closure. This is described in more detail in Chapter 30.

A nasopharyngeal swab may guide antibiotic treatment of otitis media.

RADIOLOGY

Plain radiographs are rarely used in adults but offer certain information in the assessment of adenoid size in children (Fig. 28–3).

PITFALL... Radiographs are limited by factors related to patient positioning and the inability to distinguish overlying mucus.

The demonstration of an adequate nasopharyngeal airway may be useful, for example, in supporting a clinical diagnosis of rhinitis rather than adenoidal hypertrophy as a cause of nasal obstruction in a child.

Computed tomography (CT) scanning gives detailed information of the bony anatomy of the nasopharynx and demonstrates well the

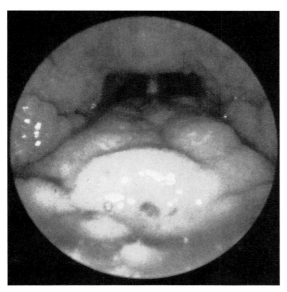

FIGURE 28–1 A 180-degree endoscopic view of normal adenoids. See Color Plate 28–1.

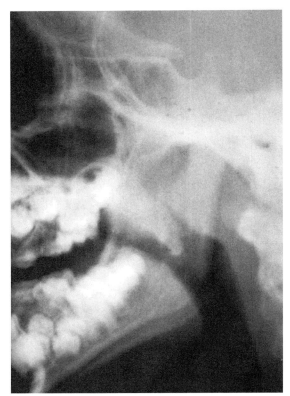

FIGURE 28-3 Plain radiograph showing enlarged adenoids.

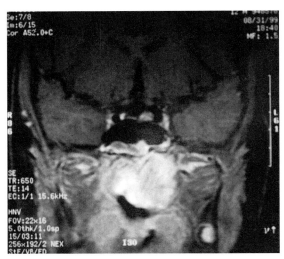

FIGURE 28-4 Magnetic resonance imaging (MRI) scan of a boy with juvenile nasopharyngeal angiofibroma.

position of soft tissue masses. It lacks the soft tissue discrimination of magnetic resonance imaging (MRI). CT scanning is the first choice of imaging for choanal atresia and for disease of the paranasal sinuses. The addition of intravenous contrast increases the detail when considering neoplasia or abscess.

MRI gives excellent soft tissue definition but is less helpful for bony detail. T1-weighted images give more anatomic detail, whereas T2-weighted images give more detailed differentiation of the pathologic processes involved in soft tissue masses. Acute and chronic inflammation gives high signal on T2-weighted images due to high water content. This may be helpful in determining the extent of a neoplasm, which has a moderate or low signal. Figure 28–4 shows an MRI of a child with juvenile nasopharyngeal angiofibroma.

SUGGESTED READING

Baden H, Waz MJ, Bernstein JM, Brodsky L, Stanievich J, Ogra PL. Nasopharyngeal flora in the first three years of life in normal and otitis prone children. *Ann Otol Rhinol Laryngol* 1991;100:612–615.

Chapter 29

CONGENITAL DISORDERS

Benjamin E. J. Hartley

CHOANAL ATRESIA

EMBRYOLOGIC BASIS

The nasal placode originates from ectoderm at around 3 weeks' gestation. This placode invaginates to form the nasal pits, which extend posteriorly to form the nasal cavity. This cavity is separated from the oral cavity by the bucconasal membrane, which ruptures at around 6 weeks' gestation to form the posterior choanae. Failure of rupture results in a persistence of the bucconasal membrane known as choanal atresia. Incidence is estimated at 1 in 8,000 births. Approximately 50 to 60% of cases are unilateral.

CLASSIFICATION

Early reports by Fraser in 1910 described the atresia as unilateral or bilateral, partial or complete, and bony or membranous. This work is probably the origin of the statement in most standard textbooks that choanal atresia is bony in 90% of patients and mixed in 10%. The advent of computed tomography (CT) scanning has given us more detailed information about the anatomy of the atresia and has lead Brown et al (1996) to suggest a new classification into pure bony, mixed bony-membranous, and pure membranous. Combining a number of studies, the relative incidence in these groups is 29% pure bony, 71% mixed bony-

membranous, and 0% pure membranous. It is suggested, therefore, that pure membranous choanal atresia is extremely rare.

CLINICAL FEATURES

> **SPECIAL CONSIDERATION**
>
> The presentation of bilateral choanal atresia is with respiratory distress and cyanosis at birth. Characteristically the cyanosis transiently improves with crying episodes (cyclical cyanosis).

There may be associated anomalies, particularly the CHARGE syndrome (coloboma, heart anomaly, atresia choanae, retardation, genital anomaly, and ear anomaly). For bilateral choanal atresia, urgent airway intervention is required, which is usually achieved either by taping an oropharyngeal airway in position or using a McGovern nipple. In the presence of other anomalies, an endotracheal tube or a tracheostomy may be appropriate.

The presentation of unilateral choanal atresia is quite different. It may not be diagnosed until later in life. Often the parents notice a child has persistent unilateral rhinorrhea. The diagnosis may be suspected clinically by the mirror test (failure to produce two mist patches on a cold metallic object when held in front of the nose). It can be confirmed by the failure to pass a suction catheter or preferably by endoscopic examination of the nose (Fig. 29–1).

CT scanning is the preferred method for defining the anatomy of choanal atresia preoperatively as it gives a clear definition of the bony component (Fig. 29–2).

OPERATIVE TREATMENT

In bilateral choanal atresia definitive surgery is usually performed in the first 1 or 2 weeks of life. The timing of surgery is dependent on the severity of any associated anomalies that may need attention first.

> **PITFALL...** Two principal approaches have been described: the transpalatal and the transnasal. Excellent access can be obtained by the transpalatal route, but concerns have been raised that division of the palate may cause maldevelopment of the dental arch and crossbite as well as the potential risk of a palatal fistula; thus the transnasal route is preferred by most surgeons.

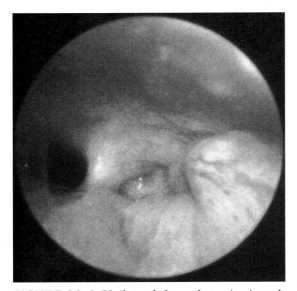

FIGURE 29–1 Unilateral choanal atresia viewed from the nasopharynx with a 120-degree endoscope. See Color Plate 29–1.

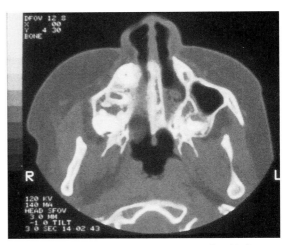

FIGURE 29–2 Computed tomography (CT) scan showing unilateral left choanal atresia.

Traditional visualization has been with the operating microscope. More recently, rigid endoscopes have been used, placed either in the nose (0-degree endoscope) or in the nasopharynx (120-degree endoscope). The choanal plate is perforated first with a urethral sound at its weakest point, which is the junction of the nasal septum with the floor of the nose. A drill may be required to enlarge bony stenosis, and the range of instruments designed for endoscopic sinus surgery complement this well. Some authors advocate the use of the carbon dioxide or the KTP laser.

It is conventional to stent the opening with modified endotracheal tube stents for 4 to 6 weeks. Some surgeons prefer not to use stents, and a range of local tissue flaps have been described, although none has gained universal popularity.

> ## SPECIAL CONSIDERATION
> There is a significant rate of restenosis with all techniques and further dilatation may be required.

TORNWALDT'S CYSTS

These cysts are derived from the pharyngeal bursa and are distinct from derivatives of Rathke's pouch. The pharyngeal bursa is a persistent embryonic communication between the roof of the nasopharynx and the notochord. Obstruction of the pharyngeal bursa leads to formation of a Tornwaldt's cyst. Added infection may lead to an abscess. This entity has long been known about, but the advent of CT and magnetic resonance imaging (MRI) has increased the identification of Tornwaldt's cysts both as a clinical entity and as an incidental finding. Classically an infected cyst may cause occipital headache, postnasal discharge, sore throat, fever, and neck stiffness. A smooth mass may be seen in the nasopharynx at about the level of the fossa of Rosenmüller. This is inferior to the site of the Rathke's pouch cyst, and so the two may be differentiated. The distinction is an academic one, as the treatment for both lesions is the same. Symptomatic lesions are excised, usually by curettage.

RATHKE'S POUCH DERIVATIVES

The anterior pituitary gland derives from the ectoderm of the stomatodeum as a pseudo-invagination caused by proliferation of surrounding mesenchyme and the folding of the embryo during the third and fourth weeks of gestation. This rostral outpouching of the primitive oral cavity is called Rathke's pouch. A number of pathologic entities have been attributed to Rathke's pouch. The commonest abnormalities are cysts, which are usually asymptomatic and situated in the roof of the nasopharynx. Extracranial pituitary tissue and tumors derived from this have also been described.

ABERRANT BLOOD VESSELS

The presence of large vascular structures in the nasopharynx has been described in the past by surgeons when severe and possibly life-threatening hemorrhage has been encountered at adenoidectomy. The advent of modern imaging now has shown that major vascular structures such as the internal carotid artery can follow an aberrant course through the nasopharynx. Any surgeon undertaking adenoidectomy should be aware of this possibility and consider not only palpation of the nasopharynx but also inspection before surgery with a mirror or endoscope.

SUGGESTED READINGS

Brown OE, Pownell P, Manning SC. Choanal atresia: a new anatomic classification and clinical management applications. *Laryngoscope* 1996;106:97–101.

Carpenter RJ, Neel HB. Correction of congenital choanal atresia in children and adults. *Laryngoscope* 1977;87:1304–1311.

Fraser JS. Congenital atresia of the choanae. *Br Med J* 1910;2:1698–1701.

Fuller GN, Batsakis JG. Pharyngeal hypophysis. *Ann Otol Rhinol Laryngol* 1996;105:671–672.

Healy GB, McGill T, Jako GT, Strong MS, Vaughan CW. Management of choanal atresia with the carbon dioxide laser. *Ann Otol Rhinol Laryngol* 1978;87:658–662.

Pirsig W. Surgery of choanal atresia in infants and children: historical notes and updated review. *Int J Pediatr Otorhinolaryngol* 1986;11:153–170.

Weissman JL. Tornwaldt's cysts. *Am J Otolaryngol* 1992;13:381–385.

Chapter 30

FUNCTIONAL DISORDERS
Benjamin E. J. Hartley

VELOPHARYNGEAL INSUFFICIENCY

Competence of the velopharyngeal valve is important for normal speech and swallowing. The assessment and management of these disorders is complex and is best managed by a team approach. The team should include an otolaryngologist, a speech and language therapist, and a prosthetist. In the pediatric population many patients will have craniofacial abnormalities, and thus a geneticist is an important member of the team.

THE NORMAL MECHANISM OF VELOPHARYNGEAL CLOSURE

During speech the palate moves upward and backward to contact the posterior pharyngeal wall. The posterior pharyngeal wall may also move forward to help achieve contact. Simultaneously the lateral pharyngeal walls move medially to form a seal with the lateral edges of the palate. Passavant's ridge consists of a muscle mass in the posterior pharyngeal wall that bulges forward during speech. Although it has traditionally been regarded as important in velopharyngeal closure, it often lies inferior to the level at which the seal is made between the palate and the lateral and posterior pharyngeal walls. Therefore, in most cases it may not be an important factor in velopharyngeal insufficiency (VPI).

Different patterns of pharyngeal closure have been observed. The most common is a coronal pattern due to a broad movement of the palate against the posterior pharyngeal wall. The next most common is a circular pattern that combines the coronal movement with a sagittal movement of the lateral pharyngeal walls. The least common is a principally sagittal movement where the lateral pharyngeal walls approximate and there is minimal posterior displacement of the soft palate.

ETIOLOGY OF VELOPHARYNGEAL INSUFFICIENCY

Structural Factors

Cleft palate is the commonest cause of VPI. The insufficiency is usually due to the palate being too short or the presence of persistent muscular defects. Submucous cleft palate may cause VPI although the majority of these patients will have normal speech.

PEARL... A submucous cleft palate is suspected if there is a bifid uvula, a bluish zona pellucida, a visible defect in the palatal masculature in the midline, or notching in the posterior border of the hard palate on palpation.

Patients with submucous cleft palates are at risk of VPI if adenoidectomy is performed. If the adenoids are not removed, these patients may present at age 5 to 9 years with speech disorders as the adenoids naturally regress.

Neuromuscular Factors

These patients have a normal structure to their velopharyngeal mechanism but have a neuromuscular discoordination. A large number of potential causes exist, but in adults the most common cause is cerebrovascular disease. Dysarthric speech with a component of VPI is not uncommon. Children with cerebral palsy or neurologic syndromes may have similar problems. A further group of patients have a functional VPI due to habitual patterns of speech formation and may respond well to speech therapy.

SPEECH PATTERNS

Typical patterns of speech disorder include hypernasality (increased sound resonance in the nasal cavity), nasal air emission, weak or omitted consonants, and short utterance length. Patients may develop compensatory patterns and secondary dysphonia possibly due to vocal cord nodules, which are common in children with VPI.

PATIENT EVALUATION

Evaluation by a speech therapist is important. The patterns of speech described above can be assessed and only with experience can their suitability for speech therapy be judged. The otolaryngologist examines the oral cavity, nasal cavity, pharynx, larynx, and relevant cranial nerve function. In the case of children, a geneticist offers help with identification of syndromes associated with VPI. Velocardiofacial syndrome is increasingly being detected by otolaryngologists. Features include a submucous cleft palate, facial abnormalities, and minor cardiac anomalies that may not have been previously detected. Identification of the syndrome may prompt a cardiology referral.

Nasopharyngoscopy is performed using a fiberoptic endoscope. This is passed transnasally and the palate is viewed from above. The adequacy of the velopharyngeal sphincter can be directly assessed during speech. Associated structural defects can be identified. The palate is assessed for evidence of a submucous cleft or hypoplastic musculus uvulae. The larynx is examined for secondary vocal nodules.

PEARL... A video recording is a useful method of documenting the exact defect. This can be played back to help the team judge the problem and plan treatment. It can also help judge improvement at subsequent visits. It also has an important role in allowing the patient to understand the problem and therefore helps them learn to correct it.

Nasometry is a computer-based assessment of the acoustic energy emanating from the oral and nasal cavities during speech. Standardized speech passages are used and the resulting "nasalance" score is compared with data from normal controls. The role of this technology in assessment and treatment of VPI in clinical practice is still being defined; however, it appears to be a useful tool.

Videofluoroscopy is a radiographic technique that is used to obtain multiple views of the velopharyngeal sphincter during speech. It gives structural and functional information and is particularly useful in the assessment of lateral pharyngeal wall motion.

TREATMENT

The treatment of VPI can be divided into three areas:

1. Speech therapy plays an important role in the management of nonstructural defects. It is also important in the postoperative period. The approach is similar to that used for articulation disorders and focuses on the reduction of compensatory articular patterns and improving oral resonance by changing the focus of articulation.

2. Prosthetic devices such as obturators or palatal lifts are used in the management of VPI.

An obturator can be useful if the palate is too short. A lift can help if a neurologic defect causes impaired movement. However, both are often poorly tolerated in children and need regular adjustment as the child grows.

3. Surgical intervention may correct structural defects and dramatically improve symptoms.

> **PEARL•••** A standard surgical approach is inappropriate; the procedure should be tailored to the patient.

Palatoplasty

The pushback palatoplasty may be appropriate for a child with a submucous cleft palate with good lateral pharyngeal wall motion. A W-shaped incision is made on the surface of the hard palate. The mucoperiosteal flap is elevated posteriorly (or pushed back), preserving the palatine arteries (Fig. 30–1). The levator palati muscles are located at their abnormal attachment at the posterior edge of the hard palate. They are detached and sutured together in the midline. The anterior palate is closed, leaving the bare surface of the hard palate to heal by secondary intention.

Pharyngeal Flap

A superiorly based pharyngeal flap is commonly used to correct VPI. Two parallel lateral

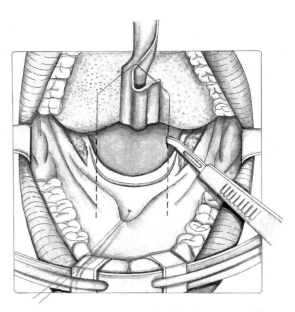

FIGURE 30–2 Incisions for the pharyngeal flap.

incisions are made in the posterior pharyngeal wall through mucosa and muscle down to the plane of the prevertebral fascia. They are then joined together inferiorly in the midline to create a pointed superiorly based flap (Fig. 30–2). Another incision is made in the nasal surface of the free edge of the soft palate and the flap is sutured to this incision, thus creating a bridge between the posterior pharyngeal wall and the soft palate (Fig. 30–3). Stents are placed through

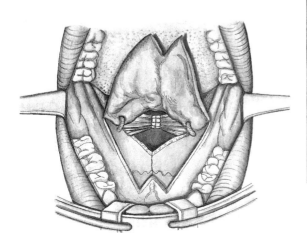

FIGURE 30–1 Pushback palatoplasty.

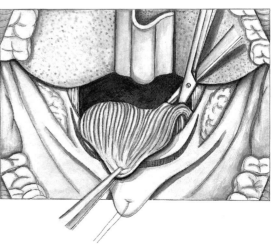

FIGURE 30–3 The pharyngeal flap is elevated.

the nose and down either side of the flap to create lateral ports, which preserve the nasal airway. They are generally removed the next day. A modification of this technique in which the palate is split allows the flap to be placed more superiorly.

> **PITFALL...** Postoperatively, nasal obstruction may be reported, requiring revision of the lateral ports. Sleep apnea has been reported, and on occasion it has been severe enough to require excision of the pharyngeal flap.

> **PEARL...** Problems with pharyngeal flaps are largely due to placement of the flap too inferiorly. In general, the higher the better.

Posterior Wall Augmentation

This approach may be considered for small gaps in the anterior-posterior diameter of the velopharyngeal opening of less than 10 mm. Augmentation must be accurately placed. This is generally at the level of the atlas promontory. Various materials have been used including cartilage, fat, fascia, silicon, and Teflon. (Teflon is not approved by the U.S. Food and Drug Administration for use in the retropharynx.)

> **PITFALL...** Posterior pharyngeal wall implantation may produce problems due to migration, undercorrection, improper placement, extrusion, or infection of the implant. The posterior pharyngeal wall is extremely mobile during the act of swallowing, and lasting accurate placement of an implant has proved technically challenging.

VPI can have a profound effect on speech, and successful treatment can significantly improve the quality of life. A team approach by professionals with a specialist interest is recommended to avoid some of the common pitfalls in treatment of this condition.

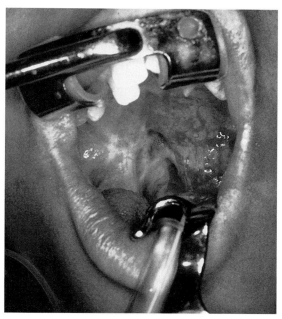

FIGURE 30–4 Nasopharyngeal stenosis secondary to adenotonsillectomy. See Color Plate 30–4.

NASOPHARYNGEAL STENOSIS

This usually occurs when there is extensive scarring following adenoidectomy or tonsillectomy (Fig. 30–4). It presents with nasal obstruction possibly associated with obstructive sleep apnea. Mild stenosis may require no treatment. Obstructive sleep apnea may be treated by continuous positive airway pressure, but most patients will request surgical correction. Dilatation may be attempted but is often unsuccessful and surgical repair is indicated. The patient is assessed preoperatively, with careful physical examination including nasopharyngoscopy. The repair procedure should be tailored to the patient's individual stenosis. Most techniques involve division of the stenosis and introducing a local tissue rotation flap derived from the posterior pharyngeal wall.

SUGGESTED READINGS

Boorman JG, Sommerlad BC. Musculus uvulae and levator palati: their anatomical and functional relationships in velopharyngeal closure. *Br J Plastic Surg* 1985;38:333–338.

Dalston RM, Warren DW, Dalston ET. Use of nasometry as a diagnostic tool for identifying patients with velopharyngeal impairment. *Cleft Palate Craniofac J* 1991;28:184–188.

McWilliams BJ, Lavoto AS, Bluestone CD. Vocal cord abnormalities in children with velopharyngeal valving problems. *Laryngoscope* 1973; 83:1745–1753.

Potsic WP, Cotton RT, Handler SD. *Surgical Pediatric Otolaryngology.* New York: Thieme; 1997: 208–211.

Stewart JM, Ott JE, Lagace R. Submucous cleft palate: prevalence in a school age population. *Cleft Palate J* 1972;9:246–250.

Willging JP, Kummer AW. Assessment and management of velopharyngeal insufficiency. In: Cotton RT, Myer CM, III, eds. *Practical Pediatric Otolaryngology*. Philadelphia: Lippincott-Raven; 1999:825–838.

Chapter 31

INFECTIOUS AND INFLAMMATORY DISORDERS

David L. Walner and Sally R. Shott

Infection and inflammation of the nasopharynx is generally part of a continuum of upper respiratory infections. These disorders are not limited to the nasopharynx and most often have nasal and oropharyngeal components.

ETIOLOGY OF NASOPHARYNGEAL INFLAMMATION

With chronic inflammation of the mucous membranes of the nose and paranasal sinuses, nasal and sinus congestion can form. The obstruction can increase both water and mucoid secretions within the nasal cavity and nasopharynx, which can lead to chronic infection and mucostasis.

> **PEARL...** In the pediatric age group the presence of nasal polyps should lead to consideration of cystic fibrosis and Kartagener's syndrome as well as ciliary motility dyskenesis syndromes.

The nasopharynx is in constant contact with inspired air, continually bathed by nasal mucus. The nasopharyngeal tissue is continually exposed to bacterial and viral as well as allergenic material and may serve as a potential reservoir of pathogens. Some authors have theorized that microorganisms release toxins and act as an antigen stimulus for exciting active immunization. This may lead to a reactive adenoidal hypertrophy.

> **PITFALL...** When chronic and severe nasopharyngeal obstruction occurs and goes untreated, it can lead to an increase in pulmonary resistance and alveolar hypoventilation. Prolongation of these symptoms can lead to cor pulmonale.

PRESENTATION

Inflammation within the naopharynx due to an acute infectious or chronic condition will often present with signs and symptoms of nasopharyngeal obstruction. These can include complaints of nasal obstruction, snoring, purulent rhinorrhea, postnasal drip, pharyngitis, referred otalgia, and halitosis. Neonates are obligate nasal breathers; therefore, when evaluating children in this age group the child's symptoms may be of greater proportion than in that of an older child or adult.

On physical exam, nasopharyngeal obstruction may be present and distinguished by a distinct airway noise known as stertor. This sound should be distinguished from stridor, which signifies laryngeal obstruction. In the outpatient clinic setting, a rigid nasal telescope or a flexible fiberoptic telescope is used to examine the nasopharynx. Inflammation can be visualized along the walls of the nasopharynx and/or adenoid region.

> **PEARL...** Radiographic examination of the nasopharynx with anteroposterior (AP) and lateral neck films may assist in providing information as to adenoidal hypertrophy, cystic structures, or masses within the nasopharynx.

When evaluating patients for nasopharyngeal infectious or inflammatory processes the differential diagnosis must include disorders of the nasal cavity as well as the oropharynx.

ADENOIDAL HYPERTROPHY

Adenoidal hypertrophy is typically more common in children. Chronic nasal obstruction may cause children to appear with "adenoid facies," due to the inability to breathe through the nose, resulting in chronic mouth breathing and possibly improper orofacial development.

> **SPECIAL CONSIDERATION**
>
> The inability to use the nasal passage is thought to result in a short hypotonic upper lip, a broad nasal arch, and an upturned nose with visible nostrils as well as a narrowed maxilla and possibly a retrognathic mandible.

Adenoidal hypertrophy has also been thought to contribute to eustachian tube dysfunction, leading to conditions such as serous or recurrent otitis media. In cases of severe adenoidal hypertrophy, the result may be sleep apnea leading to pulmonary hypertension and right heart enlargement.

> **PEARL...** In the pediatric population recurrent adenoid infections have been associated with both recurrent otitis media and recurrent sinusitis.

ACUTE INFECTIOUS PROCESSES

Nasopharyngitis is a difficult disorder to define. The nasopharynx is host to many pathogenic organisms. If, on physical examination, redness, swelling, and discharge are present in the region of the nasopharynx, the diagnosis of nasopharyngitis can be made. Acute infectious conditions are the most common conditions affecting the nasopharynx. These can be divided into bacterial and viral conditions.

Upper respiratory infections affect millions of people worldwide. It is estimated that over $37 million is spent in the antibiotic treatment of the common cold. Based on its location, the common cold is generally defined as acute nasopharyngitis. Organisms may be cultured in 50 to 60% of adult patients with upper respiratory infections. Nasopharyngeal cultures often contain respiratory pathogens and are also significantly associated with the presence of leukocytes. The most common organisms identified are *Streptococcus pneumoniae, Moraxella catarrhalis,* and *Haemophilus influenzae.* A study performed in Denmark revealed that between 91 and 98% of children with or without acute otitis media were found to have pathogenic bacteria in the nasopharynx during an episode of upper respiratory infection.

Many refer to the common cold as a viral upper respiratory infection. It is usually self-limited and often self-diagnosed. An acute mild catarrhal illness involves a nasopharyngitis lasting approximately 5 to 7 days in duration. The major viruses causing this condition include picornaviridae, coronadiridae, paramyxoviridae, orthomyxlviridae, and adenoviridae families. It is

> **SPECIAL CONSIDERATION**
>
> Numerous authors have commented on the inappropriate use of antibiotics in an attempt to treat upper respiratory infections that in fact have a viral etiology. It is felt that the overuse of antibiotics has led to the more resistant strains of *Streptococcus pneumoniae* that are now present in most cities in the United States.

estimated that viral upper respiratory infection is the most common disease of humans with a prevalence rate of six to eight colds per 1,000 persons per day during the winter months.

Syphilis is a systemic venereal disease that can present with pharyngeal and nasopharyngeal manifestations. Approximately 2 weeks after development of a chancre, the secondary or disseminated stage of syphilis occurs. Within this stage skin lesions and lymphadenopathy are seen in 90% of patients.

Pharyngotonsillitis or nasopharyngitis may also occur in secondary syphilis with mucosal involvement producing mucous patches. These patches are characterized by painless superficial erosions with a silver-gray appearance and are surrounded by raised, red peripheral margins. These are highly contagious lesions. Microscopically they resemble lesions of the primary chancre but with a less intense plasma call infiltrate, which is usually confined around vascular spaces.

Histologically, involvement of the lymphoid tissue is present, including follicular hypoplasia and noncaseating granulomas. Among these patients one-third will experience an activation of the disease with spontaneous remission, one-third will continue to have latent disease, and one-third will progress to tertiary syphilis. Resultant scarring within the nasopharynx can occur due to the chronic inflammatory nature of this disease process. A serologic test for syphilis is a fluorescent treponemal antibody absorption test, which is most sensitive (98%) and specific for tertiary syphilis. Successful treatment of syphilis consists of parental benzathine penicillin, or tetracycline for those allergic to penicillin.

CHRONIC INFLAMMATORY CONDITIONS

Chronic inflammatory conditions of the nasopharynx are rare but can include brucellosis or mycobacterial disease.

INHALANTS/IRRITANTS

Inhalants or irritants can cause a toxic nasal inflammatory response. These substances can act as chemical irritants causing vasomotor type responses. The inhalants may include agents such as oxides and nitrogen, carbon monoxide, ozone, aldehydes, ketones, chlorine, sulfur dioxide, ammonia, and hydrocarbons. Some of the more common irritants would include automotive exhaust and tobacco smoke. In addition, rhinitis medicamentosa, which is seen with the use of sympathomimetic agents, has been known to cause nasotoxic reactions due to a rebound phenomenon. Drug use including cocaine sniffing is also known to be an irritant of the nasal cavity and nasopharynx.

Researchers have investigated the role of gastroesophageal reflux on pharyngeal and nasopharyngeal inflammation. Contencin et al (1991) studied 31 infants and children, ages 1 month to 12 years, with nasopharyngeal pH monitoring; 13 had known rhinopharyngitis and gastroesophageal reflux, and 18 were controls. The authors measured the number of episodes with a pH less than 6. The patients with rhinopharyngitis had an average of 9.15 episodes of nasopharyngeal reflux versus the control patients who had an average of 2.28 episodes of nasopharyngeal reflux. In addition, they found that the rhinopharyngitis patients had a pH less than 6 for 18.7% of the exam time where the control patients had a pH less than 6 for 1.07% of the exam time.

CONTROVERSY

The effect of gastroesophageal reflux on nasopharyngeal tissue is still being discussed. One study has been performed to reveal inflammation in this area related to gastroesophageal reflux. However, there is still much controversy as to whether esophageal contents actually reach the nasopharynx.

Nasopharyngeal reflux may occur in children with oropharyngeal dysphagia or cerebral palsy, peripheral neuropathies, cleft deformities, velopharyngeal insufficiency, inherited or degenerative muscular disorders, and cricopharyngeal dysfunction. Reflux has been described in patients with delayed opening of the cricopharyngeal sphincter with familial dysautonomia. Continued study is necessary to evaluate the significance of this phenomenon and its effect on the nasopharynx.

HIV INFECTION

> **PEARL...** Nasopharyngeal lymphoid proliferation can be a presenting sign of HIV infection. In addition, this condition can produce nasal and eustachian tube obstruction.

NASOPHARYNGEAL CYSTS

INFECTION OF BENIGN CYSTS

Many cystic lesions such as a Tornwaldt's cyst of the pharyngeal bursa, a choanal polyp, and a mucosal cyst, are not uncommonly found within the nasopharyngeal space. Inflammation of the nasal cavity and nasopharynx due to acute infection, allergy, or inhalant/irritants can cause edema around these structures and occasionally lead to a secondary infection.

Tornwaldt's cyst is a common congenital lesion of the midline posterior nasopharyngeal mucosa. Other types of cysts can also be present and can be located within or outside the adenoid tissue. They often present with purulent nasal discharge, pain in the throat, and a conductive hearing loss from chronic eustachian tube dysfunction. The intraadenoidal cysts arise from the median pharyngeal recess and present as a small opening on the adenoid bud. Extraadaenoidal cysts are deep in the nasopharyngeal fossa and are derived from the pharyngeal bursa. A cuff of granulation tissue adjacent to the pharyngeal tube will be the main physical finding.

TREATMENT

Infectious disorders of the nasopharynx should be treated with supportive therapy. Those of bacterial origin should be treated with appropriate antibiotics. These include antibacterial agents commonly used for otitis media as well as sinusitis.

In disorders that cause chronic inflammation of the nasopharyngeal tissue, nasal steroid inhalers can be utilized.

When nasopharyngeal cysts are identified and become secondarily infected or inflamed, marsupialization of the cystic structures is appropriate.

> **SPECIAL CONSIDERATION**
>
> One should not hesitate to biopsy nasopharyngeal masses or asymptomatic tissue to rule out a granulomatous or neoplastic process.

> **PEARL...** When acute nasopharyngeal obstruction becomes severe enough to cause respiratory distress, an excellent temporizing measure is placement of a nasopharyngeal airway tube.

Chronic adenoid hypertrophy with recurrent infections will respond well to adenoidectomy and/or adenoid cauterization.

Rarely, and generally only in a neonate, will a tracheostomy be required due to nasopharyngeal pathology.

SUGGESTED READINGS

Belenky WM, Madgy DN. Nasal obstruction and rhinorrhea. In: Bluestone CD, Stowel SE, Kenna MA, eds. *Pediatric Otolaryngology*. 3rd ed. Philadelphia: WB Saunders; 1996:765–779.

Contencin P, Narcy P. Nasopharyngeal pH monitoring in infants and children with chronic rhinopharyngitis. *Int J Pediatr Otolaryngol* 1991;22:249–256.

Engel JP. Viral upper respiratory infections. *Semin Respir Infect* 1995;10:3–13.

Heald A, Auckenthaler R, Borst F, et al. Acute bacterial nasopharyngitis. *J Intern Med* 1993; 8:667–673.

Hendricks NK, Perez EM, Berger BJ, Mouton PA. Brucellosis in childhood in the Western Cape. *South Afr Med J* 1995;85:176–178.

Hollender AR. The lymphoid tissue of the naso-pharynx. *Laryngoscope* 1969;69:529.

Homoe P, Prag J, Farholt S, et al. High rate of nasopharyngeal carriage of potential patho-gens among children in Greenland. *Clin Infect Dis* 1996;23:1081–1090.

Horiguti S. The discovery of the nasopharyngitis and its influence on general disease. *Acta Otolaryngol Suppl* 1975;329:1–120.

Mainous AG, Hueston WJ, Clark JR. Antibiotics and upper respiratory infection. *J Fam Pract* 1996;42:357–361.

Martinez SA, Mouney DS. Treponemal infec-tions of the head and neck. *Otolaryngol Clin North Am* 1982;15:613.

Meiteles LZ, Lucente FE. Sinus and nasal mani-festations of acquired immumodeficiency syndrome. *Ear Nose Throat J* 1990;69:454–459.

Neel HB. Benign and malignant neoplasms of the nasopharynx. In: Cummings CW, Fredrickson JM, Harker LA, Krause CJ, Schuller DE, eds. *Otolaryngology–Head and Neck Surgery.* 2nd ed. St. Louis: Mosby Year Book; 1993:1355–1371.

Sprinkle PM, Hunsker DH. Bacteriology. In: Pa-parella MM, Shumrick DA, Gluckman JL, Meyerhoff WL, eds. *Otolaryngology.* 3rd ed. Philadelphia: WB Saunders; 1991:567–573.

Stern JC, Lin PT, Lucente FE. Benign nasopha-ryngeal masses and HIV infection. *Arch Oto-laryngol Head Neck Surg* 1990;116: 206.

Wood RP, Jasek DW, Eberhard R. Nasal obstruc-tion. In: Baily BJ, Johnson JT, Pillsbury HC, Kohut RI, Tardy ME, eds. *Head and Neck Sur-gery—Otolaryngology.* Philadelphia: JB Lip-pincott; 1993:302–328.

Zenni MK, Cheatham SH, Thompson JM, et al. Streptococcus pneumoniae colonization in a young child: association with otitis media and resistance to penicillin. *J Pediatr* 1995; 127:533–537.

Chapter 32

Neoplasms and Cysts

Lyon L. Gleich

The vast majority of tumors of the nasopharynx are malignant epithelial neoplasms. The second most common malignancy of the nasopharynx is malignant lymphoma. In children embryonal rhabdomyosarcoma can arise in this region.

Nasopharyngeal Carcinoma

The term *nasopharyngeal carcinoma* is used to refer to the epithelioid-derived tumors that arise in the nasopharynx. These tumors can have a varied presentation and clinical course.

Symptoms

The presentation of nasopharyngeal carcinoma is variable. Patients may present with significant nasal symptoms including nasal obstruction, epistaxis, a sensation of sinus fullness, and headache. Some patients present with minimal nasal symptoms, but complain of otalgia or decreased hearing due to eustachian tube obstruction from the mass. A majority of the patients present with a mass in the neck, and in some patients this is the only complaint.

Physical Findings

Flexible endoscopy has significantly aided in the evaluation of the nasopharynx. Nasopharyngeal carcinomas are typically erythematous and friable. The tumor arises most frequently near the fossa of Rosenmüller. At the primary site the lesion may erode the nasal septum and nasal bones and even be visible on anterior rhinoscopy. Orbital invasion can produce significant proptosis or hypertelorism. Cranial nerves may be involved at the skull base. In particular the trigeminal and abducens nerves are at risk and their function should be examined. Many patients will be anosmic from tumor obstructing the olfactory region.

Cervical nodes are present in over 70% of patients. The nodes are usually high in the neck, and posterior cervical adenopathy is common. Some patients present with cervical adenopathy only and the nasopharyngeal primary is not recognized until a biopsy is performed during the search for the primary site. Computed tomography (CT) and/or magnetic resonance imaging (MRI) scanning are useful in the evaluation of nasopharyngeal carcinoma to demonstrate the extent of the primary tumor. In particular, the relationship of the tumor to the skull base and foramina can be visualized with these scans. As with all head and neck malignancies a metastatic evaluation, including a chest X-ray and liver profile, should be performed.

Incidence and Pathology

Nasopharyngeal carcinoma is an uncommon cancer in the United States with an incidence of <1 per 100,000. In Southern China, particularly Guangdong province, it is a common tumor.

226

Prior infection with the Epstein-Barr virus (EBV) is strongly associated with nasopharyngeal carcinoma. In particular the immunoglobulin A (IgA) viral capsid antigen and IgA early antigen have been correlated with nasopharyngeal carcinoma. Some authors suggest measuring titers of these antigens prior to therapy so that they can be followed to detect recurrence. This is not done by most physicians.

Nasopharyngeal cancers occur at a younger age than other head and neck malignancies. The average age at onset is 50 and men are more frequently affected.

Nasopharyngeal carcinomas have been divided into three pathologic groups by the World Health Organization (WHO). WHO I tumors are keratinizing squamous cell carcinomas. In the United States these tumors account for approximately 25% of nasopharyngeal carcinomas. In areas of the world where nasopharyngeal carcinoma is common, such as Southern China, these tumors account for less than 5% of nasopharyngeal carcinomas. These tumors are not related to EBV infection. WHO II tumors are nonkeratinizing squamous cell carcinomas. These tumors histologically resemble transitional cell bladder cancer, and are also called transitional cell carcinoma. These tumors are related to EBV infection. WHO III tumors are undifferentiated carcinomas and include lymphoepithelioma. They account for the majority of nasopharyngeal carcinomas in the United States and worldwide. These tumors are related to EBV infection.

DIAGNOSIS AND STAGING

Once there is a suspicion of nasopharyngeal carcinoma, the suspicious lesion should be biopsied. Suspicious cervical nodes can be aspirated to aid in the diagnostic workup. Open neck biopsies should be avoided unless all other diagnostic techniques are exhausted. The pathology, however, must be clearly demonstrated before treatment can commence. Once the tumor has been evaluated both clinically and radiographically, the patient should be staged. It should be noted that because the nasopharynx is a midline structure and has such a high propensity for metastasis, even bilaterally, that the nodal staging system is different than for other regions of the head and neck (Table 32–1). In part it evaluates how far inferiorly from the nasopharynx the tumor has progressed.

TREATMENT

Nasopharyngeal carcinoma is treated primarily with radiation therapy regardless of stage. Although many patients present with significant cervical adenopathy, even these patients should

TABLE 32–1 STAGING NASOPHARYNGEAL CARCINOMA

T1	Tumor confined to the nasopharynx
T2	Tumor extends to soft tissues of oropharynx and/or nasal fossa
	T2a Without parapharyngeal extension
	T2b With parapharyngeal extension
T3	Tumor invades bony structures and/or paranasal sinuses
T4	Tumor with intracranial extension and/or involvement of cranial nerves, infratemporal fossa, hypopharynx, or orbit
N0	No regional lymph node metastasis
N1	Unilateral metastasis in lymph node(s), 6 cm or less in greatest dimension, above the supraclavicular fossa
N2	Bilateral metastasis in lymph node(s), 6 cm or less in greatest dimension, above the supraclavicular fossa
N3	Metastasis in a lymph node(s)
	N3a Greater than 6 cm in dimension
	N3b Extension to the supraclavicular fossa

be treated primarily with radiation. Neck dissection is reserved for persistent or recurrent cervical disease. The radiation field extends from above the skull base and fully encompasses the nodal basins in both necks. WHO II and WHO III tumors are more radiosensitive than WHO I tumors.

In patients with stage III or IV disease the addition of chemotherapy has been supported by recent clinical trials. Radiation with concomitant *cis*-platinum and 5-fluorouracil appears to offer improved survival as compared to radiation alone.

Recurrent or persistent nasopharyngeal carcinoma is a significant problem.

SPECIAL CONSIDERATION

If the disease recurs in any site, the nasopharynx, neck, and distant sites should be reevaluated because there may be recurrence in these sites as well.

If the recurrence is in the neck only, the patient may be salvaged with a neck dissection.

If the recurrence is only in the nasopharynx, there are advocates for a variety of forms of treatment. Some advocate reirradiation. This carries the risk of osteoradionecrosis, but can produce cures. Stereotactic radiation or brachytherapy can aid in increasing the dosage at the primary site. This reirradiation can also be combined with chemotherapy. Surgery has been used for recurrent nasopharyngeal carcinoma. This surgery can cause significant morbidity, and the cure rates are limited, but there are those that advocate this approach. Frequently, surgery for nasopharyngeal carcinoma requires carotid sacrifice, and the patient's ability to tolerate this must be evaluated. Approaches to the skull base for nasopharynx cancer include the lateral infratemporal fossa approach, transmaxillary approach, maxillary swing approach, transmandibular approach, and transcervical approach. These approaches permit access to the nasopharynx, but obtaining clear margins is difficult. An added difficulty, in addition to carotid artery involvement, is cavernous sinus invasion, which can prohibit complete resection.

OTHER NASOPHARYNGEAL MALIGNANCIES

Lymphomas can occur in the nasopharynx. To evaluate a nasopharyngeal mass for lymphoma, it is important that the biopsy tissue be sent to the pathologist fresh. Radiation therapy is generally the main form of treatment. Minor salivery tumors can occur in the nasopharynx, but are rare. Nasal tumors, such as adenocarcinoma, esthesioneuroblastoma, sinonasal undifferentiated carcinoma, and mucosal melanoma can extend to involve the nasopharynx.

PEDIATRIC NASOPHARYNGEAL MALIGNANCIES

RHABDOMYOSARCOMA

Rhabdomyosarcoma is the most common soft tissue malignancy in the pediatric age group. Almost half the cases occur when the child is younger than 5 years old. The incidence is highest in Caucasian children. The orbit is the most commonly affected head and neck site, followed by the nasopharynx.

Children with nasopharyngeal rhabdomyosarcoma may present with nasal obstruction, rhinorrhea, and symptoms secondary to eustachian tube obstruction. Diagnosis is often delayed. Metastases occur by both lymphatic and hematologic paths. Distant metastases affect the lung and bone most frequently.

PEARL... Rhabdomyosarcoma in infants and young children is usually less differentiated than in adults. It is usually the embryonal or botryoid type. The characteristic cells are small, dark, and spindle shaped. Immunohistochemistry can aid in confirming the diagnosis.

Staging for rhabdomyosarcoma, according to the Intergroup Rhabdomyosarcoma Study, is based on the extent of disease and, unlike other head and neck malignancies, whether or not resection has been accomplished. In group I all disease has been resected, in group II there is microscopic residua or regional disease, in group III there is incomplete resection, and in group IV metastases are present at diagnosis.

Current recommendations for the treatment of rhabdomyosarcoma are a combination of surgery, radiation, and chemotherapy. When the surgery will impose major functional disability, only a biopsy should be performed. For nasopharyngeal tumors, surgery would be too destructive and radiation with chemotherapy is the most common treatment. If the neck is clinically negative, it requires no treatment. If there are neck nodes, a neck dissection followed by radiation therapy should be done.

PEDIATRIC NASOPHARYNGEAL CARCINOMA

Nasopharyngeal carcinoma accounts for one-third of pediatric nasopharyngeal neoplasms. Most cases occur in adolescence. Although rhabdomyosarcoma has a higher incidence in Caucasians, nasopharyngeal carcinoma has a higher incidence in children of African descent. Presentation is similar to adult nasopharyngeal carcinoma. As with adults, most patients present with cervical metastases. WHO III tumors predominate and there is a strong association with EBV. Treatment is the same as in adults, that is, radiation therapy with or without chemotherapy.

TORNWALDT'S CYST

The nasopharyngeal bursa of Tornwaldt is a persistence of the embryonic connection between the caudal end of the notochord and the nasopharyngeal epithelium. It is normally lost, but may be retained due to inflammation or adhesions. The cyst occurs in the midline of the posterior wall of the nasopharynx. It can become infected and cause a sore throat and purulent nasal discharge. The infection will usually resolve with antibiotics but may require drainage.

JUVENILE ANGIOFIBROMA

Juvenile angiofibromas are benign neoplasms that occur almost exclusively in adolescent males. Although frequently referred to as juvenile nasopharyngeal angiofibromas, these tumors actually arise from the region of the sphenopalatine foramen. The average age of onset is 14. More than 80% of patients present with nasal obstruction and epistaxis. Headache, eustachian tube obstruction, nasal speech, and mucopurulent rhinorrhea also occur. The lesion is typically a firm, rubbery, nodular, gray-red mass. Exophthalmos and a bulging cheek may occur.

Although these tumors begin in the sphenopalatine foramen region, they grow to fill the nasopharynx and can extend to the paranasal sinuses, infratemporal fossa, orbit, and intracranially. Tumor staging, as developed by Chandler and Sessions, is related to the tumor's spread from the nasopharyngeal region (stage I) to the cranial cavity (stage IV). CT scanning is used to evaluate the extent of the tumor. Early lesions will show bony expansion, whereas advanced lesions may have bone destruction.

Histologically juvenile angiofibromas are unencapsulated and infiltrate the surrounding tissue. The major components are a fibrous stroma and intertwined vascular channels. The vessels are variable in size, lined by a single layer of endothelial cells, and lack elastic fibers in their walls. This absence of a muscular layer prevents vasoconstriction, and epistaxis prior to treatment is therefore common.

> **PEARL...** The growth of juvenile angiofibroma is hormonally influenced. Progesterone receptors, androgen receptors, and glucocorticoid receptors are present.

Juvenile angiofibromas have been treated with surgery, radiation therapy, electrocoagulation, and hormonal administration. Surgery and/or radiation therapy are the current mainstays of treatment. Most surgeons advocate complete surgical resection, especially for extracranial tumors. The tumor can be approached through the palate or by a lateral rhinotomy incision. Preoperative angiography with embolization is recommended. Radiation is a viable option, but is best reserved for cases with intracranial extension.

SUGGESTED READINGS

Al-Sarraf M, LeBlanc M, Giri S, et al. Chemoradiotherapy versus radiotherapy in patients with advanced nasopharyngeal cancer: phase III randomized intergroup study 0099. *J Clin Oncol* 1998;16:1310–1317.

Harrison DFN. The natural history, pathogenesis, and treatment of juvenile angiofibroma. *Arch Otolaryngol Head Neck Surg* 1987;113: 936–942.

Lee AWM, Poon YF, Foo W, et al. Retrospective analysis of 5037 patients with nasopharyngeal carcinoma treated during 1976–1985: overall survival and patterns of failure. *Int J Radiation Oncol Biol Phys* 1992;23:261–270.

Maurer HM, Gehan EA, Beltangady M, et al. The Intergroup Rhabdomyosarcoma Study—II. *Cancer* 1993;71:1904–1922.

Chapter 33

TRAUMA

Yoram Stern and Sally R. Shott

Acquired nasopharyngeal stenosis (NPS) is an uncommon disorder of the nasopharynx. Infectious processes, particularly syphilis, were responsible for the majority of cases in the pre-antibiotic era. Today it is most frequently seen as a complication of surgical trauma. Adenotonsillectomy was responsible for most of the reported cases. More recently, uvulopalatopharyngoplasty (UPPP) has been implicated as a cause of this problem. Most cases of NPS after UPPP appear to be related to the surgical technique, and neither electrocautery nor laser prevented the complication.

Factors implicated in the development of NPS are excessive destruction of pharyngeal mucosa, surgery in the presence of pharyngitis, exceptionally large lateral adenoid bands, revision surgery, cicatrizing or keloid diathesis, excessive removal of posterior pillar mucosa, attempts to reapproximate mucosal edges, excessive undermining of posterior pharyngeal wall mucosa, and injury to the posterior part of the palate.

The condition is characterized by partial or complete obliteration of the normal communication between the nasopharynx and the oropharynx resulting from fusion of the soft palate and the tonsillar pillars to the posterior pharyngeal wall (Fig. 33–1). The symptoms vary from mild complaints of difficulty blowing the nose

or cleaning pharyngeal secretions to severe sleep apnea.

SPECIAL CONSIDERATION

Careful preoperative examination by nasopharyngeal mirror (Fig. 33–2) nasopharyngoscopy and under anesthesia is paramount for successfully planning surgical correction.

PEARL... The general principles of surgical correction of NPS are adequate scar removal and then to resurface the denuded areas with grafts or local flap.

A variety of surgical procedures have been described. Skin or mucosal grafts or local flaps have been used to resurface the open areas and thereby prevent healing of the wound by secondary intention. The local flaps include palatobuccal flaps, palatopharyngeal flaps, and laterally based posterior pharyngeal flaps. Use of free flaps has been advocated when severe NPS is present. Z-plasty has been used to correct mild cases of NPS. Stenting is often used in

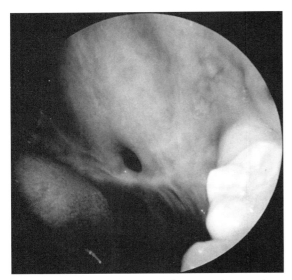

FIGURE 33–1 Severe nasopharyngeal stenosis.

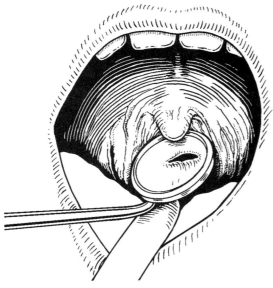

FIGURE 33–2 Mirror examination of nasopharyngeal stenosis.

conjunction with grafting or local flaps. Local infiltration of steroids can be useful in helping to prevent recurrence of scar tissue; however, it is not invariably successful.

SUGGESTED READINGS

Bennhoff DF. Current management of nasopharyngeal stenosis: indications for Z-plasty. *Laryngoscope* 1979;89:1582–1592.

Cotton RT. Nasopharyngeal stenosis. *Arch Otolaryngol* 1985;3:146–148.

Guggenheim P. Cicatricial stenosis of the nasopharyngeal isthmus. *Arch Otolaryngol* 1963; 177:13–18.

Katsantonis GP, Friedman WH, Krebs FJ. Nasopharyngeal complications following uvulopalatopharyngoplasty. *Laryngoscope* 1987; 97:309–314.

Kazanjian VH, Holmes EM. Stenosis of the nasopharynx and its correction. *Arch Otolaryngol* 1946;44:261–273.

McLaughlin KE, Jacobs IN, Todd NW, Sussack GS, Corlson G. Management of nasopharyngeal and oropharyngeal stenosis in children. *Laryngoscope* 1997;107:1322–1331.

Nichols JEH. The sequelae of syphilis in the pharynx and their treatment. *Trans Am Laryngol Assoc* 1986;18:161–168.

Stepnick DW. Management of total nasopharyngeal stenosis following UPPP. *Ear Nose Throat J* 1993;72:80–90.

Woolf RM, Broadbent TR. Nasopharyngeal stenosis following tonsillectomy and adenoidectomy. *Plast Reconstr Surg* 1970;45:352–355.

SECTION VI

LARYNX

Chapter 34

ANATOMY AND PHYSIOLOGY

Tapan A. Padhya and Keith M. Wilson

The larynx is a complex neuromuscular organ whose primary functions include (1) serving as a conduit for respiration, (2) protecting the lower respiratory tract, (3) facilitating phonation, and (4) providing sphincteric action for deglutition (closure of the glottis during Valsalva maneuver).

THE LARYNGEAL SKELETON

The laryngeal framework is composed of nine different segments of cartilage. Three cartilaginous segments are unpaired (cricoid, thyroid, and epiglottis) and three segments are paired (arytenoid, corniculate, and cuneiform). All are suspended or attached by a series of ligaments, muscles, and membranes (Fig. 34–1).

The epiglottis is composed of elastic, flexible cartilage shaped like a leaf. It is attached to the tongue base via the medial and lateral glossoepiglottic folds, which ultimately form the pouch-like depression called the vallecula. The epiglottis is connected to the hyoid and thyroid cartilage through the hyoepiglottic and thyroepiglottic ligaments, respectively.

The thyroid cartilage is composed of two quadrilateral-shaped laminae. The angle formed by these two laminae is 75 to 90 degrees in the postpubertal male and 90 to 110 degrees in the adult female. The inferior two-thirds of these

SPECIAL CONSIDERATION

The epiglottis has numerous pits, which may allow tumors on the laryngeal surface of the epiglottis to spread freely into the pre-epiglottic space.

laminae are fused in the midline, thereby forming the laryngeal prominence or Adam's apple. The superior one-third diverges from the laryngeal prominence to form the V-shaped thyroid notch.

PEARL••• The level of the true vocal cords in males is halfway between the notch and the inferior edge of the thyroid cartilage, whereas the distance in the female larynx is one-third the distance of the laminae measured from the thyroid notch.

The lateral edge of each lamina is marked by an oblique line. This line allows attachment of the inferior pharyngeal constrictor, sternothyroid, and thyrohyoid musculature.

The third unpaired cartilage of the larynx is the cricoid. The cricoid remains the only complete ring within the laryngotracheal complex.

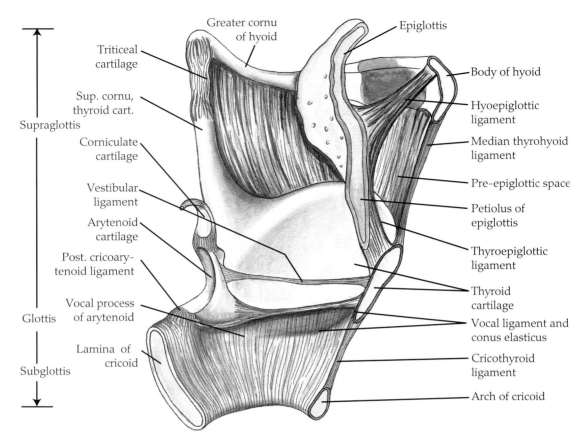

FIGURE 34–1 Sagittal section of the larynx demonstrating ligaments and cartilages.

SPECIAL CONSIDERATION

Being a complete ring, this is a common site for airway stenosis in neonates and adults.

The cricoid is shaped like a signet ring with the band facing anteriorly and the lamina (signet) part located posteriorly. The cricoid is located at C3-C4 in the child and C6-C7 in the adult.

The paired arytenoid cartilages are each shaped like three-sided pyramids that articulate with the superior border of the cricoid cartilage. Each cartilage has an apex superiorly, vocal process anteriorly, and a muscular process laterally. The apical process is attached to the aryepiglottic fold, the vocal process to the vocal ligament, and the muscular process to the posterior cricoarytenoid muscle.

The corniculate and cuneiform cartilages are the remaining group of paired cartilages. The corniculates lie on top of the arytenoid and help to elevate the height of the aryepiglottic fold. The cuneiforms lie in the aryepiglottic fold itself and help to stiffen the fold during epiglottic closure.

Only the thyroid, cricoid, and arytenoid cartilages are affected by ossification, which usually begins in the second decade and continues into the third decade. The hyoid completes ossification by age 2. Ossification of cartilage makes the larynx more susceptible to fractures when involved in direct penetrating or blunt trauma. The thyroid cartilage begins ossification from an inferior to superior direction, whereas the cricoid is ossified from posterior to anterior.

JOINTS OF THE LARYNX

There are two synovial joints in the larynx that are of particular importance—the cricothyroid joint and cricoarytenoid joint. The cricothyroid joint allows rotation and sliding of the thyroid cartilage, thereby allowing changes in the length of the vocal folds. The cricoarytenoid joint allows the arytenoids (1) to slide toward or away from one another (translation), (2) to tilt anteriorly and posteriorly, and (3) to rotate. All these movements help to manipulate the vocal fold in the needed direction.

SPECIAL CONSIDERATION

The cricoarytenoid joint can be dislocated during endotracheal intubation and can undergo arthritic changes caused by such diseases as rheumatoid arthritis.

LIGAMENTS AND MEMBRANES OF THE LARYNX

The thyroid cartilage is suspended from the hyoid bone via the medial and lateral thyrohyoid membranes. The hyoepiglottic membrane connects the hyoid and the epiglottis, whereas the trachea is attached to the cricoid by the cricotracheal ligament. The cricothyroid ligament connects the cricoid cartilage by the cricotracheal border of the thyroid cartilage.

There is an elastic membrane that supports the endolarynx itself. The upper part of this thin submucosal membrane is called the quadrangular membrane, which spans from the arytenoid to the epiglottis. The free inferior edge of this membrane is called the ventricular ligament, which is ultimately covered by loose mucosa constituting the false vocal cord/fold. The free superior edge of the quadrangular membrane ultimately forms the aryepiglottic (AE) fold.

The conus elasticus constitutes the lower half of this elastic membrane, which begins from the superior border of the cricoid and attaches to the lower anterior border of the thyroid cartilage, thus forming the cricothyroid membrane.

SPECIAL CONSIDERATION

The cricothyroid membrane is the landmark one must quickly identify in situations that warrant an emergent surgical airway.

The vocal ligament, the superior edge of the conus elasticus, is the fibrous core of the vocal fold, which extends from the anterior midline thyroid cartilage (Broyle's ligament) to the vocal process of the arytenoid cartilage.

THE INTERIOR OF THE LARYNX

The area superior to the false vocal (vestibular) folds is termed the vestibule. Between the false vocal folds and the true vocal folds lies the ventricle of Morgagni of the larynx (Fig. 34–2). The superior extension of the ventricle between the thyroid cartilage and the false vocal fold is termed the saccule. Mucus glands within the saccule provide a source of lubrication for the vocal cords.

SPECIAL CONSIDERATION

Dilation or obstruction of this space can lead to airway obstruction in neonates and present as an internal laryngocele in an adult.

The rima glottidis is the aperture between the vocal cords. The vocal cord extends from the anterior midline of the thyroid cartilage to the vocal process of the arytenoid. Broyle's ligament is the fibrous attachment of the vocal ligament to the inner perichondrium of the thyroid cartilage at the anterior commissure. The rima vestibuli is the space between the false vocal or vestibular folds. Closure of the false vocal folds acts as an airway protective mechanism to prevent penetration of food particles.

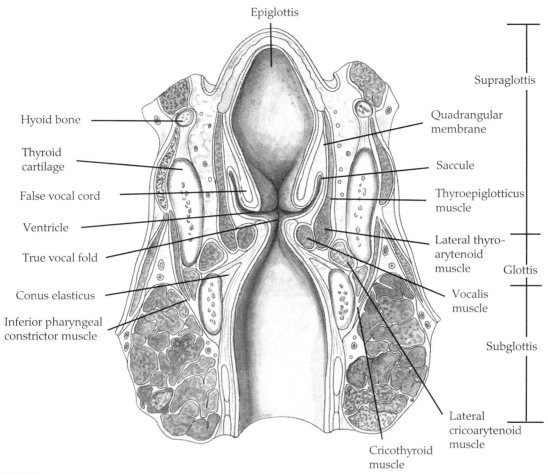

FIGURE 34–2 Coronal section of the larynx.

ANATOMIC SPACES OF THE LARYNX

The larynx is further subdivided vertically by three distinct regions: the supraglottis, the glottis, and the subglottis. The supraglottic region is defined superiorly by the epiglottis and inferiorly by a horizontal plane passing through the lateral margin of the ventricle at its junction with the superior surface of the vocal cord. The glottis is defined as the region extending from the true vocal cord to a horizontal plane 1 cm below the free edge of the vocal cord. Finally, the subglottis is the area between the horizontal plane 1 cm below the true vocal cord free edge and the lower border of the cricoid cartilage.

The pre-epiglottic space is bounded anteriorly by the thyrohyoid membrane and thyroid cartilage, posteriorly by the epiglottis and thyroepiglottic ligament, and superiorly by the hyoepiglottic ligament and vallecular mucosa. The paraglottic space is formed by the thyroid lamina, conus elasticus, and quadrangular membrane. The location where the vocal ligament attaches anteriorly to the thyroid lamina in the midline is referred to as the anterior commissure.

SPECIAL CONSIDERATION

Lymphatics and microvessels contained within Broyle's ligament at the anterior commissure allow for a possible route for tumor extension outside the larynx.

MUSCLES OF THE LARYNX (EXTRINSIC AND INTRINSIC)

The extrinsic muscles of the larynx are involved with the movement of the laryngeal complex as a whole. The following infrahyoid "strap" muscles help to depress the hyoid and the larynx: omohyoid (C2, C3), sternohyoid (C2, C3), and sternothyroid (C2, C3). These suprahyoid muscles help to elevate the hyoid and larynx: stylohyoid (VII), digastric (V, VII), mylohyoid (V), geniohyoid (C1), and stylopharyngeus (VII). The thyrohyoid (C1) muscle elevates the thyroid cartilage while it depresses the hyoid bone.

The intrinsic muscles of the larynx adjust the position and tension in the vocal folds. All intrinsic muscles of the larynx are innervated by the recurrent laryngeal nerve except the cricothyroid muscle, which is supplied by the external branch of the superior laryngeal nerve (Fig. 34–3). The posterior cricoarytenoid (PCA) muscle is the only abductor muscle of the larynx. The remaining adductor and tensor muscles of the larynx are listed in Table 34–1.

BLOOD SUPPLY OF THE LARYNX

The major blood supply to the larynx is derived from the superior and inferior laryngeal arteries, each a branch off of the superior and inferior thyroid arteries, respectively. The superior laryngeal artery joins with the internal branch of the superior laryngeal nerve near the greater cornu of the thyroid cartilage and then travels deep into the thyrohyoid muscle, ultimately passing through the thyroid membrane. The inferior laryngeal artery travels with the recurrent laryngeal nerve and penetrates the larynx behind the cricothyroid joint under the inferior pharyngeal constrictor. The superior and inferior laryngeal arteries are interconnected by multiple communicating branches.

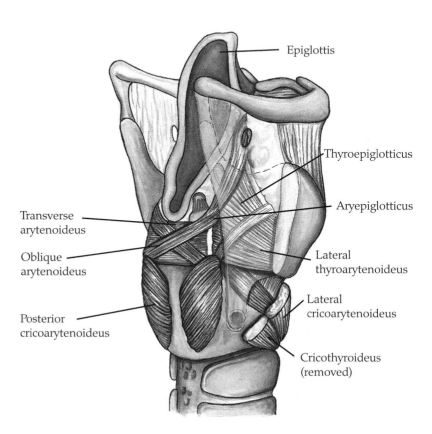

FIGURE 34–3 Intrinsic muscles of the larynx.

TABLE 34–1 MUSCLES OF THE LARYNX

Muscle	Origin	Insertion	Nerve Supply	Action
Cricothyroid	Anterolateral cricoid	Inferior thyroid cartilage	External laryngeal N	Tenses; lengthens; adducts VC
Interarytenoid	Arytenoid	Contralateral arytenoid	Bilateral RLN	
Posterior cricoarytenoid	Posterior thyroid cartilage	Muscular process of arytenoid	RLN	Abducts VC
Lateral cricoarytenoid	Arch of cricoid	Muscular process of arytenoid	RLN	Adducts VC
Transverse and oblique arytenoid	Arytenoid	Contralateral arytenoid	RLN	Adducts VC
Thyroarytenoid	Posterior thyroid cartilage	Muscular process of arytenoid	RLN	Relaxes VC
Vocalis	Midline angle of thyroid cartilage	Vocal process of arytenoid	RLN	Alters vocal fold during phonation

N, nerve; RLN, recurrent laryngeal nerve; VC, vocal cords.

Venous outflow is transported via the superior, middle, and inferior thyroid veins, all of which drain into the internal jugular vein.

NERVES OF THE LARYNX

The afferent innervation of the larynx comes from the vagus nerve through the superior and recurrent laryngeal nerves. The superior laryngeal nerve (SLN) starts at the inferior (nodose) vagal ganglion and travels inferiorly crossing medially to the internal carotid artery. The SLN divides into the internal (sensory) and external (sensory and motor) branch at the level of the greater cornu of the hyoid. The internal branch travels along with the superior laryngeal artery, finally entering the larynx through the thyrohyoid membrane. The internal branch is responsible for supraglottic mucosal sensation, which ultimately aids in airway protection. The external branch of the superior laryngeal nerve travels with the superior thyroid artery on top of the inferior pharyngeal constrictor, ultimately innervating the cricothyroid muscle and providing sensory input to the subglottis.

The recurrent laryngeal nerve provides innervation to the adductors and abductor of the larynx. The left recurrent laryngeal nerve (RLN) passes under and behind the aortic arch and enters the tracheoesophageal groove in the chest. The RLN passes to the back of the cricothyroid articulation and enters the larynx through a gap (the Killian-Jamieson area) deep in the lower border of the inferior constrictor muscle. The right recurrent laryngeal nerve (RLN) has a shorter course. It branches off the vagus nerve at the level of the right subclavian artery, passing under and behind the artery and traveling superiorly in the right tracheoesophageal groove.

SPECIAL CONSIDERATION

On rare occasions, the right RLN does not descend into the chest and loop around the subclavian artery but instead branches directly to the larynx from the vagus.

Once penetrating the larynx, the recurrent laryngeal nerve splits into an anterior division supplying the adductor muscles and a posterior division that supplies the PCA muscle. Galen's anastomoses are interconnecting fibers between the RLN and the internal branch of the superior laryngeal nerve.

LYMPHATICS OF THE LARYNX

The supraglottic larynx, due to its embryologic anlage, possesses bilateral lymphatic drainage. These lymphatics pass through the pre-epiglottic space and exit through the thyrohyoid membrane. From there, drainage goes onto the upper and middle jugular lymph nodes. The glottis is generally considered devoid of lymphatic drainage. Lymphatic drainage of the subglottis passes through the cricothyroid membrane to the lateral paratracheal nodes and medially to the Delphian node.

MUCOSA OF THE LARYNX

The vocal cords, epiglottis, free edges of the aryepiglottic fold, and the pyriform sinus are covered with squamous epithelium. Interspersed in the mucosa is respiratory epithelium composed of pseudostratified ciliated columnar epithelium with goblet cells.

AGE-RELATED CHANGES OF THE LARYNX

In the neonate, the larynx maintains a higher position in the neck. The base of the cricoid is located at the fourth cervical vertebra. The epiglottis touches the soft palate, making the neonate an obligate nasal breather during the first 4 to 6 months of life. By puberty, the larynx has descended to the level of the sixth cervical vertebra (C_6).

The length of the vocal cord increases with age. During infancy, the vocal cord is 6 to 8 mm in length, with the arytenoid accounting for about 50% of the total vocal cord length. During male puberty, there is an abrupt increase in the vocal cord length, producing a lower octave voice change. In adulthood, the vocal cord is 14 to 23 mm long, with the arytenoid accounting for approximately one-third of the total length.

The subglottic diameter in neonates is 5 to 7 mm, with a diameter less than 4 mm being considered subglottic stenosis. By age 4, the subglottic diameter is approximately 11 mm. The adult subglottis ranges from 15 to 20 mm.

SUGGESTED READINGS

Anderson JE. *Grant's Atlas of Anatomy.* 8th ed. Baltimore: Williams & Wilkins, 1983.

Armstrong WB, Netterville JL. Anatomy of the larynx, trachea, and bronchi. *Otolaryngol Clin North Am* 1995;28:685–699.

Hollingshead WH. *Anatomy for Surgeons: The Head and Neck.* Vol. 1, 3rd ed. Philadelphia: J.B. Lippincott; 1982:465–500.

Chapter 35

CLINICAL TESTS

Keith M. Wilson and Tapan A. Padhya

Diagnostic testing of the larynx elucidates details of skeletal anatomy, airway patency, and laryngeal function. All patients with laryngeal complaints should have their larynges inspected either directly or indirectly. Specific tests should be performed based on the laryngeal function that is abnormal. For example, aspiration, which demonstrates a loss of the protective function of the larynx, is best evaluated by a dynamic test such as a modified barium swallow. Similarly, disturbances in voice production or quality are best evaluated with videostroboscopy. This chapter reviews the many tests available for laryngeal evaluation.

INDIRECT LARYNGOSCOPY

Indirect laryngoscopy, the primary laryngeal screening test, provides a good view of the larynx and hypopharynx and allows for evaluation of vocal fold mobility. Subtle laryngeal pathology may be missed. Small lesions on the laryngeal surface of the epiglottis are difficult to see if the epiglottis is floppy. Anatomic variation sometimes precludes detailed examination of the anterior commissure. The apices of the pyriform sinuses usually cannot be visualized.

DIRECT LARYNGOSCOPY

When indirect laryngoscopy cannot be performed or it provides a less than adequate examination, direct laryngoscopy should be performed. Direct

PEARL... The gag reflex can often be overcome by encouraging patients to breathe easily through their mouth while keeping their eyes open. Breath holding and inadvertent touching of the base of tongue will trigger gagging. If this fails, use topical anesthesia.

laryngoscopy can be accomplished in the clinic setting or in the operating room. Flexible endoscopy provides full panoramic visualization of the larynx and pharynx in dynamic and adynamic conditions. It is the ability to examine the larynx during connected speech that makes flexible endoscopy essential in the evaluation of laryngeal complaints.

PEARL... Rigid endoscopes can be utilized in the clinic setting to provide excellent visualization of the larynx with magnification. This approach, when coupled with the appropriately curved instruments and properly placed topical anesthesia, allows for laryngeal manipulation in the office.

Direct laryngoscopy performed in the operating room is the procedure of choice when a biopsy is to be performed or precise manipulation of the vocal folds (e.g., microlaryngoscopy, bimanual manipulation) is needed.

The proper technique requires lifting of the tongue and laryngeal structures. When more visualization is desired anteriorly, the head can be lifted off the table. Proper placement of the arms with elbows on the operating table allows for easy lifting. Overwhelming strength is not necessary.

VIDEOSTROBOSCOPY

Videostroboscopy has become an integral part of the diagnostic evaluation of hoarseness. It is essentially a combination of videorecording and stroboscopy. This technique facilitates detailed evaluation of the vocal mechanism because of the ability of stroboscopy to provide a slow-motion view of the vocal folds as they vibrate.

Stroboscopy permits diagnosis of subtle pathology as well as documentation of recovery from therapeutic intervention. Slow-motion playbacks for closer scrutiny and subsequent viewing by clinicians not present at the time of the study are additional advantages afforded by this technique.

Videostroboscopy can be performed with either a rigid or a flexible scope. Flexible videostroboscopy facilitates detailed examination of fluent speech.

Rigid videostroboscopy provides better definition because of the increased light-carrying capability and better optics of the rigid system.

LARYNGEAL ELECTROMYOGRAPHY

Laryngeal electromyography (LEMG) is a technique of measuring electrical impulses generated by the muscles of the larynx. The clinical applications are still developing. There are three muscles that can be regularly tested: thyroarytenoid, posterior cricoarytenoid, and cricothyroid. LEMG can be accomplished with either monopolar or bipolar needle electrodes. When there is a need to inject and monitor electrical activity, as in Botox injections, the hollow monopolar needle is used. When monitoring electrical activity alone is needed, the bipolar electrodes will give more accurate information. Bipolar concentric needle electrodes record reliable data and eliminate the problems that face hook wire electrodes, namely sensitivities to placement and movement.

LEMG has two main clinical applications: evaluation of the immobile vocal fold and identification of the target muscle for Botox injection. Diagnostic as well as prognostic information pertaining to unilateral vocal fold paralysis is obtained with LEMG. The morphologic presentation of the paralyzed vocal fold can range from denervation with fibrillation potentials, to reinnervation with polyphasic potentials and prolonged motor units. Occasionally, normal motor unit action potentials are seen.

LEMG may provide helpful information in differentiating between paralysis and fixation. Often it is inconclusive.

Possibly the best indication for LEMG is to direct the delivery of Botox into the cricothyroid, thyroarytenoid, and posterior cricoarytenoid muscles for the treatment of spasmodic dysphonia. LEMG is utilized when a transcervical injection is performed. Botox injections performed via the transoral approach using curved needles under direct visualization do not require electromyographic guidance.

IMAGING TECHNIQUES

MODIFIED BARIUM SWALLOW

The larynx has three main functions: airway protection, airway patency, and voice production. The ability of the larynx to protect the airway is specifically detailed by the modified barium swallow.

> **PEARL•••** To get the best results, modified barium swallow is usually performed by, or with the assistance of, a competent speech pathologist.

The modified barium swallow is a fluoroscopic technique that facilitates direct observation of the upper aerodigestive tract during all stages of deglutition. The two main modifications are using less barium and placing the patient in an upright seated position. Less barium (or thin barium) is used in the event that the patient aspirates. The upright seating simulates the normal eating position and facilitates more specific analysis of the oral cavity and the pharynx.

> **PITFALL•••** Never order a standard barium swallow (upper GI) on a head and neck surgical patient. Larger quantities of barium will be used and the patient may be tested in a lying position. These situations will increase the chance of aspiration. Standard barium swallows evaluate esophageal anatomy and motility and will therefore miss the anatomic areas of concern in head and neck surgery patients.

CONVENTIONAL PLAIN FILMS

Plain film radiographs can demonstrate the soft tissues and underlying skeleton of the larynx. The lateral soft tissue film provides an overview of the entire airway from the level of the trachea entering the thoracic inlet below to the vault of the nasopharynx above. Radiopaque foreign bodies and retropharyngeal or intralaryngeal abscesses can be identified.

Mucous membrane swelling or distortion can have a characteristic appearance on plain films. A swollen epiglottis, as seen in epiglottitis, gives a "thumb" sign, so called because it looks like a thumb viewed in profile. The relationship between the cervical spine and the larynx is important.

> **PEARL•••** The soft tissue distance between the anterior aspect of any individual cervical vertebra and the posterior wall of the trachea should not exceed in distance the height of the body of the cervical vertebra at the same level. Dimensions greater than this would suggest a pathologic condition.

Retropharyngeal abscess would be a major concern in the pediatric population. Malignancy is the main diagnostic issue for adults.

COMPUTED TOMOGRAPHY (CT)

CT scanning is the major diagnostic imaging study performed for laryngeal evaluation. It elucidates the intrinsic and extrinsic laryngeal structures in an axial orientation. High-resolution or bone window settings can be utilized to enhance the soft tissue details and framework irregularities.

Laryngeal cancer evaluation requires CT scanning when the clinical and endoscopic examination is inadequate. It identifies preepiglottic and paraglottic space involvement in addition to laryngeal framework destruction. Intravenous contrast enhancement may permit improved mucosal definition. Contrast enhancement facilitates better evaluation of cervical adenopathy.

> **PEARL•••** Lymph nodes greater than 1.5 cm are considered malignant. Those measuring between 10 and 15 mm are considered to be suspicious.

CT scanning is fast and offers thin-slice (3 mm) capability with excellent spatial resolution. Cortical bone is imaged well. Disadvantages of CT include the artifacts created by dental amalgam and thick body parts such as the shoulders.

Three-dimensional CT scanning is relatively new digital technology that is used to evaluate laryngeal neoplasms and trauma. Its role is still being determined.

MAGNETIC RESONANCE IMAGING (MRI)

MRI scanning is an imaging technique that employs radiofrequency waves instead of X-rays. This study relies on the measurement of radiofrequency waves that are emitted as excited hydrogen atoms return to their steady state. Bone and calcified structures are not imaged secondary to their calcium content.

MRI imaging provides the best soft tissue detailing of all the diagnostic modalities. The utilization of gadolinium to enhance the image facilitates the differentiation of tumor from inflammatory processes. It is also helpful in determining the presence of cervical lymph nodes. Images can be acquired in multiple planes without repositioning the patient. Artifacts from dental amalgam and shoulders are eliminated. Inexperience with MRI of the larynx may be the largest impediment to gaining maximal information.

SPECIAL CONSIDERATION

MRI may be a better modality for assessing laryngeal involvement by tumors arising in adjacent sites or determining extralaryngeal extension of squamous cell carcinoma.

Magnetic resonance angiography (MRA) is a technique for a growing list of indications. It is largely used for vascular lesions. The more commonly diagnosed vascular lesions involving the larynx are arteriovenous malformations of the supraglottis and pyriform sinus (more commonly seen in adults), subglottic hemangiomas (seen more commonly in newborns and infants), and cavernous hemangiomas involving part or all of the larynx (seen more commonly in young adults).

ANGIOGRAPHY

This technique is being replaced by MRA. The major indications for laryngeal angiography are embolization of vascular lesions and direct infusion of chemotherapeutic agents in the treatment of laryngeal cancer.

RADIONUCLIDE SCANNING

The radionuclide bone scan with technetium (^{99m}Tc) methylene diphosphonate may detect arthropathies, particularly in relation to the cricoarytenoid and, occasionally, the cricothyroid joints. This technique has limited utility in assessing laryngeal pathology.

ULTRASOUND

Before CT scanning, ultrasound of the larynx was a popular method to determine thyroid cartilage invasion. Some ultrasound advocates use ultrasound to direct CT studies. Ultrasound's greatest utilization in laryngeal pathology is in determining the presence of external laryngoceles. This modality enjoys more popularity in Europe and Japan than in the United States.

SUGGESTED READINGS

Ford CN. Laryngeal EMG in clinical neurolaryngology. *Arch Otolaryngol Head Neck Surg* 1998;124:476–477.

Noyek AM, Fliss DM, Shulman HS. Diagnostic imaging of the larynx. In: Tucker HM, ed. *The Larynx.* 2nd ed. New York: Thieme; 1993:81–134.

Williams DW 3rd. Imaging of laryngeal cancer. *Otolaryngol Clin North Am* 1997;30:35–58.

Wippold FJ II, Glazer HS, Siegel MJ. Diagnostic imaging of the larynx. In: Cummings CW,

Fredrickson JM, Harker LA, Krause CJ, Schuller DE, eds. *Otolaryngology–Head and Neck Surgery.* 2nd ed. St. Louis: Mosby Yearbook; 1993:1785–1805.

Woodson GE. Clinical value of laryngeal EMG is dependent of experience of the clinician. *Arch Otolaryngol Head Neck Surg* 1998;124:476.

Yin SS, Wui WW, Stucker FJ. Major patterns of laryngeal electromyography and their clinical application. *Laryngoscope* 1997;107:126–136.

Chapter 36

CONGENITAL DISORDERS

Tapan A. Padhya and Keith M. Wilson

In today's world of advanced neonatal and perinatal medicine, there has been a renewed interest in congenital anomalies of the larynx. Symptoms that include feeding difficulty, failure to thrive, abnormal cry, and stridor often point to a more serious underlying problem. The presence of stridor is associated with several pathologic anomalies but it is the type of stridor that may indicate the level of the problem.

PEARL••• Inspiratory stridor usually points to the supraglottis, whereas biphasic (inspiratory and expiratory) suggests a glottic or subglottic site. Expiratory stridor generally involves pathology associated with the trachea.

LARYNGOMALACIA (CONGENITAL FLACCID LARYNX)

Laryngomalacia is the most common congenital anomaly of the pediatric larynx. This entity is recognized by an Ω-shaped epiglottis, foreshortened aryepiglottic folds, and redundant mucosa overlying the arytenoids and posterior supraglottis. There are two main theories for the basis of laryngomalacia. The first suggests cartilaginous immaturity, and the second supports the concept of poor neuromuscular control. Typ-

ically, inspiratory stridor presents within the first few weeks of life and is exacerbated by supine positioning and agitation. The infant's cry and swallowing are normal. Diagnosis is facilitated by flexible laryngoscopy in the office setting. This is a dynamic state that must be visualized during spontaneous respiration. Occasionally, airway fluoroscopy may also be utilized to document laryngomalacia.

SPECIAL CONSIDERATION

Not all patients require rigid endoscopic examination for the diagnosis, but this is important to rule out associated congenital anomalies and if airway intervention is needed.

Laryngomalacia is generally self-limiting and most patients improve by 2 years of age. In cases of severe/near obstructing laryngomalacia, surgical therapy is used. Tracheotomy is considered a temporizing measure but it is not without its own morbidity. Today, epiglottoplasty has become a viable option in the treatment of severe laryngomalacia. Conservative trimming of the epiglottis, aryepiglottic folds, and mucosa over the arytenoids may help avert a tracheostomy.

VOCAL CORD PARALYSIS

The second most common congenital laryngeal anomaly is vocal cord paralysis. Unilateral vocal cord paralysis generally involves peripheral lesions, whereas bilateral paralysis has a central etiology. Patients with unilateral vocal cord paralysis generally have a weak cry and no respiratory distress. Diagnosis is made by flexible laryngoscopy; however, imaging (computed tomography or magnetic resonance imaging) must be utilized to evaluate the entire course of the recurrent laryngeal nerve (brainstem to thorax). Major etiologies include cardiovascular anomaly and cervical birth trauma.

SPECIAL CONSIDERATION

Treatment is usually observation; however, in patients who aspirate, a temporary Gelfoam injection or external medialization of the affected cord must be considered.

Bilateral vocal cord paralysis presents as acute respiratory distress and requires immediate airway intervention, that is, intubation followed by tracheostomy. These patients may have a normal cry but demonstrate high-pitched inspiratory stridor during agitation. Flexible laryngoscopy reveals vocal cords in the paramedian position with an inability to abduct on inspiration. Central etiologies like Arnold-Chiari malformation, hydrocephalus, intracranial bleed, and encephalocele account for the vast majority of bilateral vocal cord paralyses. Treatment is usually tracheostomy with a long period of observation. Should vocal cord motion not return after a period of several years, one may consider arytenoidectomy or arytenoid lateralization for airway management.

CONGENITAL SUBGLOTTIC STENOSIS

The third most common congenital laryngeal anomaly is congenital subglottic stenosis. This problem arises from incomplete recanalization of the larynx during the third month of gestation. There is a continuum of this condition, ranging from complete laryngeal atresia through degrees of stenosis finally ending in thin laryngeal webs. Stenoses are considered congenital only if there is no prior history of intubation or other inducing factor. The normal subglottic luminal diameter of the newborn is 4.5 to 5.5 mm and 3.5 mm in the preterm infant. Subglottic stenosis is when the diameter is less than 4.0 mm in the newborn and 3.0 mm in the premature infant.

The typical patients with mild to moderate congenital stenosis remain asymptomatic until they experience an upper respiratory tract infection. This effectively causes mucosal inflammation, thus narrowing the subglottis, and the patient exhibits a biphasic stridor, dyspnea, and increased work of breathing.

PEARL... Flexible laryngoscopy, although not helpful in establishing the diagnosis, will give much needed information regarding the dynamic nature of the supraglottis and glottis. Definitive diagnosis is made using rigid telescopic laryngoscopy, which facilitates excellent magnification as well as a guide for sizing the stenosis (outer diameter of telescope).

A grading system has been developed to better stratify treatment. Grade 1 subglottic stenosis is a 50% luminal stenosis. Grades II and III have 51 to 70% and 71 to 99%, respectively. Grade IV has no detectable lumen. Treatment for mild stridor usually involves observation, thus allowing time for laryngeal growth. Surgical intervention for more severe forms of stenosis include tracheotomy, anterior and/or posterior cricoid split, and laryngotracheal reconstruction using costal cartilage.

SUBGLOTTIC HEMANGIOMA

Half the patients with subglottic hemangiomas present with cutaneous hemangiomas. Most patients are asymptomatic at birth but start to develop symptoms at 3 to 6 months of age. Stridor is usually inspiratory but can be biphasic.

Although lateral cervical radiographs and flexible laryngoscopy may be utilized, definitive diagnosis is made via rigid laryngoscopy and bronchoscopy.

CONTROVERSY

Due to the vascular nature of this lesion, many advocate not doing a biopsy for concern about hemorrhaging. There have been reports of minimal bleeding following biopsy.

The issue of airway intervention depends on the degree of obstruction. If there is a significant subglottic mass, a tracheotomy may be considered, allowing time for the lesion to involute. For small sessile lesions of the posterior subglottis, carbon dioxide (CO_2) laser has been used by some centers. For larger lesions, the use of oral steroids in patients younger than 1 year has been documented. The natural history of subglottic hemangiomas favor spontaneous resolution as the infant grows.

LARYNGEAL ATRESIA

Laryngeal atresia exemplifies a complete failure of laryngeal recanalization. Although rare, this entity presents as a true emergency at the time of birth. The neonate makes vigorous attempts at inspiration but quickly develops cyanosis. At this point, an emergency surgical airway (cricothyrotomy, tracheotomy) must be placed. The diagnosis is made by rigid laryngoscopy and bronchoscopy.

CONGENITAL LARYNGEAL WEB

This process represents incomplete failure of the larynx to recanalize during the third month of gestation. Depending on the site of the web, the neonate will present with some degree of respiratory obstruction, weak cry, and possibly aphonia. If the patient is in true respiratory distress, then an airway must be secured by either intubation or tracheotomy. Definitive diagnosis is again made by rigid laryngoscopy and bronchoscopy.

The majority of webs (75%) are located in the anterior glottic area.

PEARL... Thin webs are easily lysed with microlaryngeal instruments or the carbon dioxide laser. Thicker webs may require tracheotomy and open laryngeal repair with Silastic keel placement. Laryngeal dilators may be utilized in cases of recurrent formation of webs.

LARYNGOCELE/SACCULAR CYSTS

Congenital saccular cysts usually present in the supraglottis (aryepiglottic fold or lateral epiglottis) of the newborn. Symptoms include inspiratory stridor, weak cry, and varying degrees of airway obstruction. Acute respiratory distress may necessitate a secure airway by either intubation or tracheotomy. Although lateral cervical radiographs and flexible laryngoscopy may be helpful, definitive diagnosis and treatment is facilitated by rigid laryngoscopy. Surgical treatment of saccular cysts involves endoscopic marsupialization or CO_2 laser excision. For recurrent cases, a transcervical approach for excision should be considered.

Laryngoceles are considered dilation of the saccule (anterior end of ventricle). This is caused by increased intralaryngeal pressures causing the saccular space to enlarge. A classification of laryngoceles into internal, external, and combined types has been devised according to its relation to the laryngeal cartilage. Internal laryngoceles are confined within the endolarynx, whereas external laryngoceles have extended through the thyrohyoid membrane at the point of entry of the superior laryngeal nerve, and usually present as a mass in the neck. For small internal laryngoceles, endoscopic excision has been advocated. For larger internal, external, and combined laryngoceles, an external transcervical approach is used.

SPECIAL CONSIDERATION

Laryngoceles that present in adult patients with documented tobacco use should be carefully examined for possible coexisting malignancies located at the ventricular inlet.

LARYNGEAL CLEFTS

Laryngeal clefts are extremely rare, but a high index of suspicion should exist to make the diagnosis. In normal situations, the esophagus and airway are divided during weeks 5 to 7 in utero. A defect in this separation process leads to the cleft. Newborns that experienced maternal polyhydramnios have a higher incidence of laryngeal clefts. Patients with laryngeal clefts are also predisposed to have isolated tracheo-esophageal fistuals (20%).

These patients experience cyanosis with feeding, coughing, and varying degrees of respiratory distress due to the amount of aspiration and the length of the cleft. Diagnostic tests that are useful include a chest radiograph demonstrating aspiration infiltrate, barium swallow, and flexible laryngoscopy. Definitive diagnosis is made via rigid laryngoscopy/bronchoscopy.

Endoscopic examination will help classify the cleft. Type I involves a supraglottic interarytenoid cleft. Type II is a partial cricoid cleft extending below the level of the vocal cords. Types III and IV extend into the cervical trachea and thoracic trachea, respectively. Type I and II clefts may be amenable to endoscopic repair, whereas types III and IV usually require lateral pharyngotomy or anterior laryngofissure.

> **PITFALL...** In addition to surgical repair, one must attend to the recurrent aspiration risk. A gastrostomy tube with or without Nissen fundoplication must be considered.

SUGGESTED READINGS

Benjamin B. Congenital laryngeal webs. *Ann Otol Rhinol Laryngol* 1983;92:317–326.

Cohen SR, Geller KA, Birns JW, Thompson JW. Larygeal paralysis in children: a long term retrospective study. *Ann Otol Rhinol Laryngol* 1982;91:417–424.

Cotton RT, Richardson MA. Congenital laryngeal anomalies. *Otolaryngol Clin North Am* 1981;14(1):203–218.

Evans KL, Courteney-Harris R, Bailey M, Evans JNG, Parsons DS. Management of posterior laryngeal and laryngotracheoesophageal clefts. *Arch Otolaryngol Head Neck Surg* 1995; 121:1380–1385.

Hawkins DB, Crockett DM, Kahlstrom EJ, MacLaughlin EF. Corticosteroid management of airway hemangiomas: long term followup. *Laryngoscope* 1984;94:633–637.

Healy G, McGill T, Friedman EM. Carbon dioxide laser in subglottic hemangioma. *Ann Otol Rhinol Laryngol* 1984;93:370–373.

Holinger LD, Barnes DR, Smid LJ, Holinger PH. Laryngocele and saccular cysts. *Ann Otol Rhinol Laryngol* 1978;87:675–685.

Holinger LD, Holinger PC, Holinger PH. Etiology of bilateral abductor vocal cord paralysis. *Ann Otol Rhinol Laryngol* 1976;85:428–436.

Holinger PH, Brown WT. Congenital webs, cysts, laryngoceles, and other anomalies of the larynx. *Ann Otol Rhinol Laryngol* 1967; 76:744–752.

Myer CM, Cotton RT, Holmes DK, Jackson RK. Larygeal and laryngotracheoesophageal clefts: role of early surgical repair. *Ann Otol Rhinol Laryngol* 1990;99:98–104.

Myer CM, O'Connor DM, Cotton RT. Proposed grading system for subglottic stenosis based on endotracheal sizes. *Ann Otol Rhinol Laryngol* 1994;103:319–323.

Chapter 37

INFECTIOUS AND INFLAMMATORY DISORDERS

Keith M. Wilson and Tapan A. Padhya

Edema, inflammation, and exudation are the three main responses to acute injury. Chronic changes in the larynx are usually manifested by hypertrophy or metaplasia of the mucous membranes and fibrosis of the deeper tissues of the larynx. Most acute episodes occur over a period of less than 1 week, present with airway distress and fever, and are usually more prevalent and problematic in children. Chronic laryngeal infections, in general, exist for weeks before presentation. Patients usually present with airway distress, hoarseness, and pain as the major symptoms. Chronic infections are more common in adults.

The four major symptoms associated with infectious and inflammatory disorders of the larynx are dysphonia, dyspnea, dysphagia, and pain. They are variable in their onset and severity. The dyspnea may progress from simple stridor all the way to complete airway obstruction. The pain may vary from a dull ache to a severe stabbing discomfort sometimes associated with swallowing.

The history should include the severity and progression of symptoms, associated regional or systemic signs and symptoms, and precipitating factors. Additional history about family members, coworkers, and exposure to noxious substances can be helpful.

> **PEARL•••** The history is the most important tool in the diagnosis.

Physical examination should not be limited to the head and neck because many systemic illnesses may have laryngeal manifestation. Indirect or direct laryngoscopy is paramount to confirm the diagnosis. Radiographic studies and laboratory tests may also be helpful in making the correct diagnosis.

PEDIATRIC DISORDERS

ACUTE LARYNGOTRACHEOBRONCHITIS (CROUP)

Laryngotracheobronchitis is a subacute viral illness characterized by fever, barking cough, and progressive inspiratory stridor. Typically a cold-like prodrome occurs for a few days preceding the onset of symptoms. This is usually a winter illness and is occasionally epidemic. It most frequently occurs in boys aged 1 to 3 years and usually lasts 3 to 7 days. Croup can be classified as atypical when it occurs in infants younger than 1 year of age, lasts more than 7 days, or does not respond to appropriate treatment.

> **PEARL•••** In atypical cases one must think of other diagnoses such as foreign body, subglottic stenosis, or bacterial tracheitis.

The diagnosis is generally made on clinical grounds. The most important differential diagnosis in a child with suspected croup is epiglottis. Radiographs can be helpful in correctly diagnosing croup.

> **PEARL•••** X-rays of the airway will show a narrowed infraglottic airway. This is commonly referred to as a steeple sign.

Lateral airway X-rays in acute epiglottitis generally show a swollen epiglottis.

The management for acute laryngotracheobronchitis depends on the severity at presentation. A nonemergent presentation can be treated with antiinflammatory medication, humidification, and maybe antibiotics. More severe presentations may require racemic epinephrine, antibiotics, and steroids. In the more severe presentation the patients will often present with dehydration and air hunger. When medical management fails, direct airway support via intubation or tracheotomy may be necessary.

SPECIAL CONSIDERATION

Rising carbon dioxide levels, a worsening neurologic status, or a decreasing respiratory rate in the face of poor gas exchange are indications for direct airway support.

ACUTE EPIGLOTTITIS (SUPRAGLOTTITIS)

Acute epiglottitis is a specific infectious process that is usually caused by *Haemophilus influenzae* type B. The disease is much rarer than acute laryngotracheobronchitis. Although this condition is much more common in children ages 2 to 4, it can occur at any age up to and including adulthood. The child will typically present with high temperature, drooling, and sitting in an upright and forward position, demonstrating greater difficulty with inspiration than expiration. The onset is acute, often occurring in 2 to 6 hours.

The inflammatory process almost exclusively involves the supraglottic larynx with the epiglottis having a fiery, cherry-red appearance. The aryepiglottic fold and false vocal cords can also be involved. The true vocal cords are typically spared.

The diagnosis is usually straightforward.

> **PEARL•••** When the clinical findings are equivocal, a lateral soft tissue airway X-ray can be helpful. The X-ray usually shows the swollen epiglottis appearing like a large thumb seen in profile. Blood culture is much more accurate than direct culture of the supraglottic larynx.

> **PITFALL•••** Examination of the larynx should not be attempted unless the necessary personnel and equipment are available to establish an airway immediately. Therefore, the safest management of the child with suspected supraglottitis requires taking the child directly to the operating room where immediate intubation, bronchoscopy, and tracheotomy, if necessary, can be performed.

The management of supraglottitis requires the institution of appropriate antibiotic therapy. These patients often need to be intubated. Nasotracheal intubation is usually preferred over tracheotomy. The intubation allows for frequent suctioning of the airway if needed. Extubation is usually safely performed in 24 to 48 hours. Steroids may be helpful in resolving the inflammatory process. Intravenous hydration is often necessary because these patients present with dehydration.

SUPRAGLOTTIC ALLERGIC EDEMA

This process is sometimes referred to as angioedema. It usually occurs rapidly after exposure to such insults as bee stings and other allergens. This clinical picture can be very similar to acute epiglottitis. This process usually lacks an elevated temperature. The epiglottis will typically have a swollen and pale appearance in contrast to the fiery-red appearance of epiglottitis. The edema tends to respond almost immediately to a single subcutaneous dose of epinephrine or a single large dose of steroids given intravenously.

JUVENILE LARYNGEAL PAPILLOMATOSIS

The cause of laryngeal papillomatosis is considered to be viral. Although it may have an infectious etiology, papilloma is considered the most common benign tumor of the larynx. It occurs in either a juvenile- or an adult-onset form, although the distinction between the two may be difficult to make. The juvenile form, commonly designated papillomatosis because of the diffuse involvement of the larynx, usually presents in infancy or childhood as hoarseness and stridor. The causative agent is human papilloma virus, types 6 and 11 being most common. The form of papillomatosis is often aggressive and resistant to treatment, requiring frequent laryngoscopies for removal. The juvenile form often undergoes spontaneous involution at the time of puberty.

The diagnosis is made by history and direct laryngoscopy in a newborn infant or small child with progressive hoarseness or stridor. Biopsy confirmation is necessary because other lesions may present in a similar fashion. Occasionally the trachea and bronchi become involved with papillomas. Tracheotomy should be avoided if possible because of the increased incidence of tracheal involvement after tracheotomy is performed.

Management goals for juvenile laryngeal papillomatosis are maintenance of airway, maintenance of voice, and eradication of disease.

The use of microdebriders, commonly used for endoscopic sinus surgery, is gaining in popularity. It allows for a rapid, yet thorough, removal of disease without injuring the underlying laryngeal structures. Interferon is a potent antiviral agent that causes regression of disease. However, long-term therapy is not curative.

> **PEARL...** The surgical laser, CO_2 laser most often, has become the most widely accepted treatment for papillomas of the larynx. The laser is favored because of the hemostatic properties and precision of vaporization.

> **PITFALL...** Aggressive use of the laser will lead to damage of the underlying laryngeal tissues, which can secondarily cause laryngeal stenosis. Utilizing cup forceps in conjunction with laser vaporization may be a safer technique. Many other treatments have been tried, such as ultrasound treatment, cryosurgery, radiation, vaccines, and recently microdebriders. There are antiviral medications under investigation that may prove helpful. At present optimal treatment consists of serial laser laryngoscopy. Microdebriders may prove to be equally as effective and less time-consuming.

DIPHTHERIA

Diphtheria is now a very uncommon childhood disease because of the widespread use of diphtheria-pertussis-tetanus immunizations. It is caused by *Corynebacterium diphtheriae* infection. Typically a gray membrane forms in the nasopharynx. However, laryngeal involvement can occur. Patients usually develop dyspnea and stridor for 2 to 3 days after onset of a febrile illness and hoarseness. The diagnosis is based on the observation of the laryngeal membrane, but requires smear and culture for confirmation. In 10% of cases paralysis of one or more of the cranial nerves is noted. The paralysis usually resolves completely in successfully treated cases.

The treatment includes airway stabilization, antitoxin, and antibiotic therapy. When airway compromise is diagnosed, a tracheotomy is necessary.

Other infections—mumps, measles (rubeola), and chicken pox (varicella)—may cause localized laryngeal and tracheal inflammation. These diagnoses are usually made based on clinical findings. Rarely is emergency airway management necessary.

ADULT DISORDERS

ACUTE LARYNGITIS

Acute laryngitis is usually part of an upper respiratory infection and is most commonly caused by rhinoviruses. The diagnosis is generally made by history and laryngeal examination. Laryngoscopy will demonstrate diffuse erythema and patchy dry exudate. Swelling may be present and may trigger a prominent cough or hoarseness. Humidification, steam inhalation, voice rest, increased fluid intake, and the use of anti-inflammatory drugs is usually sufficient treatment. Antibiotics are not indicated for a viral upper respiratory infection.

Acute epiglottitis (supraglottitis) can occur in the adult population and is often due to *H. influenzae* type B, as it is in children. The supraglottic edema is similar to that in the pediatric patient. However, because the adult larynx is larger, the airway compromise is not as significant. Symptoms usually include muffled voice, painful dysphagia, and vague discomfort in the throat. Fever is usually present, as is a leukocytosis. The treatment of adult supraglottitis is appropriate antibiotic therapy. Adult patients often can be observed without intubation, but require close monitoring. Humidification and steroids are useful adjunctive therapy.

Sudden onset of significant laryngeal edema can result from exposure to specific allergens. The edema may be mild, leading to only slight hoarseness and a scratchy sensation. Rapid progression to airway obstruction may also develop. The usual provocateurs are bee stings, food allergies, and angioedema (Quincke's disease). Angioedema has been associated with the use of angiotensin-converting enzyme (ACE) inhibitors. In addition to laryngeal involvement, the edema may affect the uvula, tongue, and floor of mouth.

PEARL... For the treatment of angioedema, systemic steroids and antihistamines are necessary. Subcutaneous or inhaled epinephrine is also beneficial.

If airway compromise is significant, either intubation or tracheotomy should be performed.

CHRONIC LARYNGITIS

Chronic laryngitis can be caused by myriad organisms or it can be the manifestation of a systemic disorder. The symptoms usually consist of hoarseness, dyspnea, and pain. These symptoms are also the manifestations of laryngeal or hypopharyngeal cancer. If a patient has a history of tobacco or alcohol abuse coupled with weight loss, cancer must be high on the differential diagnosis. Therefore, the diagnostic challenge is to rule out cancer in the process of making the correct diagnosis.

Physical examination tends to be nonspecific. It is not uncommon for certain chronic infections to present as a submucosal mass with a normal mucosal covering. Biopsy is often necessary to make the proper diagnosis.

LARYNGOPHARYNGEAL REFLUX DISEASE

Gastroesophageal reflux disease (GERD) is the retrograde movement of gastric contents into the esophagus. Laryngopharyngeal reflux disease refers to the refluxate reaching the laryngopharynx and causing signs and symptoms. The two terms are often used interchangeably.

CONTROVERSY

Although in the past, gastroesophageal reflux was felt to be almost synonymous with heartburn and indigestion, it is evident that GERD does manifest in a myriad of head and neck symptoms including sore throat, hoarseness, chronic cough, and otalgia. These otolaryngologic symptoms occur without the presence of heartburn 50% of the time.

Other common presenting complaints include postnasal drip, dysphagia or food sticking in the throat, globus pharyngis, and frequent throat clearing. Idiopathic hoarseness tends to be the most common complaint.

On physical examination, the most common head and neck findings are erythema and edema of the posterior aspect of the larynx with interarytenoid pachyderma. Contact ulcers and granulation tissue may also be found. In as many as 50% of the patients no significant pathology is identified.

The diagnosis of laryngopharyngeal reflux disease is usually made on clinical grounds. This disease is usually the result of transient relaxation of the lower esophageal sphincter. The history and physical examination alone are usually diagnostic. However, if confirmation of the diagnosis is necessary, 24-hour double pH probe study is the gold standard. Other tests that may demonstrate abnormalities when laryngopharyngeal reflux is present are esophageal manometry and barium swallow.

The treatment of laryngopharyngeal reflux disease is usually approached in a stepwise fashion. Dietary and lifestyle modifications are usually the first measures taken. Fat ingestion and methylxanthines found in chocolate and carminatives such as spearmint or peppermint have been shown to directly lower esophageal sphincter pressure. Coffee, cola beverages, beer, and milk are potent stimuli of gastric acid secretion. A number of medications have been shown to decrease lower esophageal sphincter pressure such as theophylline, β_2-adrenergic drugs, and oral contraceptives. Alcohol and cigarette smoking decrease lower esophageal sphincter amplitude and impair normal acid clearance. Obesity, pregnancy, and tight-fitting garments all increase intraabdominal pressure and thereby decrease the gastroesophageal pressure gradient.

Elevation of the head of the bed by 6 inches has been shown to decrease the incidence of reflux episodes and increase acid clearance. Waterbeds have a negative effect. Vigorous exercise has been shown to increase reflux episodes in otherwise healthy individuals.

When lifestyle and dietary changes are not effective medical therapy is instituted. Medical therapy usually begins with antacids or H_2 blockers. If these medications are not effective, prokinetic drugs such as metoclopramide and cisapride can be used. Proton pump inhibitors such as omeprazole and lansoprazole are extremely effective in controlling acid secretions. Antireflux surgery can be safely performed endoscopically. This is usually reserved for medical failures.

INFECTIOUS TUBERCULOSIS

Tuberculosis of the larynx is still one of the most common granulomatous diseases of the larynx. It is usually the result of preexisting pulmonary involvement. Its prevalence had decreased until recently, and its upsurge is largely due to the epidemic of human immunodeficiency virus (HIV) disease. It usually presents with hoarseness, odynophagia out of proportion to the size of the lesion, cough, weight loss, night sweats, and hemoptysis. The glottis is the most common laryngeal site of involvement. The diagnosis is usually made by a combination of positive sputum samples, characteristic findings on chest X-ray, and biopsies. Biopsies are positive for acid-fast bacilli. The treatment is medical and consists of systemic use of appropriate antituberculous drugs.

> **PEARL...** Two to four drugs may be needed for an extended course of therapy based on the sensitivities of the organisms cultured.

SYPHILIS

Syphilis still must be considered in the differential diagnosis for chronic inflammatory disease and mass lesions of the larynx. Syphilis is caused by the spirochete *Treponema pallidum.* Most cases are acquired through sexual contact, although congenital syphilis has been described. Primary syphilis can occasionally present with transient lesions of the epiglottis. Secondary syphilis with laryngeal involvement is more common. This stage is usually associated with generalized lymphadenopathy and multiple lesions in the mouth as well. The larynx will demonstrate diffuse hyperemia and mucous patches. The lesions typically clear in 1 to 2 weeks even without treatment. Tertiary laryngeal syphilis is usually in the form of a diffuse nodular, gummatous infiltrate. The nodules may ulcerate or coalesce to form larger nodules. The treatment of syphilis consists of an adequate course of high-dose penicillin.

MYCOTIC INFECTIONS

Fungal infections of the larynx must be considered in the differential diagnosis of any case of chronic laryngitis that is not responding to treatment. Patients with diabetes, long-term steroid treatment, or other debilitating illnesses are prime candidates for laryngeal mycosis.

Actinomycosis is a bacterial infection that is often grouped with fungal infections. The causative agent is usually *Actinomyces israelii.* This is a gram-positive branching filamentous bacteria that is usually seen causing chronic draining infections in the submandibular area secondary to poor dental hygiene. The larynx is rarely involved except in postradiation or surgical situations. The diagnosis is usually made by biopsy. The treatment requires 3 months or longer of appropriate antibiotic therapy. Devitalized tissue must be debrided.

Blastomycosis is caused by *Blastomyces dermatitidis.* This fungus is usually found in the southeastern United States and the Mississippi River valley. It is often referred to as North American blastomycosis. It typically produces a miliary, nodular pattern with caseation, although ulcerative changes may be noted. The true vocal cords are the most commonly involved site. Diagnosis is made by biopsy. Cytologically, acute and chronic inflammation with microabscess formation is seen. Giant cells are also present.

> **PITFALL•••** Pseudoepitheliomatous hyperplasia is usually present and often misread as a malignant process, usually as squamous cell carcinoma.

Treatment is with a prolonged course of amphotericin B.

Candidiasis can cause an acute or chronic infection of the larynx. The offending organism is *Candida albicans* and is usually seen in a mild form secondary to either prolonged use of antibiotics or concomitant radiation therapy for head and neck cancers. The more serious form of this disease is seen in individuals with acquired immune deficiency syndrome (AIDS) or patients treated with systemic chemotherapy. The disease always spreads to the larynx from the oral cavity and may secondarily involve the esophagus. The diagnosis is suspected when a typical cheesy white exudate is found present on the larynx. Biopsy reveals pseudoepitheliomatous hyperplasia with yeast forms and pseudohyphae. Treatment is usually with topical antifungals. Amphotericin B is used when systemic medication is needed.

Histoplasmosis is caused by the fungus *Histoplasma capsulatum* and is endemic in the Ohio and Mississippi River valley. This disease primarily affects the lung, but the larynx and tongue can also be sites of involvement. This disease resembles tuberculosis both microscopically and clinically.

> **PEARL•••** Histoplasmosis tends to involve the epiglottis and false cords. Tuberculosis preferentially involves the posterior third of the larynx.

The diagnosis is usually made by complement fixation test and by culture of the organism. Histologically, with chronic inflammation, granuloma formation and even pseudoepitheliomatous hyperplasia may be present. The treatment is a prolonged course of amphotericin B.

Coccidioidomycosis is also called San Joaquin Valley fever and is a fungal disease endemic to the southwestern United States and northern Mexico. The infection is caused by inhaling spores, and the lungs are by far the most common site of involvement. The causative organism is *Coccidioides immitis.* The diagnosis is usually made by skin testing with complement fixation tests providing confirmation. Extrapulmonary spread of this disease is rare. Laryngeal lesions may appear as granulation tissue or ulceration and may cause airway compromise. Biopsy reveals granulomas, very similar to those of tuberculous. Histology often shows only the presence of an inflammatory infiltrate, so the diagnosis must be made using fungal stains to demonstrate the typical endospore-filled organisms. The treatment is intravenous amphotericin B.

PITFALL... All fungal infections involving the larynx can cause pseudoepitheliomatous hyperplasia. Superficial biopsies have led to erroneous diagnoses of cancer with resultant total laryngectomy. Deep biopsies are necessary in patients with atypical presentations or chronic debilitating diseases.

SYSTEMIC DISEASES AFFECTING THE LARYNX

AMYLOIDOSIS

Amyloidosis is a disease characterized by deposits of amyloid (amorphous, pink-staining material) and has primary and secondary variants. The primary variant has spontaneous development of amyloid deposits. When these deposits are present in a single organ system or even in a single location of the body, it is considered localized. Primary amyloid, where deposits are found to some extent in almost all tissues of the body, is characterized as a generalized form. Secondary amyloidosis is a condition in which amyloid is found in conjunction with some other systemic disease process such as rheumatoid arthritis.

The primary type of amyloid has a predilection for the tongue and larynx. The amyloid nodules are usually subepithelial, quite circumscribed, and are typically diagnosed by biopsy and staining with Congo red. Under light microscopy, the Congo red stain demonstrates the characteristic green birefringence when polarized. The treatment of laryngeal amyloidosis is surgical excision. Multiple excisions may be necessary for recurrent disease.

PEMPHIGUS AND PEMPHIGOID

Both these diseases produce bullous lesions of the skin and mucous membranes. Pemphigus produces intraepithelial bullae, whereas those of pemphigoid are subepithelial. The diagnosis is made when circulating antibodies can be demonstrated by immunofluorescent technique. Both disorders can affect the larynx. Chronic infection can lead to laryngeal stenosis.

The treatment of both diseases is primarily with steroids. Immunosuppressants like methotrexate are also effective.

RELAPSING POLYCHONDRITIS

Although the true etiology is unknown, relapsing polychondritis is thought to be an autoimmune disorder. It typically affects the cartilaginous structures of the ears, nose, and larynx. It is an inflammatory process characterized by exacerbations and spontaneous remissions. The diagnosis is made by history and biopsy of the involved cartilaginous structures. Cytologically there are acute and chronic inflammatory cells in association with an eosinophilic material that infiltrates and replaces the cartilaginous matrix. Early stages are characterized by fever and arthritic type symptoms. Later stages demonstrate fibrosis and chondronecrosis. Laryngeal involvement occurs often in this disorder with common symptoms being hoarseness, painful swelling of the larynx and trachea, and dysphagia. Treatment for this disease is steroid therapy.

SARCOIDOSIS

This autoimmune disease rarely involves the larynx. However, when it does, ulceration, granuloma formation, and scarring are typical. The diagnosis is made on biopsy with noncaseating granulomata being identified. The treatment is steroids.

SPECIAL CONSIDERATION

Microlaryngoscopy with laser excision is sometimes necessary for the laryngeal lesions.

SYSTEMIC LUPUS ERYTHEMATOSUS (SLE)

The laryngeal manifestations of SLE are protean. Epiglottitis, acute and chronic laryngitis, granuloma formation, and vocal cord paralysis have all been reported. The laryngeal lesions may be treated with laser excision. Steroid therapy is the treatment of choice.

WEGENER'S GRANULOMATOSIS

Wegener's granulomatosis belongs to a group of necrotizing primary systemic vasculitides of unknown etiology. This disorder is associated with antineutrophil cytoplasmic antibodies (ANCAs). This disorder is very similar in presentation to lethal midline granuloma. Laryngeal involvement is unusual with both disorders. Nasal obstruction, chronic sinusitis, and nonhealing ulcerations of the septum, often with perforation, are common. Systemic symptoms include fever, malaise, and weight loss. Laryngeal lesions may include ulcerations and pseudoepitheliomatous hyperplasia as well as subglottic stenosis. The diagnosis is made by serologic testing for ANCAs (p-ANCA and c-ANCA). Multiple biopsies are necessary. The treatment is with steroids and immunosuppressive agents such as cyclophosphamide and azathioprine. Plasmapheresis, intraveous immunoglobulin, and monoclonal antibodies may be of benefit in some cases.

SUGGESTED READINGS

Donegan JO, Wood MD. Histoplasmosis of the larynx. *Laryngoscope* 1984;94:206.

Forrest LA, Weed H. Candida laryngitis appearing as leukoplakia and GERD. *J Voice* 1998; 12(1):91–95.

Hanson DG, Kamel PL, Kahrilas PJ. Outcomes of antireflux therapy for the treatment of chronic laryngitis. *Ann Otol Rhinol Laryngol* 1995;104(7):550–555.

Jones KR, Pillsubry HC III. Infections and manifestations of systemic disease of the larynx. In: Cummings CW, Fredrickson JM, Harker LA, Krause CJ, Schuller DE, eds. *Otolaryngology–Head and Neck Surgery.* St. Louis: Mosby Year Book; 1993:1854–1863.

Koufman JA. The otolaryngologic manifestations of gastroesophageal reflux disease (GERD): a clinical investigation of 225 patients using ambulatory 24-hour pH monitoring and an experimental investigation of the role of acid and pepsin in the development of laryngeal injury. *Laryngoscope* 1991; 101(4 pt 2, suppl 53):1–78.

Tucker HM. Infectious and inflammatory disorders. In: Tucker HM, ed. *The Larynx.* 2nd ed. New York: Thieme; 1993:231–244.

Chapter 38

Neoplasms and Cysts

Keith M. Wilson

In the United States, laryngeal cancer accounts for approximately 1% of all new cancer diagnoses and 0.74% of cancer deaths. The estimated 5-year survival rate for layngeal cancer is 67%. Although this does not represent a significant change over the last 20 years, it still places laryngeal cancer as one of the most curable cancers.

Laryngeal cancer is the second most common cancer in the upper aerodigestive track, preceded in frequency only by cancer of the oral cavity. Squamous cell carcinoma (SCCa) accounts for 95% of laryngeal malignancies with the glottis being the most frequently affected subsite.

Cancer of the larynx is similar to other head and neck malignancies in that it is primarily a disease of men in the sixth and seventh decades. The male-to-female ratio in the United States has decreased from 5.6:1 to 4.3:1 from 1959 to 1999. Women are more likely to develop supraglottic cancer than glottic. The distribution of carcinoma among the supraglottis, glottis, and subglottis is 40:59:1.

ETIOLOGY

The risk factors for laryngeal cancer are multiple. Tobacco represents the primary factor. Numerous studies have demonstrated a correlation between tobacco and laryngeal cancer that seems to be a dose-dependent relationship. The relative risk was calculated at 4.4-fold for patients who smoked up to half-a-pack per day and at 10.4-fold for those smoking more than two packs per day. Smoking cessation can also decrease the smoker's risk of laryngeal cancer development. Wynder et al (1956) demonstrated that the risk diminishes dramatically after 6 years of cessation and approaches that of a non-smoker after 15 years of cessation. The risk of second-hand smoke as a cause of laryngeal cancer has not been investigated. Cigar and pipe smoking present less of a risk than cigarette smoking.

The association of alcohol with laryngeal cancer is less clear than that for tobacco. Alcohol has a synergistic affect when combined with smoking and increases the risk of laryngeal cancer by 50% over the expected additive rate.

Information about occupational risks and laryngeal cancer is somewhat confusing. Increased risk has been found for painters, construction workers, those exposed to diesel and gasoline fumes, metal working and plastic working machine operators, and those exposed to therapeutic doses of radiation therapy. Other risk factors include laryngeal papillomatosis, exposure to mustard gas, wood dust and asbestos, laryngeal keratosis, and laryngopharyngeal reflux disease. Investigations to determine the presence of dietary protective factors in fruits and vegetables have been conducted. No definite conclusions have been made. Patently, laryngeal cancer tumorigenesis is a complex interaction between host and environmental factors that remains a scientific mystery.

PATTERNS OF SPREAD

The behavior of laryngeal cancer is dependent on the site of origin of the lesion. The larynx contains several fibroelastic barriers that limit the spread of early cancer and make partial laryngeal resections, with adequate margins, possible.

SUPRAGLOTTIS

Cancers arising in the supraglottic larynx can invade the epiglottic cartilage and extend anteriorly into the pre-epiglottic space and valleculae. These lesions may also extend inferiorly within the quadrangular space to involve the pyriform sinus. Once in this location, the tumor can extend to the postcricoid area or invade the paraglottic space. Cancer in the paraglottic space can move superiorly and inferiorly as well as into the pre-epiglottic space. Supraglottic tumors typically cause pain and dysphagia.

GLOTTIC

Glottic lesions tend to remain confined to the vocal folds because of the sparse lymphatics and the anatomic configuration of the glottis.

SPECIAL CONSIDERATION

There are four barriers preventing the spread of tumor of the glottis, thus making glottic carcinoma more curable in its early stages. These barriers are the vocal ligament, anterior commissure, thyroglottic ligament, and the conus elasticus.

The vocal ligament is the first line of defense for the paraglottic space. Once it is breached, tumors will be able to spread superiorly and infe-

riorly and will impair vocal fold mobility. The thyroglottic ligament is the lateral extension of the vocal ligament along the floor of the ventricle. It resists superior spread of tumors into the ventricle.

SUBGLOTTIS

Subglottic cancer is a rare entity. It is characterized by circumferential spread and extension superiorly through the conus elasticus. Patients may present with vocal fold fixation in the absence of any mucosal abnormality. Recurrent laryngeal nerve involvement may also occur. Posterior extension of disease may result in hypopharyngeal and esophageal involvement.

DIAGNOSIS

The common symptoms produced by laryngeal cancer are hoarseness, sore throat, dysphagia, and odynophagia.

PEARL••• Hoarseness is an early symptom in cancer of the glottis but is a late finding in carcinoma of the supraglottis or subglottis.

The change in voice quality is caused by mass effect or vocal fold paralysis. Paraglottic extension can lead to impaired mobility of the vocal fold.

Sore throat and dysphagia are common findings in advanced cancer of the supraglottis but can be seen in early cancer at this site. The muffled "hot potato" voice is seen in large supraglottic tumors. Odynophagia usually indicates extension to the hypopharynx or base of tongue. Dyspnea, hemoptysis, and referred otalgia are less common symptoms.

Extralaryngeal extension of disease usually causes odynophagia, referred otalgia, and neck pain. The presence of a neck mass often indicates nodal metastasis but may result from direct extension of cancer through the thyrohyoid or cricothyroid membranes.

Physical examination of the larynx is usually accomplished with indirect mirror visualization or a fiberoptic nasolaryngoscope. Laryngeal evaluation is performed to evaluate the primary location and extent of the cancer, the degree of vocal fold mobility, and the adequacy of the airway. Palpation of the larynx may provide additional information about extralaryngeal spread of disease and cervical metastases.

> **PEARL•••** Loss of normal laryngeal crepitance against the vertebrae is indicative of postcricoid involvement.

Splaying of the thyroid cartilage as well as fixation of the larynx during swallowing can be determined by palpation.

Videostroboscopic examination has emerged as a technique that aids in our ability to assess early glottic cancers. Mucosal wave abnormalities, indicative of early invasion by premalignant or presumed benign lesions, can be evaluated best by stroboscopic evaluation. Videostroboscopy is also helpful in early detection of recurrent laryngeal carcinoma.

Direct laryngoscopy under general anesthesia remains the gold standard for pretreatment staging. Biopsies of all suspicious areas should be taken. Deep biopsies are recommended to prevent sampling of the superficial inflammation only. Typically a superficial biopsy is taken with cup forceps. Then a deeper biopsy is taken through the first biopsy site.

Panendoscopy to include bronchoscopy, esophagoscopy, and examination of the oral cavity and nasopharynx along with digital palpation complete the evaluation of the laryngeal cancer and allow for proper staging.

IMAGING

All patients with laryngeal cancer should undergo chest X-ray to exclude lung metastases or a synchronous lung cancer. Supraglottic carcinoma has a greater tendency to metastasize than glottic carcinoma.

Both computed tomography (CT) scan and magnetic resonance imaging (MRI) are capable of evaluating the larynx in terms of tumor extent, airway patency, cartilage involvement, pre-epiglottic space involvement, subglottic extension, and extralaryngeal extension. MRI generally gives better soft tissue detail, and is helpful in nodal detection especially in the clinically obese or previously operated neck.

Contrast laryngography, soft tissue plain films, and plain tomography play no role in laryngeal imaging. They are listed for historical purposes only.

STAGING

The staging of laryngeal cancer is accomplished using two major systems of classification: the Union Internationale Contre Cancer (UICC) and the American Joint Committee in Cancer (AJCC). The two systems are now identical and are less than ideal in terms of accurately predicting patient survival (see Appendix 4).

NONSQUAMOUS TUMORS

Approximately 1 to 5% of all carcinomas of the larynx are not squamous. The more common nonsquamous tumors of the larynx include those of salivary, cartilaginous, and neuroendocrine origin.

AMYLOIDOSIS

The most common head and neck sites affected by amyloid are the larynx and tongue. Amyloid is the extracellular accumulation of fibrillar proteins and may manifest in several forms, such as systemic amyloidosis, multiple myeloma-associated amyloidosis, and familial amyloidosis. Although laryngeal amyloid is not a true neoplastic process, it is included in the neoplastics section largely because its presentation is similar to that of a tumor. It tends to affect men more often than women and occurs in the fifth to sixth decades of life. Amyloid frequently presents as a mucosal covered, firm, polypoid mass causing hoarseness and, less often, dysphagia. Endoscopic resection is usually curative. Tracheotomy is necessary for large lesions causing airway obstruction. The histology is characterized by apple green birefringent staining seen under polarized light with Congo red staining.

GRANULAR CELL TUMOR

This is a tumor of Schwann cell origin that can involve the skin, tongue, breasts, larynx, gastrointestinal tract, and bronchus. This tumor has a predilection for the posterior aspect of the true vocal folds, where it causes hoarseness, but will also occur in the supraglottic and subglottic areas. It occurs more commonly in men and has an unknown etiology.

The endoscopic appearance is that of a solitary, polypoid, sessile, papillary, or cystic lesion involving the glottis. Histologically it is an unencapsulated or poorly circumscribed subepithelial lesion with a syncytial, trabecular, or nested growth pattern. Pseudoepitheliomatous hyperplasia is common. The treatment of choice is conservative but complete surgical resection. Neither chemotherapy nor radiation therapy plays a role in the treatment.

PARAGANGLIOMA

This lesion arises from the paired bilateral paraganglia within the larynx. The superior paraganglia are located at the anterior ends of the false vocal folds, associated with the internal branch of the superior laryngeal nerve. The inferior paraganglia are located anywhere between the inferior border of thyroid cartilage and the cricotracheal junction. The most common site of occurrence is the right false vocal fold/aryepiglottic region. Laryngeal paragangliomas occur most commonly in women as reddish or bluish submucosal masses. The treatment is wide excision utilizing voice-sparing procedures when possible.

CHONDROMA

This benign tumor of cartilaginous origin affects males more commonly than females. It occurs most frequently in the fourth to seventh decades. This tumor can arise from any of the laryngeal cartilages. The presenting symptoms include dyspnea, hoarseness, and stridor.

Radiologically this tumor demonstrates coarse calcification and ossification. Histologically, it appears to be normal cartilage. The treatment is conservative excision including an adequate "cuff" of normal tissue. Recurrence is rare following complete excision.

CHONDROSARCOMA

This tumor arises from the hyaline cartilages of the larynx. The cricoid is the most common site (70%), followed by the thyroid (20%) and the body of the arytenoid (10%). Chondrosarcomas of the cricoid can grow into the airway, causing progressive airway obstruction. Those that originate in the thyroid cartilage tend to grow laterally, producing a firm mass palpable through the neck.

This is the most common sarcoma of the larynx affecting men more commonly than women between 50 and 70 years of age. The symptoms of chondrosarcomas are very similar to those of carcinomas of the larynx.

Endoscopically, they appear as hard, submucosal masses. Histologically, they are graded as low grade or high grade based on the degree of cellularity, pleomorphism, and mitoses. The histologic grading has no effect on prognosis.

Laryngeal chondrosarcomas are usually treated surgically, by wide excision. Total laryngectomy is reserved for extensive cricoid involvement.

SPECIAL CONSIDERATION

Local recurrence occurs in approximately 25% of cases. In such situations, additional surgery is recommended.

Distant metastases are rare.

ADENOCARCINOMA

This carcinoma has a predilection for the supraglottic larynx, though it can occur in the subglottis. The clinical presentation is that of a submucosal, nonulcerated mass causing dysphagia, odynophagia, or referred otalgia. Adenocarcinoma of the larynx tends to present at a late stage. Cervical metastases are common. The most common sites of distant metastases are the liver and lungs. Five-year survival rates are between 12 and 17%. Aggressive surgery, including total laryngectomy and neck dissection, and postoperative radiation therapy are recommended.

ADENOID CYSTIC CARCINOMA

This is a rare malignancy of the larynx with a predilection for the subglottis. It is similar to adenoid cystic carcinoma at other locations in that it tends to produce vague symptoms of pain and fullness and has a propensity for perineural invasion.

Pulmonary metastases are common and are often present at initial presentation. Metastases are slow growing and allow for good 3-year survival rates. Therefore surgery is recommended for local regional disease even when pulmonary metastases are present. Radiation therapy is recommended postoperatively or for palliation. Adenoid cystic carcinoma is not considered radiocurable.

MUCOEPIDERMOID CARCINOMA

Mucoepidermoid carcinoma tends to affect the supraglottic larynx more often in men in the seventh decade. Histologically, it occurs in low, intermediate, and high grades. Low-grade lesions are usually treated with conservative surgery. High-grade lesions are treated like squamous cell carcinomas. Intermediate-grade tumors should be treated more like high-grade tumors. Surgery is the recommended mode of therapy, with radiation being reserved for positive or close margins.

NEUROENDOCRINE CARCINOMA

This group of malignant tumors is composed of carcinoid, atypical carcinoid, and small (oat) cell carcinoma. As a group they tend to affect males more than females and occur in the sixth to seventh decades. The most common laryngeal site is the supraglottis, and hoarseness is the most common complaint. Cigarette smoking is associated with over 60% of cases. Atypical carcinoid occurs most commonly followed by small cell carcinoma and carcinoid.

Carcinoid tumor typically behaves in a benign fashion. Complete but conservative surgical excision is the recommended treatment of choice and should produce an excellent prognosis. These tumors rarely metastasize and are rarely associated with paraneoplastic syndrome.

Atypical carcinoid is the most common neuroendocrine tumor of the larynx. It behaves in an aggressive manner, with metastases to the cervical lymph nodes, lung, bone, liver, and skin. The treatment of choice is complete surgical excision. Radiation therapy and chemotherapy are reserved for metastatic disease. In terms of prognosis, the 3-year survival exceeds 60%. When metastatic disease is present, death usually results. This disease is not usually associated with paraneoplastic syndrome.

Small cell carcinoma is an extremely aggressive disease that is almost universally fatal. Distant metastases are common to liver, lung, bone, lymph nodes, pancreas, and brain. Chemotherapy and radiation therapy are usually the treatment of choice but really have minimal impact on survival. Two-year survival rates are less than 20%. Small cell cancer is occasionally associated with paraneoplastic syndrome.

SQUAMOUS CELL CARCINOMA

SUPRAGLOTTIC

SCCa of the supraglottis accounts for approximately 35 to 40% of all laryngeal SCCa. The two most common sites of involvement are the epiglottis and the false vocal folds. As mentioned earlier, tumors at this location tend to present with pain and dysphagia initially. Advanced stages present with changes in voice, possibly airway embarrassment, and hemoptysis.

The surgical control rates for stage I and II disease are 90 to 95% and 80 to 90%, respectively. Treatment planning and prognosis are dependent on the stage of disease. Early stage (stage I and II) disease can be treated quite effectively with either surgery or radiation therapy. Radiation therapy offers control rates of 80 to 90% and 70 to 80% for stage I and II disease, respectively. Surgical salvage of radiation therapy failures raises the control rates of radiation therapy to those of surgery alone.

The traditional surgical approach to supraglottic cancer is the supraglottic (horizontal partial) laryngectomy. This procedure is onco-logically sound and produces excellent results. However, lately, endoscopic resection of supra-glottic cancers is gaining in popularity. Zeitels et al (1994) reported a 100% local control rate with endoscopic en-bloc resection of T1 or T2 supra-glottic lesions in 22 of 45 patients with supra-glottic SCCa. Further research is needed to de-termine if this technique should become the procedure of choice for these lesions.

The supraglottic larynx has an extensive lymphatic network that increases the likelihood of cervical metastases. The supraglottic lymphat-ics drain primarily to the upper and middle jugu-lar chains. The incidence of cervical metastases becomes significant at the T2 level. Therefore, the treatment of stage II supraglottic SCCa should include both necks. This can be accomplished with primary radiation therapy or partial laryn-gectomy with bilateral selective neck dissection.

Advanced-stage (T3 or T4) supraglottic SCCa carries a worse prognosis largely because of the greater incidence of cervical metastases. The treatment options include radical radiation with surgical salvage, combined chemotherapy with radiation therapy, or total laryngectomy with neck dissections as indicated with or without postoperative radiation therapy. Supraglottic la-ryngectomy can be utilized for those T3 tumors that invade the pre-epiglottic space or involve the medial wall of the pyriform sinus. Cancers that are T4 secondary to involvement of the base of tongue or hyoid bone can also be resected by supraglottic laryngectomy.

Local control for radiation therapy of T3 can-cer is approximately 60% and for T4 about 45%. Surgery provides approximately a 70% local con-trol rate for T3 disease and about 50% for T4.

THE NECK

It is universally accepted that the status of the neck at the time of presentation has the greatest impact on survival for supraglottic cancer. Wang et al (1972) noted a decrease in 3-year survival from 63 to 22% in advanced-stage supraglottic cancer when lymph nodes are palpable at initial presentation.

The metastatic rate for T1 supraglottic can-cer ranges from 15 to 40%. T2 cancers have re-

---

CONTROVERSY

There are many advocates for the con-cept of radical radiation therapy with surgical salvage. The control rates are comparable to those for surgery with postoperative radiation therapy, with the additional advantage that approxi-mately 65% of patients will retain their larynges. Opponents speak to the is-sues of the increased incidence of post-operative complications and the dif-ficulty in detecting recurrences after radiation therapy. Randomized trials are needed to resolve this issue.

---

gional metastases from 35 to 40%. Cancers that are T3 and T4 have a cervical metastatic rate be-tween 50 to 65%. Bilateral cervical metastases in supraglottic laryngeal cancer is estimated at 20 to 35%. Because of the high rate of cervical me-tastases with supraglottic cancer, the neck must be included in any treatment plan.

GLOTTIC CARCINOMA

Glottic carcinoma represents the most common laryngeal SCCa, accounting for approximately 60%. These lesions tend to arise from the ante-rior aspect of the true vocal folds, giving rise to hoarseness as the chief complaint. Carcinomas in this location are detected early because of the prompt development of symptoms secondary to impaired vocal fold mobility.

SPECIAL CONSIDERATION

The meager lymphatics of the glottis play a role in limiting the submucosal spread to adjacent laryngeal subsites and to the regional lymph nodes. These qualities of glottic cancer allow for many treatment options and a fa-vorable prognosis.

Early-stage (stage I and II) glottic carcinoma can be effectively treated by a single modality, utilizing surgery or radiation therapy. Radiation therapy will provide approximately 85 to 95% local control for T1 glottic cancer. T2 lesions can be locally controlled at about 65 to 75% with radiation therapy. The potential benefit of radiation therapy over surgery, for early glottic lesions, is better voice results, especially for T2 lesions. Complications of radiation therapy alone are few for early glottic cancer.

There are four factors that determine the overall success of radiation therapy:

1. Absolute size of cancer
2. Involvement of the anterior commissure
3. Subglottic extension
4. Decreased vocal fold mobility.

The most consistently described limitation is a decrease in vocal fold mobility.

Vertical hemilaryngectomy can achieve local control rates of about 95% for T1 lesions and about 80% for T2 lesions. Endoscopic procedures, frontolateral hemilaryngectomy, laryngofissure with cordectomy, extended vertical hemilaryngectomy for cancer involving the face of the arytenoid, anterior commissure resection, and supracricoid laryngectomy are other surgical procedures used to treat early stage glottic carcinoma. Overall, surgery provides better local control rates than radiation therapy for the patients who are eligible for conservation procedures. The local control rates are comparable when surgery is used for salvage of radiation failures.

CONTROVERSY

The management of advanced-stage SCCa of the glottis is controversial, particularly regarding the ability to preserve laryngeal function.

For more advanced disease, there are three treatment plans that yield good control rates: total laryngectomy with or without neck dissec-tion; radical radiation with surgical salvage, and induction chemotherapy with radiation using surgery for salvage. Local control rates for T3 and T4 lesions utilizing total laryngectomy with or without neck dissection have been reported at 95%. The 5-year survival rate is 53% after surgery and 63% after salvage radiation therapy. Local control rates for radiation therapy for T3 and T4 carcinoma of the glottis vary from 40 to 60%. The actuarial survival rates after surgical salvage range from 50 to 70%. The more T4 lesions present, the worse the survival rates. A protocol using induction chemotherapy with radiation therapy and surgery for salvage yields survival rates of about 70% with the additional benefit of a 65% rate of retained larynges.

THE NECK

Cervical metastases from glottic carcinoma occur infrequently. Occult metastases in T3N0 glottic carcinoma is about 10%. It is about 30% in T4N0.

Elective neck dissection is performed when the primary lesion is treated surgically. This provides important staging information. Postoperative radiation therapy is recommended for subclinical nodal disease, especially if extracapsular spread is identified.

SUBGLOTTIC CARCINOMA

Subglottic squamous cell carcinoma is a rare entity. There are no large studies comparing radiation therapy to surgery. Therefore, the best therapy is unknown. For advanced disease, combination therapy is probably best.

Metastases to levels I to IV are rare. However, paratracheal metastases may occur at 50% or greater.

STOMAL RECURRENCE

The term *stomal recurrence* refers to a carcinoma that recurs in the peristomal area after total laryngectomy. The tumor may arise from the tracheal or pharyngeal margins or the lymph nodes in the paratracheal region. The staging of stomal recurrences is done according to the Sisson classification:

Type I—Tumor involves the superior half of the stoma without esophageal involvement.

Type II—Tumor involves the superior half of the stoma with esophageal involvement.

Type III—Tumor involves the superior half of the stoma and involves the superior mediastinum.

Type IV—Tumor extends out laterally underneath the clavicles.

CONTROVERSY

Historically, emergency tracheostomy prior to definitive treatment of the laryngeal cancer was shown to increase the incidence of stomal recurrence by 10%. Cancer seeding the peristomal tissues was the presumed pathophysiology. However, more recent studies have not supported this theory. Subglottic extension of tumor greater than 1 cm appears to be the single most important factor.

The incidence of stomal recurrence can be reduced by the addition of postoperative radiation therapy to the stoma and by performing a complete paratracheal lymph node dissection in all laryngeal cancers with subglottic extension.

The treatment of stomal recurrence is primarily surgical. Chemotherapy and radiation therapy either alone or in combination are not as effective.

The surgical procedure of choice is a mediastinal dissection with extensive resection of the tracheostoma, adjacent skin, manubrium with clavicular heads if necessary, and the pharyngoesophageal tissues. Multiple flaps are often needed to close the defect. Tubed radial forearm free flaps or a free jejunal graft is often needed to close the visceral defect. Pectoralis major myocutaneous or deltopectoral flaps are often used to close the skin defect. It is possible to use only pedicled flaps for reconstruction.

The perioperative mortality is about 15%, with mediastinitis and rupture of the great vessels being the major causes. Hypocalcemia sec-

ondary to removal of the parathyroid glands is an expected postoperative result.

The survival rate for types I and II disease is 45% according to Gluckman et al (1987). The survival rate for types III and IV lesions is 9%. Mediastinal dissection with postoperative radiation therapy, if not previously used, is recommended for type I and II disease.

SPECIAL CONSIDERATION

Palliative surgery may be recommended for type III and possibly type IV disease if the patient fully understands and accepts the higher morbidity and mortality rates and can be medically cleared for surgery.

VOCAL RESTORATION

There are three general methods that are commonly used in vocal restoration after total laryngectomy. The proper choice and success of the rehabilitative effort depends on anatomic and patient factors. The extent of surgery, type of reconstruction, and utilization of radiation therapy are important anatomic factors that will influence voice rehabilitation. The patient factors include motivation, manual dexterity, and access to competent speech-language pathologists and otolaryngologists.

Esophageal voice is a type of alaryngeal voice that requires no additional surgery or prosthetic devices. The technique requires learning to inject, or swallow, air into the neopharynx and then release it in a controlled fashion. This causes the pharyngeal walls to vibrate, producing sound. This sound is then shaped by the articulators of the oral cavity to produce speech. Bulky flaps, rigid tissues, and a tight pharyngoesophageal segment make esophageal voice difficult to produce. Esophageal speech was used successfully in about one fourth of those who tried it. Currently esophageal voice is not the method of choice for vocal rehabilitation and therefore is not utilized often.

The artificial larynx is another form of alaryngeal speech. When held to the soft tissues of the neck or placed intraorally, the electrolarynx produces a vibration sound in the vocal tract. This sound is then articulated into intelligible speech. The voice that is produced is mechanical and monotone and is generally considered inferior to that produced by esophageal voice or tracheoesophageal fistula. However, it is the easiest technique for vocal rehabilitation after laryngectomy.

The third method of alaryngeal speech is produced by creating a tracheoesophageal fistula. A one-way valve is then placed in the fistula tract as a stent. The valve allows air to pass from the trachea into the esophagus when the tracheostoma is occluded, while flow from the esophagus to the trachea is prevented. The air flowing through the one-way valve causes the mucosa of the pharyngoesophageal segment to vibrate, thus producing a sound that is articulated.

The tracheoesophageal fistula can be placed primarily, at the time of total laryngectomy, or secondarily after the tracheostoma has healed and radiation therapy has been completed. Successful vocalization is reported to be 70 to 95%. Minor complications associated with prosthesis insertion occur in 25% of cases. Major complications are rare.

> **PEARL...** Failure to produce voice is most commonly caused by pharyngoesophageal spasm at a level above the fistula. Treatment of this problem includes pharyngeal plexus neurectomy, pharyngeal constrictor myotomy, and transcutaneous injection with botulinum toxin.

LARYNGEAL SURGERY

There are an increasing number of procedures utilized for laryngeal cancer (Table 38–1). Adherence to specific indications yields good cure rates with good function.

ENDOSCOPIC RESECTION

Endoscopic techniques have traditionally been employed for glottic lesions. Currently endoscopic resection is used for tumors of the supra-

TABLE 38–1 PROCEDURES FOR TREATING LARYNGEAL CANCER

Endoscopic resection
Laryngofissure and cordectomy
Partial laryngectomy
    Horizontal supraglottic laryngectomy
    Vertical hemilaryngectomy
    Supracricoid laryngectomy
    Near-total laryngectomy
Total laryngectomy

glottis, glottis, and hypopharynx. Laser and non-laser (cold) techniques are being utilized.

Endoscopic techniques are generally used for the smaller lesions and offer the advantages of equivalent cure rates (to radiation), preservation of voice, and decreased cost, while still preserving other treatment options. The goal of endoscopic procedures is the same as that for open procedures: removal of the tumor with adequate margins.

CORDECTOMY VIA LARYNGOFISSURE

This procedure is indicated for T1 and small T2 lesions. However, with the development of endoscopic laser techniques, this procedure is utilized with less frequency. Larger T2 tumors are usually treated by vertical hemilaryngectomy.

> **SPECIAL CONSIDERATION**
>
> The quality of the voice after cordectomy with laryngofissure is clearly inferior to that achieved with radiation therapy.

PARTIAL LARYNGECTOMY

Vertical Hemilaryngectomy

This procedure is indicated for T2 and limited T3 lesions of the glottis. The vertical hemilaryngectomy procedure removes:

1. One vocal fold from the anterior commissure to the vocal process of the arytenoid,
2. The ipsilateral false vocal fold,
3. The ventricle,
4. The paraglottic space,
5. The overlying thyroid cartilage.

The extended hemilaryngectomy removes all of the above structures and one arytenoid. The frontolateral hemilaryngectomy procedure implies resection of the anterior commissure and varying degrees of the contralateral vocal fold and the overlying thyroid cartilage.

Vertical hemilaryngectomy can be used for radiation failures. Thorough evaluation preoperatively and the patient's consent to extend the procedure, if necessary, are paramount. Indications for vertical hemilaryngectomy and the salvage of radiation failures are:

1. No significant contralateral vocal fold involvement.
2. Less than 5 mm anterior subglottic extension.
3. No bilateral vocal fold fixation.

Supraglottic Laryngectomy

The basic supraglottic laryngectomy resects the entire epiglottis, aryepiglottic folds, false vocal folds, preepiglottic space, and a section of the thyroid cartilage. The hyoid bone is often resected. Some authors believe that preservation of the hyoid bone stabilizes the suprahyoid musculature and therefore aids in swallowing postoperatively. The indications for this procedure are:

1. Tumor limited to supraglottic region.
2. Two-millimeter margin at anterior commissure.
3. Normal vocal fold mobility.

This procedure is contraindicated if:

1. The thyroid cartilage is invaded.
2. There is anterior neck invasion.
3. The tumor extends to the postcricoid or interarytenoid areas.

4. Prevertebral fascia invasion is present.
5. The patient has poor pulmonary function.

The supraglottic laryngectomy procedure can be extended to remove the vallecula, pyriform sinus, or base of tongue up to the circumvallate papillae.

Supracricoid Laryngectomy

This procedure is indicated for T2, T3, and selected T4 glottic and supraglottic cancers. The contraindications are:

1. Subglottic extension greater than 10 mm anteriorly and 5 mm posteriorly.
2. Arytenoid cartilage fixation.
3. Hyoid bone involvement.
4. Cancer extension into base of tongue.
5. Cricoid cartilage invasion.

This procedure removes:

1. The entire thyroid cartilage.
2. Both true vocal cords.
3. Both false vocal cords.
4. One arytenoid, if necessary.
5. The paraglottic space.
6. The epiglottis, if involved.

The reconstruction is by cricohyoidepiglottopexy (CHEP) if the epiglottis is preserved or cricohyoidopexy (CHP) if the epiglottis is removed.

NEAR-TOTAL LARYNGECTOMY

This procedure is indicated for T3 and T4 disease of the larynx where total laryngectomy would be the procedure of choice. The advantage of this procedure is that an internal speaking shunt is created, obviating the need for tracheoesophageal fistula creation and placement of a voice prosthesis. This procedure removes:

1. One entire hemilarynx and the anterior two thirds of the contralateral hemilarynx with the associated thyroid and cricoid cartilages and tracheal rings if necessary,

2. The epiglottis,

3. The hyoid,

4. The pre-epiglottic space.

The internal speaking shunt is mucosally lined and innervated. The shunt can be opened for voice and closed for airway protection. The procedure is contraindicated if there is:

1. Interarytenoid involvement,

2. Involvement of both arytenoids,

3. Postcricoid involvement.

TOTAL LARYNGECTOMY

This procedure removes the entire larynx, strap muscles, part or all of the thyroid gland, and paratracheal lymph nodes. It is indicated when conservation procedures are not feasible. It is indicated for radiation failures when the full extent of the recurrence is not apparent. When chondro-radionecrosis is present after radiation therapy, total laryngectomy is usually the procedure of choice.

SUGGESTED READINGS

Austen DF. Larynx. In: Schottenfeld D, Fraumani JF, eds. *Cancer Epidemiology and Prevention.* Philadelphia: WB Saunders; 1982.

Bocca E, Pignataro O, Oldini C. Supraglottic laryngectomy: 30 years of experience. *Ann Otol Rhinol Laryngol* 1983;92(1 pt 1):14–18.

Burch JD, Howe GR, Miller AB, Semenciw R. Tobacco, alcohol, asbestos, and nickel in the etiology of cancer of the larynx: a case-control study. *J Natl Cancer Inst* 1981;67(6):1219–1224.

Cohen J, Guillamondegui OM, Batsakis JG, Medina JE. Cancer of the minor salivary glands of the larynx. *Am J Surg* 1985;150(4): 513–518.

Gluckman JL, Hamaker RC, Schuller DE, Weissler MC, Charles GA. Surgical salvage for stomal recurrence: a multi-institutional experience. *Laryngoscope* 1987;97(9):1025– 1029.

Haberman PJ, Haberman RSD. Laryngeal adenocarcinoma, not otherwise specified, treated with carbon dioxide laser excision and post-operative radiotherapy. *Ann Otol Rhinol Laryngol* 1992;101(11):920–924.

Harrison DF. The pathology and management of subglottic cancer. *Ann Otol Rhinol Laryngol* 1971;80(1):6–12.

Johnson JT, Myers EN, Hao SP, Wagner RL. Outcome of open surgical therapy for glottic carcinoma. *Ann Otol Rhinol Laryngol* 1993; 102(10):752–755.

Laccourreye H, Laccourreye O, Weinstein G, Menard M, Brasnu D. Supracricoid laryngectomy with cricohyoidopexy: a partial laryngeal procedure for selected supraglottic and transglottic carcinomas. *Laryngoscope* 1990; 100(7):735–741.

Landis SH, Murray T, Bolden S, Wingo PA. Cancer statistics, 1999 [see comments]. *CA Cancer J Clin* 1999;49(1):8–31.

Rothman KJ, Cann CI, Flanders D, Fried MP. Epidemiology of laryngeal cancer. *Epidemiol Rev* 1980;2:195–209.

Sataloff RT, Spiegel JR, Hawkshaw MJ. Strobovideolaryngoscopy: results and clinical value. *Ann Otol Rhinol Laryngol* 1991;100(9 pt 1): 725–727.

Stephenson WT, Barnes DE, Holmes FF, Norris CW. Gender influences subsite of origin of laryngeal carcinoma. *Arch Otolaryngol Head Neck Surg* 1991;117(7):774–778.

Wang CC, Schulz MD, Miller D. Combined radiation therapy and surgery for carcinoma of the supraglottis and pyriform sinus. *Laryngoscope* 1972;82(10):1883–1890.

Wolf GT, Fisher SG, Hong WK, et al. Induction chemotherapy plus radiation compared with surgery plus radiation in patients with advanced laryngeal cancer. VA Laryngeal Cancer Study Group. *N Engl J Med* 1991;324:1685.

Wynder EL, Boss JJ, Day E. Epidemiological approach to the etiology of cancer of the larynx. *JAMA* 1956;160:1384.

Wynder EL, Covey LS, Mabuchi K, Mushinski M. Environmental factors in cancer of the larynx: a second look. *Cancer* 1976;38(4):1591–1601.

Zeitels SM, Koufman JA, Davis RK, Vaughan CW. Endoscopic treatment of supraglottic and hypopharynx cancer. *Laryngoscope* 1994; 104(1 pt 1):71–78.

Chapter 39

TRAUMA

Tapan A. Padhya and Keith M. Wilson

The incidence of blunt trauma is on the decline due to stricter seat belt and child safety legislation. Penetrating laryngeal trauma remains a major concern in light of increasing use of handguns and knives. The larynx is usually protected by the protruding mandibular arch above and the sternum below. In the event of trauma to the larynx, vital functions such as respiration, phonation, and protection of the laryngotracheal tree can be compromised. Although signs and symptoms may not be immediately apparent, diligent early intervention will help avert potentially severe short-term and long-term sequelae.

BLUNT EXTERNAL TRAUMA

Patients often present to the emergency room with a history and mechanism of injury consistent with a direct blow to the laryngeal complex. Some of the early complaints by the patient may include dyspnea, hoarseness, cervical pain, dysphagia, and odynophagia. Progression of respiratory distress with stridor may herald impending obstruction. This obstruction is brought about by increasing mucosal edema and loss of cartilaginous support of the airway. Other signs and symptoms of significance are hemoptysis, aspiration, expanding hematoma, crepitus, tenderness, and flattening of the thyroid cartilage.

> ## SPECIAL CONSIDERATION
>
> Careful attention must be given to a potential concomitant cervical spine injury. The patient's neck must be stabilized in the neutral position until it can be cleared by cervical radiography.

Palpation of the laryngeal framework may reveal floating fragments with tenderness. Subcutaneous emphysema may suggest laryngotracheal or pharyngeal disruption. Once a full head and neck exam has been completed, the next step is to visualize the endolarynx. In situations where the airway is deemed stable, flexible direct laryngoscopy provides the most information about the degree of injury. It is this step that allows a clinician to differentiate between the patient who may be observed and the patient who would benefit from thin-section axial computed tomography (CT) scan of the larynx versus the patient who requires urgent tracheotomy and subsequent surgical exploration of the larynx.

Laryngeal findings of small mucosal lacerations, hematomas, or absence of cartilaginous fractures may suggest conservative management with close observation over a 24-hour period. If flexible laryngoscopy reveals exposed cartilage, large mucosal lacerations, or disruption of the anterior commissure/true vocal cord, surgical exploration with tracheotomy should be performed.

SPECIAL CONSIDERATION

In a patient with a history of blunt trauma to the neck with increasing subcutaneous emphysema but no laryngeal tenderness or endolaryngeal findings, one must consider a hypopharyngeal or tracheal tear.

In patients who do not have severe symptoms or clinical findings requiring immediate surgical exploration, an axial CT of the larynx may yield information not clinically visualized. The thin-section CT better illuminates the anterior commissure, subglottis, and the cartilaginous skeleton. Gastrografin swallow will also yield invaluable information regarding possible pharyngeal tears. In situations of penetrating trauma, four-vessel carotid angiography should be considered to rule out vascular injury in an otherwise stable patient.

The first step in management of presumed laryngeal trauma is to decide whether the patient's laryngotracheal airway is at risk of immediate or delayed complete obstruction (Fig. 39–1). If obstruction is imminent, an emergent tracheotomy under local anesthesia should be performed in the emergency room. All other procedures should take place in the operating room.

CONTROVERSY

Controversy still remains regarding the role of intubation in the face of possible laryngeal trauma. One may consider intubation only under direct visualization with a small tube with skilled personnel present. In almost all cases, tracheotomy provides the safest means of airway control.

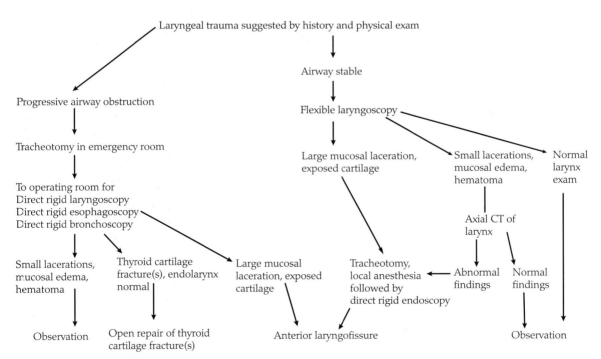

FIGURE 39–1 Treatment pathways for suspected laryngeal trauma.

In cases where tracheotomy must be performed in the emergency room, a decision must be made to either perform a CT scan or proceed directly to surgical exploration. The best time for surgical exploration is within the first 24 hours. It usually involves a horizontal transcervical incision overlying the laryngeal skeleton. The strap musculature is carefully retracted and the cartilaginous skeleton inspected for fractures. If there are mobile pieces, the fragments can be stabilized by wire or absorbable suture. A laryngofissure may be required to inspect and repair any mucosal injuries.

It is generally felt that primary repair of lacerations and coverage of exposed cartilage affords the best long-term healing and voice function. Grafts are to be considered when there are great areas of tissue loss. All endolaryngeal repair should be done with absorbable suture, thus allowing the best hope for full voice recovery. Soft stents may be of use when there is extensive mucosal injury. The loose stent serves as a lumen keeper while keeping granulation tissue and fibrosis to a minimum. All stents must be firmly anchored to the cervical skin and should be removed endoscopically 2 to 3 weeks post injury.

PEARL••• Whenever surgical exploration of the larynx is performed, direct rigid laryngoscopy and direct rigid esophagoscopy should also be done. A horizontal cervical incision also allows direct repair and drainage of any potential pharyngeal tear. Bilateral carotid sheaths may also be explored via this incision.

In cases where flexible laryngoscopy or CT scan mandates surgical exploration, a tracheotomy in the operating room setting is considered the safest option. Finally, in cases where clinical findings suggest minimal or no endolaryngeal damage, overnight observation is indicated. Humidified inspired oxygen, head of bed elevation, and intravenous steroids are mainstays of therapy.

PENETRATING LARYNGEAL TRAUMA

The treatment algorithm for this trauma mimics that of blunt trauma to the larynx. Special attention must be given to possible vascular and pharyngeal injuries. Antibiotics and tetanus toxoid should be given at the initial encounter.

SUGGESTED READINGS

Feliciano DV, Bitondo CG, Mattox KL, et al. Combined tracheoesophageal injuries. *Am J Surg* 1985;150:710–715.

Gussack GS, Jurkovich GJ, Luterman A. Laryngotracheal trauma: a protocol approach to a rare injury. *Laryngoscope* 1986;96:660–665.

Line WS, Stanley RB, Choi JH. Strangulation: a full spectrum of blunt neck trauma. *Ann Otol Rhinol Laryngol* 1985;94:542–546.

Lucente FE, Mitrani M, Sacks SH, Biller HF. Penetrating injuries of the larynx. *Ear Nose Throat J* 1985;64:13–28.

Myer CM, Orobello P, Cotton RT, Bratcher GO. Blunt laryngeal trauma in children. *Laryngoscope* 1987;97:1043–1048.

Schaefer SD. The acute management of external laryngeal trauma. *Arch Otolaryngol Head Neck Surg* 1992;118:598–604.

Schaefer SD. Primary management of laryngeal trauma. *Ann Otol Rhinol Laryngol* 1982;91:399–402.

Schaefer SD. The treatment of external laryngeal injuries. *Arch Otolaryngol Head Neck Surg* 1991;117:35–39.

Schaefer SD, Close LG. Acute management of laryngeal trauma update. *Ann Otol Rhinol Laryngol* 1989;98:98–104.

Stanley RB, Hanson DG. Manual strangulation injuries of the larynx. *Arch Otolaryngol* 1983;109:344–347.

SECTION VII

TRACHEA
AND
BRONCHI

Chapter 40

ANATOMY AND PHYSIOLOGY

Daniel J. Kelley, Mark E. Gerber, and Charles M. Myer III

ANATOMY

The trachea begins at the inferior aspect of the larynx below the cricoid cartilage and enters the superior mediastinum through the superior aperture of the thoracic cavity. At the inferior extent of the superior mediastinum it divides into right and left bronchi at the level of the carina. The right and left mainstem bronchi course to their respective lungs via secondary and tertiary bronchioles. The diameter of the tracheal lumen is maintained by a series of incomplete cartilage rings forming part of its wall. These U-shaped rings of hyaline cartilage are present anteriorly and laterally but are incomplete posteriorly. The trachea varies in length in adults from 3½ to 5 inches and is approximately ¾ inch in diameter.

The wall of the trachea is composed (from medial to lateral) of mucosa, submucosa, a fibrocartilaginous layer, and adventitia or fascia. The mucosa consists of pseudostratified ciliated columnar epithelium and goblet cells. The submucosa contains loose connective tissue and tubuloalveolar glands, which open into the lumen of the trachea. The lamina propria is made up of connective tissue interspersed with lymphatic tissue and occasional nests of solitary lymph nodules. A longitudinal elastic membrane can be found in the deepest layer of the lamina propria. Tracheal muscles insert into the perichondrium, which surrounds each cartilage ring and communicates with the inner submucosa and outer fascia. An extensive neurovascular network can be found within the tracheal fascia.

The smooth musculature of the human trachea is composed of both circular and longitudinal fibers. The trachealis muscle is found within the posterior wall of the trachea, which lacks cartilaginous support, and functions to control variations in the diameter of the lumen of the trachea. Other longitudinal muscle fibers outside the constrictor musculature have also been observed in humans. In addition, annular muscles that may also serve to constrict the diameter of the trachea have been identified. These outer tracheal muscle groups function as constrictors, are often rudimentary, and are of little to no functional importance. The main function of the outer musculature of the trachea and the elastic cartilaginous arches is to maintain the stability of the tracheal wall.

The fascia of the trachea is attached to the upper rim and oblique line of the thyroid cartilage and continues inferiorly on the anterior surface of the trachea. It is fused with the adventitia of the aortic arch, the posterior aspect of the pulmonary artery, and the pericardium. Laterally it is attached to the cartilaginous part of the trachea. The fascia pretrachealis is clinically important in tracheotomy, mediastinoscopy, and the management of tracheal and bronchial trauma.

Many structures are found anterior to the trachea, including the brachiocephalic veins and tributaries, thymus gland, superior vena cava, aortic arch and its brachiocephalic branch, and branches of the vagus nerve coursing inferiorly to join the deep cardiac plexus found anterior to the trachea near its bifurcation into two primary bronchi. To the right of the trachea is the azygous vein and pleura and to the left is the arch of the aorta, left subclavian artery, and the common carotid artery. Posteriorly and laterally, the trachea is bounded by the esophagus, recurrent laryngeal nerves, several intercostal arteries, and thoracic duct.

EMBRYOLOGY

The precursor to the larynx and trachea is the endodermally lined laryngotracheal tube or pharyngeal groove, which develops from the foregut and surrounding mesenchyme between the fourth and sixth branchial arches. The foregut first appears around day 20 (Carnegie stage 9). Over the next 2 days, the primitive pharynx develops along with several pharyngeal pouches and arches. The laryngeal sulcus and pulmonary primordium develop, and by 24 days the pulmonary primordium divides into right and left lung buds, which eventually form the lobes of the lung. By day 26, the pulmonary primordium has begun to migrate caudally into the mesenchyme ventral to the foregut. At this point, the tracheoesophageal septum is formed, which divides the respiratory system from the digestive system and allows them to develop separately. The tracheoesophageal septum, which eventually forms the common wall between the trachea and esophagus, remains relatively constant as the lung buds migrate inferiorly. It is the elongation of the lung buds relative to the tracheoesophageal septum that forms the trachea, which is evident by day 28 of development. The trachea elongates and enlarges for the remainder of gestation and continues to increase in size during the postnatal period of respiratory development.

During development of the respiratory tract, embryonic cells are instructed to organize themselves along an axis and differentiate, such that proximal structures (trachea) greatly differ from those in distal alveoli. Pattern formation relates to this process of organization, and it is believed to be transcriptionally regulated in many developmental systems. Although the lung is the site of expression of many transcription factors, such as Hox, retinoid receptors, hepatocyte nuclear factors, little information is available on how they influence respiratory development. Functional studies so far have directly implicated the product of the proto-oncogene N-*myc* and the retinoic acid receptors as transcriptional regulators of lung patterning, and it is likely that tissue-specific homeobox genes, such as the thyroid transcription factor-1, play an important role in distal lung formation.

Ciliogenesis of the respiratory epithelium starts at 7 weeks of gestation and follows a predetermined pattern of distribution. It starts exclusively in the upper segment of the membranous trachea and spreads distally. Cartilage development is evident within the trachea by 10 weeks. Ciliation of the cartilaginous trachea does not take place until after the 12th week of gestation. Epithelial cell differentiation patterns in both the cartilaginous and membranous trachea are different as well. During the pseudoglandular phase, between 13 and 16 weeks' gestation, tracheal gland morphogenesis occurs. This involves the penetration of epithelial cells into the submucosa, a process that requires digestion of the basal lamina and the surrounding extracellular matrix. Gelatinase A is a specialized product of the tracheal gland epithelial cell and most likely plays an important role in this process. Ciliation of the entire trachea is complete by 16 weeks of development.

Innervation from the autonomic nervous system also occurs during this period. In addition to autonomic innervation, undifferentiated precursors present in the endodermal pulmonary epithelium begin to differentiate into neuroendocrine small-granule cells within the upper trachea and expand into pulmonary airways as they develop. Innervated small-granule cell clusters are reached first by ganglion cells derived from pulmonary neuroblasts and later by processes from extrinsic sensory nerves. The latter convey information to the central nervous system. Dissociated cells that are not reached by ganglion cells exhibit physiologic characteristics of oxygen sensors despite the lack of innervation.

INNERVATION

The trachea receives its motor nerve supply from the autonomic nervous system. The sympathetic portion arises from preganglionic neuron cell bodies contained within the first four thoracic segments of the spinal cord. The axons of these cell bodies pass through the ventral roots to form white communicating rami and synapse with the first four sympathetic ganglia located on either side of the vertebral column. Within the sympathetic ganglia, preganglionic fibers can either synapse within the ganglion, pass up or down the sympathetic chain to synapse with ganglion cells at other levels, or pass through to other ganglia located outside the sympathetic chain. Postganglionic fibers travel with intercostal nerves to the cardiac plexus located at the bifurcation of the trachea. These postganglionic sympathetic fibers innervate the trachea and cause vasoconstriction, decreased mucous secretion, and relaxation of smooth muscle within the trachea.

The parasympathetic innervation of the trachea arises within the dorsal motor nucleus of the vagus in the brainstem. These fibers exit through the jugular foramen and travel with the vagus within the carotid sheath. They continue through the superior aperture of the thoracic cavity and form part of the cardiac plexus. Stimulation of parasympathetic fibers causes vasodilation, secretion of mucous glands, and contraction of the smooth muscles in the trachea. The trachealis muscle itself contracts with an inspiratory rhythm that closely parallels the phrenic nerve.

VASCULAR SUPPLY

The vascular supply to the trachea is composed of several sources that interconnect to form a rich network. One of the main arterial sources

of the trachea is branches of the inferior thyroid artery, which is a branch of the thyrocervical trunk of the subclavian artery.

SPECIAL CONSIDERATION

Tracheomalacia or stenosis following thyroid surgery may be related to disturbances in local blood supply, which can cause changes in tracheal tissue. The inferior thyroid artery and its branches also seem to play an important role in the success or failure of tracheal reconstructions following resection of stenoses and end-to-end anastomoses.

Bronchial arteries, the nutrient vessels of the lung, which arise from the intercostal arteries and the aorta, and their side branches supply the trachea as well as many other mediastinal structures including the esophagus, lymph nodes, pericardium, aorta, and mediastinal parietal pleura. They are small-diameter vessels despite being part of the systemic circulation. Bronchial arteries connect with each other via the rich vascular network located within the tracheal fascia. Longitudinal tracheoesophageal arteries and veins, as well as segmental branches running circumferentially in the intercartilaginous spaces, have also been observed.

Within the tracheal fascia is both a subepithelial capillary network and a submucous venous plexus. The subepithelial capillary network is normally unfenestrated except for those vessels close to neuroepithelial bodies and submucosal glands, but it is fenestrated in asthmatics. Deeper within the tracheal mucosa, the submucous venous plexus acts as a capacitance system of vessels. The extensive subepithelial capillary network drains into venous networks at different levels of the mucosa and collects into circumferentially arranged veins that run between the cartilages. The veins terminate in the plexus of veins around the thyroid gland and into the inferior thyroid vein.

CONTROVERSY

Some advocate that saving the blood supply to the trachea is possible with careful preservation of the intercostobronchial arteries and the tracheal sheath during radical dissection of the central compartment of the neck and upper mediastinum. However, this is based largely on anecdotal evidence.

LYMPHATICS

The lymph nodes associated with the trachea are relatively constant and classified into three groups: anterior and posterior tracheal lymph nodes, superior and inferior tracheobronchial lymph nodes, and bronchomediastinal lymph nodes. In addition, the recurrent lymph node chain drains laterally from the trachea, posterior to the carotid sheath, and into either deep cervical nodes situated on the scalenus anterior, or directly into the venous angle. The bronchomediastinal lymphatic system collects lymphatic drainage from the trachea as well as other structures, including the great vessels, esophagus, and mediastinal pleura. On the right side, the trunks of the bronchomediastinal lymphatic system are located on both the right brachiocephalic vein and the subserous surface of the mediastinal pleura. On the left side, the drainage pattern of the bronchomediastinal lymphatic system is much more variable. The collecting vessels can be divided into two pathways on each side: the anterior and posterior mediastinal trunks on the right side and the superior and inferior mediastinal trunks on the left side.

Communications exist between the lymphatic drainage systems on either side of the trachea. The large transverse superficial communicating vessel between the right and left sides is usually found anterior to the trachea and superior to the aortic arch. Deep communications are also present anterior and posterior to the trachea at the level of the carina.

PHYSIOLOGY

VENTILATION

The function of the trachea and bronchi is to direct inspired air to the gas-exchanging regions of the lung. Because they do not participate in gas exchange, the trachea and bronchi are considered anatomic dead space. Ventilation of the trachea and bronchi involves complex relationships between lung resistance, elasticity, and compliance. During inspiration, the volume of the thoracic cavity increases due to contraction of the diaphragm and intercostal muscles, and air flows through the trachea and bronchi. Active shortening and lengthening of contractile elements within airway smooth muscle helps modulate changes in airway diameter. Increased negative intrathoracic pressure acts independently to draw the trachea into the thorax and increase the patency of the upper airway. The lung is elastic and it returns passively to its preinspiratory volume after relaxation of the diaphragm and intercostal muscles.

Airway smooth muscle must overcome the elastic load provided by cartilage and lung to relax and contract. In fact, maximal muscle shortening is limited by the afterload provided by the tracheal cartilaginous rings. Cartilage is also responsible for the stability of the large airways, and yet very little is known about its mechanical properties. The outermost layer of cartilage is usually the most rigid, and deeper layers are progressively less rigid. Tensile stiffness correlates inversely with water and hydroxyproline content. Both water and hydroxyproline content decrease with age, causing airways to become less compliant. Total tissue content of glycosaminoglycans does not change with age, although changes in glycosaminoglycan type and proteoglycan structure with age have been described. Thus, age-related changes in the biomechanical properties and biochemical composition of airway cartilage influence airway dynamics. Age-related changes occur in parallel within airway smooth muscle: both passive and active stress increase from preterm to adult. These changes are thought to be due to a progressive increase in contractility and sensitivity to acetylcholinesterase (ACh) throughout maturation.

INNERVATION

In the trachea and mainstem bronchi, the autonomic nervous system regulates a variety of functions, including blood flow, smooth muscle tone, and defense mechanisms such as seromucinous secretion and ciliary activity. The trachea and bronchi are richly innervated with adrenergic nerve fibers, which contain noradrenaline. When adrenergic fibers derived from the superior cervical ganglia are stimulated, there is relaxation of airway smooth muscle. Contraction and secretion are inhibited by muscarinic receptor blockers like atropine and enhanced by acetylcholine breakdown inhibitors.

The central respiratory rhythm produces a continuous cycle of inspiration and expiration by coupling sympathetic and parasympathetic innervation of the airways. For example, medullary neurons from the respiratory center in the brainstem project to both phrenic motor neurons and airway-related vagal preganglionic cells, modulating cholinergic outflow to the tracheal smooth muscle through the parasympathetic nerves. The electrical activity of tracheal smooth muscle consists of slow oscillatory potentials, which result in intermittent contraction and relaxation. There is a difference in timing of contraction between the trachea and bronchial smooth muscle, suggesting distinct motor control within the central nervous system.

Stimulation of chemoreceptors, irritant receptors, mechanoreceptors, and pulmonary C-fiber receptors constricts airway smooth muscle, alters ventilation, and can affect other respiratory systems through reflex arcs as well. Other reflex effects include mucous secretion in the trachea, vasoconstriction both in the nose (with reduction in airflow resistance) and trachea, and pulmonary vasoconstriction. The larynx and pharynx dilate during peripheral chemoreceptor stimulation. Most of these changes affect airway caliber, which, in turn, affect lung ventilation and blood-gas tensions.

The receptors responsible for eliciting respiratory protective reflexes are not uniformly distributed in the airways, and responses to airway irritation, such as cough, vary depending on the site and nature of the stimulation. Reflex arcs also exist between the esophagus and the respiratory system. Changes in airway smooth muscle tone and pulmonary circulation can be caused by mechanical or acid (pH 2) stimulation of esophageal afferents. Other effects on the trachea and bronchi, such as how cold air causes vasoconstriction, and how hypercapnia and hypoxia both relax airway smooth muscle, remain poorly understood.

NEUROPEPTIDES

During the last decade, the concept of the cholinergic and adrenergic systems as the only two regulatory systems acting to balance each other within the autonomic nervous system has been revised. In general, parasympathetic nerves cause vasodilation and sympathetic nerves cause vasoconstriction. Other nonadrenergic, noncholinergic mechanisms, such as neuropeptides, are thought to play a more important role in the relaxation of human airway smooth muscle. Bioactive peptides, including vasoactive intestinal peptide (VIP), substance P, leucine enkephalin, bombesin, and calcitonin, also have effects on airway smooth muscle tone. Neuropeptides are present in both afferent and efferent fibers innervating the bronchial arteries.

Vasoactive intestinal peptide and peptide histidine methionine are the primary mediators of nonadrenergic, noncholinergic peptidergic nerves. These peptides produce vasodilation in the tracheobronchial circulation and contribute to the regulation of secretion by respiratory epithelium by causing relaxation of airway smooth muscle. VIP may modulate release of acetylcholine from cholinergic nerves and neuropeptides from sensory nerves. Afferent or sensory nerves that contain tachykinins, such as substance P and neurokinins A and B, are potent vasodilators in the tracheobronchial circulation and also induce bronchoconstriction and postcapillary permeability. Substance P and neurokinins A (NKA) and B (NKB) have been implicated in mediating neurogenic inflammation of the airways. Asthma is associated with hyperplasia of airway smooth muscle, and substance P may induce airway smooth muscle cell proliferation by transmembrane signaling coupled to selective activation of the NK1 receptor.

Another important nonadrenergic noncholinergic mediator of airway relaxation (bronchodilation) is nitric oxide (NO). NO-containing nerve fibers are found in airway smooth muscle, around submucosal glands and blood vessels, and in the lamina propria. The density of airway smooth muscle innervated by nitric oxide synthase (NOS)-containing nerve fibers varies according to airway diameter. It is greatest within the trachea and decreases significantly in small-diameter bronchi. NO is probably generated by de novo synthesis at the nerve terminal during neural activation by the action of the enzyme NOS, although the location of the NOS enzyme or the site of production of NO remains unclear. NO is a crucial mediator in the response of mucosal arterioles to a hypertonic stimulus presented to the epithelial surface of the trachea and is considered one of the most important nonadrenergic, noncholinergic bronchodilator neural relaxant pathways in human airways.

MUSCLE CONTRACTION

Smooth muscle cells within the trachea contain myofibrils, which are composed of actin, myosin, and tropomyosin. Myosin is the primary component of thin filaments, whereas actin and tropomyosin make up thick filaments. Thin and thick filaments overlap to create the basic muscle units that contract in response to a variety of stimuli.

Cholinergic stimuli acting via muscarinic receptors stimulate airway smooth muscle to contract and β-adrenergic stimuli induce it to relax. Cholinergic agonists stimulate intracellular Ca^{2+} release and Ca^{2+} influx, and β-adrenergic agonists stimulate adenosine $3',5'$-cyclic monophosphate (cAMP) production. Because it was found that cAMP alters cholinergic agonist-induced changes in cellular Ca^{2+} metabolism, it was postulated that cAMP brought about a relaxation of this smooth muscle primarily by decreasing intracellular Ca^{2+}. A key feature of this model of airway smooth muscle function is the presence of reciprocal pathways by which the Ca^{2+} and cAMP messenger systems modulate each other's expression.

CONTROVERSY

The decrease in intracellular Ca^{2+} may be the primary event that causes relaxation of tracheal smooth muscle.

The mechanical performance of smooth muscle decreases progressively down the tracheobronchial tree. This fact allows division of airway smooth muscle into extrapulmonary and intrapulmonary groups. The extrapulmonary group includes muscle from the trachea, mainstem bronchi, and secondary bronchi, and is characterized by higher maximum shortening capacity and lower sensitivity to stimulation. The intrapulmonary group, which contains tertiary and smaller bronchioles, has a lower maximum shortening capacity but higher sensitivity to stimulation. The relatively lower mechanical performance of intrapulmonary bronchial smooth muscle may represent a safety device that prevents excessive smooth muscle shortening. The bronchi are probably the main sites of airway narrowing in exercise-induced bronchoconstriction, whereas the trachea undergoes simultaneous dilatation. Results to date suggest that different mechanisms are responsible for regulating the patency of the upper and lower airways.

MUCOCILIARY FUNCTION

Mucociliary transport is critical for normal function of the tracheobronchial system. The surface of each ciliated cell contains approximately 200 cilia. Each cilium contains two central microtubules surrounded in a circular fashion by nine doublets that join at the tip and are attached to the cell body by a basal body. Movement of the cilia is accomplished by dynein arms that bridge the space between the doublets of the peripheral microtubules and cause bending of the cilia. The energy source for cilia motion is adenosine triphosphate (ATP) provided by the cell body. The cephalad direction in which cilia beat is coordinated into a single orientation with a power stroke followed by a slower recovery stroke. The mechanism that controls the synchronous movement of the ciliated cells remains unknown. Ciliary beat frequency (CBF) is extremely sensitive to changes in temperature: low temperature decreases CBF and high temperatures enhance CBF.

In the central airways, the epithelium is lined by two layers of liquid. The cilia are surrounded by a periciliary fluid layer (sol) and are covered by a mucous layer (gel), which may be discontinuous and contain mucin glycoproteins. Other proteins are found within the proximal airways that contribute to the physiology of the respiratory system. Aquaporins are water transport proteins and are involved in humidification, glandular secretion, and clearance of fluid from distal airways. Collagenous lectins (collectins) bind to influenza virus and display antiviral activity. Glycosaminoglycans, such as hyaluronan, are present in human respiratory epithelial cells and submucosal gland serous cells and are exocytosed in response to parasympathetic stimulation. These proteins may play a role in packaging cationic proteins in serous cells, cellular adhesion to basement membranes, and activation of macrophages in airway lumens. Secretory proteins, such as secretory immunoglobulin A (IgA), transferrin, and lysozyme, participate in the airway antibacterial defense. Other biochemical components found in secretions, such as antiinflammatory and antioxidant agents, as well as antiproteases, contribute significantly to the protection of the underlying epithelium. The epithelium is a relatively weak barrier for lipophilic agents but plays a major role as a diffusion barrier to hydrophilic substances.

A variety of external stimuli alter the function of the mucociliary transport system within the trachea and bronchi to reduce the impact of potential toxins, chemical irritants, or alterations in normal homeostasis, such as dry-air inhalation. For example, gastric juice causes hyperpermeability across human airway epithelium probably through the additive effects of gastric acid, pepsin activity, and lower osmolarity. The production of mucins increases due to enhanced expression of a tracheobronchial

mucin (TBM) gene. Reactive nitrogen species stimulate the secretion of mucin, which suggests that intracellularly generated radical species of nitrogen and oxygen may be important modulators of the response of airway epithelial cells to external oxidant stress. When these responses cannot adequately protect the mucosa, stimulation of mucociliary transport occurs. Increases in tracheal ciliary beat frequency, mucus velocity, and mucociliary clearance can be demonstrated in response to inhaled substances.

Extravasation of plasma from the abundant subepithelial microvessels can also protect the airways. A plasma exudate has important actions through its volume, its specific and nonspecific binding proteins, its enzyme systems, and its potent peptides (kinin, complement, coagulation, fibrinolysis, and other systems). Plasma exudation can be considered part of the first line of respiratory defense operating with other systems of the mucosal surface. Tracheal mucus transport velocity correlates with tracheal surface area. As tracheal size increases, the rigidity of airway secretions decreases, and rigidity is inversely correlated with mucociliary transportability.

Airway secretion can be modified by alterations in autonomic regulation and gene expression as well as in response to inhaled toxins. The ventral medulla contains cells near its surface that influence tracheal fluid secretion and modulate reflex responses of airway submucosal glands, probably by altering the level of general excitation within the central respiratory integrating circuits. Cholinergic stimulation is a very effective means of enhancing mucociliary clearance. Recent data from mammals suggest that mucociliary clearance is also regulated by neuropeptides either directly (substance P) or by facilitating the stimulatory effect of cholinergic agents. Retinoic acid appears to alter mucin gene expression in tracheal epithelial cells.

One of the major roles of the upper respiratory mucosa is to humidify inspired air. This function requires the coordinated activity of respiratory epithelium and mucosal vasculature. Changes in solution osmolarity on the epithelial surface of the trachea can regulate diameter of mucosal blood vessels. Alterations in mucosal blood flow, in turn, influence the magnitude and duration of airway smooth muscle contraction in the trachea. Increased respiratory blood flow leads to distention of the airway vasculature and thickening of the mucosa, probably both by vascular distention and edema formation. The latter can lead to exudation into the airway lumen.

Proteins and lipids synthesized by airway secretory cells are involved in the control of mucus hydration as well.

CYTOKINES AND SECONDARY MESSENGERS

Epithelial cells lining the respiratory airways classically are considered to be "target" cells, responding to exposure to a variety of inflammatory mediators by altering one or several of their functions, such as mucin secretion, ion transport, or ciliary beating. Recent studies have indicated that airway epithelial cells also can act as "effector" cells, responding to a variety of exogenous and/or endogenous stimuli by generating and releasing additional mediators of inflammation, such as eicosanoids, reactive oxygen species, and cytokines. Many of these epithelial-derived substances can affect neighboring cells and tissues, or act via autocrine or paracrine mechanisms to affect structure and function of epithelial cells themselves.

Prostaglandins and leukotrienes are produced by the enzymatic degradation of arachidonic acid. Prostaglandin E_2 (PGE_2) may be an important inhibitory modulator of airway inflammation by causing tracheobronchial smooth muscle relaxation. The effect of leukotrienes on tracheal smooth muscle is both direct and indirect. Inhalation or application to tracheal mucosa causes an intense contraction of the underlying smooth muscle. Leukotrienes also cause a significant decrease in ciliary beat frequency within the trachea.

Other factors that may serve to regulate airway smooth muscle contraction include the balance between the cyclooxygenase pathway and leukotriene pathway in arachidonic acid metabolism. Platelet-activating factor (PAF) is a phospholipid mediator of inflammation and vascular leakage that may be important in the etiology of asthma. PAF causes rapid and prolonged neutrophil accumulation in the canine trachea and an increase in vascular permeability that is partially mediated by neutrophils. Exposure to epidermal growth factor (EGF) causes tracheal epithelium to become taller and contain a greater proportion of secretory cells and a smaller proportion of intermediate cells. Rhinovirus infection causes an increase in intercellular adhesion molecule-1 (ICAM-1), which, in turn, increases the production of inflammatory cytokines such as interleukin (IL)-1β, IL-6, IL-8, and tumor necrosis factor (TNF)-α. IL-5 induces eosinophil infiltration, which precedes the development of airway hyperreactivity and mucosal exudation. Endothelins are recently discovered peptides that cause vasoconstriction and bronchoconstriction in addition to significant mucociliary stimulatory effects. The significance of endothelins in the airway is unclear, but they are thought to play an important role in respiratory homeostasis and inflammatory conditions.

SUGGESTED READINGS

Baker D.G. Parasympathetic motor pathways to the trachea: recent morphologic and electrophysiologic studies. *Clin Chest Med* 1986;7(2):223–229.

Belvisi MG, Ward JK, Mitchell JA, Barnes PJ. Nitric oxide as a neurotransmitter in human airways. *Arch Int Pharmacodyn Ther* 1995;329(1):97–110.

Butler JE, McKenzie DK, Crawford MR, Gandevia SC. Role of airway receptors in the reflex responses of human inspiratory muscles to airway occlusion. *J Physiol (Lond)* 1995;487(pt 1):273–281.

Cohn LA, Adler KB. Interactions between airway epithelium and mediators of inflammation. *Exp Lung Res* 1992;18(3):299–322.

Crafts RC. *A Textbook of Human Anatomy.* New York: Churchill Livingstone; 1985.

Daniel EE, O'Byrne P. Effect of inflammatory mediators on airway nerves and muscle. *Am Rev Respir Dis* 1991;143(3 pt 2):S3–S5.

Funami Y, Okuyama K, Shimada Y, Isono K. Anatomic study of the bronchial arteries with special reference to their preservation during the radical dissection of the upper mediastinum lymph nodes. *Surgery* 1996;119(1): 67–75.

Godden DJ. Reflex and nervous control of the tracheobronchial circulation. *Eur Respir J Suppl* 1990;12:602S–607S.

Hakansson CH, Mercke U, Sonesson B, Toremalm NG. Functional anatomy of the musculature of the trachea. *Acta Morphol Neerl Scand* 1976;14(4):291–297.

Haxhiu MA, Erokwu BO, Cherniack NS. The brainstem network involved in coordination of inspiratory activity and cholinergic outflow to the airways. *J Auton Nerv Syst* 1996;61(2): 155–161.

Jacquot J, Hayem A, Galabert C. Functions of proteins and lipids in airway secretions. *Eur Respir J* 1992;5(3):343–358.

Le Merre C, Kim HH, Chediak AD, Wanner A. Airway blood flow responses to temperature and humidity of inhaled air. *Respir Physiol* 1996;105(3):235–239.

Lutchen KR, Gillis H. Relationship between heterogeneous changes in airway morphometry and lung resistance and elastance. *J Appl Physiol* 1997;83(4):1192–1201.

Moscoso GJ, Driver M, Codd J, Whimster WF. The morphology of ciliogenesis in the developing fetal human respiratory epithelium. *Pathol Res Pract* 1988;183(4):403–411.

Nishino T, Kochi T, Ishii M. Differences in respiratory reflex responses from the larynx, trachea, and bronchi in anesthetized female subjects. *Anesthesiology* 1996;84(1):70–74.

Ohrui T, Yamaya M, Suzuki T, et al. Mechanisms of gastric juice-induced hyperpermeability of the cultured human tracheal epithelium. *Chest* 1997;111(2):454–459.

Panitch HB, Deoras KS, Wolfson MR, Shaffer TH. Maturational changes in airway smooth muscle structure-function relationships. *Pediatr Res* 1992;31(2):151–156.

Persson CG, Erjefalt I, Alkner U, et al. Plasma exudation as a first line respiratory mucosal defense. *Clin Exp Allergy* 1991;21(1):17–24.

Picado C. Response of nose and bronchi to exercise in asthma and rhinitis: similarities and differences. *Clin Exp Allergy* 1996;26(suppl 3):36–38.

Rains JK, Bert JL, Roberts CR, Pare PD. Mechanical properties of human tracheal cartilage. *J Appl Physiol* 1992;72(1):219–225.

Reading PC, Morey LS, Crouch EC, Anders EM. Collectin-mediated antiviral host defense of the lung: evidence from influenza virus infection of mice. *J Virol* 1997;71(11):8204–8212.

Russell JA. Tracheal smooth muscle. *Clin Chest Med* 1986;7(2):189–196.

Salonen RO, Webber SE, Widdicombe JG. Effects of neurotransmitters on tracheobronchial blood flow. *Eur Respir J Suppl* 1990;12: 630S–636S.

Sanjar S. Measurement and pharmacology of mucociliary clearance. *Agents Actions Suppl* 1991;34:457–470.

Shen X, Wu MF, Tepper RS, Gunst SJ. Mechanisms for the mechanical response of airway smooth muscle to length oscillation. *J Appl Physiol* 1997;83(3):731–738.

Smith TL, Prazma J, Coleman CC, Drake AF, Boucher RC. Control of the mucosal microcirculation in the upper respiratory tract. *Otolaryngol Head Neck Surg* 1993;109(4):646–652.

Staindl O, Lametschwandtner A. The pathogenesis of tracheal stenosis following thyroidectomy. *HNO* 1979;27(8):260–266.

Terajima M, Yamaya M, Sekizawa K, et al. Rhinovirus infection of primary cultures of human tracheal epithelium: role of ICAM-1 and IL-1beta. *Am J Physiol* 1997;273(4 pt 1): L749–L759.

Tewfik TL, Der Kaloustian VM. *Congenital Anomalies of the Ear, Nose, and Throat.* New York: Oxford University Press; 1997.

Uddman R, Sundler F. Innervation of the upper airways. *Clin Chest Med* 1986;7(2): 201–209.

Van Oosterhout AJ, Fattah D, Van Ark I, Hofman G, Buckley TL, Nijkamp FP. Eosinophil infiltration precedes development of airway hyperreactivity and mucosal exudation after intranasal administration of interleukin-5 to mice. *J Allergy Clin Immunol* 1995;96(1):104–112.

Wanner A, Chediak AD, Csete ME. Airway mucosal blood flow: response to autonomic and inflammatory stimuli. *Eur Respir J Suppl* 1990; 12:618S–623S.

Widdicombe JG. Chemoreceptor control of the airways. *Respir Physiol* 1992;87(3):373–381.

Chapter 41

CLINICAL TESTS

Daniel J. Kelley, Mark E. Gerber, and Charles M. Myer III

Diagnostic evaluation of the trachea and mainstem bronchi can be divided into five main categories of investigation: physical examination, pulmonary function testing, radiography, nuclear medicine, and endoscopy.

PHYSICAL EXAMINATION

Tracheal sounds originate from turbulent flow within the upper and central airways. Turbulent flow characteristics are influenced by a number of factors, such as the physical dimensions of the trachea and bronchi. Sound generation occurs as a result of air flow separation, downstream movement of air flow eddies, and collision of fast-moving cores of the inflowing air with the carina, occurring primarily during inspiration. Tracheal dimensions are a function of age and body height.

Stridor and wheezing are probably the two most common physical signs noted in patients with tracheobronchial abnormalities. Stridor originating at the tracheobronchial level is most commonly expiratory, although it can be biphasic. Voice quality is typically unaffected. Hoarseness in combination with stridor is a sign of a more diffuse process, such as a serious opportunistic infection in an immunocompromised patient involving both the larynx and trachea. Extrinsic conditions, such as innominate artery compression, as well as intrinsic pathol-

ogy, such as foreign bodies, tracheomalacia, or neoplasms, can all cause stridor, wheezing, or altered breath sounds. Chronic cough is a symptom that has diagnostic significance but is nonspecific.

Lung sound analysis is a potential source of objective, noninvasive information on the status and function of the pulmonary system. Both extrathoracic and intrathoracic lesions can be correlated with changes in the spectral acoustic pattern of breath sounds. Tracheal sounds are recorded during spontaneous breathing, digitized with an analog-to-digital converter, and analyzed using fast-Fourier transform. Alterations in inspiratory tracheal sound intensity in patients with obstructive sleep apnea suggest a potential value for daytime acoustic screening. Digital sound analysis is able to detect episodes of bronchoconstriction in asthmatic patients during sleep.

SPECIAL CONSIDERATION

Children often have difficulty performing spirometric tests reliably. Therefore, spectral analysis of lung sounds can be used to assess bronchial responsiveness to bronchodilator therapy in children.

Changes in lung sounds correspond well with spirometry. The combination of spirometry and lung sounds analysis improves the ability to detect mild pulmonary disease and may provide an early sign of lung disease that was not detected by spirometry alone.

PULMONARY FUNCTION TESTS

The goals of pulmonary function testing are to detect occult disease, diagnose and characterize the type and degree of dysfunction, and monitor response to therapy. Pulmonary function testing is also useful in evaluating dyspnea, wheezing, and cough, and in assessing preoperative pulmonary risk.

Spirometry reveals both obstructive and restrictive airway disease.

> **PEARL...** Accurate office spirometry requires routine preventive maintenance, cleaning, and calibration of equipment and quality control measures.

The determination of normal range for individual patients is achieved by using regression equations based on physiologic parameters such as age, height, weight, and sex. Results are usually presented as a percentage of the predicted value. Values less than two standard deviations from the normal range are suggestive of pulmonary disease (Table 41–1).

Spirometry, which measures air volume over time, is used to assess both maximal expiratory flow rates from total lung capacity (TLC) and certain lung volumes (Fig. 41–1).

> **SPECIAL CONSIDERATION**
>
> Forced expiratory volume in one second (FEV$_1$) is the most reproducible flow parameter and is used often to measure response to treatment in patients with obstructive disease, such as asthma. FEV$_1$ is often expressed as percentage of vital capacity or the ratio of FEV$_1$ to peak expiratory flow rate (PEFR), also referred to as Empey's index.

TABLE 41–1 PARAMETERS PREDICTIVE OF PULMONARY DISEASE

Parameter	Percent of Predicted Value
Vital capacity (VC)	75
Functional residual capacity (FRC)	70
Residual volume (RV)	65
Total lung capacity (TLC)	80
Forced expiratory volume in 1 second (FEV$_1$)	80
Forced expiratory flow (FEF)	65
Maximum inspiratory pressure (MIP)	65

> **PEARL...** Obstructive conditions, such as asthma, emphysema, and intratracheal neoplasms or stenosis, are characterized by reduced FEV$_1$, reduced FEV$_1$ forced vital capacity (FEV$_1$/FVC), and normal to increased TLC and residual volume. Restrictive disorders typically reduce TLC with preservation of flow rates.

The most common causes of restrictive lung disorders include pleural, alveolar, or interstitial conditions, neuromuscular weakness of the ventilatory muscles, and thoracic cage abnormalities, such as kyphoscoliosis or obesity. Spirome-

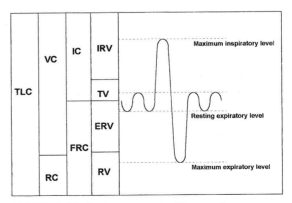

FIGURE 41–1 Assessment of lung volumes. TLC, total lung capacity; VC, vital capacity; RC, residual capacity; IC, inspiratory capacity; FRC, functional residual capacity; IRV, inspiratory residual volume; TV, total volume; ERV, expiratory reserve volume; RV, residual volume.

try may also reveal abnormalities in other sites of the upper airway, including the nasopharynx and vocal cords. Changes in spirometry following the administration of bronchodilators are suggestive of reactive airway disease. Peak expiratory flow (PEF) and peak inspiratory flow (PIF) are the most appropriate parameters to assess airway mechanics before and after surgical or endoscopic procedures.

Experimental evidence indicates that laryngotracheal obstruction below 50 mm^2 surface area (diameter of circular opening <8 mm) compromises respiratory function enough to be clinically evident. Spirometry can occasionally be misleading, particularly in cases of tracheomalacia.

> **PEARL...** Spirometry can be used as an objective assessment before and after treatment in patients with tracheal stenosis.

Unlike spirometry, flow volume loops measure air flow versus lung volume during maximum inspiration and expiration. Flow volume loops offer improved assessment of air flow versus lung volume. To obtain a flow-volume loop, the seated or standing patient is instructed to inspire maximally to TLC, exhale as hard, fast, and completely as possible (FVC), and inhale quickly and deeply to TLC (Fig. 41–2).

> **PITFALL...** A high resistance to airflow and absence of expiratory flow limitation is usually suggestive of a fixed obstruction, but can be seen in cases of tracheomalacia.

> **PEARL...** Marked blunting of peak flow rates is suggestive of fixed obstruction in the upper airways, such as tracheal stenosis.

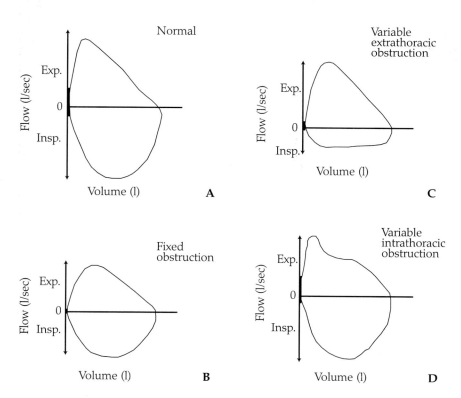

FIGURE 41–2 (A). Normal flow volume loop. Pattern demonstrating (B). a fixed obstruction, (C). a variable extrathoracic obstruction, and (D). a variable intrathoracic obstruction. Exp., expiration; insp., inspiration.

Exercise testing uses a combination of electro-cardiography, spirometry, arterial blood gases, and expired gas concentrations to assess the degree of cardiopulmonary dysfunction. Exercise testing is very useful in treatment planning and evaluation of treatment response.

Recent advances in the diagnosis and treatment of sleep disorders have had a major impact on pulmonary medicine, otolaryngology, and head and neck surgery. An early version of a cutaneous oximeter was originally developed in 1947 by Milikan, but it was the combination of the pulse signal with spectroscopy by Aoyagi in the 1970s that transformed oximetry into the monitor used currently. Cutaneous or pulse oximeters use infrared light, which penetrates human tissues. The infrared light interacts with the chromophore oxyhemoglobin, and the attenuated light is detected by a photodetector. The amount of attenuation reflects the amount of oxyhemoglobin present and allows monitoring of oxygenation. Nasal thermistors, chest wall movement detectors, electrocardiography, and electroencephalography are combined with pulse oximetry to help assess the presence, type, and degree of sleep disorder.

> **PEARL...** Pulse oximetry has become the standard of care in the operating room and intensive care unit as well as during procedures performed under sedation, such as endoscopy and interventional radiology and cardiology.

Other pulmonary function tests include gas dilution, body plethysmography, radiographic planimetry, and recoil/compliance assessment. Gas dilution techniques, which use helium dilution and nitrogen washout of inspired air, are used to accurately measure absolute lung volume. Body plethysmography measures the compressible gas volume within the thoracic cavity and is particularly useful in measuring TLC in patients with chronic obstructive pulmonary disease. Radiographic planimetry uses conventional chest radiographs to estimate TLC. Carbon monoxide diffusion capacity is a relatively nonspecific measure of respiratory function and is not commonly used. Assessments of elastic re-

coil and static compliance of the lung are somewhat impractical because they require measurement of esophageal pressure, are time and labor intensive, and have a wide range of normal values. Closing volume and dynamic compliance can be measured by a variety of techniques, but their clinical relevance has yet to be defined.

Gas exchange abnormalities are caused by the mismatch of ventilation and perfusion within the lung. Areas of the lung that are adequately ventilated by gas but are not perfused by blood because of shunts within pulmonary circulation result in hypoxemia and hypercapnia. Pulmonary shunting will also occur in areas within the lung that are perfused by blood but not ventilated. The degree of shunt can be estimated by the difference in the amount of oxygen found in alveoli relative to arterial blood. Assessment of ventilation-perfusion mismatch can also be determined by nuclear medicine techniques as will be discussed.

RADIOGRAPHY

Radiographic evaluation is complementary to pulmonary function testing in the evaluation of the trachea and bronchi. Adult and pediatric tracheobronchial anatomy is well defined, and careful radiographic analysis can yield considerable information. Standard anteroposterior and lateral chest radiographs remain the initial imaging study for most pulmonary symptoms. In many instances of acute blunt and penetrating trauma, chest radiographs provide the first evidence of the extent of injury.

Many chronic intrinsic and extrinsic tracheal disorders eventually cause an alteration in the diameter of the airway lumen to some degree. New-onset wheezing in the young child may be a sign of an airway foreign body, and chest radiography can demonstrate air-trapping and tracheal deviation. The chest radiograph is often normal, however, and posteroanterior and lateral neck roentgenograms may also suggest the diagnosis.

> **PEARL...** When compared to angiography, bronchoscopy, and echocardiography, barium swallow is the most sensitive indicator of vascular compression of the trachea.

Computed tomography (CT) of the chest is probably the radiographic test of choice after plain radiographs in the assessment of tracheobronchial pathology. CT facilitates quantitative assessment of a cross-sectional area of the trachea. Large retrosternal goiters, which can cause significant compression of the airway, can be easily demonstrated on CT. In the past, computed axial tomography has been limited by respiratory-induced motion artifacts and misregistration, which limited its accuracy. Spiral CT differs from conventional CT in that the entire thorax can be rapidly imaged in the axial plane after a single breath-hold. Selective windowing allows air within the tracheobronchial tree to be used as a negative contrast agent. Helical CT produces very high quality images of the trachea, is particularly suited to the study of the tracheobronchial tree, and can now be utilized instead of endoscopy in many instances.

> **PEARL...** CT remains the modality of choice for evaluating patients with a tracheobronchial or intrathoracic malignancy.

Magnetic resonance imaging (MRI) is complementary to other imaging techniques in the assessment of stridor in the pediatric population. MRI can distinguish between various types of congenital vascular anomalies, such as double aortic arch and a right aortic arch with an aberrant left subclavian artery. In cases of pulmonary artery sling, MRI enables a detailed evaluation of the vascular anatomy and may also demonstrate the tracheobronchial anomalies. MRI is very sensitive in demonstrating intrinsic segmental tracheomalacia as well as innominate artery compression of the trachea. Finally, MRI distinguishes between tracheal stenosis and tracheomalacia, and is especially helpful in cases of isolated stenosis. Three-dimensional reconstructions also provide critical information about the relationships between the trachea and adjacent structures. Multiplanar capability helps resolve problem areas for CT, such as the aortopulmonic window, subcarinal region, and lesions at the cervicothoracic or thoracoabdominal junction.

> **PEARL...** MRI is an excellent alternative to angiography when delineation of a vascular abnormality is required.

Other imaging techniques that are less commonly used in the evaluation of the trachea and bronchi include ultrasound and xeroradiography. Ultrasonography has been limited by the two-dimensional quality of the images. Techniques that use multiple contiguous frontal planes in combination with Doppler color flow imaging can successfully delineate vascular anomalies and patent ductus arteriosus.

> **PITFALL...** Advocates of ultrasound point to avoidable complications associated with surgical tracheostomy related to anatomic variations overlying the trachea.

Ultrasound, however, is not commonly utilized for evaluation of the trachea and bronchi. Xeroradiography is a radiologic technique that easily records images in rapid sequence and, due to the phenomenon of edge enhancement, provides excellent visualization of mucous membrane anatomy and abnormalities. Alternative techniques, such as MRI, provide comparable image resolution without the need for ionizing radiation and have limited the recent use of xeroradiography.

New experimental technologies offer the possibility of even greater image resolution of the trachea and bronchi. Current medical imaging technologies offer resolutions ranging from 100 μm to 1 mm. Greater resolution is required to detect early-stage disease, such as premalignant lesions and atherosclerosis. Optical coherence tomography utilizes high-speed visualization of tissue with a specially designed endoscopic catheter. Cross-sectional images on the order of 10 μm may allow this technique to be used as an "optical biopsy."

Magnetic resonance (MR) spectroscopy is a research technique that may soon have clinical application. Similar to optical coherence tomography, MR spectroscopy has the potential for tissue characterization and assessment of disease activity.

NUCLEAR MEDICINE

Nuclear medicine testing is commonly used in the diagnostic evaluation of pulmonary embolic disease and is based on the recognition of unmatched segmental perfusion defects during ventilation-perfusion scanning (VPS).

Approximately 500,000 thromboembolic events occur per year in the United States. The most important risk factors for pulmonary embolism include age, cancer, previous surgery, trauma, coagulation disorders, and immobilization.

> **PITFALL•••** Despite the high mortality of pulmonary embolism, venous thromboembolism is probably underdiagnosed.

Typical symptoms include chest pain, dyspnea, and tachypnea in the absence of preexisting cardiorespiratory disease. The interpretation of defects requires a thorough knowledge of the segmental anatomy of the lungs and are usually classified into small, medium, and large sizes. VPS is most helpful when there is high or low probability of an embolism.

> **PITFALL•••** Unfortunately, 70% of cases are interpreted as indeterminate.

Patients with a low probability scan are at minimal risk for an embolic event, even in the absence of therapeutic anticoagulation. The use of artificial intelligence and computerized image analysis to interpret VPS scans has met with some success.

One source of variability in the accuracy of VPS occurs when estimating the size of a defect. Acceptable sensitivity and specificity have been an elusive goal despite the use of virtual scinti-

graphic lung models and lung segmental reference charts. Although the lung bases are the most common site of embolic disease, the accuracy of lung scans is lowest in these areas. Another disadvantage of ventilation-perfusion testing is contamination of working areas by aerosolized radiopharmaceuticals. Both the patient and the equipment can act as a source of radioactive contamination. There is also considerable variability in the policies and procedures used in the administration and interpretation of VPS.

Color Doppler ultrasound (US) of the lower extremities can be used to complement VPS in the diagnosis of deep vein thrombosis. In fact, Doppler sonography yields the most diagnostic information per dollar spent when compared to other tests for pulmonary embolism.

> **PEARL•••** The combination of clinical assessment, VPS, and color Doppler US lowers by about 20% the number of indeterminate cases.

Patients with undiagnosed cardiorespiratory insufficiency despite VPS and US require pulmonary angiography or spiral CT. Pulmonary arteriography should consist of a biplanar selective pulmonary angiogram with subselective injections as needed. The risks of pulmonary arteriography are less than the consequences of untreated pulmonary embolic disease.

> **CONTROVERSY**
>
> Noninvasive testing, including VPS and Doppler US of the lower extremities, remains the most cost-effective strategy for the evaluation of pulmonary emboli.

At present, effective therapies are available for thromboembolism. Standard heparin and low molecular weight heparin fractions, fibrinolytic agents, surgery, and, recently, caval filters are playing a major role in secondary prophylaxis of pulmonary embolism.

Assessment of increased pulmonary microvascular permeability in patients at risk for acute respiratory distress syndrome (ARDS) is a newer indication for pulmonary nuclear medicine testing.

> **PEARL...** Radiolabeled gallium-transferrin can accurately detect increased permeability and may be an early marker of acute lung injury and progression to ARDS.

Abnormalities in lung ventilation and alveolar permeability can also be determined in chronic renal failure patients on hemodialysis who are at risk for respiratory dysfunction. Bedside nuclear medicine testing, including pulmonary scintigraphy for embolism, can be accomplished with low levels of radiopharmaceuticals with minimal radiation exposure to patients and staff in the intensive care setting.

Nuclear medicine techniques are also helpful in the diagnosis of impaired mucociliary clearance of the tracheobronchial tree. The diagnosis of primary ciliary dyskinesia (PCD) requires the demonstration of either anatomic or physiologic abnormalities within the ciliated cells of the upper respiratory tract.

> **PITFALL...** Endoscopic biopsy of respiratory epithelium and electron microscopic evaluation is invasive, time-consuming, and expensive.

The low incidence of this abnormality, the large number of infants and children with suggestive symptoms, and the lack of a reliable screening test make the decision to perform a diagnostic biopsy a common problem in recurrent or chronic respiratory pediatric conditions. Inhaled radioisotopes can detect altered tracheobronchial sputum production, a technique used to diagnose *Pneumocystis carinii* pneumonia in patients with acquired immune deficiency syndrome (AIDS). Evaluation of nasal mucociliary transport using technetium 99m (Tc-99m)-labeled seroalbumin can demonstrate alterations in transport velocity, particularly in newborns with Kartagener's syndrome. The technique is simple, safe, and well tolerated in this age group and can be used as a screening test for PCD.

Important innovations in pulmonary nuclear medicine have been made in the instrumentation and radiopharmaceuticals used in diagnostic testing. Technegas, a new monodisperse aerosol, provides higher quality images in ventilation studies. Indium 111–diethylenetriamine pentaacetic acid immunoglobulin G (^{111}In-IgG) is a new radiopharmaceutical that has been developed for the detection of infection without the need for in vitro cell labeling. Antifibrin monoclonal antibodies and radioactive peptides specific for activated platelet receptors have been developed for the evaluation of acute thromboembolism. Primary lung cancer and its metastases can now be visualized with tracers used for the study of myocardial perfusion (sestamibi, tetrofosmin) or labeled octreotide, a molecule able to recognize lung tumors with somatostatin receptors. Positron emission tomography (PET) provides information about cellular metabolism and is useful in the assessment of solitary pulmonary nodules. It has applications in the initial staging and response assessment to lung cancer therapy. PET also has potential uses in the study of vascular lung physiology, receptor physiology, and drug transport in the lung. Measurements of regional lung density (LD), extravascular density (EVD), and the pulmonary transcapillary escape rate (PTCER), an index of vascular permeability, may be useful in the assessment of patients with ARDS.

ENDOSCOPY

Endoscopic evaluation remains an integral part of the assessment of abnormalities of the trachea and bronchi.

> **SPECIAL CONSIDERATION**
>
> Rigid endoscopy is the gold standard for assessment of the airway and continues to offer the advantage of maintaining ventilation during general anesthesia.

The development of flexible fiberoptic equipment has expanded the indications for endoscopic evaluation of the large airways and allows improved visualization and documentation of some pathologic conditions. Bronchoscopy is complementary to noninvasive tests such as pulmonary function testing, radiographs, and nuclear medicine scans. The diagnosis of many conditions, ranging from tracheomalacia to neoplasms, often depends on visual inspection and diagnostic biopsy.

Indications for bronchoscopy generally fall into two large groups: 60% of patients have evidence of lower airway disease, and 30% of patients have evidence of upper airway obstruction. In most situations, bronchoscopy will contribute to the diagnosis and alter therapy.

SPECIAL CONSIDERATION

The most common diagnostic indication for bronchoscopy is sampling the lower respiratory tract for suspected or persistent infection. The most common therapeutic indication is removal of retained secretions. The complication rate of bronchoscopy ranges from 0.5 to 3% of cases and mortality is rare.

Complications include transient hypoxia, epistaxis, hemoptysis, and pneumothorax. The incidence of major complications is higher with therapeutic bronchoscopy, particularly when a biopsy is performed, and thoracotomy may be required.

One indication for endoscopic evaluation is bronchoalveolar lavage and biopsy. Tissue sampling can provide information about cell populations and inflammatory mediators involved in the pathogenesis of chronic airway and lung inflammatory disorders, such as chronic obstructive pulmonary disease (COPD) and asthma. Cultures of secretions can help guide antibiotic therapy in both community- and hospital-acquired pneumonia. Transbronchial lung biopsies are useful to establish the etiology of pulmonary pathology, including lung infiltrates, peripheral lung lesions, and hilar adenopathy. It

can be performed in the intensive care unit on critically ill patients to diagnose opportunistic infection or localize and tamponade the site of pulmonary hemorrhage.

PEARL••• In patients with hemoptysis and a normal chest roentgenogram, male sex, age more than 40 years, and greater than 40-packs-a-year smoking history, there is an increased likelihood that bronchoscopy will establish the diagnosis.

There is a direct correlation between the number of samples obtained at bronchoscopy and the diagnostic yield.

Other bronchoscopic interventions include carbon dioxide and neodymium:yttrium-aluminum-garnet (Nd-YAG) laser photoresection, balloon dilatation, stent placement, and brachytherapy for areas of benign or malignant obstruction. Both rigid and flexible endoscopic treatment of malignant central airway obstructions can be accomplished with minimal morbidity and mortality. Cryotherapy may be useful before some laser resections to minimize bleeding. Flexible bronchoscopy can be used to place self-expandable metallic stents to maintain airway patency and give immediate symptomatic relief. Endobronchial high-dose rate (HDR) brachytherapy can deliver high levels of radiation to treat malignancies of the trachea and bronchi. These treatments, which are often palliative, can be combined to provide symptomatic improvement in patients with advanced airway malignancies.

Flexible fiberoptic bronchoscopy can now be performed in children using topical anesthesia and light sedation and, in many institutions, has replaced rigid bronchoscopy for diagnostic purposes. Even preterm neonates and intubated infants can undergo successful endoscopy with the new generation of miniature bronchoscopes.

Common findings include bronchopneumonia, intubation trauma, tracheomalacia, laryngomalacia, foreign body aspiration, obstructing tracheal or bronchial granulation or stricture, mucous plug, tracheobronchitis, tracheoesophageal H-fistula, laryngeal perforation, laryngeal steno-

SPECIAL CONSIDERATION

Indications for bronchoscopy include noisy breathing, recurrent pneumonia, suspected pneumonia, atelectasis, possible foreign body aspiration, stridor or weak cry, and persistent wheezing or cough unresponsive to medical therapy.

sis, and laryngotracheoesophageal cleft. Microlaryngoscopy and bronchoscopy are highly sensitive in the diagnosis of vascular compression of the airway when compared to MRI, barium esophagram, and aortogram.

Probably the clearest indication for bronchoscopy is in the diagnosis and treatment of airway foreign bodies. If there is clinical evidence of foreign body aspiration from physical and radiographic findings, such as radiopaque foreign body on chest X-ray, unilateral decreased breath sounds, or obstructive emphysema, rigid bronchoscopy should be performed. Other patients suspected of foreign body aspiration can undergo diagnostic flexible bronchoscopy. If a foreign body is found, rigid bronchoscopy should be performed for extraction.

PEARL... One of the most important factors in the diagnosis of airway foreign bodies is a high index of suspicion by the clinician.

Finally, bronchoscopy can be used to assess and manage a compromised or tenuous airway, particularly in patients in whom oral intubation may be difficult. Patients can be successfully intubated and indwelling endotracheal tubes changed over a flexible bronchoscope. Double-lumen endotracheal tubes are used frequently in intensive care units to maintain independent lung ventilation, in the face of bronchopleural fistula, massive hemoptysis, and other asymmetrical pulmonary disorders. In addition, double-lumen tubes are very useful during thoracic surgical procedures when ventilation to one lung may be interrupted. Fiberoptic bronchoscopy is the most efficient and reliable method to position a double-lumen tube when the anatomy is distorted.

SUGGESTED READINGS

Bisset GS 3d, Strife JL, Kirks DR, Bailey WW. Vascular rings: MR imaging. *AJR* 1987;149(2): 251–256.

Dellinger RP, Bandi V. Fiberoptic bronchoscopy in the intensive care unit. *Crit Care Clin* 1992; 8(4):755–772.

Erwin EA, Gerber ME, Cotton RT. Vascular compression of the airway: indications for and results of surgical management. *Int J Pediatr Otorhinolaryngol* 1997;40(2–3):155–162.

Esclamado RM, Richardson MA. Laryngotracheal foreign bodies in children. A comparison with bronchial foreign bodies. *Am J Dis Child* 1987;141(3):259–262.

Fitzgerald DJ, Speir WA, Callahan LA. Office evaluation of pulmonary function: beyond the numbers. *Am Fam Physician* 1996;54(2): 525–534.

Galli G, Giordano A. The role of nuclear medicine in pulmonary embolism. *Rays* 1996;21 (3):363–377.

Godfrey S, Avital A, Maayan C, Rotschild M, Springer C. Yield from flexible bronchoscopy in children. *Pediatr Pulmonol* 1997;23(4):261–269.

Groeneveld AB, Raijmakers PG. The 67 gallium-transferrin pulmonary leak index in patients at risk for the acute respiratory distress syndrome. *Crit Care Med* 1998;26(4):685–691.

Henschke CI, Yankelevitz DF, Mateescu I, Whalen JP. Evaluation of competing tests for the diagnosis of pulmonary embolism and deep vein thrombosis, part 1. *Clin Imaging* 1994;18(4):241–247.

Hermans R, Verschakelen JA, Baert AL. Imaging of laryngeal and tracheal stenosis. *Acta Otorhinolaryngol Belg* 1995;49(4):323–329.

Hoeve LJ, Rombout J. Pediatric laryngobronchoscopy. 1332 procedures stored in a data base. *Int J Pediatr Otorhinolaryngol* 1992;24(1): 73–82.

Holbert JM, Strollo DC. Imaging of the normal trachea. *J Thorac Imaging* 1995;10(3):171–179.

Leigh TR, Jones BE, Ryan P, Collins JV. The use of inhaled radioisotopes for measuring the effect of sputum induction on tracheobronchial clearance rates. *Nucl Med Commun* 1994;15(3):156–160.

LoCicero J 3rd, Costello P, Campos CT, et al. Spiral CT with multiplanar and three-dimensional reconstructions accurately predicts tracheobronchial pathology. *Ann Thorac Surg* 1996;62(3):811–817.

Macha HN, Wahlers B, Reichle C, von Zwehl D. Endobronchial radiation therapy for obstructing malignancies: ten years' experience with iridium-192 high-dose radiation brachytherapy afterloading technique in 365 patients. *Lung* 1995;173(5):271–280.

Magnussen JS, Chicco P, Palmer AW, et al. Variability of perceived defect size in virtual lung scintigraphy. *J Nucl Med* 1998;39(2):361–365.

Martinot A, Closset M, Marquette CH, et al. Indications for flexible versus rigid bronchoscopy in children with suspected foreign-body aspiration. *Am J Respir Crit Care Med* 1997; 155(5):1676–1679.

Murdison KA, Andrews BA, Chin AJ. Ultrasonographic display of complex vascular rings. *J Am Coll Cardiol* 1990;15(7):1645–1653.

Nussbaum E. Usefulness of miniature flexible fiberoptic bronchoscopy in children. *Chest* 1994;106(5):1438–1442.

Pasterkamp H, Sanchez I. Tracheal sounds in upper airway obstruction. *Chest* 1992;102(3): 963–965.

Pasterkamp H, Schafer J, Wodicka GR. Posture-dependent change of tracheal sounds at standardized flows in patients with obstructive sleep apnea. *Chest* 1996;110(6):1493–1498.

Perkins AC, Yeoman P, Hindle AJ, et al. Bedside nuclear medicine investigations in the intensive care unit. *Nucl Med Commun* 1997;18(3): 262–268.

Pue CA, Pacht ER. Complications of fiberoptic bronchoscopy at a university hospital. *Chest* 1995;107(2):430–432.

Rietveld S, Rijssenbeek-Nouwens LH. Diagnostics of spontaneous cough in childhood asthma: results of continuous tracheal sound recording in the homes of children. *Chest* 1998;113(1):50–54.

Salvatori M. Advances in pulmonary nuclear medicine. *Rays* 1997;22(1):51–72.

Simoneaux SF, Bank ER, Webber JB, Parks WJ. MR imaging of the pediatric airway. *Radiographics* 1995;15(2):287–298.

Slinger PD. Fiberoptic bronchoscopic positioning of double-lumen tubes. *J Cardiothorac Anesth* 1989;3(4):486–496.

Tearney GJ, Brezinski ME, Bouma BE, et al. In vivo endoscopic optical biopsy with optical coherence tomography. *Science* 1997;276 (5321):2037–2039.

Tello R, Kruskal J, Dupuy D, Costello P. In vivo three-dimensional evaluation of the tracheobronchial tree. *J Thorac Imaging* 1995;10(4): 291–293.

Wahr JA, Tremper KK. Noninvasive oxygen monitoring techniques. *Crit Care Clin* 1995; 11(1):199–217.

Weiss K. Pulmonary thromboembolism: epidemiology and techniques of nuclear medicine. *Semin Thromb Hemost* 1996;22(1):27–32.

Wiseman NE, Sanchez I, Powell RE. Rigid bronchoscopy in the pediatric age group: diagnostic effectiveness. *J Pediatr Surg* 1992;27 (10):1294–1297.

Chapter 42

CONGENITAL DISORDERS

Mark E. Gerber, Daniel J. Kelley, and Charles M. Myer III

Congenital abnormalities of the tracheobronchial tree can result in life-threatening airway obstruction at birth or can be more subtle, presenting with expiratory wheezing or atelectasis. This chapter reviews some of the more common congenital anomalies that affect the tracheobronchial tree, including primary and secondary tracheomalacia, tracheal stenosis, and tracheal atresia.

TRACHEOMALACIA

Primary and secondary tracheomalacia together account for nearly half of all congenital tracheal anomalies (see also Chap. 43). In primary tracheomalacia, the anatomic abnormality is intrinsic to the trachea, without other contributing factors. The normal cartilaginous trachea to membranous trachea ratio is approximately 4.5:1. In primary tracheomalacia, there is an elongation of the membranous trachea, decreasing that ratio to approximately 2:1 or 3:1. Secondary tracheomalacia may have the same abnormal ratio, but in addition there are other factors contributing to the tracheobronchial distortion, such as a tracheoesophageal fistula or vascular compression.

Symptoms of tracheomalacia may include expiratory stridor, a brassy cough, recurrent lower respiratory infections, and reflex apnea. The severity of symptoms depends on the degree of collapse and length of involved trachea, as well as if there are other contributing factors (secondary tracheomalacia).

The diagnosis of tracheomalacia can be suggested initially by a narrowing of the trachea on a lateral chest radiograph taken in expiration. Further confirmation can be obtained with airway fluoroscopy. When performing bronchoscopy, maintenance of spontaneous respiration is necessary to visualize the length of the involved segment and the severity of malacia. This can be accomplished by examination with either a flexible or rigid endoscope.

> **PITFALL•••** Clinically significant pathology can be missed if endoscopy is performed without spontaneous ventilation.

Rarely is surgical intervention needed in the treatment of primary tracheomalacia. When necessary, intrinsic support of the tracheal walls can be obtained with a tracheotomy. Positive pressure ventilation can be added if necessary, when severe tracheomalacia extends to the carina and into the bronchial tree.

TRACHEOBRONCHIAL VASCULAR COMPRESSION

Vascular compression of the tracheobronchial tree has an overall incidence of 3%. The most common symptomatic true vascular ring is the double aortic arch, which occurs if the fourth branchial arches and the dorsal aortic root persist on both sides. In 1 in 2,500 persons, the left arch has an atretic segment, but the right arch persists. A right-sided arch with a descending right aorta does not cause airway compromise. However, if there is an associated left ductus or an aberrant left subclavian artery, a loose vascular ring is formed that generally results in less airway compromise than a true double aortic arch.

The pulmonary artery sling is the most symptomatic of the noncircumferential vascular anomalies and occurs when the left sixth arch resorbs and the left pulmonary artery arises as a large collateral artery from the right pulmonary artery, and passes between the esophagus and trachea to perfuse the left lung. This anomaly commonly results in significant compromise of the right mainstem bronchus and airway symptoms. In addition, 30% of patients with pulmonary artery slings have associated complete tracheal rings.

The aberrant right subclavian artery is the most common mediastinal vascular anomaly. However, because of its retroesophageal course, affected individuals may present with dysphagia but rarely with symptomatic airway compromise.

Innominate artery compression of the trachea is not actually a true vascular anomaly. The innominate artery normally passes from its origin on the aortic arch left of the midline, across the anterior trachea to the right side. However, occasionally the artery will cause significant compression of the right anterolateral trachea as it crosses the midline.

There are three possible explanations for why these patients are symptomatic from innominate artery compression of the trachea: (1) the innominate artery is more taut than normal; (2) the tracheal cartilages are unusually compliant and more easily compressed; or (3) dilatation of other structures such as the heart, esophagus, or thymus cause mediastinal crowding.

Respiratory compromise from tracheobronchial vascular compression is potentially life threatening, but can present with subtle symptoms. Frequently, a high index of suspicion is required to make the diagnosis. Patients with significant vascular compression usually present early, with stridor, chronic cough, recurrent bronchitis and pneumonia, difficulty feeding and failure to thrive, and occasionally reflex apnea.

Chest radiographs may provide some evidence of tracheal compression, and a barium esophagram can show relatively characteristic filling defects that correspond to the various types of vascular compression. However, once vascular compression is suspected, the diagnostic modality of choice is magnetic resonance imaging, which will clearly demonstrate the mediastinal vascular anatomy as well as the size of the lower airway. Although today the diagnosis of vascular compression is usually known prior to undergoing endoscopy, bronchoscopy also reveals characteristic findings of compression depending on the type of vascular ring or sling. It provides an immediate visual assessment of the surgical results on relieving the compression and the degree of residual tracheomalacia present.

Nonsurgical management may be effective for the majority of innominate artery compression and loose vascular rings and slings that are mildly symptomatic. In contrast, moderately to severely symptomatic patients usually require surgical repair. Absolute indications for surgical treatment include reflex apnea, failure of medical management of severe respiratory distress after 48 hours, and prolonged intubation. Relative criteria include repeated episodes of lower respiratory tract infections, exercise intolerance, significant dysphagia with failure to thrive, and coexisting subglottic stenosis, asthma, cystic fibrosis or previous tracheoesophageal repair.

Innominate artery compression is relieved by aortopexy or reimplantation, with success rates of 93% to 100% and no reports of operative mortality or long-term morbidity.

> **PITFALL...** Occasionally, aortopexy sutures can loosen and the procedure needs to be repeated.

Results of surgical treatment of vascular rings are also encouraging, with 70% to 92% obtaining complete resolution of symptoms. Double aortic arch requires surgical division of the smaller of the two arches. The ductus arteriosus or aberrant subclavian artery is divided in the case of right aortic arch with left ductus arteriosus or aberrant left subclavian artery. In cases of severe tracheobronchial compression, residual tracheomalacia may persist for a variable period of time, and occasionally a tracheotomy is required to stent the malacic segment. The pulmonary artery sling is corrected by dividing the aberrant left pulmonary artery at its origin and reimplanting it anterior to the trachea. There is a significantly increased morbidity and mortality rate in these cases, usually due to the associated complete tracheal rings.

CONGENITAL TRACHEAL STENOSIS

Congenital tracheal stenosis is a rare, potentially life-threatening anomaly that usually involves complete cartilaginous tracheal rings and over the years has proven to be difficult to treat. Cantrell and Guild in 1964 classified congenital tracheal stenosis into three categories: long segment stenosis with generalized hypoplasia (22%), funnel-like stenosis (37%), and segmental stenosis (41%). Associated anomalies in children with congenital tracheal stenosis are common, with 24% having coexistent vascular anomalies, most commonly pulmonary artery sling.

Congenital tracheal stenosis can present with a history of biphasic stridor and possibly acute respiratory distress.

> **PITFALL...** Symptoms such as persistent wheezing, atypical croup, chronic cough, and bronchiolitis can be more subtle, resulting in a delay in the diagnosis.

Definitive diagnosis is often first obtained with endoscopy. However, even by an experienced surgeon and expert anesthesia, endoscopy is potentially dangerous. Minimal edema in an already critically small lumen can become impassable by a ventilating tracheoscope or endotracheal tube. When the condition is suggested by finding segmental or diffuse narrowing on plain radiographs, magnetic resonance imaging or computed tomography can delineate the nature and extent of the narrowing, as well as facilitate the identification of possible associated anomalies.

Over recent years, tremendous progress has been made in the treatment of congenital tracheal stenosis. Segmental resection and primary anastomosis have been shown to be the treatment of choice for stenosis involving up to 50% of the trachea. However, a large number of procedures have been advocated in long-segment stenosis because none has proven to be universally successful. In fact Benjamin et al in 1981 recommended a nonsurgical approach because the 57% survival in this group of patients was higher than in the operated group. Anterior tracheoplasty using pericardium was first described by Idriss et al in 1984. Since then, reported results of this technique reveal survival rates of 47 to 76% in the larger series. Costal cartilage grafting for augmentation has had similar results in a smaller number of patients. Other augmentation materials that have been tried include esophageal wall, rib, dura, and periosteum. Slide tracheoplasty involves a transverse division of the trachea in the middle of the stenosis, longitudinal incisions of the anterior portion on one end and the posterior portion on the other, then sliding the two ends over each other, halving the length and doubling the diameter, with successful results reported so far in three of four cases. More recently, tracheal homograft reconstruction was described for use in cases of severe long-segment and recurrent stenosis with a survival rate of 83%.

TRACHEAL ATRESIA

Congenital tracheal agenesis is a rare anomaly that in general is incompatible with life. In this condition, the esophagus communicates with either the mid-trachea or distal trachea, or to the mainstem bronchi directly. The neonate with this condition presents at birth with immediate respiratory distress. Laryngeal anomalies are frequently present, and attempts at laryngeal intubation will not be successful. Esophageal intubation with decompression of the stomach with a nasogastric tube will provide some degree of airway control; however, long-term successful management has not been described.

SUGGESTED READINGS

Adler SC, Isaacson G, Balsara RK. Innominate artery compression of the trachea: diagnosis and treatment by anterior suspension. A 25-year experience. *Ann Otol Rhino Laryngol* 1995;104(12):924–927.

Backer CL. Vascular rings, slings, and tracheal rings. *Mayo Clin Proc* 1993;68:1131–1133.

Backer CL, Ilbawi MN, Idriss FS, et al. Vascular anomalies causing tracheoesophageal com-

pression. *J Thorac Cardiovasc Surg* 1989;97: 725–731.

Benjamin B, Pitkin J, Cohen D. Congenital tracheal stenosis. *Ann Otol Rhinol Laryngol* 1981; 90(4 pt 1):364–371.

Blumer JR, Bauman NM, Kearns DP, et al. Distal tracheal stenosis in neonates and infants. *Otolaryngol Head Neck Surg* 1992;107(4):583–590.

Cantrell JR, Guild HG. Congenital stenosis of the trachea. *Am J Surg* 1964;108:297–305.

Dunham ME, Holinger LD, Backer CL, et al. Management of severe congenital tracheal stenosis. *Ann Otol Rhinol Laryngol* 1994;103(5 pt 1):351–356.

Grillo HC, Mathisen DJ. Surgical management of tracheal strictures. *Surg Clin North Am* 1988;68:511–524.

Holinger LD, Green CG, Benjamin B, et al. Tracheobronchial tree. In: Holinger LD, Lusk RP, Green CG, eds. *Pediatric Laryngology and Bronchoesophagology.* Philadelphia: Lippincott-Raven; 1997:187–213.

Idriss FS, DeLeon SY, Ilbawi MN, et al. Tracheoplasty with pericardial patch for extensive tracheal stenosis in infants and children. *J Thorac Cardiovasc Surg* 1984;88(4):527–536.

Jacobs JP, Elliott MJ, Haw MP, et al. Pediatric tracheal homograft reconstruction: a novel approach to complex tracheal stenoses in children. *J Thorac Cardiovasc Surg* 1996;112(6): 1549–1558; discussion 1559–1560.

Jacobs JP, Haw MP, Motbey JA, et al. Successful complete tracheal resection in a three-month-old infant. *Ann Thorac Surg* 1996; 61(6):1824–1826; discussion 1827.

Lierl M. Congenital abnormalities. In: Hilman B, ed. *Pediatric Respiratory Disease: Diagnosis and Treatment.* Philadelphia: WB Saunders; 1993:477–487.

Tsang V, Murday A, Gillbe C, et al. Slide tracheoplasty for congenital funnel-shaped tracheal stenosis. *Ann Thorac Surg* 1989;48(5): 632–635.

Weber TR, Eigen H, Scott PH, et al. Resection of congenital tracheal stenosis involving the carina. *J Thorac Cardiovasc Surg* 1982;84(2): 200–203.

Chapter 43

FUNCTIONAL DISORDERS

David L. Walner and Charles M. Myer III

Functional disorders of the tracheobronchial tree can create serious respiratory difficulties in both infants and children.

TRACHEOMALACIA

Tracheomalacia refers to tracheal collapse on expiration, causing expiratory stridor. It may occur concomitantly with or independently of laryngomalacia. The condition generally presents with a history of audible expiratory stridor that is sometimes high-pitched and reminiscent of asthmatic wheezing.

> **PITFALL•••** These patients may be misdiagnosed as having asthma or reactive lower airway disease.

Oftentimes, a harsh, barking cough, recurrent infections, and, possibly, a history of reflex apnea can be present.

Tracheomalacia may be classified as primary or secondary. The former results from tracheal rings that are abnormal in shape and consistency. The latter is due to some form of external compression.

PRIMARY TRACHEOMALACIA

In primary tracheomalacia, the mobility of the trachea and bronchi with respiration is markedly exaggerated so that the posterior membranous wall of the tracheobronchial tree can nearly approximate the anterior cartilaginous tracheal wall with forced expiration. This condition is generally worsened with crying, coughing, or activity. The onset may be at birth, but the stridor and respiratory distress often become more obvious as the child becomes more active. In the majority of cases, no treatment is needed and the condition improves gradually with growth of the tracheobronchial tree and disappears by 18 to 24 months of age.

> **PEARL•••** Mucolytic agents can often help to thin secretions in these children and humidity is very helpful, especially during the winter months.

Continuous positive airway pressure has been utilized in some infants with fairly good success. For the most severe cases, a tracheotomy may be necessary until the child has established more rigidity of the tracheobronchial tree.

Recently, an expandable metallic angioplasty stent (Palmaz) has been utilized and placed within the trachea and/or bronchi.

CONTROVERSY

The long-term effects of stenting and airway growth are a concern. Problems with granulation tissue formation and difficulty removing or expanding the stent must be given consideration prior to its use. Continued experimentation with these stents as well as the development of new materials may make these stents more attractive for use in the future.

SECONDARY TRACHEOMALACIA

External compression of the trachea can be due to vascular or cardiac causes. Innominate artery compression of the trachea can cause children to demonstrate expiratory and, sometimes, biphasic wheezing, or stridor, with a croupy, barking cough and reflex apnea. Endoscopy will confirm the diagnosis with compression of the right anterolateral wall of the upper trachea.

PEARL••• Placing the pulse oximeter on the right hand and using the tip of the bronchoscope to gently compress this pulsatile artery will diminish the right brachial pulse.

The majority of the time, conservative observation can be utilized in treating these children. When symptoms are severe, surgical intervention in the form of innominate artery suspension or reimplantation can be utilized.

Another vascular anomaly that can cause compression is the double aortic arch. This condition implies that a complete ring that encircles the trachea and esophagus is present and compresses both structures. The most common type of ring anomaly is one in which the ascending aorta bifurcates to encircle both the trachea and esophagus and then joins the descending aorta. In the majority of these patients, the right side of the arch is dominant. These children generally are symptomatic at birth or within the first few months of life. Biphasic stridor as well as feeding problems and recurrent respiratory tract infections can occur. Endoscopic findings generally include lateral compression of the tracheal walls. However, a barium esophogram and/or magnetic resonance imaging (MRI) of the chest will confirm the diagnosis. Treatment usually consists of surgical division of the complete vascular ring.

The pulmonary artery sling can cause similar symptoms to those described previously with a double aortic arch. In this anomaly the normal left pulmonary artery is absent and the aberrant vessel arises from the right pulmonary artery. This vessel then encircles the right bronchus and passes between the trachea and esophagus. Endoscopy in these cases generally shows compression of the right mainstem bronchus. A barium esophogram and/or MRI can confirm the diagnosis. Treatment involves division and reimplantation of the pulmonary artery.

TABLE 43-1 CLASSIFICATION OF TRACHEOMALACIA AND BRONCHOMALACIA

I. Primary
   A. In preterm infants
   B. In term infants
II. Secondary
   A. External compression
      1. Vascular
         a. Innominate artery compression
         b. Double aortic arch and right aortic arch
         c. Pulmonary artery sling
         d. Aberrant right subclavian artery
      2. Cardiac: enlarged left atrium or pulmonary vessels
      3. Congenital cyst
      4. Neoplasm
      5. Abscess
   B. Tracheoesophageal fistula and esophageal atresia
   C. Dyschondroplasia

Adapted from Holinger LD, Lusk RP, Green CG. *Pediatric Laryngology and Bronchoesophagology.* Philadelphia: Lippincott-Raven; 1997. Reprinted by permission of Lippincott Williams & Wilkins, Philadelphia, PA.

An aberrant right subclavian artery is another condition that can cause compression of the trachea and bronchus. This condition similarly requires diagnosis with a barium esophogram and/or MRI.

Cardiac enlargement generally at the left atrium can cause compressive symptoms in the left mainstem bronchus. These conditions need close evaluation by the cardiothoracic surgeon. Other causes of secondary tracheomalacia are listed in Table 43–1.

TRACHEOESOPHAGEAL FISTULA

Congenital tracheoesophageal fistula (TEF) presents immediately after birth with respiratory difficulty, feeding problems, excessive mucus, and persistent aspiration. It is estimated to occur in approximately 1 in 3000 to 5000 live births. Commonly, a maternal history of polyhydramnios has been present.

PEARL... Due to the excessive mucosa that is present in the posterior aspect of the airway, tracheomalacia is commonly seen in these children, both before and following repair.

The characteristic collapse, weakness, and instability of the tracheal wall leads to the findings of a widened semicircular-shaped cartilage with ballooning of the posterior membranous wall and collapse or partial loss of the tracheal lumen. These children can generally be managed conservatively and rarely go on to require a tracheotomy.

SPECIAL CONSIDERATION

Associated congenital anomalies of other organ systems are present in approximately 50% of these children, and a thorough evaluation of the cardiovascular system, gastrointestinal system, and genito/urinary tract should be performed.

SPECIAL CONSIDERATION

The most common type of TEF involves proximal esophageal atresia with the distal esophagus communicating with the trachea (86%).

A more frequently talked about but less commonly occurring form is the H-variety in which a small communication exists between the upper trachea and the upper third of the esophagus. Management of this condition is with surgical correction, and there is a greater than 90% survival rate (see also Chap. 50).

BRONCHIAL DISORDERS

BRONCHOMALACIA

Bronchomalacia may be unilateral, bilateral, and, in some children, associated with tracheomalacia. On inspiration the lumen is of normal caliber, but on expiration there is marked diminution of lumen size. This generally results in an expiratory wheeze, and symptoms become worse when secretions are increased or thickened due to respiratory infections. The wall rigidity may be abnormal due to intrinsically weak or malformed bronchial wall cartilages. These children are often intubated due to ventilator dependence with the need of high airway pressures. Endoscopy can generally confirm this disorder.

SPECIAL CONSIDERATION

Tracheostomy allows these children to be free of sedation and intensive care unit needs.

Many of these children have associated reactive airway disease. The natural history of primary bronchomalacia is that of gradual improvement. With time even more severely affected patients do not appear to have abnormal exercise tolerance.

BRONCHIECTASIS

This condition occurs due to progressive bronchial dilation with damage and weakening of the bronchial walls. It is seen in children with cystic fibrosis, immunoglobulin deficiencies, foreign body aspiration, and hamartomatous malformations, as well as in children with bronchomalacia. Treatment involves medical control of any infection that is present as well as reducing the viscosity of secretions, improving clearance of secretions by postural drainage, physiotherapy, and, occasionally, surgical removal of diseased areas.

KARTAGENER'S SYNDROME

Kartagener's syndrome is an autosomal-recessive trait that involves bronchiectasis, situs inversus, sinusitis, and absent frontal sinuses. This syndrome is a subgroup within the condition of immotile cilia syndrome. The ciliary motility is abnormal due to defects in ciliary microtubules. Treatment is generally the same as that for bronchiectasis.

ATELECTASIS

Atelectasis is the collapse of one or more segments or lobes of the lung. There is imperfect expansion of the lung segments. The condition may be due to extrinsic compression or intrinsic occlusion of a bronchial lumen. Emphysema can then result from partial bronchial obstruction that allows air to enter but impedes the egress of air on expiration. Treatment of atelectasis is directed toward correction of the underlying disease. If pulmonary infection is present, this should be treated appropriately.

> **PEARL...** Chest physiotherapy and postural drainage will aid in clearing the mucus from obstructed bronchioles. Bronchoscopy and removal of mucus plugs is indicated if atelectasis impedes the child's recovery or persists after clearing of an infection.

SUGGESTED READINGS

Benjamin B. Tracheomalacia in infants and children. *Ann Otol Rhinol Laryngol* 1984;93:438.

Ein SH, Friedberg J. Esophageal atresia and esophageal fistula. *Otolaryngol Clin North Am* 1989;14:219–249.

Filler RM, Forte V, Fraga JC, Matute J. The use of expandable metallic airway stents for tracheobronchial obstruction in children. *J Pediatr Surg* 1995;30:1050–1055.

Finder JD. Primary bronchomalacia in infants and children. *J Pediatr* 1997;130:59–66.

Holinger LD, Green CG, Benjamin B, Sharp JK. Tracheal bronchial tree. In: Hollinger LD, Lusk RP, Green CG, eds. *Pediatric Laryngology and Bronchoesophogology*. Philadelphia: Lippincott-Raven, 1997:187–213.

Schild JA. Congenital malformations of the trachea and bronchi. In: Bluestone CD, Stewell SE, Kenna MA, eds. *Pediatric Otolaryngology*. 3rd ed. Philadelphia: WB Saunders; 1996: 1307–1328.

Chapter 44

INFECTIOUS AND INFLAMMATORY DISORDERS

Yoram Stern and Charles M. Myer III

Infections of the respiratory tract are very common and still constitute a major cause of morbidity and mortality, especially in the pediatric age group. This chapter provides an overview of the more common tracheobronchial infections and discusses etiology, clinical features, diagnosis, and management.

LARYNGOTRACHEOBRONCHITIS

Laryngotracheobronchitis, or croup, almost always has a viral cause, most commonly parainfluenza types I and II. Other possible pathogens include influenza virus and respiratory syncytial virus (RSV).

Croup usually occurs in the fall and early winter. Although it may occur in all pediatric age groups, it is most common before 3 years of age with peaks in the first and second year. The patient usually has a low-grade fever, rhinorrhea, and a characteristic barky cough. Other common symptoms are hoarseness and variable degrees of inspiratory stridor. Retractions, tachypnea, restlessness, and tachycardia are signs of significant airway obstruction and hypoxia.

> **PEARL...** The history and physical examination are the most important part of the evaluation.

Anteroposterior and lateral neck films are helpful in differentiating croup from other forms of obstruction. The anteroposterior view may demonstrate a nonspecific "pencil" or "steeple" sign in the subglottic region (Fig. 44–1). Flexible nasopharyngoscopy is helpful in making a positive diagnosis of subglottic edema and excluding other obstructive problems. Treatment is usually supportive, as the majority of children need no specific therapy and can be managed as outpatients.

> **SPECIAL CONSIDERATION**
>
> Children with signs of significant airway obstruction require hospital admission for careful observation in an environment in which skilled airway intervention is immediately available.

The short-term efficacy of racemic epinephrine is generally accepted. A single dose of steroids (dexamethasone sodium phosphate 0.6 mg/kg up to 20 mg) may be efficacious if given within 12 to 24 hours.

The final therapy in patients who progress to respiratory failure is intubation. The need for intubation should be judged on clinical grounds only.

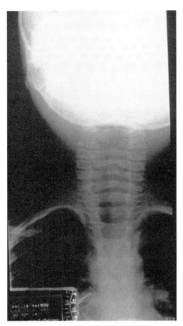

FIGURE 44–1 Laryngotracheobronchitis—edema of the subglottis.

CONTROVERSY

Because the course of the illness is likely to be short and the need for airway intervention is rare, it has been difficult to determine the role of steroids in the management of croup.

PITFALL••• Airway intervention should be performed before the child becomes significantly hypoxic or has a respiratory arrest.

Intubation should be performed in a controlled fashion by an experienced practitioner who is skilled in that technique. The size of the endotracheal tube should be chosen carefully, and the tube should be checked periodically for leaks. Administration of steroids may shorten the duration of intubation and decrease the incidence of reintubation. Usually the duration of intubation is short unless the course is complicated or the child has underlying laryngo-

tracheal stenosis. In such cases, a tracheotomy may be necessary to prevent long-term laryngeal damage.

SPECIAL CONSIDERATION

In children with recurrent croup, direct laryngoscopy and bronchoscopy are indicated to rule out anatomic problems.

BACTERIAL TRACHEITIS

Bacterial tracheitis (membranous or pseudomembranous croup, membranous tracheitis) is caused by a bacterial infection of the upper airway resulting in profuse production of mucopurulent secretions. The bacteria associated with this infection are varied, but *Staphylococcus aureus* is by far the most frequent. Other common bacterial agents include *Moraxella catarrhalis, Streptococcus pneumoniae,* and *Haemophilus influenzae.*

PEARL••• Bacterial tracheitis frequently may develop following viral infection such as croup. It was also reported to develop during an outbreak of parainfluenzae and influenza virus infections.

The age range when this disease presents is broad and generally older than with croup. The symptoms of bacterial tracheitis include croup-like stridor and barking cough. The children usually appear more toxic and often have a higher fever. However, symptoms depend on the stage of the disease and the extent of airway obstruction and may vary from mild symptoms to very severe obstruction. Evaluation should include upper airway lateral and posteroanterior radiographs, looking for irregular tracheal densities (Fig. 44–2).

Flexible nasopharyngoscopy may reveal thick secretions below the level of the cords. The white blood cell count is usually elevated and shows a left shift. The first concern must be the patient's airway. In patients with severe ob-

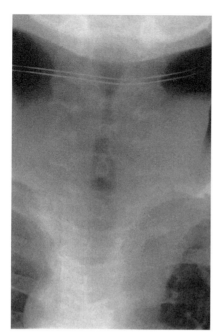

FIGURE 44–2 Bacterial tracheitis—irregular tracheal densities.

structive symptoms, laryngoscopy and bronchoscopy should be performed as soon as possible. The procedure is both diagnostic and therapeutic. The tracheal membranes and crusts are removed and sent for culture. If the patient has a large amount of thick secretions and especially if the subglottis is edematous, the airway should be secured by an endotracheal tube, allowing deep suctioning as needed. Antibiotic therapy should be broad-spectrum and effective against *S. aureus.* More specific therapy can be guided by the results of the tracheal culture. The leak around the endotracheal tube should be checked periodically and together with the clinical course should determine the time of extubation. If not intubated, the patient should be observed in the intensive care unit for 24 to 48 hours.

DIPHTHERIA

The causal agent for this disease is *Corynebacterium diphtheriae,* a gram-positive, club-shaped non–acid-fast aerobic bacterium. This bacterium produces exotoxin, which causes the systemic

manifestations. The disease is characterized by a gray pseudomembrane that may be visible in the nose or over the tonsils, soft palate, larynx, or tracheobronchial tree. Removal of this pseudomembrane usually results in bleeding.

> **PITFALL...** Another process that may produce a pseudomembrane and mimic diphtheria is infectious mononucleosis. Atypical lymphocytes in the peripheral blood and a positive heterophil test differentiate it from diphtheria.

Fever is low grade, and malaise, headaches, vomiting, and nausea are common. Systemic symptoms relating to involvement of the heart, liver, kidney, and brain occur 10 to 14 days after the onset of the disease. The diagnosis should be based initially on the physical findings. These can be confirmed by specific bacterial smears and cultures.

The treatment for airway obstruction is by tracheostomy or endotracheal intubation and systemic antibiotics. Procaine penicillin and erythromycin are the agents of choice.

> ## SPECIAL CONSIDERATION
>
> Supportive and antimicrobial care should be instituted once the diagnosis is suspected on the basis of the physical findings and should not be delayed by the results of specific smears or cultures.

The prevention of diphtheria is accomplished best by immunization. If there is any question about the presence of immunity, a Schick test should be administered. Little or no reaction indicates that immunity exists.

> **PEARL...** The presence of immunity is a negative result on the Schick test, whereas a positive test indicates the absence of immunity.

PERTUSSIS

Pertussis or whooping cough is caused by the gram-negative coccobacillus *Bordetella pertussis.* Most patients affected by the disease are in the pediatric age group.

SPECIAL CONSIDERATION

The incidence of pertussis has been increasing and it is becoming more common in adults. Adult pertussis occurs despite a prior history of immunization and in individuals with a prior history of having had the disease.

The disease usually occurs in three phases: catarrhal, paroxysmal, and convalescent. After an incubation period of 2 weeks, a patient develops symptoms of upper respiratory tract infection and low-grade fever. This stage progresses to a paroxysmal stage, in which the cough becomes more frequent and prolonged. The paroxysms of coughing can be associated with cyanosis or vomiting or both. The paroxysmal stage is usually followed by a prolonged convalescent stage.

PITFALL••• In neonates paroxysmal cough is not noted and they may present with only choking and apneic spells.

The diagnosis is ultimately made by clinical history and nasopharyngeal culture.

PITFALL••• The culture of Bordetella pertussis may be positive only if taken early in the course of disease.

The blood count usually reveals significant leukocytosis although this may be absent in young infants.

The best way to manage this disease is through immunization.

PITFALL••• Unlike the natural disease, which generally confers lifelong immunity, the pertussis vaccine provides a high degree of protection for only 3 years, after which resistance to infection gradually decreases over the next 10 to 15 years.

CONTROVERSY

Because of the associated morbidity of the vaccine, questions have been raised about the risk-to-benefit ratio.

Antibiotic treatment includes erythromycin, which shortens the course of disease and decreases its transmission.

BRONCHIOLITIS

Bronchiolitis is most commonly seen in children less than 2 years of age. Most cases are caused by respiratory syncytial virus (RSV), followed by parainfluenza viruses types 1, 2, 3, adenovirus, and rhinovirus. The disease is most commonly seen in the winter months. It usually begins with slow onset of upper respiratory tract symptoms such as cough, coryza, low-grade fever, and irritability. In more severe disease, tachypnea, intercostal retractions, hypoxemia, and cyanosis may appear. Auscultation usually reveals fine rales, a prolonged expiration, and wheezes.

SPECIAL CONSIDERATION

At risk for more severe disease are infants younger than 3 months of age, premature infants, infants with bronchopulmonary dysplasia (BPD), infants with congenital heart disease, and children with immunodeficiencies.

The diagnosis is based on the clinical symptoms and signs and cell cultures of nasal secretions obtained by washings. Immunofluorescent staining of epithelium contained in nasopharyngeal specimens can also provide a rapid diagnosis of RSV. A chest radiograph is usually normal but may reveal hyperinflation, possibly with segmental atelectasis. Appropriate isolation in cases in which RSV infection is suspected should be maintained.

Treatment depends on the severity of illness and is usually supportive.

Ribovirin is a nucleoside analog that is used in an aerosolized form for treatment of severe RSV bonchiolitis, especially in infants in established risk groups.

CONTROVERSY

The utility of ribovirin in RSV bronchiolitis is controversial. A recent study failed to show benefit in the morbidity and mortality by using ribovirin.

Recently, high-titered anti-RSV intravenous immunoglobulin has been successfully used to prevent severe RSV infection in high-risk infants.

BRONCHITIS

ACUTE

The principal viruses responsible for acute bronchitis are adenoviruses, influenza viruses, respiratory syncytial virus, parainfluenza viruses, and rhinoviruses. Bacterial pathogens include *Mycoplasma pneumoniae* as well as *Streptococcus pneumoniae* and *Staphylococcus* species. *Chlamydia* species also may be an important causative agent, especially in young infants. The disease usually occurs during the winter months and it is characterized by cough, rhonchi, malaise, coryza, and fever. Chest radiographs may be necessary to distinguish it from pneumonia.

Treatment is initially supportive and includes warm mist and mucolytic agents. Antibiotics are indicated when bacterial infection is suspected because of recurrence of fever, thickened secretions, and prolongation of symptoms. A culture of sputum may be helpful in guiding antibiotic therapy.

CHRONIC

Chronic bronchitis is a condition associated with excessive tracheobronchial mucus production causing productive cough for at least 3 months of the year for more than 2 consecutive years. The disease is more common in males, and cigarette smoking is considered the most important etiologic factor. In a child with chronic bronchitis, cystic fibrosis and immunodeficiency status must be considered in the differential diagnosis.

The patient has a history of cough and sputum production, which usually presents initially only in winter months but progresses over the years with mucopurulent relapses increasing in frequency, duration, and severity. Increasing purulence, viscosity, or volume of secretions usually signals the onset of an infection.

On physical examination, there is usually no apparent distress at rest and the respiratory rate is normal or slightly increased. By auscultation, coarse rhonchi and wheezes can be heard. On radiographic examination, the bronchovascular markings are increased in the lower lung fields. Pulmonary function tests usually reveal mildly diminished vital capacity and low maximal expiratory flow rates.

SPECIAL CONSIDERATION

Sputum culture is indicated if there are chills, fever, or chest pain.

The patient should be strongly advised about cessation of smoking. Tetracycline or amoxicillin should be given for a 7- to 10-day course if bacterial infection is suspected. Bronchodilator drugs (methylxanthines, sympathomimetic, and anticholinergic agents) often are quite helpful in alleviating symptoms, especially in those patients who respond to them in the laboratory. When arterial hypoxia is persistent and severe (PaO_2 of 55 to 60 mm Hg), oxygen therapy is indicated.

NONINFECTIOUS INFLAMMATORY DISEASES OF TRACHEA AND BRONCHI

RELAPSING POLYCHONDRITIS

Relapsing polychondritis (RP) is a rare disease characterized by recurrent inflammation and destruction of cartilage of the nose, larynx, trachea, and peripheral joints.

The disease peaks in patients in the fifth decade of life. Laryngeal or tracheal involvement occurs in 50 to 79% of patients and may be the presenting symptom. Laryngotracheal manifestations include hoarseness, choking, nonproductive cough, laryngeal tenderness, dyspnea, apnea, wheezing, and stridor. Tracheal stenosis is usually a late manifestation of the disease.

> **PEARL...** The diagnosis of RP should be suspected in patients with recurrent inflammation of cartilaginous structures such as the auricle, nose, or upper airway.

The sedimentation rate is elevated in most patients, and anemia and leukocytosis occur in 30 to 60% of the patients. Bronchoscopy with biopsies may assist in making the diagnosis. Treatment of RP involves agents (particularly corticosteroids) that ablate the acute inflammatory process. Because of the episodic nature of the disease, corticosteroids are often reserved for acute flares or clinical exacerbation of disease.

Nonsteroidal antiinflammatory agents may have an adjuvant role. Immunosuppressive/cytotoxic agents have been tried with unsatisfactory results. Dapsone, an agent that inhibits lysosomal enzymes, has been tried in an attempt to suppress lysosomal enzyme-mediated cartilage degradation, but data affirming its therapeutic efficacy are limited.

Surgical management may be required for patients with severe laryngotracheal involvement.

WEGENER'S GRANULOMATOSIS

Wegener's granulomatosis (WG) is a necrotizing granulomatous vasculitis with multisystem involvement. Classically, it affects the upper and lower respiratory tract and the kidneys. WG involvement of the trachea or tracheobronchial tree occurs in 10 to 20% of cases and may cause hoarseness, dyspnea, stridor, and progressive airway obstruction. Tracheal symptoms usually develop only after the disease has affected other sites. However, tracheal obstruction may be the presenting feature of the disease or manifestation of relapse (Fig. 44–3).

> **PEARL...** When airway symptoms occur in a patient with known or suspected WG, it is necessary to rule out this complication. Soft-tissue radiographs of the neck may assist in delineating the site and extent of stenosis but direct endoscopy should be performed to assess the extent of tracheobronchial pathology and mucosal inflammation.

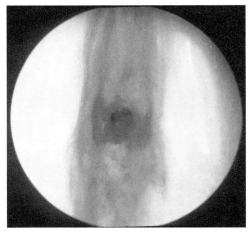

FIGURE 44–3 Grade III subglottic stenosis due to Wegener's granulomatosis. See Color Plate 44–3.

Recently, antibodies that react to cytoplasmic components of neutrophils have been identified in several patients with WG. The titer of these circulating antineutrophil cytoplasmic antibodies (ANCAs) correlate with activity of disease.

Due to the potentially life-threatening nature of tracheobronchial disease, aggressive therapy is essential. In most cases, satisfactory results can be achieved with cyclophosphamide and corticosteroids. However, for severe or progressive stenosis, urgent tracheotomy may be required. Surgical procedures also may be required for treatment of severe tracheal or bronchial stenosis refractory to medical therapy.

SUGGESTED READINGS

Boss JW, Stephenson ST. The return of pertussis. *Pediatr Infect Dis J* 1987;6:141–144.

Cohen Tevaert JW, Vander Woude FJ, Fauci AS, et al. Association between active Wegener's granulomatosis and anticytoplasmic antibodies. *Arch Intern Med* 1989;149:2461–2465.

Denney TC, Handler SD. Membranous laryngotracheobronchitis. *Pediatrics* 1982;70:705–707.

Denny FW, Murphy TF, Clyde WA, Collier AM, Henderson FW. Croup: an 11-year study in a pediatric practice. *Pediatrics* 1983;71:871–876.

Devaney KO. Interpretation of head and neck biopsies in Wegener's granulomatosis: a pathologic study of 126 biopsies in 70 patients. *Am J Surg Pathol* 1990;74:555–564.

Groothuis JR, Simoes EAF, Levin MJ, et al. Prophylactic administration of respiratory syncytial virus immune globulin to high risk infants and young children. *N Engl J Med* 1993; 329:1524.

Kairys SW, Olmstead EM, O'Connor GT. Steroid treatment of laryngotracheitis: a meta-analysis of the evidence from randomized trials. *Pediatrics* 1989;83:683–693.

Korvorsky J. Otorhinolaryngologic complications of rheumatic disease. *Semin Arthritis Rheum* 1984;14:141–150.

Liston SL, Gehrz RC, Siegel LG, Titelli J. Bacterial tracheitis. *Am J Dis Child* 1983;137:764–767.

Smith DW, Frankel LR, Mathers LH, et al. A controlled trial of aerosolized ribovivin in infants receiving mechanical ventilation for severe respiratory syncytial virus infection. *N Engl J Med* 1991;325:24–29.

Wheeler JG, Wafford J, Turner RB. Historical cohort evaluation of ribovivin efficacy in respiratory syncytial virus infection. *Pediatr Infect Dis J* 1993;12:209–213.

Chapter 45

NEOPLASMS AND CYSTS

J. Scott McMurray and Sally R. Shott

Primary tumors of the trachea are exceedingly rare. This explains the relatively small experience that exists regarding their management, even among the major institutions of the world. It has been estimated that only 2.7 new cases per million per year will present for treatment. Of 546 cases presented by Gilbert et al (1953), only 7.9% occurred in infants. Although 50% of evaluated lesions in the trachea of adults were malignant, Gilbert et al also found that 93% were benign in pediatric patients. Other large series include 53 primary cancers of the trachea over a 30-year period at the Mayo Clinic, 41 patients over a 33-year period at Memorial Hospital for Cancer and Allied Disease in New York, and 38 primary tracheal tumors at Toronto General Hospital. The largest most recently reported experience comes from Massachusetts General Hospital, with 198 patients with both benign and malignant tumors of the trachea between the years of 1962 and 1989.

The paucity of experience with primary tumors of the trachea precludes the development of definitive treatment guidelines. More experience with advanced surgical techniques and combined modality treatments is necessary.

The approach to neoplasms of the cervical trachea is similar to that of the distal trachea, although the cervical trachea is more readily approached surgically. In the pediatric population, nearly 50% of the trachea can be delivered into the neck with cervical extension. This is less true with advancing age. Although there is a difference in the distribution of certain tumors from the proximal to the distal trachea, the behavior of specific tumor types does not alter with location. Finally, benign neoplasms of the trachea are usually amenable to local resection and primary reanastomosis.

Adult tracheal tumors generally present in the distal one-third of the trachea, whereas tracheal tumors in children generally present in the proximal one-third of the trachea.

PEARLS... Tumors in the proximal one-third of the trachea can present with impaired vocal fold mobility, causing hoarseness or stridor. Distal tracheal tumors can obstruct the bronchi causing atelectasis, pneumonitis, and wheezing. Tumors of the middle one-third of the trachea may not produce symptoms until late in their course, with near-complete obstruction of the trachea, causing indolent progressive dyspnea.

EVALUATION

A high index of suspicion for these rare tumors is required for early diagnosis and successful treatment. All too often there is already a high degree of airway obstruction with insidious symptoms of shortness of breath.

> **PEARL...** Complaints often are misdiagnosed as asthma after a chest X-ray fails to detect the tracheal mass. Asthma refractory to treatment should be a red flag for further workup.

Often patients are placed on steroids for a prolonged period while symptoms of progressive exertional dyspnea remain resistant to therapy. In order of decreasing frequency, the symptoms of tracheal tumors are dyspnea, hemoptysis, cough, wheeze, dysphagia, change in voice or hoarseness, stridor, and pneumonia, as seen in the series reported by Weber and Grillo (1978).

Careful examination by chest radiographs is indicated if the presence of any of the above symptoms cannot be adequately explained. Radiographic studies will usually define the presence and extent of tracheal tumors.

> **PEARL...** High-quality posteroanterior and lateral chest radiographs along with anteroposterior and lateral neck films are often the most useful studies obtained.

Chest computed tomography (CT) is also useful for determining the extraluminal extent of tracheal tumors. Barium contrast esophagram is helpful in identifying compression and invasion of the trachea from esophageal tumors. Magnetic resonance imaging has not been fully investigated for the evaluation of tracheal tumors but offers the advantage of sagittal and coronal views that may be useful in determining the extent of disease.

At some point, endoscopy will be required for diagnosis, evaluation, and perhaps treatment. Care should be taken when approaching obstructing lesions bronchoscopically if preparations for concomitant surgical excision have not been made.

> **PITFALL...** Biopsy is useful for diagnosis unless the lesion appears vascular. Frequently, a tracheal hemangioma may only be the tip of the iceberg of a larger mediastinal hemangioma.

In some instances, tracheoscopy and bronchoscopy are required for airway management. A rigid bronchoscopy can almost always be passed through a near-complete obstruction. Once the complete extent of the lesion has been determined, the tumor can frequently be cored out via biopsy forceps or laser for diagnosis and temporary relief of airway obstruction. If bleeding ensues, direct pressure can be applied by the ventilating bronchoscope. Topical epinephrine can be applied with soaked pledgets to control oozing. An insulated cautery can also be used down the bronchoscope if necessary.

CLASSIFICATION

Neoplasms of the trachea and bronchi can be divided into benign, intermediate, and malignant lesions. Although rare, and many neoplasms may be considered one of a kind, each subclass of lesion will be reviewed individually. Specific diagnostic studies and treatment plans will be outlined for each subclass as warranted.

Excluding adenoid cystic and squamous cell carcinoma, tracheal tumors occur evenly distributed by age (Table 45–1). The most common of the pediatric tracheal tumors are recurrent respiratory papillomas, hemangiomas, and fibromas. Adenoid cystic carcinoma has a fairly even distribution between 20 and 70 years of age. Squamous cell carcinoma has a peak occurrence between 50 and 60 years of age. An association with synchronous or preceding squamous cell carcinoma of the upper aerodigestive tract has been reported. Forty percent of patients seen in the Boston series with tracheal squamous cell carcinoma had a previous history, concurrent finding, or later presentation of a squamous cell carcinoma in the respiratory tract. Recurrent respiratory papilloma occurs more frequently at junction areas between squamous mucosa and respiratory mucosa.

TABLE 45–1 INCIDENCE OF PRIMARY TRACHEAL TUMORS IN 198 PATIENTS BY AGE

Age (years)	Number of Tumors		
	Squamous Cell	Adenoid Cystic	Other
1–10	0	0	4
11–19	0	0	8
20–29	1	13	11
30–39	1	16	9
40–49	9	19	5
50–59	29	15	6
60–69	24	13	4
70–79	6	5	1

Adapted from Grillo HC, Mathisen DJ. Primary tracheal tumors: treatment and results. *Ann Thorac Surg* 1990; 49:69–77. Reprinted by permission of The Society of Thoracic Surgeons.

There is a tendency toward malignancy with tumors of the trachea seen in adults (50%), whereas pediatric tumors are mostly benign (93%). The majority of tracheal tumors are seen in adults, with only 7.9% of 546 cases presenting in the pediatric population. It has been reported that adult tracheal tumors are seen more frequently in the distal trachea, whereas pediatric tumors are found frequently in the proximal trachea. These tumors can interfere with vocal fold function, causing dysphonia and airway obstruction.

Tumors of the distal trachea may cause wheezing and asthma symptoms or pneumonitis and atelectasis. Proximal tumors of the trachea may present with stridor and voice changes. Middle-third tumors of the trachea may be asymptomatic for prolonged periods until near-total airway obstruction presents.

Adenoid cystic carcinoma is the most common of the primary tracheal tumors, as seen in the series from Boston (Table 45–2). It is followed closely by squamous cell carcinoma. The other tumors reported in the trachea have varying malignant potentials. Malignant tumors reported in the trachea include small cell undifferentiated carcinoma, lymphoma, Hodgkin's disease, plasma cell myeloma, and leiomyosarcoma.

Adenoid cystic carcinoma is relatively common in the proximal trachea and relatively rare in the main bronchi. Carcinoids, on the other hand,

TABLE 45–2 PRIMARY TRACHEAL TUMORS IN A SERIES OF 198 PATIENTS

Type	Number of Patients
Benign	
Squamous papilloma	
Multiple	4
Solitary	1
Pleomorphic adenoma	2
Granular cell tumor	2
Fibrous histiocytoma	1
Leiomyoma	2
Chondroma	2
Chondroblastoma	1
Schwannoma	1
Paraganglioma	2
Hemangioendothelioma	1
Vascular malformation	2
Intermediate	
Carcinoid	10
Mucoepidermoid	4
Plexiform neurofibroma	1
Pseudosarcoma	1
Malignant	
Adenoid cystic carcinoma	80
Squamous cell carcinoma	70
Adenocarcinoma	1
Adenosquamous carcinoma	1
Small cell carcinoma	1
Atypical carcinoid	1
Melanoma	1
Chondrosarcoma	1
Spindle cell sarcoma	2
Rhabdomyosarcoma	1

Adapted from Grillo HC, Mathisen DJ. Primary tracheal tumors: treatment and results. *Ann Thorac Surg* 1990; 49:69–77. Reprinted by permission of The Society of Thoracic Surgeons.

are found more commonly in the main and distal bronchi and are exceedingly rare in the proximal trachea. Briselli et al (1978) reported 10 carcinoids in the primary trachea and carina and another that was recurrent from a proximal main bronchus lesion. Finally, cartilaginous tumors, rare in the larynx, are even rarer in the trachea.

Neoplasms may also involve the trachea secondarily. Carcinomas of the lung, esophagus, thyroid, and larynx may invade the trachea by direct extension or metastasis. Undifferentiated pulmonary lesions such as oat cell carcinoma may metastasize to paratracheal nodes and invade the trachea. Carcinoma of the esophagus may directly invade the trachea through the common wall. Thyroid neoplasms may invade the trachea and present as hemoptysis.

> **PEARL•••** Complete endoscopy and physical exam are required when evaluating a tracheal tumor.

BENIGN

Papilloma

Recurrent respiratory papilloma of the trachea, although more common in the larynx, is the most common tracheal neoplasm in children. Caused by a viral infection, the papilloma can grow to large dimensions, potentially causing complete airway obstruction.

> **PEARL•••** There have been reports that different viral strains predict early virulence. Human papilloma virus HPV-11 has been associated with early aggressive disease, although the ultimate outcome is no different.

Treatment is the same as for laryngeal papilloma. Interval bronchoscopic removal of the papilloma to maintain a patent airway is the most common form of therapy (Fig. 45–1).

> **SPECIAL CONSIDERATION**
>
> Surveillance biopsy should periodically be performed due to infrequent but sporadic malignant degeneration.

Tracheotomy should be avoided if possible. Distal tracheal spread has been reported at the ciliated and squamous mucosa junction. A stable airway takes precedence over all other forms of

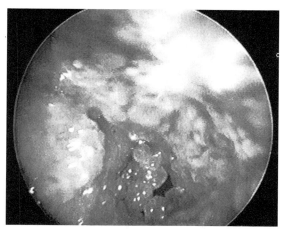

FIGURE 45–1 Papilloma of the trachea almost totally occluding the tracheal lumen. See Color Plate 45–1.

treatment, however. If tracheotomy is required, the length of time the child is tracheotomy dependent should be kept to a minimum.

Laser ablation of obstructing papilloma has been the mainstay of therapy, although more recent investigators have explored the use of microdebriders. Interferon should be explored in patients with disseminated papillomatosis. Leventhal et al (1991) recommend interferon treatment in patients requiring surgical treatment every 2 to 3 months to maintain a patent airway. Photodynamic therapy is also being investigated as a tool to direct cytotoxicity to the affected cells. Initial results are encouraging, but the delivery of the argon light to the distal trachea is problematic.

Chondroma, Osteochondroma, and Osteoma

Cartilaginous and bony lesions of the trachea and bronchi are exceedingly rare. In reviewing the literature, Neis et al (1989) found 250 lesions of the larynx of which 28% were chondrosarcomas and the remainder chondromas. Only eight chondrosarcomas and four chondromas have been reported in the trachea and bronchi. Their firm composition can make biopsy diagnosis difficult. They may present as enlargements of the normal cartilaginous structures of the trachea or bronchi or may present in the trachea separately. This benign lesion grows slowly but may cause extensive bronchopulmonary destruction. The benign lesions are amenable to local resection either bronchoscopically or through tracheotomy with resection and primary anastomosis. Sarcomatous degeneration can occur.

Tracheopathia Osteoplastica

This relatively rare condition may present with airway obstruction or chronic wheezing and may mimic asthma. Diagnosis may be achieved at endoscopy, with multiple hard masses projecting into the tracheal lumen. These masses are found only on the anterior and lateral walls of the trachea, as they originate from the cartilaginous rings of the trachea.

SPECIAL CONSIDERATION

If symptoms are severe, the obstructing lesions may be removed by shearing them off with the bronchoscope or through laser ablation with either the holmium:yttrium-aluminum-garnets (YAG) laser or the CO_2 laser.

Serum calcium levels are normal, and the appearance of other bony and cartilaginous structures is normal on radiographs.

Fibrous Histiocytoma

The histologic diagnosis of this rare tumor is difficult. Differentiation between malignant and benign tumors has also not been clearly defined. These tumors resemble inflammatory pseudotumor and fibromatosis, with the histologic features of proliferating fibroblasts with moderate nuclear pleomorphism and low mitotic activity. They present most commonly in the distal trachea of children. Resection with primary reanastomosis is the best form of treatment although recurrence can occur. Malignant neoplasms require resection and benefit little from radiotherapy.

Granular Cell Tumor

Rare in the larynx, granular cell tumor is even rarer in the trachea. Granular cell tumor may present anywhere in the body. In the head and neck, it presents most commonly in the tongue followed by the larynx. The tumor is seen more commonly in the bronchi, but has also been reported as a primary tumor of the trachea.

CONTROVERSY

The origin of the tumor is still under debate but generally it is thought to arise from neural derivatives.

The tumor may present as a solitary, polypoid, sessile, papillary, or cystic mass that is rarely ulcerated. Histologically it is an unencapsulated subepithelial lesion with syncytial, trabecular, or nested growth patterns.

PITFALL... Polygonal cells with round vesicular nuclei and coarse granular cytoplasm may be covered by an epithelium with pseudoepitheliomatous hyperplasia. This exuberant epithelium may lead to the misdiagnosis of squamous cell carcinoma.

The granular cells are S-100 protein and neuron specific enolase positive. Conservative but complete excision is considered curative. Tumors in the trachea may be treated with excision and reanastomosis. Malignant transformation is exceedingly rare but has been reported in approximately 1% of granular cell tumors.

Inflammatory Pseudotumor

Proliferating reticuloendothelial cells can cause a mass lesion that is easily mistaken for a malignant neoplasm. It is easily distinguished from a malignant neoplasm histologically, however. It is most commonly seen in children, and it has been reported in children as young as 10 months. It is a benign process that can be locally invasive. Successful treatment requires complete removal either bronchoscopically, if amenable, or through open resection.

Hamartomas

Hamartomas are a collection of normal benign tissue in an inappropriate proportion or arrangement. Hamartomas may present in the trachea or bronchi, as seen in 38 cases in a series of 128 benign tumors between 1951 and 1981 reported by Hurt (1984). Hamartomas can also present as an extraluminal mass. Gross et al (1996) reported a fixed paratracheal mass in a 21-month-old, which was successfully treated with resection.

SPECIAL CONSIDERATION

A triad of tumors has been identified in young women consisting of pulmonary hamartomas, extraadrenal paraganglioma, and gastric smooth muscle tumors. If a young woman presents with one of these tumors, the other two should be searched for as well.

Fibroma

Tracheal fibroma is the second most common benign neoplasm of the trachea and bronchi. It may present as a smooth, firm, round mass that may be pedunculated or sessile. Histologically, it is a fatty tumor densely packed with spindle-shaped cells. Pedunculated tumors may be removed endoscopically. Open surgical resection may be required for sessile or broad-based tumors. Partial pneumonectomy may be required if the fibroma has caused severe atelectasis or bronchiectasis.

Lipoma

Occurring more commonly in the fifth through eighth decades of life, tracheal and endobronchial lipomas may cause airway obstruction through intraluminal growth. If the tumor is pedunculated, it may be removed endoscopically.

Larger tumors within the wall of the trachea may require an open procedure. The tumor generally does not extend beyond the cartilaginous bronchial wall. Histologically, lipomas consist of lobules of fat cells between a fine interlacing and delicate fibrous stroma.

INTERMEDIATE
Carcinoid

Most commonly seen as a bronchial carcinoid, this neoplasm may also present infrequently in the trachea as well. It is classified in the intermediate group as it has a low-grade malignant character with local invasion and indolent growth. However, carcinoids also have the capability of lymphatic metastasis. Carcinoid syndrome may also be associated with pulmonary carcinoid, but this is more common with intestinal carcinoid or with florid hepatic metastasis.

The classic triad at presentation for bronchial carcinoid is cough, pneumonitis, and hemoptysis. The tumor may appear as a polypoid mass either partially or completely obstructing the bronchus. The diagnosis is made by histologic analysis at biopsy. Complete excision with removal of any affected lymphatics is the treatment of choice. Repeat bronchoscopy and interval CT scan are recommended to detect early recurrence. The prognosis with complete excision is very good with reported survival better than 90% (Fig. 45–2).

Mucoepidermoid

Tracheobronchial mucoepidermoid tumors represent 0.2% of all pulmonary tumors. They arise from elements of the minor salivary glands present in the trachea and bronchi. Mucoepidermoid tumors of the tracheobronchial tree are identical to those of the salivary glands. As such, the biologic behavior of these lesions may be divided into high- and low-grade neoplasms. The grade of the lesion is determined on the basis of mitotic activity, cellular necrosis, and nuclear pleomorphism. High-grade tracheal or bronchial mucoepidermoid lesions are thought to behave

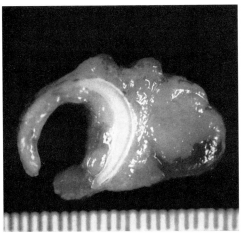
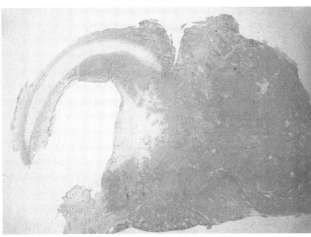

A   B

FIGURE 45–2 (A). Carcinoid tumor of the trachea. (B). Microscopic evaluation of carcinoid tumor in the same patient. See Color Plate 45–2.

like adenosquamous carcinoma. The term *adenosquamous carcinoma* is reserved for lesions peripheral to identifiable bronchi, whereas high-grade mucoepidermoid carcinoma is reserved for the tracheobronchial tree.

Low-grade mucoepidermoid carcinoma is amenable to local resection, with an excellent survival rate. Twelve patients with low-grade mucoepidermoid carcinoma were free of disease at a mean follow-up of 4.7 years. High-grade mucoepidermoid carcinoma conveys a poor prognosis with a uniform mortality. Complete resection of the tumor is the treatment of choice.

SPECIAL CONSIDERATION

The efficacy of adjuvant radiotherapy has not been completely defined. Advanced high-grade tumors with incomplete excision did not appear to respond to radiotherapy.

MALIGNANT

Adenoid Cystic Carcinoma

Billroth first described adenoid cystic carcinoma in 1859. It is the most common primary tumor of the trachea. Histologically, adenoid cystic carcinoma has been characterized as a group of small, dark-staining cells arranged in solid or cystic cords with an adenoid appearance. Grossly, the tumor is smooth, firm, and well circumscribed. Adenoid cystic carcinoma is a slow-growing and slow-metastasizing tumor. Patients have been known to live for 10 to 15 years with multiple lung metastases. Spread tends to be similar to that at other anatomic sites, with both submucosal and perineural advancement with skip lesions.

Primary resection with reanastomosis is the treatment of choice for adenoid cystic carcinoma. Grossly negative margins may be microscopically involved with tumor, however, and so a margin of at least 1 cm is recommended. Intraoperative frozen section analysis of the surgical margin is invaluable.

CONTROVERSY

Postoperative irradiation has not been addressed in large randomized trials in tracheal tumors, although most authors recommend postoperative irradiation.

Extended follow-up is imperative for patients after resection.

SPECIAL CONSIDERATION

Bronchoscopy should be performed at least once a year for the life of the patient in an effort to detect early recurrence.

The natural history of adenoid cystic carcinoma differs from many other malignant neoplasms. It spreads most commonly by direct extension, submucosal and perineural invasion, or hematogenous metastasis. Pulmonary metastasis is the most common and may remain silent for many years. Local recurrence of tracheal adenoid cystic carcinoma is common and occurs an average of 51 months after primary treatment. The course of adenoid cystic carcinoma is indolent. The presence of small synchronous pulmonary metastases, therefore, may not be a factor in treatment. Many patients will live for years with asymptomatic lesions.

Squamous Cell Carcinoma

Squamous cell carcinoma has a poorer prognosis than adenoid cystic carcinoma. It occurs twice as often in men than in women. The patient population is found to be older than that of the adenoid cystic group, and patients are generally current or former cigarette smokers.

SPECIAL CONSIDERATION

Rare pediatric cases have been reported, but with a poor prognosis.

Primary squamous cell carcinoma of the trachea generally presents with hemoptysis or progressive airway obstruction. It may be found as a well-circumscribed exophytic lesion or as a large spreading ulcerated mass involving a considerable length of the trachea. Direct extension and mediastinal metastasis are frequently seen. Nearly 40% of patients seen with primary tracheal squamous cell carcinoma are deemed unresectable due to direct extension into sur-

rounding structures or due to lymphatic metastases.

The histologic character of squamous cell carcinoma has been well described. Grossly at bronchoscopy, the lesions are either exophytic or ulcerated. If the tumor is found on the posterior tracheal wall, it may be a primary carcinoma of the esophagus with direct extension.

PEARL... Complete endoscopy of the aerodigestive tract is required prior to surgical extirpation to rule out synchronous lesions.

Complete surgical resection when possible is the treatment of choice. Radiotherapy is indicated in inoperable patients and in patients at high risk for recurrence. Radiotherapy is more effective in the treatment of adenoid cystic carcinoma than in the treatment of squamous cell carcinoma.

Other Malignant Tumors

There have been sporadic case reports of other malignant tumors of the trachea and bronchi. Diagnosis is made through biopsy, and successful treatment requires early intervention and an individualized approach. Reported malignancies include leiomyosarcoma, rhabdomyosarcoma, and myxosarcoma.

Limited experience exists with these individually reported tumors. The principles of complete surgical excision with adjuvant therapy when appropriate are the guidelines that may lead to successful treatment.

SUGGESTED READINGS

Abramson AL, Shikowitz MJ, Mullooly VM, Steinberg BM, Hyman RB. Variable light-dose effect on photodynamic therapy for laryngeal papillomas. *Arch Otolaryngol Head Neck Surg* 1994;120:852–855.

Azar T, Abdul-Karim FW, Tucker HM. Adenoid cystic carcinoma of the trachea. *Laryngoscope* 1998;108:1297–1300.

Billroth T. Beobachtungen über Geschwülste der Speicheldrüsen. *Virchows Arch [A]* 1859; 17:357–375.

Birzgalis AR, Farrington WT, O'Keefe L, Shaw J. Localized tracheopathia osteoplastica of the subglottis. *J Laryngol Otol* 1993;107:352–353.

Briselli M, Mark GJ, Grillo HC. Tracheal carcinoids. *Cancer* 1978;42:2870–2879.

Burton DM, Heffner DK, Patow CA. Granular cell tumors of the trachea. *Laryngoscope* 1992; 102:807–813.

Caldarola VT, Harrison EG Jr, Clagett OT, et al. Benign tumors and tumorlike conditions of the trachea and bronchi. *Ann Otol Rhinol Laryngol* 1964;73:1042.

Chen TF, Braidley PC, Shneerson JM, Wells FC. Obstructing tracheal lipoma: management of a rare tumor. *Ann Thorac Surg* 1990;49:137–139.

Contencin P, Gumpert LC, Cortez A, Livarek S. Squamous cell carcinoma of the trachea in an infant: a case report. *Int J Pediatr Otorhinolaryngol* 1998;43:163–173.

Dewar AL, Connett GJ. Inflammatory pseudotumor of the trachea in a ten-month-old infant. *Pediatr Pulmonol* 1997;23:307–309.

Gilbert JG, Mazzarella LA, Feit LJ. Primary tracheal tumors in the infant and adult. *Arch Otolaryngol* 1953;58:1.

Gleich LL, Rebeiz EE, Pankratov MM, Shapshay SM. The holmium:YAG laser-assisted otolaryngologic procedures. *Arch Otolaryngol Head Neck Surg* 1995;121:1162–1166.

Grillo HC. Tracheal tumors: surgical management. *Ann Thorac Sugr* 1978;26:112–125.

Grillo HC, Mathisen DJ. Primary tracheal tumors: treatment and results. *Ann Thorac Surg* 1990;49:69–77.

Gross E, Chen MK, Hollabaugh RS, Joyner RE. Tracheal hamartoma: report of a child with a neck mass. *J Pediatr Surg* 1996;31:1584–1585.

Hajdu SI, Huvos AG, Goodner JT, Foote FW Jr, Beattie EJ Jr. Carcinoma of the trachea. Clinicopathologic study of 41 cases. *Cancer* 1970; 25:1448–1456.

Heitmiller RF, Mathiesen DJ, Ferry JA, Mark EJ, Grillo HC. Mucoepidermoid lung tumors. *Ann Thorac Surg* 1989;47:394–399.

Houston HE, Payne WS, Harrison EG Jr, Olsen AM. Primary cancers of the trachea. *Arch Surg* 1969;99:132–140.

Hulka GF, Rothschild MA, Warner BW, Bove KE. Carcinoid tumor of the trachea in a pediatric patient. *Otolaryngol Head Neck Surg* 1996;114:822–825.

Hurt R. Benign tumours of the bronchus and trachea, 1951–1981. *Ann R Coll Surg Engl* 1984;66:22–26.

Kashima H, Mounts P, Leventhal B, Hruban RH. Sites of predilection in recurrent respiratory papillomatosis. *Ann Otol Rhinol Laryngol* 1993;102:580–583.

Leventhal BG, Kashima HK, Mounts P, et al. Long-term response of recurrent respiratory papillomatosis to treatment with lymphoblastoid interferon alfa-N1. Papilloma Study Group. *N Engl J Med* 1991;325:613–617.

Mathisen DJ. Tracheal tumors. *Chest Surg Clin North Am* 1996;6:875–898.

Maziak DE, Todd TR, Keshavjee SH, Winton TL, Van Nostrand P, Pearson FG. Adenoid cystic carcinoma of the airway: thirty-two-year experience. *J Thorac Cardiovasc Surg* 1996;112: 1522–1531; discussion 1531–1532.

Neis PR, McMahon MF, Norris CW. Cartilaginous tumors of the trachea and larynx. *Ann Otol Rhinol Laryngol* 1989;98:31–36.

Pearson FG, Todd TR, Cooper JD. Experience with primary neoplasms of the trachea and carina. *J Thorac Cardiovasc Surg* 1984;88:511–518.

Regnard JF, Fourquier P, Levasseur P. Results and prognostic factors in resections of primary tracheal tumors: a multicenter retrospective study. The French Society of Cardiovascular Surgery. *J Thorac Cardiovasc Surg* 1996;111:808–813; discussion 813–814.

Rimell FL, Shoemaker DL, Pou AM, Jordan JA, Post JC, Ehrlich GD. Pediatric respiratory papillomatosis: prognostic role of viral typing and cofactors. *Laryngoscope* 1997;107: 915–918.

Sculerati N, Mittal KR, Greco MA, Ambrosino MM. Fibrous histiocytoma of the trachea: management of a rare cause of upper airway obstruction. *Int J Pediatr Otorhinolaryngol* 1990;19:295–301.

Sennaroglu L, Sozeri B, Ataman M, Gokoz O. Malignant fibrous histiocytoma of the trachea. Case report. *Acta Otorhinolaryngol Belg* 1996;50:147–149.

Tan-Liu NS, Matsubara O, Grillo HC, Mark EJ. Invasive fibrous tumor of the tracheobronchial tree: clinical and pathologic study of seven cases. *Hum Pathol* 1989;20:180–184.

Thedinger BA, Cheney ML, Montgomery WW, Goodman M. Leiomyosarcoma of the trachea. Case report. *Ann Otol Rhinol Laryngol* 1991;100:337–340.

Vazquez E, Enriquez G, Castellote A, et al. US, CT, and MR imaging of neck lesions in children. *Radiographics* 1995;15:105–122.

Weber AL, Shortsleeve M, Goodman M, Montgomery W, Grillo HC. Cartilaginous tumors of the larynx and trachea. *Radiol Clin North Am* 1978;16:261–267.

Weber AL, Grillo HC. Tracheal tumor: radiological, clinical and pathological evaluation *Adv Otorhinolaryngol* 1978;24:170–176.

Chapter 46

TRAUMA

Mark E. Gerber, Daniel J. Kelley, and Sally R. Shott

Traumatic injuries of the tracheobronchial tree can be divided into two groups: cervical (extrathoracic) and intrathoracic. Although these types of injuries are relatively uncommon, their exact incidence is difficult to ascertain. Etiologies include blunt and penetrating trauma as well as internal injury from endotracheal intubation.

Penetrating injuries are more common than blunt injuries, with both types occurring more commonly in the extrathoracic trachea. They can be low velocity, such as stabbings, or high velocity, such as gunshot wounds. A low-velocity stab wound results in laceration, perforation, or transection injuries. High-velocity gunshot wounds are more common, with the resultant injury dependent on the trajectory and kinetic force of the missile involved.

SPECIAL CONSIDERATION

Higher kinetic energy missiles create a larger temporary cavity with more surrounding tissue damage. This results in a more severe tracheal injury as well as a greater frequency of injury to surrounding structures.

Blunt or nonpenetrating injury is due to a direct blow to the neck or thorax. The cervical trachea may be injured by hyperextension, causing traction/distraction, or a direct blow, such as occurs with an unrestrained driver hitting the neck on the steering wheel. Blunt thoracic injuries can cause disruption of the intrathoracic trachea or mainstem bronchi by direct compression or acceleration-deceleration, causing shear force injury. Most patients with tracheobronchial trauma have associated injuries. Associated vascular injuries are more common with cervical penetrating injuries.

PEARL••• Esophageal injuries frequently occur with tracheal injuries, whether the cause is blunt or penetrating trauma.

Iatrogenic trauma to the tracheobronchial tree can occur during endotracheal intubation. This can be a result of cuff overinflation, but more commonly occurs at the time of intubation, often with an inappropriately used stylet.

DIAGNOSIS

Typical signs and symptoms of tracheobronchial injury include cough, pain, dyspnea, hemoptysis, subcutaneous emphysema, pneumothorax, and pneumomediastinum.

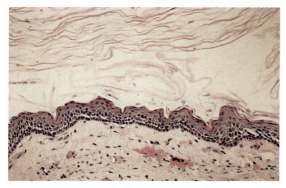

COLOR PLATE 18–1 Keratocyst. See Figure 18–1, p. 146.

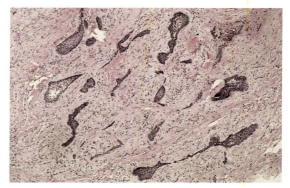

COLOR PLATE 18–2 Ameloblastoma. See Figure 18–2, p. 147.

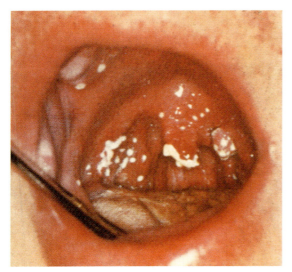

COLOR PLATE 24–1 Pseudomembranous form of *Candida albicans* showing yellow-white plaques. See Figure 24–1, p. 188.

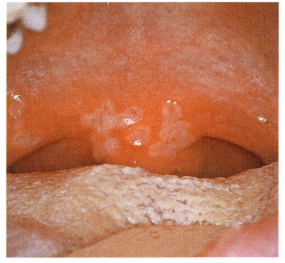

COLOR PLATE 24–2 Erythematous form of *Candida albicans.* Yellow-white plaques visible in the pseudomembranous form have disappeared. See Figure 24–2, p. 188.

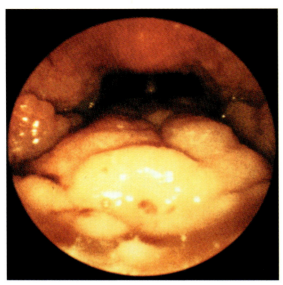

COLOR PLATE 28–1 A 180-degree endoscopic view of normal adenoids. See Figure 28–1, p. 211.

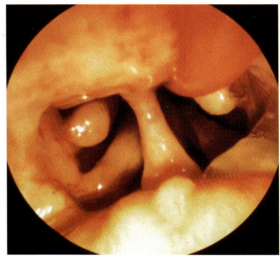

COLOR PLATE 28–2 A 120-degree endoscopic view of the nasopharynx and posterior choanae. A red rubber catheter is seen on the left and is used to elevate the palate. See Figure 28–2, p. 211.

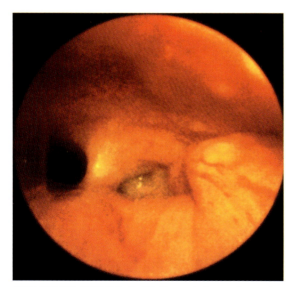

COLOR PLATE 29–1 Unilateral choanal atresia viewed from the nasopharynx with a 120-degree endoscope. See Figure 29–1, p. 214.

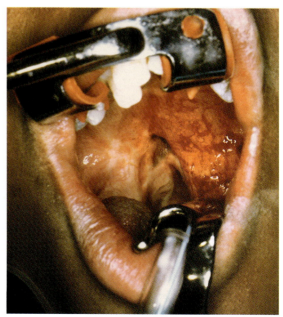

COLOR PLATE 30–4 Nasopharyngeal stenosis secondary to adenotonsillectomy. See Figure 30–4, p. 219.

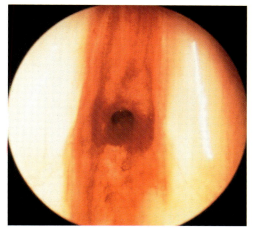

COLOR PLATE 44–3 Grade III subglottic stenosis due to Wegener's granulomatosis. See Figure 44–3, p. 308.

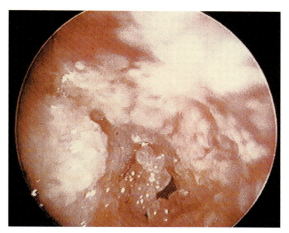

COLOR PLATE 45–1 Papilloma of the trachea almost totally occluding the tracheal lumen. See Figure 45–1, p. 313.

A

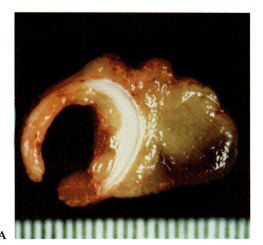

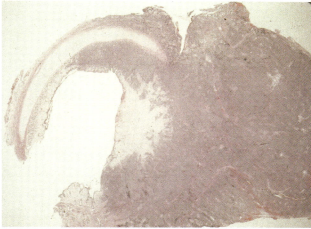

B

COLOR PLATE 45–2 (A). Carcinoid tumor of the trachea. (B). Microscopic evaluation of carcinoid tumor in the same patient. See Figure 45–2, p. 316.

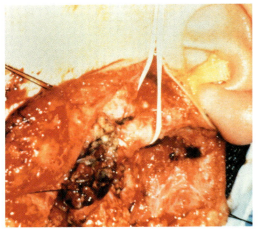

COLOR PLATE 72–6 First branchial cleft cyst (type I) loop at cartilage. See Figure 72–6, p. 493.

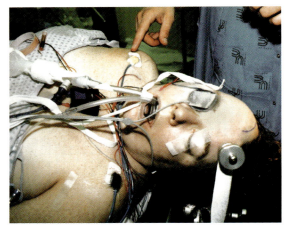

COLOR PLATE 82–2 The choice of electrode array is important. Needle electrodes allow for a fixed reference point and are quite stable. See Figure 82–2, p. 554.

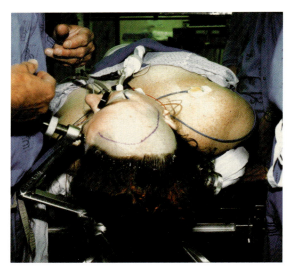

COLOR PLATE 82–1 Immediately following intubation and positioning of the patient, the electrode array for intraoperative monitoring is set. Often with multiple nerves being concomitantly followed, the neurophysiologist monitoring the patient must set the wires and electrodes in a fashion so as not to be caught by drapes, anesthesia equipment, or field equipment. See Figure 82–1, p. 553.

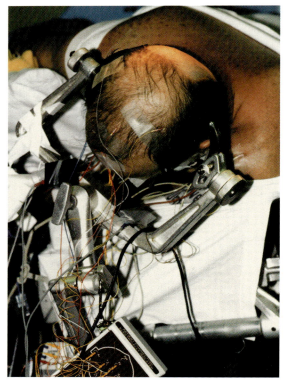

COLOR PLATE 82–3 With electrodes set, only one reference electrode is employed despite the number of nerves being assessed. Impedance is checked relative to both interelectrode and field impedance before proceding. See Figure 82–3, p. 554.

The severity of clinical signs usually correlates
with the severity of injury. Respiratory difficulty
can range from hoarseness to complete obstruction. Bleeding may be significant secondary to
associated vascular injuries. Intrathoracic tracheobronchial injuries may result in a pneumothorax that will not completely resolve after
thoracostomy tube placement. A persistent air
leak may be present through the tube. Alternatively, a small amount of mediastinal emphysema may worsen significantly after mechanical
ventilation is initiated.

CONTROVERSY

Imaging techniques are not diagnostic
of tracheobronchial injuries. However,
a plain chest radiograph can show
suggestive findings such as pneumothorax or pneumomediastinum.

Also, in all multitrauma patients, cervical spine
radiographs are clearly indicated to evaluate for
possible associated cervical spine injury.

Once tracheobronchial injury is suspected,
bronchoscopy is the most useful tool to establish the diagnosis. The findings at bronchoscopy
may be subtle and can be easily missed. Esophagoscopy should be considered as well to rule
out associated injury.

MANAGEMENT

As with all multitrauma patients, the ABC of resuscitation (airway, breathing, and circulation)
needs to be followed at the time of presentation. If needed, an airway must be established
with in-line stabilization of the cervical spine
until this associated injury can be ruled out with
cervical spine radiographs.

CONTROVERSY

Tracheostomy or cricothyrotomy (in
adults) is often recommended for
emergent airway management. However, orotracheal intubation can be accomplished in the vast majority of
cases, even when there is total tracheal
or laryngotracheal or tracheobronchial
separation.

When the injury is to the extrathoracic trachea, management is similar to that for laryngeal trauma. Patients with impending airway
obstruction may require urgent tracheotomy
under local anesthesia. However, when the
degree of airway compromise allows, tracheal
intubation may be performed at the time of
bronchoscopy. Often this can be done simultaneously by passing the endotracheal tube over
the flexible bronchoscope, ensuring placement
distal to the site of injury. In some rare instances,
the quickest way to secure the airway with open
cervical wounds is intubating the distal trachea
through the wound itself.

Intrathoracic injury to the tracheobronchial
tree is also initially managed with bronchoscopy
to assess the severity of injury and ensure placement of the endotracheal tube distal to the site
of injury. Once the airway has been established,
associated injuries should be assessed and
managed as indicated.

Nonoperative management can be considered for patients with small tracheobronchial
lacerations without a large air leak or other associated injuries requiring surgical exploration.
Most injuries with greater than one-third of the
circumference involved require surgical intervention. The cervical trachea can be approached
through a standard collar incision that can be
extended to a median sternotomy if needed. A
right posterolateral thoracotomy is the preferred
approach for repair of intrathoracic tracheal and
tracheobronchial lacerations. Even those involving the first 2 cm of the left mainstem
bronchus can be approached in this manner.
More distal left bronchial lacerations require a
left thoracotomy approach.

The general approach is adequate debridement to healthy tissue and primary airtight repair with mucosal closure posteriorly and pericartilaginous closure anterolaterally. Most tracheobronchial repairs can be extubated at the time of repair or require stenting with an endotracheal tube for only a short time thereafter. In more severe injuries, longer term endoluminal stenting may be considered to control stricture formation.

SUGGESTED READINGS

Devitt JH, Boulanger BR. Lower airway injuries and anaesthesia. *Can J Anaesth* 1996;43(2): 148–159.

Huh J, Milliken JC, Chen JC. Management of tracheobronchial injuries following blunt and penetrating trauma. *Am Surg* 1997;63:896–899.

Kaloud H, Smolle-Juettner FM, Prause G, List WF. Iatrogenic ruptures of the tracheobronchial tree. *Chest* 1997;112:774–778.

Lee RB. Traumatic injury of the cervicothoracic trachea and major bronchi. *Chest Surg Clin North Am* 1997;7(2):285–304.

Rossbach MM, Johnson SB, Gomez MA, Sako EY, Miller OL, Calhoon JH. Management of major tracheobronchial injuries: a 28-year experience. *Ann Thorac Surg* 1998;65:182–186.

Chapter 47

SPECIAL CONSIDERATIONS: TRACHEOTOMY

David L. Walner and Sally R. Shott

Frequently disorders of the larynx, trachea, and bronchi require the placement of a tracheotomy tube either temporarily or permanently. This chapter discusses special considerations involved with tracheotomy.

INDICATIONS FOR TRACHEOTOMY

Tracheotomy is indicated for emergent or elective management of acute and chronic upper airway obstruction. In cases where prolonged intubation is anticipated, tracheotomy should be considered early in the decision-making process to avoid potential complications of prolonged intubation.

SPECIAL CONSIDERATION

In adults, tracheotomy is generally recommended once a patient has been intubated for 10 to 14 days. In children, use of uncuffed endotracheal tubes has lengthened this period of time. However, in patients requiring multiple traumatic intubations a tracheotomy should be done without delay.

TECHNIQUES

TRANSTRACHEAL NEEDLE VENTILATION

Transtracheal needle ventilation is an option in an emergency situation in the face of airway obstruction. A 12- or 14-gauge angiocatheter attached to a syringe filled with saline or water can be inserted through the cricothyroid membrane or trachea. Entrance into the airway is confirmed by negative pressure and bubbling. This method is only a temporizing measure in the most emergent of situations. Pneumothorax has been described following this procedure.

PERCUTANEOUS TRACHEOTOMY

Over the past decade there has been an increased interest in this technique. It is generally performed by inserting an introducer needle into the trachea or through the cricothyroid membrane. A guidewire is passed through the inducer followed by a series of tracheal dilators, which allow placement of the tracheostomy tube. The most important factor in reducing complications is adequate training of the physician performing the procedure as well as careful patient selection.

CRICOTHYROIDOTOMY

This procedure is generally performed in emergent situations for upper airway obstruction where intubation cannot be performed. It would rarely be indicated in patients with severe spinal deformities that do not allow an opening to be made within the trachea. The procedure is performed with the patient in the supine position. A horizontal or vertical skin incision can be utilized. Once the cricothyroid membrane is encountered a horizontal incision is made through the cricothyroid membrane and the cricoid cartilage elevated caudally using a tracheal hook. A tracheotomy tube or small endotracheal tube is then immediately inserted for ventilation.

TRACHEOTOMY

Tracheotomy is the most common method for obtaining access to the airway when endotracheal tube intubation is not possible or is dangerous, and for patients with prolonged ventilatory demands. The procedure is performed in a supine position with the neck extended. A shoulder roll helps to achieve better extension of the neck. The procedure can be performed in an awake patient under local anesthetic or under general anesthesia. A vertical or horizontal incision can be made over the anterior tracheal wall. The strap muscles are separated in the vertical midline, and if necessary the thyroid isthmus is divided such that the anterior tracheal wall can be visualized. The tracheal hook is then placed in the midline under the cricoid cartilage and a tracheotomy incision is performed, usually between the second and third or third and fourth tracheal rings. Many techniques are used on the anterior tracheal wall including removal of an anterior square of cartilage, a vertical incision, or an inferiorly based flap. Once the incision is made, the endotracheal tube is partially removed to a point just superior to the tracheal incision and the tracheotomy tube is inserted. If there is any problem inserting the new tube, the endotracheal tube can then easily be advanced inferiorly again. The endotracheal tube should not be totally removed until adequate ventilation through the tracheotomy tube is confirmed.

For the pediatric population, the technique of tracheotomy has several important differences. Because of the small size of the trachea, about the size of a drinking straw in an infant, and because of the soft, malleable cartilage of the trachea in this age group, it can be more difficult to identify the trachea on palpation of the neck. It is therefore best to perform the procedure with the trachea intubated with either an endotracheal tube or a bronchoscope. In the pediatric population tracheal cartilage is not removed. Once adequate exposure of the anterior trachea is achieved, a vertical midline incision is made through tracheal rings three and four. Just prior to this incision, 4-0 Prolene vertical stay sutures are placed just lateral to both sides of the planned tracheal incision. These are labeled "right" and "left" and taped to the child's chest. If the tracheotomy inadvertently dislodges before the tract has healed, these sutures facilitate quick identification of the tracheal opening. In addition, chromic sutures can be used to secure the anterior tracheal wall to the skin in four quadrants. This is of particular importance in cases of airway stenosis or obstruction where intubation from above is not possible and the tracheotomy represents the patient's only viable airway. These sutures quickly establish a more permanent stoma.

> **PEARL...** Although a common technique in the adult tracheotomy, removal of tracheal cartilage is not done in the pediatric population as this will most likely lead to anterior tracheal wall collapse.

COMPLICATIONS OF TRACHEOTOMY

Complications of tracheotomy can be divided into intraoperative, early, or delayed. The most common complications related to tracheotomy include hemorrhage (3.7%), tube obstruction (2.7%), and tube displacement (1.5%). Pneumothorax, atelectasis, aspiration, tracheal stenosis, and tracheoesophageal fistula occur with less than 1% frequency each. However, in the pediatric population, pneumothorax can be more common. Death occurs in 0.5 to 1.6% of the cases and is most often caused by hemorrhage or inadvertent tube displacement. Emergent tracheotomy carries a two- to fivefold increase in the incidence of complications over an elective procedure.

INTRAOPERATIVE COMPLICATIONS

Intraoperative complications during tracheotomy are unusual. However, attention must be focused on the anatomic landmarks and on recognizing anatomic variations. Complications are related to the skill of the surgeon, the organization of the patient care team, adequacy of lighting and instruments, and the proper securing of the airway prior to tracheotomy.

These complications may include unanticipated or premature airway obstruction, false passage formation, pneumomediastinum, pneumomediathorax, esophageal perforation, hemorrhage, recurrent laryngeal nerve injury, or intraoperative fire. It is best to remove all esophageal instruments during the procedure. A postoperative chest X-ray should be ordered in the immediate postoperative period to rule out pulmonary complications due to the tracheotomy.

Hemorrhage is the most common intraoperative complication and is usually from the thyroid or local soft tissues. If major intraopera-tive hemorrhage occurs it may rarely be due to injury to the innominate artery.

EARLY POSTOPERATIVE COMPLICATIONS

Postoperative care can help avoid complications and should include humidification, pulmonary toilet, prevention of infection, maintenance of the airway, and ensuring that caregivers are familiar with the care of tracheostomy tubes and problems that can be related to them.

Hemorrhage is the most common postoperative complication following tracheotomy. This can be related to spasmodic coughing, which causes irritation of small blood vessels. Bleeding that is present in the early postoperative period is usually minor in comparison to late hemorrhage. Infection can also occur around the stoma site in the immediate postoperative period due to contamination from saliva with the subsequent formation of stomal cellulitis. Wound care with appropriate packing and cleaning with 0.25% acetic acid and systemic antibiotics directed at staphylococci and gram-negative rods are the recommended treatment.

Subcutaneous emphysema, pneumomediastinum, and pneumothorax can be recognized in the early postoperative period.

> **PEARL...** Some mild degree of subcutaneous crepitance is not unexpected, but if air trapping occurs, it can become quite extensive and progress into a pneumomediastinum or pneumothorax. It is therefore important that skin incisions are allowed to heal secondarily without suturing, and any wound packing that may be needed should be placed loosely.

The incidence of pneumothorax in children may approach 10%.

Accidental decannulation can be a devastating early postoperative complication due to the fact that the stoma is not completely formed yet. Prompt replacement of the tube is necessary, and caregivers should be aware that in the majority of cases mouth-to-mouth or mask ventilation is possible via the nose and mouth in this situation.

SPECIAL CONSIDERATION

In patients with complete upper airway obstruction it is advisable not only to suture the incised tracheal wall to the skin to provide a more complete stoma but also to have a sign at the patient's bedside notifying all potential medical caregivers that intubation from above is not possible. In these cases, a tracheotomy surgical set should be at the bedside in case early decannulation occurs.

Postobstructive pulmonary edema can occur when preoperative airway obstruction is significant and is relieved with the placement of the tracheotomy tube. Negative pleural pressure is thought to be transmitted to the pulmonary interstitium, reducing the hydrostatic pressure around pulmonary vessels and resulting in an increased hydrostatic pressure and interstitial water accumulation. Generally there will be frothy material emanating from the tracheotomy tube. Treatment is generally with Lasix, which, if used aggressively, will relieve the problem.

Tube obstruction can occur within the first 24 hours, most likely due to a blood clot, partial displacement, or tube impingement on the posterior tracheal wall.

PEARL... Alternative tracheotomy tubes should be available at the patient's bedside and it is best to always have a one-size-smaller tube present to allow for an easier replacement.

DELAYED COMPLICATIONS

Delayed complications are those that occur later than 7 days postoperatively. Hemorrhage is the most catastrophic delayed complication and can occur due to erosion of the innominate artery as it crosses anterior to the trachea at the superior thoracic inlet. For this reason, any bleeding from the tracheotomy requires careful examination in the postoperative period. The incidence of massive hemorrhage as a late complication has been reported as high as 4.5% and as low as 0.4%.

Infection as a delayed complication can occur due to breakdown around the tracheostomy tube. Generally antimicrobial agents that cover *Staphylococcus aureus, Pseudomonas,* and *Candida* should be utilized if tracheitis or peristomal cellulitis is suspected.

Delayed tracheoesophageal fistulas can occur due to erosion of the posterior tracheal wall. An indwelling nasogastric tube predisposes the patient to this complication. Mortality associated with tracheoesophageal fistula has been estimated as high as 70 to 80%.

Tracheal granulomas can occur commonly just at the superior aspect of the tracheotomy stoma. These are likely due to chronic low-grade inflammation resulting from secretions pooling just above the tracheotomy tube.

SPECIAL CONSIDERATION

If the granulomas are large and obstructive, they should be removed to allow for an airway above the tracheotomy tube in the event of accidental decannulation. Small granulomas that are relatively nonobstructing can be followed observantly.

When tracheotomy tubes have been in for a long period of time, the suprastomal region may lose support, resulting in collapse of the anterior wall of the airway. This anterior tracheal wall collapse may be mild or severe such that reconstruction with a cartilage graft to this region to add support is needed to achieve decannulation. Persistent tracheocutaneous fistulas can occur after decannulation at an estimated rate of 19 to 45%. If this occurs, a procedure can be performed to close the anterior cartilaginous structures as well as the strap muscles over the region of the open airway.

TRACHEOTOMY TUBES

In years past the majority of tracheotomy tubes were of the metal variety. Pediatric-sized tubes were originally simply miniaturized adult versions. In the mid-1960s siliconized polymer or Silastic tracheotomy tubes became available. These tubes provide both sufficient rigidity and increased flexibility. In 1965 Aberdeen and Holinger first emphasized the differences in the anatomy between a child's and an adult's trachea. This led to the development of specialized pediatric tubes. The inner diameter, outer diameter, and length of the tube are critical components in deciding which tracheotomy tube size to utilize. These must be taken into careful consideration based on the patient's age, size, and requirements.

DECANNULATION

In the majority of cases a formal microlaryngoscopy and bronchoscopy should be performed prior to decannulating patients.

> **PEARL...** It must be established that no other airway pathology or suprastomal granulomas exist before decannulating the patient.

It is most often advisable to downsize the tracheotomy tube sequentially followed by plugging the tracheotomy tube for a variable period of time prior to decannulation. In the majority of cases, in-hospital observation should be performed for downsizing, plugging, and decannulation. Once it is established that a patient tolerates plugging, decannulation can be performed with close in-hospital observation for a period of 48 hours.

SUGGESTED READINGS

Flint PW. Complications of tracheostomy. In: Eisele DW, ed. *Complications in Head and Neck Surgery.* St. Louis: Mosby Year Book; 344–358.

Graham JS, Malloi RH, Southerland FR, Rose S. Percutaneous vs open tracheostomy: a retrospective cohort outcome study. *J Trauma* 1996;41:245–248.

Haller JA, Talbert JL. Clinical evaluation of a new Silastic tracheotomy tube for respiratory support of infants and young children. *Ann Surg* 1970;171:915–922.

Hill BB, Sweng TN, Maley RH, Charish WE, Toursarkissian B, Kearney PA. Percutaneous dilational tracheostomy: report of 356 cases. *J Trauma Injury Infect Crit Care* 1996;40:238–243.

Johnson JT, Rood SR, Stool SE, Myers EN, Thearle PB. Tracheotomy. Self instructional package from the American Academy of Otolaryngology-Head and Neck Surgery, 1984:38–48.

Myers WO, Lawton BR, Santter RD. An operation for tracheal innominate artery fistula. *Arch Surg* 1972;105:269–274.

Reilly H, Sasaki CT. Tracheotomy complication. In: Krespi YP, Ossoff RH, eds. *Complications in Head and Neck Surgery.* Philadelphia: WB Saunders; 1993:257–274.

Shott SR. Pediatric tracheostomy. In: Myer CM, Cotton RT, Shott SR, eds. *Pediatric Airway: An Interdisciplinary Approach.* Philadelphia: JB Lippincott; 1995:151–169.

Wetmore RF, Handler SD, Potsic WP. Pediatric tracheostomy: experience during the past decade. *Ann Otol Rhinol Laryngol* 1982;91: 628–632.

Weymuller EA. Laryngeal injury from prolonged endotracheal tube intubation. *Laryngoscope* 1988;98:1–15.

SECTION VIII

ESOPHAGUS

Chapter 48

ANATOMY AND PHYSIOLOGY

Allen M. Seiden

EMBRYOLOGY

The primitive gut forms during the fourth week of embryogenesis and is divided into the foregut, midgut, and hindgut. The derivatives of the foregut include the digestive tract from the pharynx to the duodenum and the lower respiratory tract. At day 26, a small pit develops in the caudal end of the pharyngeal floor known as the laryngotracheal groove, and this deepens to form a diverticulum. Grooves that produce internal tracheoesophageal folds form on either side of this diverticulum. These folds gradually fuse in the midline to form the tracheoesophageal septum, as the diverticulum elongates caudally to form the respiratory tract. This septum then partitions the foregut into the ventral respiratory tract and dorsal esophagus.

SPECIAL CONSIDERATION

Incomplete fusion of the tracheo-esophageal fold leads to a defective tracheoesophageal septum, resulting in a tracheoesophageal fistula.

The epithelium and glands of the digestive tract are derived from the endoderm of the primitive gut. This endoderm proliferates and essentially obliterates the lumen, but by the end of the embryonic period, recanalization occurs. Esophageal smooth muscle is derived from the surrounding splanchnic mesenchyme, while the striated muscle develops from the lower branchial arches and is therefore innervated by the vagus nerve.

HISTOLOGY

The digestive tract and esophagus are composed of four layers: an inner mucosa, a submucosa, a muscularis externa, and an adventitia.

INNER MUCOSA

The inner mucosa is generally 500 to 800 μm thick and is itself composed of three layers: an epithelial membrane, a supportive connective tissue layer or lamina propria, and a thick smooth layer or muscularis mucosa.

The epithelial lining is a tough, nonkeratinizing stratified squamous epithelium that gives way to columnar epithelium at the gastroesophageal junction. This transition is generally 1.5 cm proximal to the true anatomic border with the stomach and is readily seen as an irregular line between the pale esophageal mucosa and reddened gastric mucosa. The latter appears so because of the more superficial and transparent columnar cells. This irregular transition has a saw-toothed pattern and is often referred to as the Z line.

The lamina propria is a loose areolar connective tissue layer containing collagenous and elastic fibers, as well as neurovascular elements.

The muscularis mucosa is composed of smooth muscle oriented longitudinally and is continuous with the elastic layer of the pharynx at the level of the cricoid cartilage. It is thickest at the lower end of the esophagus.

SUBMUCOSA

The submucosal layer is composed largely of dense collagenous connective tissue that is pulled up into longitudinal folds when the esophagus is at rest and the lumen is collapsed. Autonomic fibers and parasympathetic ganglion cells within this layer form the myenteric plexus of Meissner.

MUSCULARIS EXTERNA

The external muscular layer, or coat, has classically been described as having an inner layer of circular fibers and an outer layer of longitudinal fibers. In fact, the circular layer is not directly horizontal but is angled 10 to 20 degrees, and the longitudinal layer is not directly vertical but spirals around one-quarter of the esophageal circumference. This creates a screw-like configuration that facilitates peristalsis.

The circular layer assumes a more horizontal position in the area of the upper and lower esophageal sphincter, where the longitudinal layer largely blends in. Neither one is an anatomically defined sphincter, but the muscular bundles behave as such. This external muscular layer is composed of largely striated muscle within the upper third of the esophagus, mixed striated and smooth muscle within the middle third, and smooth muscle within the lower third. The fluid transition that occurs between these segments demonstrates a remarkable degree of coordination, innervated in part by the myenteric plexus of Auerbach, also located within this layer.

ADVENTITIA

The outermost adventitial layer contains neurovascular structures and, more importantly, elastic fibers that are continuous with fibers interspersed within the inner layers of the esophagus. This complex network allows the esophagus to distend in response to bolus feeding and resume its normal shape after deglutition.

ANATOMY

The esophagus begins just below the cricoid cartilage at the level of the sixth cervical vertebra (Fig. 48–1). Endoscopically, this is 15 to 20 cm from the upper incisor teeth. During its vertical descent anterior to the spine, it shifts to the left, opposite the suprasternal notch.

> **PEARL...** Surgical access to the cervical esophagus is usually best through a left neck incision because of its anatomic location.

Opposite the sternal angle and fourth thoracic vertebra, the esophagus is pushed back to the midline by the aorta. The aortic arch lies at the junction of the proximal and middle third of the esophagus, while the distal third passes just behind the heart. Opposite the seventh thoracic vertebra, it once again shifts to the left to pass through the esophageal hiatus in the diaphragm, which is opposite the 10th thoracic vertebra. Here the phrenoesophageal ligament inserts into the circular muscular layer. In addition, fibers from the right crus of the diaphragm pass around the esophagus to form a sling.

Once passing through the diaphragm, the abdominal portion of the esophagus is 2 to 4 cm long. The gastroesophageal junction is opposite the 11th thoracic vertebra, lying within the esophageal groove of the left lobe of the liver.

Although the esophagus is already the narrowest portion of the digestive tract, three areas of further narrowing present along its length, which become important when dealing with foreign body or caustic ingestion.

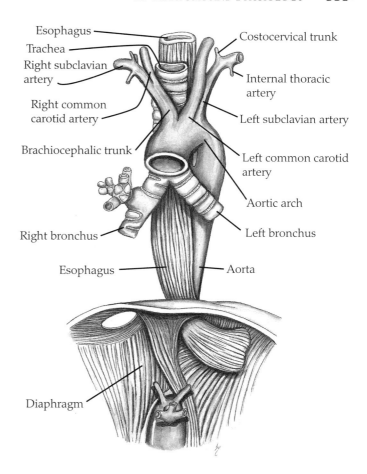

FIGURE 48–1 Gross anatomy of the esophagus.

SPECIAL CONSIDERATION

The esophagus has three areas of anatomic narrowing that become important when confronted with a foreign body or caustic ingestion: (1) the upper esophageal sphincter, corresponding to the cricopharyngeus muscle and cricoid cartilage at 15 to 20 cm from the upper incisors; (2) the anterior compression by the aortic arch and left mainstem bronchus, at 20 to 25 cm from the upper incisors; and (3) the gastroesophageal junction, at 40 to 45 cm from the upper incisors.

ARTERIAL SUPPLY

The blood supply and lymphatic drainage of the esophagus can be broken up into thirds. Blood supply in the upper third is from the inferior thyroid artery off of the thyrocervical trunk on either side. Similarly, venous drainage occurs via the inferior thyroid veins. Lymph nodes of the cervical esophagus drain into the internal jugular chain as well as the paratracheal nodes.

The middle third of the esophagus is supplied with blood by several direct branches from the thoracic aorta, and outflow occurs through venous plexuses along the surface into the hemiazygos vein on the left and the azygos vein on the right, both of which drain into the superior vena cava. Lymph nodes drain into the tracheobronchial and posterior mediastinal nodes.

Blood supply to the lower third of the esophagus is from branches of the left gastric artery, which originates from the celiac trunk off the abdominal aorta. Lower esophageal veins are tributaries of the left gastric vein, but also anastomose with the azygos system. The left gastric vein drains to the portal vein, which passes through the hepatic circulation and into the inferior vena cava. The portal system is essentially valveless, and portal hypertension and hepatic cirrhosis may lead to shunting upward through the esophageal plexus, leading to the development of varicosities. Lymph nodes of the lower esophagus drain into nodes following the left gastric vessels and the celiac nodes.

UPPER ESOPHAGEAL SPHINCTER

The anatomy of the upper esophageal sphincter has been variously described. The inferior constrictor muscle extends from the oblique line of the thyroid cartilage to insert into the posterior midline pharyngeal raphe (Fig. 48–2). This raphe is a fibrous band that extends from the base of the skull to which all of the constrictor muscles are attached. The cricopharyngeus muscle is attached to either side of the cricoid cartilage without a midline raphe, forming a muscular sling.

CONTROVERSY

Some reports consider the cricopharyngeus muscle to have two parts: the pars fundiformus, or transverse portion, which forms the sling, and the pars obliqua, which is continuous with the lower end of the inferior constrictor muscle. Others describe completely separate muscular units, while still other reports describe the cricopharyngeus muscle as actually being the lower portion of the inferior constrictor. The confusion stems largely from disagreement as to the precise physiologic arrangement of the upper esophageal sphincter.

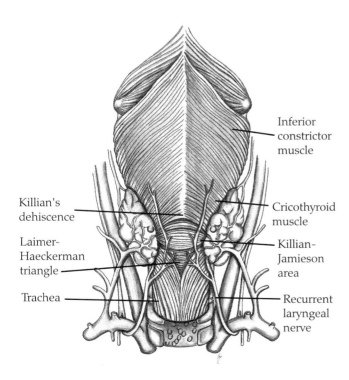

Killian's dehiscence

Laimer-Haeckerman triangle

Trachea

Inferior constrictor muscle

Cricothyroid muscle

Killian-Jamieson area

Recurrent laryngeal nerve

FIGURE 48–2 Posterior pharyngeal segment.

SPECIAL CONSIDERATION

The muscular configuration in the area of the upper esophageal sphincter results in several areas of inherent weakness, where diverticula may potentially develop (Fig. 48–2): *Killian's dehiscence*, or *triangle*, is located between the inferior pharyngeal constrictor muscle and its raphe, and the cricopharyngeus muscle, site of Zenker's diverticulum. The *Laimer-Haeckerman triangle* is located in the upper posterior esophageal wall covered only by the circular muscular fibers. The longitudinal muscle fibers diverge in this area to insert laterally and anteriorly around the esophagus. The *Killian-Jamieson area* is a lateral dehiscence between the cricopharyngeus muscle and circular esophageal fibers through which the recurrent laryngeal nerve passes.

PHYSIOLOGY

The esophagus is a conduit 20 to 25 cm long, capable of propelling almost a limitless variety of food, regardless of posture and opposing thoracic and abdominal pressures. In addition, it prevents reversal of this flow except when emesis becomes necessary. The average adult swallows 600 times per day, 35 times per hour while awake and 6 times per hour while asleep.

SWALLOWING

The swallowing sequence can be divided into three phases.

SPECIAL CONSIDERATION

The oral, or preparatory, phase is under voluntary control; the pharyngeal and esophageal phases are controlled by reflex.

Oral Phase

The oral phase is preparatory, mixing the food with saliva and forming it into an appropriately sized bolus. This is largely under voluntary control and utilizes a variety of functions such as olfaction, gustation, mastication, and salivation. The tongue is then responsible for delivering the bolus into the pharynx, by compressing it against the hard palate. This activity very much depends on the intrinsic musculature of the tongue.

Pharyngeal Phase

Once the bolus passes into the oropharynx, the pharyngeal phase and reflex portion of deglutition begins. Receptors that initiate the reflex appear to be scattered over the base of the tongue, tonsillar pillars and fossa, uvula, and posterior pharyngeal wall. Receptors are also located within the larynx, but probably serve a more protective or backup function, responding more to water than to mechanical stimulation. In addition, some stimuli seem to provoke coughing and gagging rather than swallowing. Although this mechanism is not completely understood, studies seem to indicate that strong stimuli producing higher neuronal firing rates are more likely to yield a gag response.

These receptors belong to the maxillary division of the trigeminal nerve, the glossopharyngeal nerve, and the superior laryngeal nerve. Afferent impulses converge in the tractus solitarius of the brainstem, and then are transmitted to the swallowing center within the reticular substance of the upper medulla. Efferent impulses travel to appropriate cranial nerve nuclei, including V_3, VII, IX, X, and XII, that control ipsilateral deglutitory muscles, except for the middle and inferior pharyngeal constrictor muscles, which are contralaterally innervated. During both the pharyngeal and esophageal phases, other activities such as chewing, breathing, coughing, or vomiting are consequently inhibited.

The pharyngeal phase of swallowing includes four important goals: (1) initiate the swallowing reflex, (2) propel food through the pharynx into the esophagus, (3) protect the airway, and (4) prevent regurgitation into the oral cavity and nasopharynx. Propulsion of the food bolus depends on posterior tongue thrust and pharyngeal persistalsis, and to a lesser degree gravity. Pharyngeal peristalsis begins with apposition of the soft palate against a ridge created by the contracting superior constrictor muscle (Passavant's ridge). The pharyngeal constrictor muscles then fire in overlapping sequence, innervated by the surrounding pharyngeal plexus. The peristaltic wave that is created travels down the pharynx at approximately 15 cm/second, reaching the esophageal inlet in 0.67 seconds, regardless of the nature of the bolus.

Apposition of the tongue to the palate and of the soft palate to the pharyngeal wall prevents regurgitation of food into the mouth or nasopharynx. Protection of the airway is accomplished by glottal closure and laryngeal elevation, both of which occur as the swallowing reflex begins.

Although anatomically there is no clearly defined upper esophageal sphincter, manometrically there is an intraluminal area of elevated pressure centered around the cricopharyngeus muscle, measuring 3 to 5 cm. The cricopharyngeal sling is only 1 cm wide, so that this area of increased pressure most likely incorporates a portion of the lower inferior constrictor muscle and the upper circular muscle fibers of the esophagus. This area remains tonically contracted via vagal stimulation to protect the airway from refluxed gastric contents, but relaxes during swallowing. Manometric studies indicate that a pressure of 10 mm Hg remains after relaxation due to the inherent elasticity of the sphincter. However, this is fully abolished by elevation of the larynx, which serves to dilate this area, thereby facilitating bolus passage into the esophagus.

This period of upper esophageal sphincter relaxation lasts less than 1 second and must be precisely coordinated with pharyngeal contraction. As the peristaltic wave reaches the upper esophageal sphincter, the cricopharyngeus muscle contracts in sequence to carry the wave distally. The esophageal phase then begins.

Esophageal Phase

The primary peristaltic wave travels more slowly in the esophagus, at approximately 3 cm/second, and therefore takes 8 to 12 seconds to reach the gastroesophageal junction. Vagal somatic efferents from the nucleus ambiguus innervate the striated muscles of the esophagus. The smooth muscles receive autonomic innervation via vagal fibers that form a plexus over the body of the esophagus and sympathetic fibers from the cervical and thoracic chains. An intramural network of autonomic fibers (Auerbach's and Meissner's plexuses) provides afferent input that gauges the speed and force of contraction to the nature of the bolus. Thus, unlike the pharynx, a large bolus in the esophagus will precipitate a more forceful contraction, and higher temperatures will accelerate its propagation.

Spontaneous secondary peristalsis may occur seven to ten times per hour and is important for clearing refluxed gastric acid. Tertiary contractions comprise approximately 5% of swallows in normal individuals, but tend to increase with age. They are usually mild in amplitude and can be seen as a ripple effect on a barium swallow. A significant increase in frequency and amplitude of these contractions leads to one of the spastic motility disorders.

SPECIAL CONSIDERATION

Primary esophageal peristalsis is induced by the swallowing reflex; secondary peristalsis occurs in response to esophageal distention, as might occur from a residual bolus or refluxed material, independent of any pharyngeal component; tertiary contractions are nonperistaltic, simultaneous contractions that are therefore nonfunctional.

Similar to the upper esophageal sphincter, the lower esophageal sphincter is not demarcated anatomically, but corresponds to an intraluminal zone of high pressure approximately 3 cm long. It separates the esophagus, which is surrounded by negative intrathoracic pressure, from positive intragastric pressure. However, the lower sphincter is not maintained by tonic neural activity. Rather, sphincter competence depends on (1) the gastroesophageal angle, (2) positive intraabdominal pressure compressing the intraabdominal portion of the esophagus, (3) hormonal activity (gastrin), (4) mucosal rosette caused by redundant folds of gastric mucosa at the gastroesophageal junction, (5) diaphragmatic support from the right crus and phrenoesophageal ligament, and (6) inherent smooth muscle tone within the circular muscle layer.

The lower esophageal sphincter relaxes 2 seconds after initiation of the swallowing reflex and remains so for 8 to 10 seconds. Once reached by the peristaltic wave, it too contracts and returns to normal resting tone after 10 to 15 seconds.

SUGGESTED READINGS

Dobie RA, Pillsbury HC, Postma DS, Lanier B. *Otolaryngologic Approach to Swallowing Disorders.* Washington, DC: AAO-HNS; 1984.

Ellis FH. Upper esophageal sphincter in health and disease. *Surg Clin North Am* 1971;51:553–565.

Goyal RK, Cobb BW. Motility of the pharynx, esophagus, and esophageal sphincters. In: Johnson ER, ed. *Physiology of the Gastrointestinal Tract.* New York: Raven Press; 1981: 359–391.

Hurwitz AC, Duranceau A, Haddad JK. *Disorders of Esophageal Motility.* Philadelphia: WB Saunders; 1979.

Palmer ED. Disorders of the cricopharyngeus muscle: a review. *Gastroenterology* 1978;71: 510–519.

Seiden AM. Esophageal disorders. In: Paparella MM, Shumrick DA, Gluckman JL, Meyeroff WL, eds. *Otolaryngology.* 3rd ed. Philadelphia: WB Saunders; 1991:2439–2481.

Chapter 49

CLINICAL TESTS

Allen M. Seiden

Although the clinical history is certainly important, symptoms related to esophageal disease can be very nonspecific. For example, patients presenting with esophageal dysphagia will often localize their problem above the sternal notch. As such they will often present to an otolaryngologist, who must then consider the need for further objective testing. This chapter reviews the various testing methods available to evaluate the esophagus. Essentially these tests can be divided into imaging techniques and intubation procedures.

IMAGING TECHNIQUES

BARIUM ESOPHAGRAM

Traditionally, the most accessible technique for examining the esophagus has been the barium swallow. The patient is placed in a horizontal position to eliminate the effect of gravity, and swallows a large amount of barium. Spot films are then taken under fluoroscopic control. This approach readily demonstrates any intraluminal or extraluminal process that grossly distorts the contour of the esophagus, such as a large carcinoma or stricture. In fact, careful fluoroscopy is reported to be the most sensitive test for a fixed

structural stenosis of the esophagus provided maximal distention is achieved, whereas endoscopy can miss up to 42% of lower esophageal rings.

In addition, fluoroscopic observation of multiple, single swallows of barium may accurately assess esophageal motility, and has been shown to have a high correlation with manometry. In fact, recent studies suggest that radiologic examination has better than a 90% sensitivity for detecting abnormal motility.

> **PITFALLS...** A normal barium swallow does not exclude an esophageal motor defect. On the other hand, false-positive and false-negative diagnoses for esophageal carcinoma as high as 21% and 37%, respectively, have been reported.

To enhance the detection of subtle mucosal defects, the double-contrast technique is used. The patient is in the upright position, and is given both an effervescent agent and high-density barium. This serves to distend the esophagus and coat the mucosal epithelium, and can detect small ulcers, esophagitis, and early carcinoma.

SPECIAL CONSIDERATION

When used to confirm an esophageal perforation, the barium study should be performed with a water-soluble contrast material such as meglumine diatrizoate (Gastrografin). Conversely, patients suspected of aspiration should be given thin suspensions of barium, because the water-soluble materials are more irritating to the tracheobronchial tree.

It is generally agreed that a barium study is not very sensitive for the detection of gastroesophageal reflux. The brief period of time that the test entails simply does not allow useful diagnostic information in this regard. Even the presence of a hiatal hernia, while it may be associated with reflux, is not diagnostic.

PEARL... A modified barium swallow utilizes varying consistencies and quantities of barium to functionally evaluate the oral and pharyngeal phases of swallowing. Input from a speech pathologist is often helpful. A solid bolus, such as a barium tablet or a barium-impregnated marshmallow, can be used to aid in the detection of various structural esophageal abnormalities.

Various provocative maneuvers that can be used during a barium study to elicit more diagnostic information include the administration of acid barium (90% of patients with reflux esophagitis will demonstrate abnormal esophageal motility during this maneuver), test feeding techniques, bolus modification, and altering patient position.

COMPUTED TOMOGRAPHY (CT) AND MAGNETIC RESONANCE IMAGING (MRI)

The use of CT and MRI for evaluating esophageal disease has revolved largely around the pretreatment staging of esophageal carcinoma.

Otherwise, such tests are rarely indicated in the initial workup of esophageal disease.

RADIONUCLIDE SCINTIGRAPHY

Esophageal scintigraphy was first introduced in 1972 in an attempt to provide a noninvasive, quantitative measurement of esophageal transit. The patient is given 15 mL of water mixed with technetium (Tc) 99m-sulfur colloid in a single swallow, and then swallows at 15-second intervals for 10 minutes. Counts are recorded by a gamma camera and processed by computer. In some cases, the radioisotope may be bound to specific foods.

Esophageal transit time is determined by the amplitude of and coordination between esophageal contractions. Transit is delayed when contractions are nonperistaltic, such as in diffuse esophageal spasm (DES), where repetitive retrograde-antegrade movement of the bolus can be seen. Other major esophageal motility disorders, such as achalasia and scleroderma, can be readily detected because of bolus retention.

PITFALLS... Other less severe motility disorders may be more difficult to detect. For example, although nutcracker esophagus is associated with prolonged and high-amplitude contractions, peristaltic activity is maintained and radionuclide transit time may be normal. Similarly, nonspecific esophageal motility disorder (NSEMD), a relatively common problem, is frequently missed by esophageal scintigraphy alone.

SPECIAL CONSIDERATION

Esophageal scintigraphy provides no anatomic information, and this along with its relative insensitivity precludes it from being a first-line test in the evaluation of dysphagia. Its primary advantage is in providing quantitative information that may be used to gauge response to therapeutic intervention. It may also be useful when manometry is either unavailable or its findings equivocal.

Radionuclide scintigraphy has been utilized to diagnose gastroesophageal reflux but relies upon provocative maneuvers and is not considered to be as definitive as 24-hour intraesophageal pH monitoring. However, it may be useful in patients who remain symptomatic despite being on suppressive medications. In such cases, if the gastric pH is buffered to above 4, reflux events would not be detected by an esophageal pH probe, whereas scintigraphy records volume of refluxed material. Gastroesophageal reflux scintigraphy has also been described in pediatric patients to investigate reflux in relation to pulmonary disorders, vomiting, and failure to thrive, and to determine patients at risk for sudden infant death.

INTUBATION PROCEDURES

MANOMETRY

Esophageal manometry is primarily used to assess peristaltic activity within the body of the esophagus, and lower esophageal sphincter (LES) pressure and relaxation. Some information regarding relaxation of the upper esophageal sphincter (UES) may also be generated.

Intraluminal pressure measurements are made by a series of pressure-sensitive transducers that may be of two designs. A water-perfused multilumen catheter is connected to external volume displacement pressure transducers, recording pressure based on relative obstruction to flow of water through the side holes of the catheter. The advantage of this system is its relatively low cost. Disadvantages are the need for skilled personnel to maintain the equipment and its inability to accurately record pharyngeal pressures. The other system places small strain gauge transducers at fixed points directly on the manometric catheter. This system has an enhanced frequency response and is less cumbersome; however, it is very expensive and fragile and is a less flexible system to use.

Due to laryngeal elevation and peristaltic activity, both the UES and LES move upward approximately 2 to 3 cm during swallowing relative to the manometric probe. Therefore, to achieve accurate recording of sphincter pressure, a sleeve sensor that can span the sphincter is currently the most effective technique. This sensor utilizes a 6-cm silicone membrane under which water is perfused, and pressure changes anywhere along the membrane are recorded. This device can only be incorporated with the water-perfused system. It is not sensitive to radial pressure asymmetry that occurs within the UES due to the laryngeal cartilages, making UES pressure measurements very difficult to evaluate.

In the clinical setting, esophageal manometry is used to determine whether primary peristalsis is weak, absent, or disordered, and whether LES relaxation is impaired. Such findings are sensitive for detecting esophageal motor disturbances, but are nonspecific.

SPECIAL CONSIDERATION

The American Gastroenterological Association advocates the use of manometry to establish the diagnosis of achalasia or diffuse esophageal spasm, or to detect esophageal motor abnormalities associated with systemic diseases. However, more common disorders should first be excluded with barium study or endoscopy.

It has been suggested that defects of secondary peristalsis occur more frequently than those of primary peristalsis in patients with unexplained dysphagia or reflux disease. In many cases the primary peristaltic wave travels too fast to completely carry a solid bolus all the way to the stomach. Secondary peristalsis, responding to esophageal distention, must finish the job. Secondary peristalsis can be tested by using air insufflation or balloon distention along with manometry.

INTRALUMINAL pH STUDIES

Esophageal pH monitoring is considered the gold standard for detecting clinically significant gastroesophageal reflux. Spontaneous reflux events and the duration of esophageal acid exposure are recorded. A reflux event is defined as a drop in esophageal pH below 4, the level considered clinically relevant because heartburn generally occurs below this point. Whereas some reflux naturally occurs, approximately 2% of the time while a person is upright and 0.3% while supine, the normal esophagus will quickly rid itself of this material and be able to maintain esophageal pH between 6 and 7.

Ambulatory pH monitoring is usually performed over a 24-hour period, thus providing more comprehensive and reproducible information. Patients must stop all histamine receptor antagonists at least 24 hours before the study and proton pump inhibitors 72 hours before the study. In some cases the drugs may be continued if the test is being utilized to evaluate their efficacy.

The electrode is generally positioned 5 cm above the proximal border of the LES. In patients with respiratory or aerodigestive symptoms thought to relate to reflux, it may be helpful to record from the proximal esophagus, placing the electrode just below the UES. During the test, patients are encouraged to continue normal activity but to avoid eating particularly acidic foods. It is very important that they maintain an accurate diary as to timing of meals, sleep, and symptoms.

> **PEARL...** Most reflux occurs during the day, and the magnitude of daytime reflux appears to correlate with the severity of esophagitis.

The most widely used parameter, and the one most consistent with a diagnosis of esophagitis, is the percentage of time that esophageal pH is below 4. The total duration of esophageal acid exposure in normal subjects generally does not exceed 7% for a 24-hour period. The number of reflux episodes has not been found to be a reliable indicator; however, the percentage of reflux episodes associated with symptoms is referred to as the symptom sensitivity index and is considered positive if over 50%.

> **PITFALL...** Intraluminal pH measurements are very much dependent on equipment and technique. Studies of accuracy demonstrate reproducibility ranging from 75 to 86%.

Patients with symptoms suggestive of gastroesophageal reflux may appropriately be given a trial of medical therapy prior to investigational tests. Endoscopy is considered to be the most sensitive in making the diagnosis and assessing its severity. Patients who continue to have symptoms despite medical therapy and negative endoscopy should be considered for pH monitoring, as well as those patients with atypical symptoms. In addition, this test is helpful to assess the adequacy of therapy.

The acid infusion or Bernstein test is an attempt to reproduce the patient's symptoms by infusing 0.1 N hydrochloric acid directly into the distal esophagus. The acid clearance test measures the patient's ability to bring esophageal pH back to normal following an acid infusion, a prolonged clearance time being indicative of esophagitis.

ENDOSCOPY

Esophagoscopy is the best method for assessing mucosal integrity, inflammation, and malignancy of the esophagus, and provides access for direct tissue examination. Patients with persistent symptoms, such as dysphagia, the cause of which has not been determined by other means, should be considered for endoscopic examination. In many instances when the diagnosis is established, endoscopy will be necessary for a full evaluation. Disorders that have been associated with malignant degeneration, such as Barrett's epithelium, lye stricture, achalasia, or the Plummer-Vinson syndrome, should be considered for regular endoscopic follow-up.

When a motility disorder is suspected, endoscopy is not very helpful. Peristaltic contractions and sphincter competence are not easily visualized. On the other hand, if complications such as reflux esophagitis and stricture secondary to scleroderma were to occur, or if the clinical picture were atypical, then direct visualization may add useful information.

Gastroenterologists generally prefer flexible fiberoptic instruments that allow better optics, air insufflation for distention, and better access to the distal esophagus. Otolaryngologists are usually trained with rigid telescopes that allow better facility for instrumentation and provide a more accurate view of the esophageal inlet and postcricoid area.

SUGGESTED READINGS

American Gastroenterological Association. Medical position statement on the clinical use of esophageal manometry. *Gastroenterology* 1994; 107:1865.

Dent J, Holloway RH. Esophageal motility and reflux testing: state-of-the-art and clinical role in the twenty-first century. *Gastroenterol Clin North Am* 1996;25:51–73.

Grishaw EK, Ott DJ, Frederick MG, et al. Functional abnormalities of the esophagus: a prospective analysis of radiographic findings relative to age and symptoms. *Am J Radiol* 1996;167:719–723.

Kahrilas PJ, Clouse RE, Hogan WJ. American Gastroenterological Association technical review on the clinical use of esophageal manometry. *Gastroenterology* 1994;107:1865–1884.

Klein HA. Esophageal transit scintigraphy. *Semin Nucl Med* 1995;25:306–317.

Parkman HP, Miller MA, Fisher RS. Role of nuclear medicine in evaluating patients with suspected gastrointestinal motility disorders. *Semin Nucl Med* 1995;25:289–305.

Seiden AM. Esophageal disorders. In: Paparella MM, Shumrick DA, Gluckman JL, Meyerhoff WL, eds. *Otolaryngology.* 3rd ed. Philadelphia: WB Saunders, 1991;2439–2481.

Chapter 50

CONGENITAL DISORDERS

Allen M. Seiden

Most congenital malformations of the esophagus manifest early in life due to associated feeding or respiratory difficulties. Occasionally, more subtle abnormalities are not recognized until later childhood. An accurate diagnosis can be elusive and requires familiarity with the clinical presentation of these disorders and the most appropriate diagnostic tests.

Major anomalies generally occur between the third and sixth weeks of gestation, usually as a result of faulty separation of the esophagus from the trachea or from faulty recannulation of the esophageal lumen. The former leads to various types of fistulous tracts, whereas the latter yields various degrees of closure from web formation and stricture to atresia.

ESOPHAGEAL ATRESIA AND TRACHEOESOPHAGEAL FISTULA

Esophageal atresia, with or without tracheoesophageal fistula, is the most common congenital esophageal anomaly, occurring once in every 3000 to 5000 live births. A gestational history of hydramnios has been frequently reported in these patients, as well as prematurity. Although a variety of classification schemes have been described, the specific abnormalities are best remembered by their anatomic descriptions.

Esophageal atresia with a distal tracheoesophageal fistula occurs most often, accounting for 86% of these cases (Fig. 50–1). With this anomaly, infants tend to aspirate as fluids pool within the esophageal atretic sac during feeding. Between feedings, excessive drooling occurs, and the stomach frequently becomes distended with air. Regurgitation of gastric contents through the fistula may lead to recurrent pneumonias.

Atresia without associated fistula is the second most commonly encountered anomaly (7.7%), and is characterized by similar symptoms. Therefore, the distinction may need to be made radiographically. An isolated tracheoesophageal fistula without atresia (4.2%) may present with a fistula anywhere between the cricoid and tracheal bifurcation. Because the continuity of both the trachea and the esophagus is intact, these patients may have minimal symptoms and the abnormality may go undetected for months or years. Regurgitation during feeding may cause flow through the fistula into the trachea, causing paroxysmal coughing, choking, and perhaps subsequent pneumonia. Unexplained periods of abdominal distention may also occur.

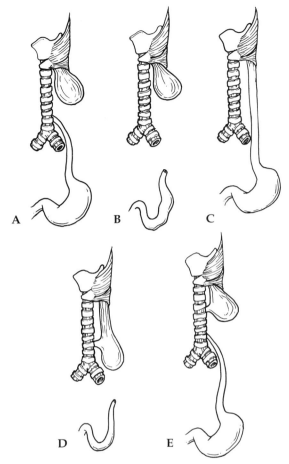

FIGURE 50–1 The most common types of combined esophageal atresia (EA), in descending order of frequency. (A). EA with distal tracheoesophageal fistula (TEF) (86.5%). (B). Isolated EA (7.7%). (C). Isolated TEF (4.2%). (D). EA with proximal TEF (0.8%). (E). EA with double TEF (0.7%).

PEARL••• Recurrent pneumonia unresponsive to antibiotic therapy should suggest the possibility of an underlying tracheoesophageal fistula.

Early diagnosis can be made if a soft 8- or 10-French catheter cannot be passed to the stomach. Such a maneuver should be considered in the newborn with excessive mucus or signs of respiratory distress, although some would recommend this procedure be performed routinely.

PITFALL••• Coiling of the tube within the atretic esophageal segment may create the false impression of successful passage into the stomach. Coiling of the tube can be demonstrated on chest X-ray and is pathognomonic for esophageal atresia. (Fig. 50–2).

Also on chest X-ray, the presence or absence of air in the stomach indicates the presence or absence, respectively, of a distal tracheoesophageal fistula.

If necessary, barium contrast can be used to confirm the diagnosis. Such procedures must be performed with great caution because of the propensity for aspiration; 0.5 mL of thin barium should be used.

PITFALL••• Water-soluble contrast media need to be avoided, as they will cause a fulminant pneumonitis if aspirated.

Up to 48% of these patients have been described as having other associated anomalies, particularly cardiovascular or gastrointestinal, and this will certainly impact their management. Therefore, a thorough search for such anomalies must be made.

Therapy initially needs to be supportive. To prevent respiratory complications, regular suctioning of the esophageal pouch is performed to prevent aspiration, and prophylactic antibiotics are provided. To maintain adequate nutritional support, a gastrostomy will be necessary. This also allows gastric decompression, which helps prevent further pulmonary compromise and helps to avoid gastric reflux.

Surgical correction should be scheduled as soon as the child's condition allows. Definitive repair includes division and closure of the fistula and direct esophageal anastomosis. In 15% of infants with esophageal atresia, the gap between the segments will be too long to close primarily, and an interposition graft such as colon will be needed. Esophageal stricture is the most common postoperative complication. The sudden appearance of choking or pneumonia

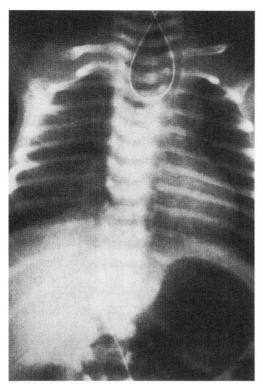

FIGURE 50-2 Nasogastric tube coiled in blind upper esophageal atretic pouch, pathognomonic for EA. (From Ein SH, Friedberg J. Esophageal atresia and tracheoesophageal fistula: review and update. *Otolaryngol Clin North Am* 1981;14:221. Reprinted by permission of the publisher.)

after surgery may indicate the recurrence of the tracheoesophageal fistula. Survival has improved with earlier detection and better perioperative care, and is reported to be between 75 and 82%. Survival usually depends on any associated congenital anomalies and the severity of associated pulmonary disease.

ESOPHAGEAL STENOSIS

This is the least common congenital tracheoesophageal anomaly, occurring once in every 25,000 live births. It also seems to result from faulty separation of the trachea and esophagus. Unlike tracheoesophageal fistula and atresia, stenosis is often not diagnosed until later childhood or even adulthood. Symptoms include dysphagia, regurgitation, prolonged eating time, and recurrent solid bolus impaction.

> **PEARL...** A barium esophagram generally best demonstrates the stenosis, usually within the middle third of the esophagus. Treatment involves either dilatation or segmental resection.

DUPLICATIONS

The ileum is the most common site for duplication of the gastrointestinal tract to occur; the esophagus is the second most common and accounts for 15% of cases. The cause is uncertain but most likely relates to failure of recanalization of the esophageal lumen. During embryonic development, the esophageal lumen is formed by the development of scattered vacuoles that ultimately coalesce. If one or more of these vacuoles fails to join the lumen, it may remain as an isolated cyst attached to the esophageal wall.

Esophageal duplications may be tubular or more commonly cystic, and may or may not communicate with the esophageal lumen. They occur within the wall of the esophagus and are surrounded by two layers of smooth muscle. They are the second most common benign esophageal tumor, leiomyoma being the most

> **SPECIAL CONSIDERATION**
>
> Lining epithelium may be squamous, respiratory, intestinal, or mixed. The presence of a secretory epithelium may cause cystic expansion with compression of surrounding structures, and this usually accounts for presenting symptoms. Esophageal compression may cause dysphagia or regurgitation. Tracheal compression may cause dyspnea, stridor, cough, and pneumonia. A lining of gastric epithelium may cause acid secretions that can lead to ulceration, bleeding, and perforation. Occasionally mild lesions remain asymptomatic for many years and are only detected incidentally on a later chest X-ray.

common; 60% occur in or along the lower third of the esophagus, 23% occur in the upper third, and 17% occur in the middle third. There is a high incidence of associated vertebral abnormalities, as occurs with other foregut anomalies.

The diagnosis is usually made radiographically, demonstrating either a cystic mass in the posterior mediastinum or a barium-filled tubular duplication. Endoscopy usually demonstrates only extraesophageal compression, and as such is not diagnostic. The preferred treatment is surgical excision.

DYSPHAGIA LUSORIA

This term refers to dysphagia resulting from compression of the esophagus by an aberrant right subclavian artery, a fourth branchial arch anomaly. Rather than passing ventral to the trachea, the artery passes obliquely upward behind the esophagus after arising from the descending aorta. In 15% of cases it passes between the esophagus and trachea. Although other anomalies of the great vessels within the superior mediastinum may occur to cause dysphagia, this is by far the most common.

The incidence of this abnormality is relatively low. Estimates suggest 3% of the population have a congenital abnormality of the aortic arch vessels, and 1% have an aberrant right subclavian artery, but only 10% of these patients develop compressive symptoms. There is a higher incidence in association with congenital heart disease.

In severe cases, the infant may display dysphagia from birth, with regurgitation and aspiration. However, more often symptoms present later as the diet begins to incorporate solid food. Signs of tracheal compression may also appear, with episodes of stridor and cyanosis.

> **PEARL...** Symptoms of tracheal compression secondary to an aberrant subclavian artery will typically improve when the head is hyperextended.

The diagnosis of dysphagia lusoria is best made on barium swallow, demonstrating an in-

dentation of the posterior esophageal wall near the level of the aortic arch at the third and fourth thoracic vertebrae. Endoscopy may serve to exclude other causes, at the same time often revealing a pulsatile nature to the compression.

> **PEARL...** Applying pressure with the tip of the endoscope to the area of compression will tend to obliterate the right radial pulse.

Angiographic confirmation is usually not necessary unless surgery is required, and this may be the case if significant aspiration occurs or nutritional intake is inadequate. Surgery involves ligating the aberrant subclavian artery in the presence of adequate collateral circulation, or reanastomosis to the ascending aorta.

CHALASIA

Chalasia refers to an incompetent lower esophageal sphincter without the presence of a hiatal hernia, thus resulting in persistent reflux. Most healthy infants occasionally regurgitate small amounts of food or formula, and some esophageal reflux may be seen after a barium meal in as many as 25% of infants.

> **CONTROVERSY**
>
> Some consider chalasia in infants simply a normal phenomenon rather than a true disease entity.

Typically these infants show persistent regurgitation and vomiting within the first week of life, particularly in the supine position. The infant may feed more normally in the upright position. In severe cases the infant demonstrates poor weight gain.

A barium study is diagnostic, demonstrating free reflux of barium into a dilated esophagus. Motility studies show a patulous lower esophageal sphincter.

The abnormality usually disappears by 6 weeks of age, until which time the infant will need to be fed sitting up. Frequent, thickened feedings should be initiated. Significant reflux needs to be treated aggressively to avoid complications such as esophagitis and stricture. The problem has also been linked to respiratory arrest and sudden infant death syndrome.

Studies for gastroesophageal reflux should be considered in any child with symptoms of recurrent or chronic pulmonary disease, anemia, or failure to thrive. Once reflux has been demonstrated, esophagoscopy is usually indicated.

SUGGESTED READINGS

Adkins JC. Congenital malformations of the esophagus. In: Bluestone CD, Stool SE, eds. *Pediatric Otolaryngology.* 2nd ed. Philadelphia: WB Saunders, 1990:973–984.

Boyce GA, Boyce HW. Esophagus: anatomy and structural anomalies. In: Yamada T, ed. *Gastroenterology.* Philadelphia: JB Lippincott, 1995: 1156–1174.

German JC, Mahour GH, Woodley MM. Esophageal atresia and associated anomalies. *J Pediatr Surg* 1976;11:299–306.

Jafek BW, Berney JL, Spoffard BT. Congenital esophageal disorders. *Ear Nose Throat J* 1984; 63:43–54.

Seiden AM. Esophageal disorders. In: Paparella MM, Shumrick DA, Gluckman JL, Meyerhoff WL, eds. *Otolaryngology.* 3rd ed. Philadelphia: WB Saunders, 1991;2439–2481.

Chapter 51

FUNCTIONAL DISORDERS

Allen M. Seiden

Proper esophageal function relies on proper timing and strength of muscle contraction to generate effective peristalsis. Broadly stated, a failure of esophageal transfer can usually be attributed to one of two problems: (1) a motility disorder, characterized as a failure of peristalsis or sphincter function, or both; or (2) a structural defect that causes obstruction.

The primary symptoms associated with esophageal motility disorders include dysphagia, heartburn, regurgitation, and chest pain.

> **PEARL...** Dysphagia secondary to esophageal dysmotility tends to be intermittent, progresses very slowly if at all, and occurs with both liquids and solids right from the outset. On the other hand, obstructive disorders tend to produce constant and progressive dysphagia, beginning first with solids and then progressing to liquids as the disease worsens.

Esophageal motility disorders are a frequent cause of noncardiac chest pain. High-pressure nonperistaltic contractions may produce episodic chest pain that may be severe enough to simulate the pain of myocardial infarction. Symptoms that may distinguish an esophageal etiology include other related symptoms, such as heartburn, dysphagia, chest pain

associated with the ingestion of hot or cold foods, and pain relief with antacids.

In addition to dysphagia, globus pharyngis is a common complaint in patients presenting to the otolaryngologist. The etiology of this complaint remains controversial and is probably multifactorial.

> **CONTROVERSY**
>
> Farkkila (1994) found a local pathologic reason for globus symptoms in only 6% of patients, whereas evidence of gastroesophageal reflux was found in 24% and abnormal esophageal motility in 67%. Other studies have both supported and refuted these findings, but such diagnoses need to be carefully considered in patients presenting with globus symptoms.

It is important to note that functional abnormalities of the esophagus tend to increase with age. That is, older individuals will have a higher incidence of nonperistaltic contractions and incomplete peristalsis. Such findings may be incidental and not associated with true symptoms. Therefore, clinical correlation becomes important.

Esophageal motility disorders are classified as either primary, affecting just the esophagus, or secondary, in which esophageal dysfunction is part of a systemic illness or specific injury.

Primary Motility Disorders

Achalasia

Achalasia is characterized by incomplete relaxation of the lower esophageal sphincter (LES) with absent esophageal peristalsis, leading to stasis and esophageal dilatation. It is one of the most common of the primary motor disorders and appears to relate to degenerative changes within the dorsal vagal nucleus, vagal trunks, and myenteric ganglia of the esophagus.

Dysphagia is the most prevalent symptom, usually slowly progressive over a number of years. Patients will often point to the xiphoid as the point of obstruction. Retained material within the esophagus may cause halitosis, and subsequent regurgitation may lead to chronic aspiration with resulting chronic bronchitis or recurrent pneumonia.

In advanced cases a plain chest X-ray may reveal an air-fluid level in a dilated esophagus. However, the diagnosis is best made with a barium study that will classically show marked esophageal dilatation tapering to a so-called bird's beak deformity or narrowing at the LES. Manometry may be used to confirm the diagnosis, demonstrating high resting pressure of the LES, usually more than 35 mm Hg above gastric pressure with failure of relaxation during swallowing.

SPECIAL CONSIDERATION

Endoscopy should be performed in all patients believed to have achalasia to rule out the possibility of an underlying malignancy or benign stricture. Long-standing achalasia has been associated with a 5 to 10% incidence of secondary carcinoma, which should be suspected in patients also complaining of odynophagia and chest pain.

Therapy has centered primarily around decreasing lower esophageal sphincter pressure, either by forceful balloon dilatation or surgical myotomy (Heller procedure). Both approaches reportedly achieve similar results, with 80 to 90% of patients reporting satisfactory swallows provided the LES pressure is brought below 10 mm Hg.

Diffuse Esophageal Spasm

Diffuse esophageal spasm (DES) is characterized by repetitive, nonperistaltic, high amplitude contractions of the smooth muscle portion of the esophagus that are associated with more than 30% of swallows. The proximal striated portion and LES generally maintain normal function.

Similar to achalasia, there appear to be degenerative changes in esophageal branches of the vagus nerve, along with muscular hypertrophy. In fact, it has been suggested that DES and achalasia may be part of the same spectrum of abnormal esophageal motility, related to varying degrees of neurogenic damage to the esophagus.

The prevailing symptoms are substernal chest pain and dysphagia. The pain may radiate to the arms and back, and may occur with or without swallowing, thereby often simulating cardiogenic pain. However, there should be no exertional pain, and the occasional relationship with swallowing along with associated dysphagia help in the diagnosis. Frequent precipitating factors include the ingestion of hot or cold liquids, gastroesophageal reflux, and emotional stress.

A barium esophagram demonstrates segmentation of the barium column in the distal two-thirds of the esophagus due to the simultaneous contractions, producing a so-called corkscrew or rosary-bead appearance. Manometry demonstrates prolonged, high-amplitude nonperistaltic or tertiary contractions.

Treatment begins by avoiding factors that trigger symptoms and controlling any associated gastroesophageal reflux. Clinical improvement has been reported with sublingual nitroglycerin for acute attacks and longer acting nitrates for prophylaxis. Patients who are incapacitated and do not respond to conservative therapy may be candidates for surgical myotomy, to include the entire smooth muscle portion of the esophagus.

NUTCRACKER ESOPHAGUS

This disorder is characterized by high-amplitude esophageal contractions that produce chest pain and dysphagia. However, in contrast to DES, the contractions remain peristaltic.

A barium esophagram is often normal or may demonstrate some nonspecific tertiary contractions. Esophageal transit will also usually be normal. On the other hand, while manometry will indicate normal peristalsis, distal peristaltic pressure amplitudes will exceed 180 mm Hg. Normal mean distal esophageal pressure amplitude is 100 mm Hg.

Treatment is generally aimed at reducing the amplitude of peristaltic contractions, and therefore smooth muscle relaxants and calcium channel blockers have been tried but with only mixed results. There seems to be a poor correlation between reduction of contraction amplitude and resolution of chest pain, and recent studies suggest a high incidence of gastroesophageal reflux in these patients. Omeprazole or ranitidine was effective in alleviating the chest pain in many cases.

NONSPECIFIC MOTILITY DISORDER

Not uncommonly, patients may present with dysphagia and chest pain and will be noted to have abnormal esophageal motility, yet not characteristic of any of the preceding disorders. Manometric findings are generally nonspecific but include intermittent absence of peristalsis on 20% or more of swallows, low-amplitude contractions, and prolonged or repetitive contractions.

The severity of these findings will vary and, in fact, may be incidental as many of these patients are asymptomatic. Therefore, clinical correlation is important, and treatment needs to be individualized based on symptoms. A barium study may demonstrate disruption of primary peristalsis and nonperistaltic contractions. Many of these patients have associated gastroesophageal reflux, the correction of which may alleviate the underlying dysmotility.

SECONDARY MOTILITY DISORDERS

COLLAGEN VASCULAR DISEASES

The collagen vascular diseases include a number of inflammatory disorders that tend to have multisystem involvement, and while it may be unusual for dysphagia to be the presenting symptom, significant functional impairment of the esophagus may be present during the later stages of disease. Esophageal involvement is seen most often with scleroderma, polymyositis, and dermatomyositis.

SPECIAL CONSIDERATION

Approximately 80% of patients with scleroderma have head and neck manifestations, and 52% report some type of dysphagia as a primary symptom. Esophageal involvement is found in 75 to 90%.

Scleroderma is characterized by a generalized small vessel arteritis with excessive collagen deposition. Raynaud's phenomenon is closely correlated with esophageal involvement. While the proximal striated portion of the esophagus remains normal, smooth muscle atrophy and collagen deposition within the submucosa of the distal esophagus have been found. The result is aperistalsis within the distal esophagus.

A decrease in LES pressure allows significant reflux to occur, while distal aperistalsis prevents the esophagus from clearing the acid. This leads to severe esophagitis and ultimately to complications such as stricture.

SPECIAL CONSIDERATION

Lower esophageal stricture has been found in as many as 48% of patients with scleroderma. This compares to 11% in patients with idiopathic reflux.

Therefore, dysphagia may be due to abnormal motility, reflux esophagitis, or stricture. A barium esophagram typically shows diminished peristalsis or tertiary contractions of the distal two-thirds of the esophagus with a patulous LES. In more advanced cases, a stricture with proximal esophageal distention may be noted. Endoscopy is usually indicated to assess the severity of esophagitis and to rule out the possibility of malignancy.

OTHER SECONDARY MOTILITY DISORDERS

A number of metabolic and endocrine disorders, as well as various neuromuscular diseases, may affect esophageal motility. Both diabetes and alcoholism can produce a peripheral neuropathy that may result in disordered peristalsis.

Presbyesophagus is the term used to describe esophageal dysmotility that occurs with aging. However, the findings are very similar to those in *nonspecific motility disorder,* and this now is the preferred term. Clinically significant esophageal dysfunction as a consequence of age alone is rare.

SUGGESTED READINGS

Bak YT, Lorang M, Evans PR, et al. Predictive value of symptom profiles in patients with suspected oesophageal dysmotility. *Scand J Gastroenterol* 1994;29:392–397.

Farkkila MA, Ertama L, Katila H, et al. Globus pharyngis, commonly associated with esophageal motility disorders. *Am J Gastroenterol* 1994;89:503–508.

Grishaw EK, Ott DJ, Frederick MG, et al. Functional abnormalities of the esophagus: a prospective analysis of radiographic findings relative to age and symptoms. *Am J Radiol* 1996;167:719–723.

Ott DJ. Motility disorders of the esophagus. *Radiol Clin North Am* 1994;32:1117–1134.

Patti MG, Pellegrini CA, Arcerito M, et al. Comparison of medical and minimally invasive surgical therapy for primary esophageal motility disorders. *Arch Surg* 1995;130:609–616.

Seiden AM. Esophageal disorders. In: Paparella MM, Shumrick DA, Gluckman JL, Meyerhoff WL, eds. *Otolaryngology.* 3rd ed. Philadelphia: WB Saunders; 1991:2439–2481.

Chapter 52

INFECTIOUS AND INFLAMMATORY DISORDERS

Allen M. Seiden

Infection or inflammation of the esophagus typically produces dysphagia and odynophagia, so these patients may frequently present to the otolaryngologist. Physical findings are often lacking, and therefore diagnosis often depends on a thorough history and an understanding of the epidemiology of these disorders.

> **PEARL...** One recent study found that esophageal candidiasis was the most common cause of dysphagia and odynophagia in a series of patients with AIDS, while estimates suggest that 75% of AIDS patients will have symptoms attributable to esophageal infection at some time during the course of their disease.

INFECTIOUS ESOPHAGITIS

In an otherwise immunocompetent individual, primary esophageal infection is rare without some predisposing factor. Typically this involves a disruption of normal esophageal defenses. For example, impaired peristalsis may lead to stasis of esophageal contents, providing a milieu for pathogenic infection. Conditions that may alter peristalsis include diabetes, scleroderma, and achalasia. The use of antimicrobial agents may alter the normal esophageal flora and allow colonization by pathogenic organisms, most frequently *Candida* species.

More often esophageal infection is seen in patients who are immunocompromised, such as those with cancer, AIDS, or posttransplant immunosuppression. The incidence of infectious esophagitis in patients with cancer ranges from 2.8 to 13%, those with myeloproliferative disorders being at greater risk.

FUNGAL INFECTION

The most common fungal infection of the esophagus is caused by *Candida albicans*, typically as a result of antibiotic therapy suppressing bacterial commensals, immunosuppression, or the development of hematologic malignancies. Symptoms may range from mild dysphagia to refusing all oral intake because of associated pain. The dysphagia tends to be more pronounced after ingesting solids rather than liquids. Although manifestations of oral thrush may aid in the diagnosis, many of these patients have fungal infection limited to the esophagus.

> **PITFALL...** The absence of oral lesions does not rule out the possibility of esophageal candidiasis.

The diagnosis should be suspected in any high-risk patient complaining of dysphagia or odynophagia and can be verified by either barium swallow or endoscopy.

> **PITFALL...** In esophageal candidiasis, a barium swallow classically demonstrates a so-called shaggy or cobblestone appearance due to diffuse mucosal inflammation and ulceration. However, focal lesions have also been described. A false-negative rate of 25% has been reported.

Endoscopy is the most sensitive diagnostic technique and generally reveals raised white plaques with or without ulceration. Brushings may be obtained from these lesions.

Oral imidazole derivatives such as fluconazole or ketoconazole generally provide effective treatment and are preferred over nystatin suspension. Amphotericin B is rarely necessary and is reserved for those patients who otherwise don't respond to less toxic therapy. If possible, it is also desirable to correct any predisposing factors.

Although less common, esophagitis may also occur secondary to aspergillosis, histoplasmosis, and blastomycosis.

VIRAL INFECTION

Second to *Candida* species, the most common organism causing esophagitis is herpes simplex virus type I (HSV-1). Although it is more common in immunocompromised patients or those with predisposing factors, it may also occur in otherwise healthy individuals.

HSV-1 esophagitis generally starts as a cluster of vesicles within the lower third of the esophagus. In immunocompromised patients these lesions may progress to a diffuse ulcerative esophagitis. Patients typically present with extremely severe pain with swallowing. Labial herpes may precede or coincide with the esophageal infection. In immunocompetent patients the infection usually resolves within 2 weeks, whereas in those patients who are immuno-

compromised the disease may progress to severe hemorrhage, perforation, or dissemination.

A barium esophagram may demonstrate focal areas of ulceration in the distal esophagus, or, if the infection is more diffuse, it may look very much like *Candida* esophagitis as described above. Endoscopy enables the collection of brushings or biopsy material for culture and characteristically will reveal discrete, punched-out ulcers. Therapy is with acyclovir, while at the same time maintaining adequate hydration.

BACTERIAL INFECTION

Bacterial infection of the esophagus accounts for approximately 10 to 15% of cases of infectious esophagitis. It seems to largely reflect colonization after esophageal injury, for example, from nasogastric tubes, radiation therapy, or gastroesophageal reflux, and once again tends to occur in immunocompromised patients. Organisms are generally consistent with oral flora; however, therapy should be culture directed.

GASTROESOPHAGEAL REFLUX DISEASE

The term *gastroesophageal reflux disease* (GERD) is used to describe any condition in which symptoms or histopathologic change results from refluxed gastric acid. This includes esophagitis as well as extraesophageal manifestations. Estimates suggest that GERD affects 7 to 10% of the population on a daily basis, and 40% on a monthly basis.

A certain amount of acid reflux is considered physiologic and generally occurs after meals. Whether it becomes pathologic depends on the frequency, volume, and duration of exposure. For example, although reflux episodes occur more often during the day, damage is more significant at night. This is because swallowing occurs much less frequently during sleep, averaging seven times an hour as opposed to 72 times an hour when awake. Refluxed material is therefore not cleared as rapidly and tends to pool in the lower esophagus. Defense mechanisms to gastroesophageal reflux, or the so-called antireflux barrier, include (1) the lower esophageal sphincter (LES), (2) peristaltic clearance of esophageal acid, (3) esophageal epithelial resistance, and (4) the upper esophageal sphincter.

Lower esophageal sphincter pressure tends to be adversely affected by fatty foods, caffeine, chocolate, alcohol, and tobacco. Drugs such as theophylline, β-agonists, α-antagonists, birth control pills, and calcium channel blockers can have the same effect.

CONTROVERSY

It is often suggested that a hiatal hernia predisposes to reflux. However, opinion varies as to whether a hiatal hernia sufficiently lowers LES pressure.

Although the pH of the refluxate is important, it is the pepsin concentration that seems to be responsible for the mucosal injury. Pepsin requires an acidic environment for its activity and retains 75% of its activity at a pH of up to 4.5.

The most common symptom of GERD is heartburn, a retrosternal and epigastric burning pain that may radiate to the back, arm, pharynx, and ear when severe. Occasionally it must be distinguished from cardiac pain; however, if it dissipates rapidly with nitroglycerin, it is unlikely to be esophageal in origin. The severity of pain often does not correlate histologically with the amount of esophageal inflammation. Pain that is aggravated by hot or cold liquids, coffee, citrus juices, or alcohol suggests ulcerative esophagitis.

PEARL••• A sour (acid) or bitter (bilious) taste in the mouth may suggest reflux. Excess salivation known as waterbrash may occur secondary to lower esophageal irritation. Nocturnal aspiration, choking, and coughing may be presenting symptoms.

DIAGNOSIS

The diagnosis of GERD can often be made by history, after which it is reasonable to institute empirical therapy and gauge the patient's response. If the patient fails to respond or has atypical symptoms, or complications are suspected, a number of tests are available for verification.

The 24-hour pH probe is currently considered the definitive test for reflux. It quantitates the number and magnitude of reflux episodes over a 24-hour period, as well as the time for esophageal clearance. A barium swallow is readily available but has a sensitivity of only 25 to 35%. Radionuclide scintigraphy has a sensitivity of about 68%, although it has been reported to be only 11% sensitive in patients with head and neck manifestations of reflux.

Endoscopy may be helpful but is not essential in most cases. If symptoms do not respond to therapy, or the patient complains of associated dysphagia, odynophagia, or bleeding, then endoscopy is indicated. However, the presence of normal-appearing mucosa does not rule out the possibility of reflux disease because as many as 55% of patients with symptomatic reflux have a normal endoscopic examination. Aside from esophagoscopy, bronchoscopy with cytology may also be helpful, particularly in children. The presence of lipid-laden macrophages would suggest reflux aspiration with a sensitivity of 85%, although other inflammatory conditions can produce similar findings.

TREATMENT

Generally, the treatment for gastroesophageal reflux should proceed in a stepwise fashion. Initially this should include conservative measures such as dietary management, bed elevation, avoiding bedtime snacking, weight loss if indicated, and reducing alcohol and tobacco consumption. Over-the-counter antacids are also helpful.

For those patients who fail conservative treatment, the second step involves more aggressive medical therapy. The H_2-receptor antagonists have been shown to effectively reduce gastric acid output, with a therapeutic gain of 10 to 24% relative to placebo.

Proton pump inhibitors are the newest class of agents for treating GERD, and they block the hydrogen potassium adenosine triphosphatase (ATPase) pump responsible for the final step in the release of gastric acid. These agents have demonstrated a therapeutic gain of 57 to 74% relative to placebo, and have been shown to be effective in more than 80% of severe esophagitis cases resistant to H_2-receptor antagonists.

When medical therapy fails, and particularly if complications develop, antireflux surgery should be considered. The development of laparoscopic approaches has greatly reduced the morbidity of surgical intervention, and in well-selected patients these approaches have demonstrated a 90% efficacy rate. The two most common procedures are the Nissan fundoplication and the Toupet partial fundoplication, both of which aim to restore competence of the LES.

HIATAL HERNIA

The esophagus passes through a hiatus in the diaphragm before reaching the stomach, at which point it is stabilized by the diaphragmatic crura and the attachment of the phreno-esophageal membrane. The latter is simply a coalescence of the thoracic and abdominal fasciae that line the diaphragm. A sliding hiatal hernia occurs when the gastric cardia herniates through the hiatus (Fig. 52–1). The phreno-esophageal membrane remains attached, though lax, so the herniated segment is not a free peritoneal sac. In contrast, a paraesophageal hiatal hernia occurs when a portion of the gastric fun-

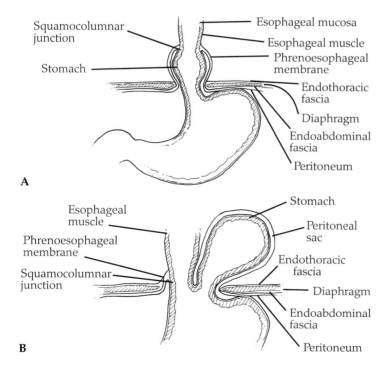

FIGURE 52–1 Type I, sliding (A) and type II, paraesophageal (B) hiatal hernias.

dus herniates through the hiatus adjacent to the esophagus. It generally occurs through a weakened portion of the phrenoesophageal membrane, while the LES remains in its subdiaphragmatic position. Eventually the gastroesophageal junction may be pulled upward through the defect, producing a combined sliding and paraesophageal hiatal hernia.

The sliding type of hiatal hernia is more common, although the specific cause remains unknown. Estimates suggest that 10% of adults will demonstrate varying degrees of a sliding hiatal hernia during a routine barium swallow, whereas only 5% of these patients will have symptomatic gastroesophageal reflux.

CONTROVERSY

A sliding hiatal hernia has long been implicated as a causative factor in GERD. However, more recent investigations indicate that it is the competency of the lower esophageal sphincter, independent of its relationship to the diaphragm, that determines whether reflux will occur. The presence of a hiatal hernia does not necessarily predispose to the development of symptomatic reflux.

A sliding hiatal hernia generally does not require any specific therapy. However, as a paraesophageal hernia continues to dilate, complications such as volvulus, infarction, and perforation may ensue. Therefore, surgical correction of paraesophageal hernias is recommended.

COMPLICATIONS

The most common complications of gastroesophageal reflux are ulceration, hemorrhage, stricture, and Barrett's esophagus.

Esophageal ulceration tends to occur in those patients with delayed esophageal and gastric emptying. Such patients typically complain of dysphagia and odynophagia but may experience a deep, boring pain that radiates to the back and is relieved with antacids. Significant bleeding from esophagitis or a penetrating esophageal ulcer is unusual, but, when it occurs, it must be distinguished from varices. Therefore, endoscopy is indicated.

Chronic reflux esophagitis that leads to ulceration ultimately causes scarring that may result in stricture formation. Approximately 10 to 15% of patients with reflux esophagitis develop a stricture. Progressive dysphagia is characteristic, although patients may not always present with a prolonged history of heartburn.

Continued acid exposure of the squamous epithelium that lines the esophagus may lead to replacement by metaplastic columnar epithelium, known as Barrett's esophagus. This tends to occur by upward migration of gastric epithelium, although isolated islands of columnar epithelium may be found elsewhere in the esophagus and are believed to be congenital in origin. Barrett's esophagus can be recognized endoscopically by its salmon red appearance. The significance is its association with a 10% incidence of adenocarcinoma, and it is therefore considered to be a premalignant condition. Management includes controlling the underlying reflux and closely monitoring the risk of cancer.

OTOLARYNGOLOGIC MANIFESTATIONS

Otolaryngologic manifestations of GERD are being recognized with increasing frequency and generally result from spillage of gastric juice into the larynx or pharynx, although some symptoms may relate to secondary spasticity or hypertrophy of the upper esophageal sphincter.

SPECIAL CONSIDERATION

It has recently been demonstrated that pepsin, and not hydrochloric acid, is the agent largely responsible for the mucosal injury.

When there is a prior mucosal injury, such as from intubation, damage from reflux is much more likely to occur.

Symptoms that have been linked to acid reflux include hoarseness, chronic cough, chronic throat clearing, globus sensation, dysphagia, otalgia, dysgeusia, and laryngospasm. Recent studies have also suggested an association with laryngeal cancer. In the pediatric patient manifestations include burping, choking, gagging, emesis, failure to thrive, airway obstruction, and sudden infant death syndrome.

Many of these patients do not have the classic symptoms normally associated with GERD and esophagitis. Such symptoms have been reported in only 20 to 50% of patients with head and neck manifestations of GERD, and therefore the diagnosis requires a high index of suspicion.

PEARL... While not pathognomonic for GERD, erythema and edema of the posterior larynx, referred to as pachydermia laryngitis, is highly suggestive.

Other physical findings might include varying degrees of laryngeal and subglottic edema, and even granulation tissue.

H_2 blockers are frequently ineffective in this group of patients. Full suppression over a prolonged period with proton pump inhibitors is usually required to achieve mucosal recovery.

SUGGESTED READINGS

Cote DN, Miller RH. The association of gastroesophageal reflux and otolaryngologic disorders. *Compr Ther* 1995;21:80–84.

Kahrilas PJ. Gastroesophageal reflux disease. *JAMA* 1996;276:983–988.

Koufman JA. The otolaryngologic manifestations of gastroesophageal reflux disease (GERD): a clinical investigation of 225 patients using ambulatory 24-hour pH monitoring and an experimental investigation of the role of acid and pepsin in the development of laryngeal injury. *Laryngoscope* 1991; 101(suppl):1–64.

Olson NR. Laryngopharyngeal manifestations of gastroesophageal reflux disease. *Otolaryngol Clin North Am* 1991;24:1201–1213.

Raufman JP. Esophageal infections. In: Yamada T, Alpers DH, Owyang C, Powell DW, Silverstein FE, eds. *Gastroenterology*. 2nd ed. Philadelphia: JB Lippincott, 1995:1243–1255.

Seiden AM. Esophageal disorders. In: Paparella MM, Shumrick DA, Gluckman JL, Meyerhoff WL, eds. *Otolaryngology*. 3rd ed. Philadelphia: WB Saunders; 1991:2439–2481.

Chapter 53

Neoplasms and Cysts

Allen M. Seiden

Esophageal neoplasms are not very common but are potentially quite lethal. Squamous cell carcinoma is the most common malignancy of the esophagus and has one of the worst prognoses of any cancer in the United States, with an average 5-year survival of 8%. Leiomyomas are the most common benign neoplasm of the esophagus.

BENIGN NEOPLASMS

Benign tumors account for only 0.5 to 0.8% of all esophageal neoplasms. Because they tend to be asymptomatic, many go undetected and are only discovered incidentally on X-ray, endoscopy, or autopsy. They can be classified as nonepithelial, epithelial, and heterotopic tumors.

NONEPITHELIAL TUMORS

Of the nonepithelial tumors leiomyoma is by far the most common, accounting for 36% of the benign neoplasms. It occurs more often in men, at a ratio of 2:1. Because it arises from smooth muscle, it generally is found within the distal two-thirds of the esophagus. The majority of patients are asymptomatic, but those who do have symptoms complain of dysphagia and retrosternal discomfort. If the tumor grows to a large size, tracheal or bronchial compression may occur with secondary cough, wheezing, or dyspnea. Because the tumor usually remains intramural and the overlying mucosa remains intact, ulceration and bleeding are uncommon.

A barium esophagram is diagnostic, revealing a smooth, round, well-circumscribed mass and no irregularity of the surrounding mucosa. Esophagoscopy reveals a rounded, freely movable mass with normal overlying mucosa.

> **PITFALL...** Biopsy is contraindicated because it may lead to bleeding, infection, and perforation. In addition, it may impede subsequent surgical enucleation, which becomes the procedure of choice should treatment be necessary.

Granular cell tumors of the esophagus are not common but may occasionally be incidental findings at endoscopy. They are believed to arise from neural or Schwann cell elements and appear endoscopically as smooth, sessile polypoid lesions. The vast majority occur in the distal esophagus and are usually asymptomatic unless they reach a large size.

The fibrovascular polyp is composed of fibrous and vascular tissue covered by smooth mucosa. It is intraluminal and usually pedunculated, most frequently arising within the upper portion of the esophagus. It may occasionally reach a very large size and actually prolapse into the larynx. Surgical removal is therefore indicated, and this may be done endoscopically with little chance of recurrence.

Lipomas and fibromas occur as sessile, submucosal nodules of fat and fibrous tissue, respectively. They compose less than 5% of benign esophageal tumors. Again, they are usually asymptomatic unless reaching a large size, at which point dysphagia may occur.

EPITHELIAL TUMORS

Similar to other benign tumors of the esophagus, squamous cell papillomas are usually found incidentally during endoscopy. They appear as small, sessile polypoid lesions usually located within the distal third of the esophagus. They may be removed endoscopically, and they rarely recur. No association has been noted with human papillomavirus.

MALIGNANT NEOPLASMS

Although esophageal cancer accounts for only 1.1% of all cancers, tumors of the esophagus are much more often malignant rather than benign. Approximately 90 to 95% are squamous cell carcinoma, whereas primary adenocarcinoma is responsible for most of the remainder. Patients generally present with advanced disease as symptoms become more pronounced.

SQUAMOUS CELL CARCINOMA

Esophageal squamous cell carcinoma has demonstrated a predilection for certain geographic areas, notably Japan, Iran, and certain regions of China. In the United States, it is more common in men, and African Americans demonstrate four to five times the risk of Caucasians. However, there is little evidence of any genetic predisposition; rather, environmental factors seem to be largely responsible, particularly excessive tobacco and alcohol use.

Chronic esophagitis of any cause seems to predispose to squamous cell carcinoma of the esophagus. Therefore, increased risk has been noted with caustic injury, long-standing achalasia, and some of the connective tissue disorders. However, the magnitude of such risk is difficult to estimate. For example, the mean duration from the onset of achalasia to the development of carcinoma has been estimated to be 20 years. Esophageal cancer has also been linked to prior radiation exposure, celiac sprue, Plummer-Vinson syndrome (postcricoid and cervical esophagus), and esophageal diverticula.

Patients presenting with squamous cell carcinoma elsewhere in the head and neck usually undergo endoscopy to rule out the possibility of a second primary, including esophagoscopy. The incidence of a coexisting esophageal primary has been estimated to be between 0.7 and 6%.

Symptoms

Initially, symptoms tend to be mild, nonspecific, and easily ignored, explaining why most lesions are advanced when finally discovered. Progressive dysphagia is the most common presenting symptom, the average time between onset of symptoms and diagnosis being 6 months. It typically begins with solid food and may progress to include liquids.

PEARL... Dysphagia usually indicates that more than 50% of the esophageal lumen has been compromised.

Approximately 50% of patients complain of pain with swallowing. Anorexia and weight loss are generally significant and an iron-deficiency anemia may be found secondary to occult bleeding. Cough secondary to chronic aspiration or an erosive tracheoesophageal fistula may occur, leading to further pulmonary complications. Involvement of the recurrent laryngeal nerve may produce hoarseness.

Diagnosis

Esophageal carcinoma may develop as a polypoid, intraluminal mass, or it may infiltrate and circumferentially constrict the esophageal lumen. There is generally extensive submucosal spread.

There appears to be a predilection for the middle third of the esophagus, at the level of the tracheal bifurcation and aortic arch, with prevalence in the upper and lower thirds being about equal.

A barium esophagram is helpful in making the diagnosis, although it may miss early lesions. Accuracy may be enhanced by the double-contrast technique and has been reported to be 73%, with a 27% false-negative rate and a 37% false-positive rate. More advanced tumors may appear as an exophytic mass creating a filling defect, a narrowed, irregular segment suggesting ulceration, or an annular constricting mass ("apple core" defect).

When there is suspicion of esophageal malignancy, endoscopy is essential for direct inspection and histologic confirmation. Esophagoscopy, particularly flexible esophagoscopy, is reported to be more sensitive than radiology for detecting early lesions. If the endoscope can be passed beyond the point of narrowing, then the tumor's proximal and distal extent should be assessed.

> **PITFALLS...** To prevent perforation, it is important never to force the instrument. If the lesion is largely submucosal and stenotic, then direct biopsy may prove difficult and should be combined with brushings for cytology.

An accuracy rate of 90 to 100% has been reported when cytology is combined with multiple endoscopic biopsies.

It is important to stage the extent of disease, and computed tomography (CT) scanning is generally the procedure of choice. Studies that have compared CT with magnetic resonance imaging (MRI) have found them to be comparable in terms of accuracy. Endoscopic ultrasound has also been recommended, particularly for assessing the depth of invasion of early tumors.

Treatment

As stated previously, most patients with esophageal carcinoma tend to present with advanced disease. Therefore, palliation frequently becomes an important goal of therapy rather than cure. This outlook is perhaps somewhat different in high-risk countries, such as China and Japan, where surveillance programs are in place for earlier detection.

> **CONTROVERSY**
>
> Surgical resection remains the most effective treatment for cure, although the best surgical approach, extent of resection, and most effective reconstruction are still debated.

For lesions of the cervical esophagus, a total laryngectomy with esophagectomy is required, whereas for more distal lesions an esophagectomy with gastric pull-up is generally performed. Lesions smaller than 5 cm in length or limited to the mucosal layer of the esophagus, and without lymph node involvement, are more likely to benefit from surgical resection. A bypass procedure using interposition grafts from the stomach, jejunum, or colon may be palliative in some unresectable patients. In addition, endoscopic placement of an indwelling stent, laser therapy, and bipolar electrocoagulation therapy may help to temporarily recannulate the esophageal lumen.

> **CONTROVERSY**
>
> Postoperative adjuvant radiotherapy is often recommended; however, two recent randomized trials failed to show any survival advantage. Adjuvant chemotherapy also seems to be of little benefit, although clinical trials are ongoing.

ADENOCARCINOMA

Most adenocarcinomas of the esophagus arise from areas of Barrett's metaplasia and therefore more often involve the distal esophagus. Of note is that adenocarcinoma of the gastric cardia also develops from Barrett's metaplasia. Although once thought to be uncommon, during the past two decades the incidence of Barrett's associated adenocarcinoma of both the esophagus and gastric cardia have risen more than any other cancer in the United States, making it one of the 15 most common malignancies in this country.

In contrast to squamous cell carcinoma, adenocarcinoma is more common in Caucasian men and has been related to chronic gastroesophageal reflux causing Barrett's metaplasia. During the early stages of malignancy, most patients have symptoms of gastroesophageal reflux. However, the severity of symptoms does not correlate with the risk for cancer. As the lesion progresses, patients develop dysphagia, weight loss, odynophagia, fatigue, vomiting, and occult gastrointestinal bleeding.

> **PEARL...** A high index of suspicion is important, and in patients known to have Barrett's esophagus regular endoscopic follow-up with biopsy is imperative.

The 5-year survival for patients with esophageal adenocarcinoma is generally similar to those with squamous cell carcinoma, and hovers around 7%. However, surveillance in patients with known Barrett's esophagus can catch early tumors and improve the prognosis. Once again,

surgical resection is the preferred treatment provided the lesion is resectable and there is no evidence of metastatic disease. The entire columnar-lined segment needs to be removed because Barrett's adenocarcinoma is often multicentric and surrounded by high-grade dysplasia.

OTHER MALIGNANT TUMORS

Other malignancies may develop in the esophagus but are exceedingly rare. These include carcinosarcoma, spindle cell sarcoma, leiomyosarcoma, adenoid cystic carcinoma, and lymphoma. Leiomyosarcoma is the most common nonepithelial malignant tumor of the esophagus. Primary melanoma may occur but is more often a metastatic lesion. Adenocarcinoma of the breast may also metastasize to the esophagus.

SUGGESTED READINGS

Girling DJ, Clark PI. Randomized trials in the treatment of cancer of the esophagus. *J Clin Oncol* 1992;10:1031.

Reid BJ, Thomas CR. Esophageal neoplasms. In: Yamada T, Alpers DH, Owyang C, Powell DW, Silverstein FE, eds. *Textbook of Gastroenterology.* 2nd ed. Philadelphia: JB Lippincott; 1995:1256–1283.

Seiden AM. Esophageal disorders. In: Paparella MM, Shumrick DA, Gluckman JL, Meyerhoff WL, eds. *Otolaryngology.* 3rd ed. Philadelphia: WB Saunders; 1991:2439–2481.

Chapter 54

TRAUMA

Allen M. Seiden

Trauma to the esophagus may be either internal, such as from caustic ingestion or iatrogenic perforation, or external, such as from blunt or penetrating injury. The diagnosis can be difficult because symptoms do not always correlate with the extent of injury. Therefore, a high index of suspicion is required, and a delay in diagnosis may result in catastrophic complications. The otolaryngologist is frequently called on to evaluate such patients.

CAUSTIC INGESTION

Beginning with the work of Chevalier Jackson in 1927, the United States federal government has increasingly regulated the packaging and labeling of caustic products. Nevertheless, there continue to be as many as 5000 accidental lye ingestions per year by children under the age of 5. Such injury is also seen in adults attempting to commit suicide and in adults with mental retardation. The most common agents are alkaline (60%), such as sodium or potassium hydroxides that are found in many household cleaners, and acid corrosives. The resultant degree of injury is dependent on the pH of the product, as well as the quantity ingested, its viscosity, and mucosal contact time (esophageal transit).

SPECIAL CONSIDERATION

Alkalis tend to penetrate more rapidly than acids, causing a liquefaction necrosis that may extend rapidly through the submucosa to the underlying muscle of the esophagus. On the other hand, acids produce a coagulation necrosis with superficial eschar that helps prevent deeper penetration, leading to greater damage within the stomach.

Liquid products are more apt to burn the esophagus because they are more easily swallowed. The most damage tends to occur at normal anatomic narrowings within the esophagus where there is greater mucosal contact time, including the level of the cricopharyngeus, the aortic arch, the left mainstem bronchus, and the gastroesophageal junction. Crystalline substances may attach to the oral mucosa and are more difficult to swallow, thereby more often causing damage to the oral cavity and pharynx. First-degree burns are superficial, causing mucosal hyperemia and edema but no significant scarring. Second-degree burns are associated with penetration through the submucosa into the muscle, producing necrosis, an exudate, and deep ulcerations that may be seen on esophagoscopy. Stenosis may occur over the ensuing weeks. Third-degree burns are transmural, eroding into the mediastinum, pleural cavity, or peritoneal cavity.

The immediate goal in these cases is to accurately assess the location and extent of injury and to prevent the development of complications such as stricture or perforation.

CONTROVERSY

Unfortunately, it is difficult to develop well-controlled, randomized studies to explore these issues, and so the most effective means to achieving this goal remains somewhat controversial.

CLINICAL FINDINGS

It is important to recognize that the severity of injury often cannot be determined by the history alone. It is helpful to identify the type of substance that was ingested, recognizing that even small amounts can cause severe damage. It is also important to ascertain whether the patient vomited after ingestion because this would increase mucosal contact time.

Acutely, patients may complain of burning of the lips, tongue, or pharynx, odynophagia, and dysphagia. Excessive salivation with drooling is frequently noted, and wheezing and stridor suggest airway involvement.

PEARL... Fifty percent of patients complaining of two of the three following symptoms—drooling, vomiting, and stridor—will have serious esophageal burns. The presence of only one of these symptoms tends to be associated with very little esophageal injury.

Hematemesis and abdominal pain suggest gastric injury. Should esophageal perforation occur, patients may suffer severe chest pain, subcutaneous emphysema, sepsis, and shock.

Esophageal spasm and edema, as well as supraglottic edema, peak within the first 48 hours. As the edema then subsides, swallowing generally improves and patients may enter a quiescent period lasting 3 to 6 weeks during which there are relatively few symptoms. If there has been extensive injury, fibroplastic and collagen proliferation with scar contracture now occurs, leading to gradual stenosis and increasing dysphagia.

PITFALL... There is no correlation between the presence or absence of oropharyngeal burns and esophageal injury.

DIAGNOSTIC EVALUATION

The most sensitive method for establishing the extent of injury and the need for further therapy is endoscopy. Most recommend endoscopic examination within the first 48 to 72 hours due to the advantages of instituting early therapy.

CONTROVERSY

If extensive esophageal injury is encountered during endoscopy, particularly a circumferential second- or third-degree burn, it is generally recommended that further passage of the endoscope be avoided due to the risk of perforation. However, some point out that this may preclude detection of a more distal, life-threatening burn that might require open debridement and repair.

A chest X-ray and abdominal film may help rule out pneumonitis, pleural effusion, or possibly free air in the mediastinum or peritoneum. The early use of barium studies is of limited value because they are not sensitive for establishing the depth of injury, although they may detect a perforation. However, they are recommended routinely at 3 weeks and during regular follow-up to assess the development of stenosis.

THERAPY

The main focus of therapy for caustic ingestion has been to prevent subsequent complications. Acute measures are largely supportive, such as airway management and volume replacement. Efforts to neutralize or dilute ingested caustics has not been effective and may add to injury. By the same token, emesis and gastric lavage should be avoided because of the risk of repeated esophageal exposure.

The greatest concern is to prevent the development of esophageal stricture or perforation. The most useful prognostic factor in this regard is the depth of injury, hence the importance of endoscopy. First-degree burns are rarely associated with such complications, but if second- and third-degree burns are found at endoscopy, prompt administration of antibiotics and steroids is indicated. Antibiotics have been shown to decrease the bacterial load, and they thereby minimize granulation tissue as well as help to prevent intramural spread and possibly mediastinitis. Steroids have been found to help prevent stricture formation if administered within 24 to 48 hours of injury, but are most effective in cases of moderately severe alkaline injuries. As stated previously, acid ingestion is less likely to result in severe esophageal injury. Therapy should be continued for at least 3 to 4 weeks.

Although some recommend early prophylactic dilatation in patients with severe burns, this is associated with a greater risk of perforation. Therefore, most advocate delaying dilatation for 2 to 4 weeks. Indwelling tubes or esophageal stents have met with little success.

CONTROVERSY

The early placement of a nasogastric tube has been advocated by some groups to prevent stenosis. However, the data are insufficient to universally support this approach, and it is not widely practiced.

MEDICATION-INDUCED ESOPHAGEAL INJURY

One source of caustic ingestion that is often overlooked is that of medication-induced esophagitis. A variety of medications when retained in the esophagus can cause a localized irritation and even ulceration. In fact, over 70 medications have been implicated as causative agents.

In younger patients, drug-induced esophagitis is most often caused by antibiotics, whereas in older patients potassium chloride, nonsteroidal antiinflammatory drugs (NSAID), and vitamin C are often responsible. Of note is that complications such as bleeding and stricture occur in one-third of patients suffering esophagitis secondary to NSAID.

Although preexisting esophageal disease may affect esophageal transit and thereby put patients at increased risk for this sort of injury, most cases of drug-induced esophagitis occur in patients without prior esophageal problems. Taking medications at night, in the supine position, and with little or no water clearly predisposes to drug retention within the esophagus, and the ensuing esophagitis only exacerbates the problem. The esophageal site most often injured is that portion compressed by the aortic arch. This also marks the site of transition from striated to smooth muscle, so that the peristaltic wave is reduced in amplitude.

Symptoms may occur several hours after ingestion or may be delayed for days or weeks. Complaints usually are consistent with esophagitis, including odynophagia in 74%, persistent retrosternal pain in 72%, and dysphagia in 20%. A barium esophagram may be helpful depending on the degree of inflammation and may demonstrate ulceration or stricture. Endoscopy usually demonstrates areas of discrete ulceration and esophagitis, and occasionally remnants of the medication may be found. Biopsies show inflammation with regenerative hyperplasia, and must be distinguished from neoplasm.

Treatment includes stopping as many of the medicines as possible or replacing them with liquid preparations. Patients need to be instructed to take medications in the sitting or standing position with adequate liquids, and not just before bedtime. Symptoms usually subside within days to several weeks.

ESOPHAGEAL PERFORATION

Esophageal perforation may occur from a variety of causes, but most commonly it is iatrogenic, resulting from endoscopic manipulation or dilatation. In their series, Michael and coworkers (1981) found that 68% of their patients' perforations were iatrogenic, 13% were spontaneous, 11% were secondary to foreign body ingestion, and 8% were secondary to external trauma. In a more recent series (Flynn et al, 1989), 48% of the perforations were iatrogenic, 33% were caused by external trauma, and 8% were spontaneous. Successful management of these patients depends on early diagnosis and prompt intervention.

IATROGENIC PERFORATIONS

Although most esophageal perforations are iatrogenic, the incidence of such injury after diagnostic endoscopy is actually quite low, reported to be from 0.1 to 1% with rigid instruments and 0.01% with flexible endoscopes. The most common sites of injury are the cervical esophagus at the cricopharyngeus and the thoracoabdominal esophagus at the diaphragmatic hiatus.

> **PEARL•••** Injury at the cricopharyngeus occurs because of inadvertent introduction of the scope into the pyriform sinus, narrowing of the upper esophageal sphincter, or prominent cervical osteophytes. Injury at the diaphragmatic hiatus tends to occur as the esophagus angles anteriorly toward the diaphragm, which is often not appreciated by the endoscopist.

Esophageal dilatation carries a much greater risk of perforation, depending on the type of stricture and method of dilatation. Pneumatic dilatation for achalasia carries the highest risk, ranging from 1 to 5%, whereas the Maloney and Hurst dilators have the lowest risk, at 0.1 to 0.4%. Chronic lye strictures and malignant strictures are generally associated with a higher likelihood of perforation.

Other less common causes of iatrogenic perforation include placement of nasogastric tubes and traumatic endotracheal intubation.

EXTERNAL TRAUMA

Penetrating trauma to the neck, chest, or upper abdomen should alert the physician to the possibility of associated esophageal injury. In addition, by producing a sudden change in esophageal transmural pressure, blunt trauma may sometimes cause esophageal rupture. Typically this occurs in the cervical and upper thoracic esophagus.

> **PITFALL•••** The Heimlich maneuver has been reported to cause an esophageal rupture by rapidly raising intrathoracic pressure.

SPONTANEOUS RUPTURE

Spontaneous esophageal rupture was first described by Boerhaave in 1724, when he reported a patient who died suddenly after an episode of severe vomiting, hence Boerhaave's syndrome. Autopsy revealed an esophageal rupture with food contaminating the thorax.

> ## SPECIAL CONSIDERATION
>
> The majority of spontaneous esophageal perforations occur in the distal esophagus, where there appears to be an inherent weakness within the left posterolateral wall. Some reports have suggested an anatomic predisposition in some patients with an absence of the muscularis mucosa.

In 1929 Mallory and Weiss described a similar syndrome in alcoholics after severe emesis, resulting in hematemesis. This is associated with mucosal tears within the distal esophagus or proximal stomach, and not true perforations. Although it has been most often reported in alcoholics, it may occur after any activity that suddenly raises intraabdominal pressure, including coughing, seizures, hiccups, and heavy lifting. The bleeding usually stops spontaneously, but occasionally more aggressive intervention is required. In such cases endoscopic therapy with the use of hemostatic agents or cautery is the preferred approach, as balloon tamponade may extend the tear or lead to rupture.

DIAGNOSIS

When an esophageal perforation does occur, it is important to make the diagnosis rapidly. Although symptoms vary depending on the location of injury, persistent pain and fever after esophagoscopy should alert the clinician as to its possibility.

> **PITFALL...** As many as 50% of patients with iatrogenic perforations will be asymptomatic for the first 8 hours following injury.

Perforations of the cervical and upper esophagus generally cause neck pain (95%) and subcutaneous emphysema (55%). Dysphagia, odynophagia, and hematemesis may also occur, with fever and leukocytosis developing over the first 24 hours. More distal perforations in the thoracoabdominal esophagus produce retrosternal or pleuritic chest pain, and shoulder pain if there is diaphragmatic irritation. Abdominal rigidity and splinting of respirations may be noted. Again, fever and leukocytosis will occur.

A plain chest X-ray or abdominal film may show a thin streak of prevertebral air, subcutaneous or cervical emphysema, mediastinal widening, pneumomediastinum, or pneumothorax.

> **PITFALL...** Plain films may initially be normal in up to 33% of patients.

Over the ensuing 12 to 24 hours, a left pleural effusion and pulmonary infiltrates may develop.

In most cases, a contrast study will be diagnostic. A water-soluble contrast medium, such as Gastrografin, is preferable because it causes less mediastinal inflammation. However, if negative, a barium esophagram should be considered because it remains more sensitive. A computed tomography scan with contrast is helpful if an abscess is suspected.

Endoscopy in many cases may simply miss small defects and risks enlarging the perforation. However, in the case of penetrating injuries to the cervical region, it is usually an indispensable means for evaluating the esophagus at the time of surgery.

THERAPY

It has been clearly shown that delays in diagnosis and treatment are associated with an increase in mortality. Therefore, medical therapy should begin even before the perforation is verified.

> ### CONTROVERSY
>
> There remains considerable controversy as to whether medical therapy alone is adequate or whether all esophageal perforations need to be surgically addressed. Documentation can be found in the literature to support either approach. Generally, appropriate treatment depends on the site and size of the perforation, the time since the injury occurred, and the health status of the patient.

Perforations of the cervical esophagus are associated with less morbidity and mortality and can often be treated conservatively. Medical therapy includes allowing nothing by mouth, intravenous hydration and alimentation, cardiorespiratory support, and high-dose antibiotics. Nasogastric suction may be helpful and may be used as a route for nutritional support provided the tube can be safely passed. Treatment needs to be individualized and patients closely monitored. Any deterioration in overall status or signs of sepsis will necessitate surgical drainage.

Conservative therapy for perforations of the middle and lower esophagus has been less favored due to the higher complication rate. Some reports have suggested the safety of medical therapy alone after instrumental perforations because these tend to be recognized early. However, most authors seem to advocate surgical drainage and, if less than 24 hours after injury, surgical closure of the perforation.

SUGGESTED READINGS

Bozymski EM, Isaacs KL. Miscellaneous diseases of the esophagus. In: Yamada T, Alpers KH, Owyang C, Powell DW, Silverstein FE, eds. *Textbook of Gastroenterology.* 2nd ed. Philadelphia: JB Lippincott; 1995:1256–1283.

Dolgin SR, Kumar NR, Wykoff TW, Maniglia AJ. Conservative medical management of traumatic pharyngoesophageal perforations. *Ann Otol Rhinol Laryngol* 1992;101:209–215.

Flynn AE, Verrier ED, Way LW, et al. Esophageal perforation. *Arch Surg* 1989;124:1211.

Michael L, Grillo HC, Malt RA. Operative and nonoperative management of esophageal perforation. *Ann Surg* 1981;194:57–63.

Riding KH, Bluestone CD. Burns and acquired strictures of the esophagus. In: Bluestone CD, Stool SE, eds. *Pediatric Otolaryngology.* 2nd ed. Philadelphia: WB Saunders; 1990: 998–1008.

Seiden AM. Esophageal disorders. In: Paparella MM, Shumrick DA, Gluckman JL, Meyerhoff WL, eds. *Otolaryngology.* 3rd ed. Philadelphia: WB Saunders; 1991:2439–2481.

Shockley WW, Tate JL, Stucker FJ. Management of perforations of the hypopharynx and cervical esophagus. *Laryngoscope* 1985;95:939–941.

Chapter 55

SPECIAL CONSIDERATIONS

Allen M. Seiden

This chapter covers additional topics on the esophagus that were not covered in the preceding chapters. While they may be associated with inflammatory conditions, they are separate entities.

FOREIGN BODIES IN THE ESOPHAGUS

Suffocation from foreign body ingestion and aspiration remains one of the leading causes of mortality in infants and young children. Nevertheless, ingestions are far more common than aspirations, and the esophagus is the most common site of foreign body impaction within the gastrointestinal tract.

Impaction is generally seen in children from 6 months to 6 years of age. Objects are often being placed in the mouth and the swallowing function is still somewhat immature. Coins tend to be the most common foreign body ingested by children. The problem is also seen in adults, but the foreign body tends to be food products, particularly fish and chicken bones. The most common sites of impaction are areas of inherent narrowing within the esophagus, specifically, just distal to the cricopharyngeus, the level of compression by the aortic arch and mainstem bronchus, and the gastroesophageal junction.

> **PEARL...** Food bolus impaction usually occurs in the distal esophagus, and is almost always associated with an esophageal abnormality.

Adults usually describe a history of having eaten fish or chicken and present with dysphagia, odynophagia, a choking sensation, and sometimes drooling. On the other hand, most foreign body ingestions in children go unnoticed and the history may be very misleading.

> **SPECIAL CONSIDERATION**
>
> Foreign body ingestion needs to be considered in any child with dysphagia, weight loss, or airway symptoms, particularly when there is a history of choking, gagging, coughing, or vomiting.

Physical findings are usually absent or nonspecific. Patients may present with drooling and occasionally stridor secondary to tracheal compression. Radiographs should be obtained in all patients, and include both anteroposterior and lateral neck films, as well as a chest X-ray. Dense foreign bodies such as coins should be plainly evident.

> **PEARL•••** Less radiopaque materials such as bones are usually best seen on lateral views.

Radiolucent materials may be suspected by the presence of soft tissue swelling or evidence of complications such as subcutaneous air, aspiration pneumonia, or mediastinitis.

> **PITFALL•••** The stylohyoid ligament is often calcified, as are the laryngeal cartilages. Very often this may be mistaken for a foreign body such as a fish or chicken bone, particularly on a lateral neck X-ray.

It is important to remember that a negative X-ray does not rule out a foreign body.

In general, all foreign bodies in the esophagus should be removed and not allowed to pass. Although sharp objects are more apt to cause complications such as perforations, chronic inflammation and erosion can also occur with smooth objects. If a disk battery is ingested and becomes lodged in the esophagus, it should be emergently removed, as it will release a caustic solution that may cause significant injury to the esophageal mucosa. It can be recognized radiographically by its rounded, "double density" appearance. If the battery has passed to the stomach, it can generally be observed by serial radiographs and endoscopically removed only if it does not continue to progress through the gastrointestinal system.

Postoperatively, after endoscopic removal of a foreign body, patients need to be observed for any signs of perforation. Many practitioners avoid the use of antibiotics or steroids so as not to mask the appearance of fever within the first 24 hours. Clear liquids may then be started and the patient advanced to a regular diet.

RINGS AND WEBS

Although the terms *rings* and *webs* are often used interchangeably, strictly speaking a ring occurs only at the gastroesophageal junction with squamous epithelium on its upper surface and columnar epithelium on its lower surface. Conversely, webs may be found anywhere in the esophagus but usually occur in the upper and mid-esophagus, are generally thinner, and may not always be concentric. Very often these lesions are found incidentally and may not be causing symptoms. Therefore, it is important to correlate such findings with the patient's history.

LOWER ESOPHAGEAL (SCHATZKI'S) RING

Described by Schatzki and Gary in 1953, a lower esophageal ring is one of the most common causes of dysphagia, yet is often an incidental finding. It is present in as many as 14% of routine barium studies; however, only a third of these patients will be symptomatic. Most symptomatic patients tend to be male and over the age of 40.

Lower esophageal rings may be either muscular (A rings) or mucosal (B rings). The former consists of a concentric ring of hypertrophied muscle covered with normal squamous epithelium. It occurs 1.5 cm proximal to the squamocolumnar junction corresponding to the upper portion of the lower esophageal sphincter, and occurs most often in patients with esophageal motor disorders, gastroesophageal reflux, and hiatal hernia. Mucosal rings are devoid of muscle and are less than 3 mm in thickness, usually containing a variable amount of connective tissue.

The diameter of the ring largely determines whether symptoms will occur. If the intraluminal diameter of the ring is less than 13 mm, solid food dysphagia is inevitable, whereas if the diameter is larger than 20 mm symptoms are unlikely. Characteristically the dysphagia is intermittent, with attacks often being separated by weeks or months. A bolus tends to become stuck when the patient is distracted, excited, and eating a hurried meal. Hence the term *steak-house syndrome* because poorly chewed steak is often the culprit, and steak houses are frequently the site of hurried business lunches.

PEARL... The patient may relieve the obstruction with vomitting or forceful swallowing of liquids after which eating may occur normally. This is typical of no other disorder.

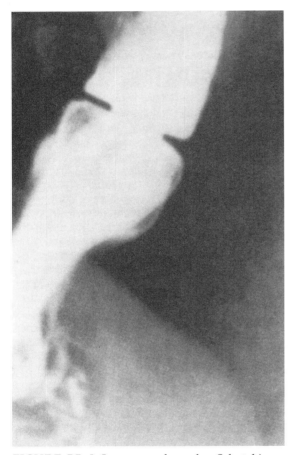

FIGURE 55–1 Lower esophageal or Schatzki ring easily seen as the esophagus is sufficiently dilated. Note that it is narrow in width and, unlike an esophageal web or malignancy, it appears symmetric. The patient also has a hiatal hernia. (From Seiden AM. Esophageal Disorders. In: Paparella et al, ed. *Otolaryngology.* Vol. 3, *Head and Neck.* Philadelphia: WB Saunders; 1991:2465. Reprinted by permission of the publisher.)

On barium esophagram a lower esophageal ring appears symmetric, as opposed to an esophageal web (Fig. 55–1). The gastroesophageal junction needs to be adequately dilated with barium to detect the ring, but symptomatic rings should be reproducible and should not disappear during X-ray examination. Endoscopically it is probably better seen with a flexible scope due to that scope's larger caliber and ability to insufflate air.

Because the dysphagia is intermittent, weight loss is unusual. Conservative treatment includes slower eating habits and perhaps a better pair of dentures. If the patient remains symptomatic, dilation is indicated.

ESOPHAGEAL WEBS

Esophageal webs are thin, membranous bands projecting into the esophageal lumen and are covered by squamous epithelium. They are more commonly single, but may be multiple. Although the majority are asymptomatic, intermittent solid food dysphagia is the most frequent complaint when symptoms are present.

Upper esophageal webs typically occur in the postcricoid area or along the anterior wall of the cervical esophagus. The association of upper esophageal webs with iron deficiency anemia is known as the Plummer-Vinson or Paterson-Kelly syndrome. These patients are typically of Scandinavian descent and are also found to have achlorhydria, atrophic gastritis, and hiatal hernia. Ninety percent are women, usually between the ages of 20 and 50.

SPECIAL CONSIDERATION

There is an increased incidence of cervical esophageal carcinoma in patients with Plummer-Vinson syndrome. Therefore, endoscopic evaluation is essential, and long-term follow-up must be maintained.

Cervical esophageal webs may be detected on barium study, but are best seen in lateral projection with the esophagus fully distended (Fig. 55–2).

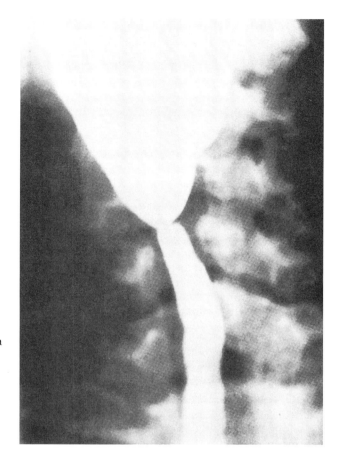

FIGURE 55–2 Upper esophageal web, seen here in anteroposterior projection as a narrowing at the mouth of the esophagus below a distended hypopharynx. More often the web is better seen in lateral projection, but in either case it is easily missed. (From Seiden AM. Esophageal Disorders. In: Paparella et al, ed. *Otolaryngology*. Vol. 3, *Head and Neck.* Philadelphia: WB Saunders; 1991:2464. Reprinted by permission of the publisher.)

PITFALL··· On barium study, an upper esophageal web must be differentiated from indentations caused by the cricopharyngeus muscle or the postcricoid venous plexus.

PEARL··· The radiographic appearance of mid-esophageal webs is that of a sharp, thin indentation of the barium column. On the other hand, a stenosis tends to have tapered edges, a muscular spasm or tertiary contraction is transient, and a carcinoma presents as a broader, more irregular narrowing.

Mid-esophageal webs are much less common and may occur anywhere along the middle length of the esophagus. When congenital, they tend to become symptomatic at 5 to 10 months of age when the infant begins to eat solid food and may subsequently spit up. Such webs may also be acquired from some inflammatory process, such as reflux esophagitis or caustic ingestion.

If patients are symptomatic, dilatation usually suffices as adequate therapy. Rarely, endoscopic lysis may be useful, and resection through an external approach has been reported.

ESOPHAGEAL DIVERTICULA

Esophageal diverticula may occur at the pharyngoesophageal junction, in the midesophagus just below the level of the carina, and in the distal esophagus. They tend to result from pulsion forces and consist of mucosa that has herniated through the muscularis propria, rather than containing all layers of the esophageal wall. Therefore, they are, in fact, false diverticula.

PHARYNGOESOPHAGEAL (ZENKER'S) DIVERTICULUM

This is the most common of the esophageal diverticula. It occurs as a protrusion of posterior hypopharyngeal mucosa between the oblique and transverse fibers of the cricopharyngeus muscle in the posterior midline, an inherently weakened area of the esophagus known as Killian's triangle. The pathophysiology remains controversial.

CONTROVERSY

Because Killian's triangle lies just above the transverse fibers of the cricopharyngeus muscle, it has long been postulated that spasm or poor compliance of this muscle results in a proximal high pressure zone as the pharyngeal constrictor muscles contract, leading to mucosal herniation. However, manometric studies have not consistently supported this theory.

Patients typically present after the age of 50, with 70 percent of patients being older than 60 years. The most prevalent symptom is dysphagia to both solids and liquids, usually of gradual onset, and a sense of food sticking in the throat. Regurgitation of undigested food may occur, with associated cough and halitosis. This regurgitation may be worse at night, causing aspiration and a picture of recurring pneumonitis.

As the sac distends, it typically projects into the left side of the neck posterior and inferior to the sternocleidomastoid muscle. Because the cervical esophagus bulges to the left, this seems to be the path of least resistance. Rarely, it may become palpable and produce compressive symptoms.

A barium study is usually diagnostic, demonstrating a fluid-filled sac (Fig. 55–3).

PITFALL... Endoscopy is generally quite hazardous because the sac has no muscular component and is easily perforated. In any event, it adds little to the diagnosis unless there is a concern about malignant degeneration, and this is distinctly uncommon, having a reported incidence of only 0.31%.

Treatment usually requires surgical excision, but there is no consensus as to the best surgical approach. Diverticulectomy, diverticulectomy with cricopharyngeal myotomy, cricopharyngeal myotomy alone, and diverticular inversion with myotomy have all been described with varying results.

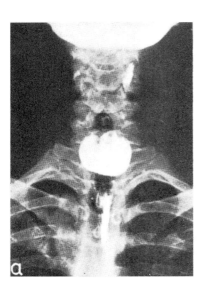
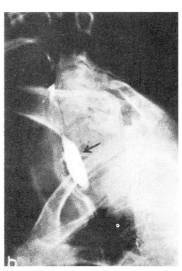

FIGURE 55–3 Zenker's diverticulum (arrow) in a 40-year-old man. (A) Anteroposterior view demonstrates barium retention in the rather distended pouch. (B) Right recumbent position. (From Mesh-Kinpoui H. Esophageal diverticula. In: Berk JE, ed. *Bockus Gastroenterology.* Vol. 2. Philadelphia: WB Saunders; 1985:810. Reprinted by permission of the publisher.)

In the earlier part of the 20th century, an endoscopic approach to resection of the party wall between the esophageal lumen and the diverticulum was described but abandoned due to associated morbidity. It was later revived by Dohlman and Mattson in the 1960s (Dohlman procedure) and has been described more recently with improved endoscopic techniques. However, the external approach is generally still preferred.

MID-ESOPHAGEAL AND EPIPHRENIC DIVERTICULA

Diverticula may also occur in the middle and lower esophagus and are usually due to underlying motility disorders. They may also occur in patients with long-standing lower esophageal stricture.

Mid-esophageal diverticula generally incorporate the entire esophageal wall and therefore tend not to reach a very large size. Associated symptoms are uncommon and more often relate to the abnormal motility. Diagnosis is often made incidentally on X-ray, and surgical excision is rarely necessary.

Epiphrenic diverticula are most often associated with diffuse esophageal spasm, achalasia, reflux esophagitis, and hiatal hernia. They typically develop posteriorly and extend toward the right thorax. If distention of the sac occurs, dysphagia may result. Again, treatment is usually directed at the underlying motility problem.

SUGGESTED READINGS

Bonafede JP, Lavertu P, Wood BG, Eliachar I. Surgical outcome in 87 patients with Zenker's diverticulum. *Laryngoscope* 1997;107(6):720–725.

Bozymski EM, Isaacs KL. Miscellaneous diseases of the esophagus. In: Yamada T, ed. *Textbook of Gastroenterology.* 2nd ed. Philadelphia: JB Lippincott; 1995:1283–1302.

Crysdale WS, Sendi KS, Yoo J. Esophageal foreign bodies in children: 15-year review of 484 cases. *Ann Otol Rhinol Laryngol* 1991;100(4 pt 1):320–324.

Holinger LD. Management of sharp and penetrating foreign bodies of the upper aerodigestive tract. *Ann Otol Rhinol Laryngol* 1990; 99(9 pt 1):684–688.

Holinger PH, Johnston KC. Endoscopic surgery of Zenker's diverticula. Experience with the Dohlman technique. 1961 [classic article]. *Ann Otol Rhinol Laryngol* 1995;104(10 pt 1): 751–757.

Laccourreye O, Menard M, Cauchois R, et al. Esophageal diverticulum: diverticulopexy versus diverticulectomy. *Laryngoscope* 1994;104 (7):889–892.

Macpherson RI, Hill JG, Othersen HB, Tagge EP, Smith CD. Esophageal foreign bodies in children: diagnosis, treatment, and complications. *AJR* 1996;166(4):919–924.

Migliore M, Payne H, Jeyasingham K. Pathophysiologic basis for operation of Zenker's diverticulum. *Ann Thorac Surg* 1994;57:1616–1612.

Schatzki R, Gary JE. Dysphagia due to a diaphragm-like localized narrowing in the lower esophagus ("lower esophageal ring"). *AJR* 1953;70:911–922.

Scher RL, Richtsmeier WJ. Long-term experience with endoscopic staple-assisted esophagodiverticulosotomy for Zenker's diverticulum. *Laryngoscope* 1998;108(2):200–205.

Seiden AM. Esophageal disorders. In: Paparella MM, Shumrick DA, Gluckman JL, Meyerhoff

WL, eds. *Otolaryngology.* 3rd ed. Philadelphia: WB Saunders; 1991:2439–2481.

Singh B, Kantu M, Har-El G, Lucente FE. Complications associated with 327 foreign bodies of the pharynx, larynx, and esophagus. *Ann Otol Rhinol Laryngol* 1997;106(4):301–304.

Stool SE, Manning SC. Foreign bodies of the pharynx and esophagus. In: Bluestone CD, Stool SE, eds. *Pediatric Otolaryngology.* 2nd ed. Philadelphia: WB Saunders; 1990:1009–1019.

van Overbeek JJ. Meditation on the pathogenesis of hypopharyngeal (Zenker's) diverticulum and a report of endoscopic treatment in 545 patients. *Ann Otol Rhinol Laryngol* 1994;103(3):178–185.

Von Doersten PG, Byl FM. Endoscopic Zenker's diverticulotomy (Dohlman procedure): forty cases reviewed. *Otolaryngol Head Neck Surg* 1997;116(2):209–212.

Watemberg S, Landau O, Avrahami R. Zenker's diverticulum: reappraisal [see comments]. *Am J Gastroenterol* 1996;91(8):1494–1498.

Westrin KM, Ergun S, Carisoo B. Zenker's diverticulum—a historical review and trends in therapy. *Acta Otolaryngol (Stockh)* 1996;116(3):351–360.

SECTION IX

SALIVARY GLANDS

Chapter 56

ANATOMY AND PHYSIOLOGY

David L. Steward and Thomas A. Tami

There are three paired major salivary glands: parotid, submandibular, and sublingual. Additionally, there are hundreds of minor salivary glands throughout the oral cavity and pharynx. Saliva, the secretory product of these exocrine glands, is delivered into the oropharynx through neurologic input from sympathetic and parasympathetic innervation. The relevant anatomy and physiology are reviewed in this chapter.

ANATOMY OF THE PAROTID GLAND

The parotid, the largest of the salivary glands, is encased within the superficial layer of the deep cervical fascia. Inferiorly, a thickening of this fascia forms the stylomandibular ligament, which separates the parotid from the submandibular gland. The parotid is dumbbell shaped with the deep portion abutting the parapharyngeal space, and the superficial portion is covered by facial skin and subcutaneous fat (Fig. 56–1). The parotid contains predominantly serous secreting acinar cells.

The parotid is bounded superiorly by the zygomatic arch. Anteriorly, it overlies the masseter superficially, and the mandible and medial pterygoid more deeply. Posteriorly, it overlies the sternocleidomastoid superficially and the posterior belly of the digastric more deeply. Me-

> **SPECIAL CONSIDERATION**
>
> When enlarged by tumor, the deep portion may invade the parapharyngeal space and present in the oropharynx as a peritonsillar mass.

dially, it is bounded by the styloid and its muscular attachments (stylohyoid, stylopharyngeus, and styloglossus).

The parotid (Stensen's) duct arises from the anterior border of the gland as a termination of various extraglandular ductules. It traverses the masseter muscle about 1.5 cm below the zygoma and then penetrates the buccinator muscle to empty into the oral cavity opposite the upper second molar.

> **PITFALL•••** Stensen's duct runs in close proximity with the buccal branch of cranial nerve VII. When repairing a facial laceration involving the duct, a concerted effort must be made to clearly identify this branch of the nerve.

The parotid gland is supplied by the external carotid artery, specifically the transverse

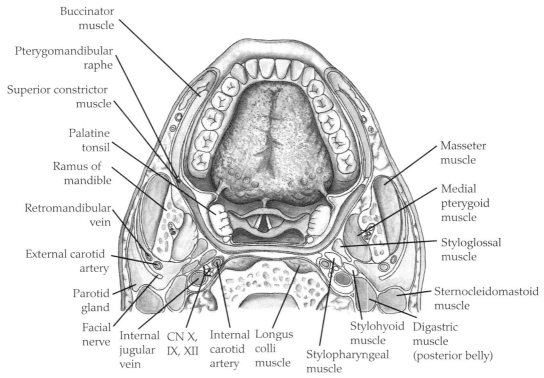

FIGURE 56–1 Medial relations of the parotid gland.

facial, which is a branch of the superficial temporal. Venous drainage is via the internal and external jugular veins. The retromandibular vein, which drains the superficial temporal vein, joins the postauricular vein to form the external jugular vein. Frequently, a posterior facial joins the anterior facial vein to form the common facial, which empties into the internal jugular system (Fig. 56–2).

> **PEARL•••** By delaying ligation of the posterior facial vein during parotidectomy, venous congestion and bleeding from the gland may be decreased.

Lymphatic drainage is via superficial and deep cervical systems. Periparotid nodes drain the face and scalp, external auditory canal and middle ear, nasopharynx and soft palate, as well as the parotid gland itself.

SPECIAL CONSIDERATION

Unlike other salivary glands, lymph nodes are contained within the parenchyma of the parotid. Because these nodes have infectious, neoplastic, and metastatic potential, they must be included in surgical lymphadenectomy if they are part of the drainage pathways for head and neck tumors.

FACIAL NERVE

The facial nerve, cranial nerve (CN) VII, emerges from the stylomastoid foramen in the region of the tympanomastoid suture line, to enter the parotid gland superficial to the retromandibular vein and the deeper external carotid artery. After exiting the foramen and prior to entering the gland, the nerve gives branches to the stylo-

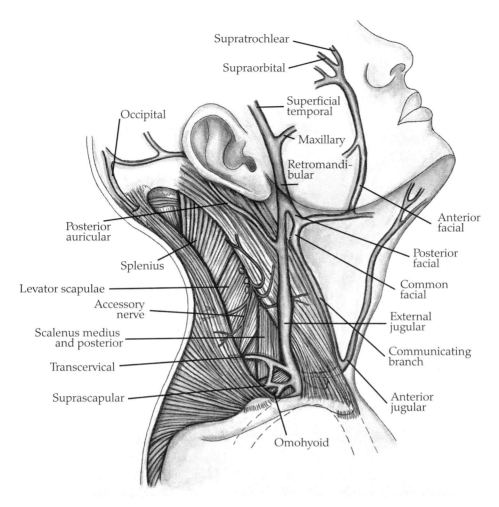

FIGURE 56–2 Superficial veins of the neck.

hyoid, postauricular, and posterior belly of the digastric muscles. For surgical discussion, the parotid is described as being separated into a superfical and a deep lobe by the facial nerve.

> **PITFALL...** When tumors arise in the deep portion of the parotid gland, the facial nerve will be displaced superficially and be vulnerable to iatrogenic injury.

The facial nerve divides at the pes anserinus to form the temporofacial and cervicofacial branches, which usually give rise to the temporal, zygomatic, and buccal branches, and mandibular and cervical branches, respectively. The marginal mandibular branch exits the gland distally to pass superficial to the facial vein. The buccal branch courses parallel to Stensen's duct. The zygomatic branch crosses the zygoma just over the periosteum. The temporal branch can be located crossing the zygoma parallel, anterior, and superficial to the superficial temporal vessels.

ANATOMY OF THE SUBMANDIBULAR GLAND

The submandibular (submaxillary) gland, the second largest of the salivary glands, is enveloped in the superficial layer of the deep cervical fascia. The gland is C-shaped with the larger, superficial portion lateral to the mylohyoid muscle and the smaller, deep portion wrapped around the posterior border of this muscle. The gland is contained within the submandibular triangle (the anterior and posterior bellies of the digastric and the mandible). The submandibular gland contains both serous and mucous secreting acinar cells.

The submandibular (Wharton's) duct emerges from the deep portion to course anteriorly between the hyoglossus and mylohyoid muscles, adjacent to the sublingual gland, to enter the oral cavity just lateral to the lingual frenulum.

The marginal mandibular branch of the facial nerve also lies within the superficial layer of the deep cervical fascia and may course as low as the hyoid bone (another second branchial arch derivative).

PEARL••• Because the marginal mandibular nerve lies superficial to the facial vein, it may be protected during submandibular gland resection by ligating the vein at the level of the hyoid and dissecting in a place deep to the vein.

The hypoglossal nerve (CN XII) remains deep to the digastric tendon. The lingual nerve, a branch of CN V3, courses along the hyoglossus muscle where it gives two branches to the submandibular ganglion and then crosses the submandibular duct twice.

ANATOMY OF THE SUBLINGUAL GLAND

The sublingual gland, the smallest of the paired, major salivary glands, is not enveloped in a fascial capsule. Rather, it lies submucosally in the anterolateral floor of mouth bounded by the mandible and genioglossus laterally and the mylohyoid inferiorly. The submandibular duct and lingual nerve travel between the genioglossus and the sublingual gland. The sublingual gland contains predominantly mucous secreting acinar cells.

Unlike the parotid and submandibular glands, the sublingual gland has small ductules (ducts of Rivinus), which open from the superior surface of the gland directly into the oral cavity along the lingual fold. Occasionally, a separate ductule empties into the submandibular duct.

MINOR SALIVARY GLANDS

There are hundreds (500 to 1000) of minor salivary glands within the oral cavity and pharynx. Predominantly located along the hard and soft palate, they may also be found in the buccal, labial, lingual, and tonsillar locations. Each gland has a simple duct opening directly into the mouth or pharynx. Minor salivary glands contain predominantly mucus but may also contain serous secreting acinar cells.

PHYSIOLOGY OF THE SALIVARY GLANDS

The major secretory product of salivary glands is saliva, with between 500 and 1500 mL produced daily. Saliva aids in taste transmission, mastication, deglutition, and digestion (starch by α-amylase). Additionally, saliva prevents dental carries and enhances enamel formation. Saliva contains antimicrobial compounds such as lysozymes, secretory immunoglobulin A (IgA), and peroxidase.

Salivary production is an active process beginning in the acinus and distally modified by the ductal cells (Fig. 56–3). The acini and proximal ducts secrete preformed saliva through contraction of myoepithelial cells. The more distal ductal cells modify the tonicity through active sodium and passive water transport. The degree of modification is dependent on the rate of salivary flow, with slower flow rates corresponding to more hypotonic saliva. The net effect of ductal transport is a decrease in sodium and an increase in potassium concentrations.

As parotid glands consist predominantly of serous acini, the secretory product is high in enzymes and low in mucin. The converse is true for the sublingual glands.

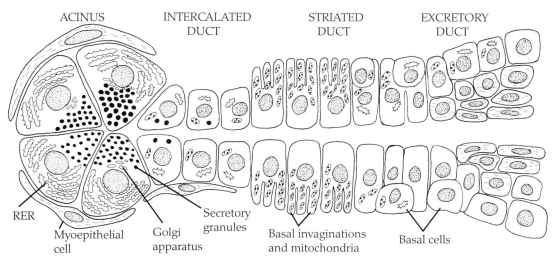

ACINUS   INTERCALATED DUCT   STRIATED DUCT   EXCRETORY DUCT

RER
Myoepithelial cell
Golgi apparatus
Secretory granules
Basal invaginations and mitochondria
Basal cells

FIGURE 56-3 The salivary gland.

AUTONOMIC INNERVATION

Although a minimal basal secretory rate exists (mostly from the submandibular gland), as does a diurnal variation (decreased flow at night and in the morning), salivary secretion is predominantly under autonomic control. In fact the parasympathetic system is most important in regulation of the secretory rate, whereas the sympathetic system may have a role for modulation of salivary composition. Thus, salivary secretion is dependent on parasympathetic stimulation.

PAROTID INNERVATION

The parotid gland receives parasympathetic innervation from Jacobson's nerve, a branch of the glossopharyngeal (CN IX), which after traversing the tympanic cavity as the tympanic plexus becomes the lesser superficial petrosal nerve, synapsing at the otic ganglion. Postganglionic fibers travel to the parotid gland via the auriculotemporal nerve, a branch of CN V3 (Fig. 56–4). Unstimulated the parotid gland contributes about 25% to total salivary flow, which increases to 70% once stimulated.

Acetylcholine (ACh) is the primary neurotransmitter of the parasympathetic system. Muscarinic, rather than nicotinic, receptors are involved in salivary gland stimulation. Stimulation is by passive diffusion of neurotransmitter, rather than nerve synapse.

Sympathetic fibers leave the ventral roots of the thoracic spinal cord to ascend the cervical sympathetic chain and synapse at the superior cervical ganglion. Postganglionic fibers then travel along the external carotid artery to the parotid gland. Norepinephrine is the major neurotransmitter of the sympathetic system, and all synapses are adrenergic.

SPECIAL CONSIDERATION

Gustatory sweating, Frey's syndrome, a problem often encountered following superficial parotidectomy, results from ACh released from parasympathetic fibers stimulating acetylcholine receptors on sweat glands normally stimulated by sympathetic fibers.

SUBMANDIBULAR AND SUBLINGUAL INNERVATION

The submandibular and sublingual glands receive parasympathetic innervation from the chorda tympani nerve, a branch of the facial (CN VII), which after traversing the tympanic cavity joins the lingual nerve, a branch of CN V3, to synapse in the submandibular ganglion. From the submandibular ganglion, postgan-

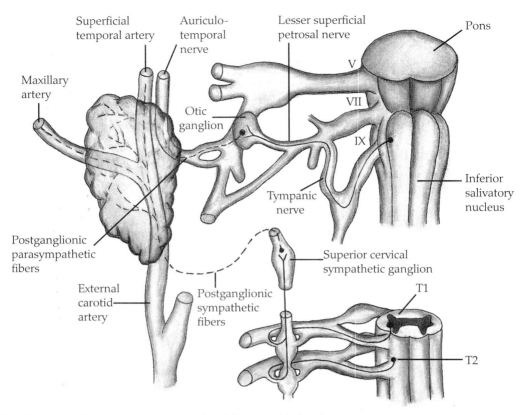

FIGURE 56–4 Autonomic nerve supply of the parotid gland.

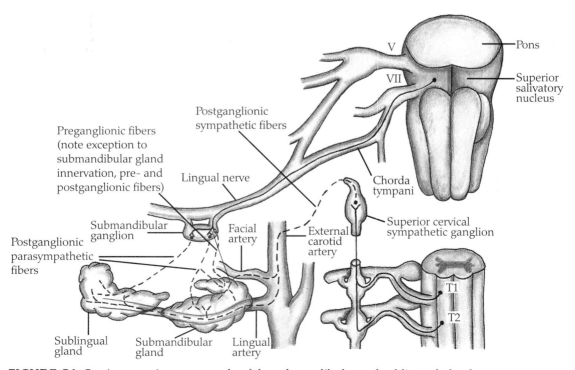

FIGURE 56–5 Autonomic nerve supply of the submandibular and sublingual glands.

glionic fibers travel to the submandibular and sublingual glands (Fig. 56–5). The submandibular gland is unique in that some preganglionic fibers synapse within small ganglia contained within the gland itself. Unstimulated the submandibular gland contributes about 70% of the total salivary flow, which decreases to 25% once all glands are stimulated.

Sympathetic fibers ascend along the external carotid to the facial artery and then continue to the submandibular gland. The sublingual gland is supplied by fibers that traverse the lingual artery.

SUGGESTED READINGS

Batsakis JG. Physiology, salivary glands. In: Cummings CW, Fredrickson JM, Harker LA, Krause CJ, Schuller DE, eds. *Otolaryngology—Head and Neck Surgery.* 2nd ed. St. Louis: Mosby Year Book; 1993:986–996.

Graney DO, Jacobs JR, Kern R. Anatomy, salivary glands. In: Cummings CW, Fredrickson JM, Harker LA, Krause CJ, Schuller DE, eds. *Otolaryngology—Head and Neck Surgery.* 2nd ed. St. Louis: Mosby Year Book; 1993:977–985.

Grant JC. *Grant's Atlas of Anatomy.* 6th ed. Baltimore: Williams & Wilkins; 1972:466–552.

Johns ME. The salivary glands: anatomy and embryology. *The Otolaryngologic Clinics of North America—Symposium on Salivary Gland Diseases* 1977;10(2):261–271.

Kontis TC, Johns ME. Anatomy and physiology of the salivary glands. In: Bailey BJ, Kohut RI, Pillsbury HC III, Tardy ME Jr, eds. *Head and Neck Surgery—Otolaryngology.* Vol. 1. Philadelphia: JB Lippincott; 1993:447–454.

Rice DH. Salivary gland physiology. *The Otolaryngologic Clinics of North America—Symposium on Salivary Gland Diseases* 1977;10(2):273–285.

Chapter 57

CLINICAL TESTS

David L. Steward and Thomas A. Tami

Clinical tests of the salivary glands can be classified as laboratory (hematology, sialochemistry, antibody serology, or microbiology), imaging (radiography, sialography, computed tomography, ultrasonography, radionucleotide, or magnetic resonance), pathology (cytology, frozen or permanent histology), and functional (salivation or lacrimation). The best clinical test is one that is specific, sensitive, and cost-effective, and the decision to obtain a clinical test should be based on an expectation that the information obtained will change the course of patient management. This chapter reviews the more common clinical tests, with unusual disease-specific tests being described in Chapters 59 to 63, which discuss specific disease states.

LABORATORY TESTS

Laboratory tests may be helpful in selected cases of salivary pathology, generally cases of inflammatory disease. Hematologic tests, such as complete blood count and erythrocyte sedimentation rate (ESR), are not very sensitive or specific for salivary disease and are only rarely helpful in making a diagnosis. Serologic chemistry tests, with the possible exception of fasting glucose, are also not clinically helpful in most cases. Sialochemistry, the measurement of endogenous and exogenous factors in saliva, is likewise not clinically useful.

SERUM ANTIBODIES

An autoimmune workup for Sjögren's disease often includes SS-A (Ro) and SS-B (La) autoantibodies. These are elevated in 70% and 50%, respectively, of primary Sjögren's syndrome. The sensitivity is less for secondary Sjögren's syndrome, where rheumatoid factor (RF) and antinuclear antibodies (ANAs) are more commonly elevated. Although ESR is elevated in 70% of patients with Sjögren's disease, it is nonspecific (see Chapter 60).

Viral antibody titers can be useful to identify the specific cause of viral sialadenitis, although these tests are necessary in only a minority of cases. In adolescent or postpubescent boys who are at risk for developing orchitis, acute and convalescent mumps S and V antiviral titers should be obtained from blood or urine to confirm the diagnosis (see Chapter 60). Cytomegalovirus (CMV), Epstein-Barr virus (EBV), and human immunodeficiency virus (HIV) sialadenitis can be diagnosed using specific antibody tests when suspected.

MICROBIOLOGY

Cultures are most commonly obtained in cases of bacterial sialadenitis. These are recommended to direct antibiotic therapy in immunocompromised patients and may be obtained by culturing purulent saliva from the involved salivary duct or by performing needle aspiration of the involved salivary gland. Though rarely needed, viral cultures may be obtained in a similar manner.

PEARL... As a general rule, swab cultures are least likely to demonstrate positive growth on culture, especially anaerobes. Aspiration of a collection of fluid is much more sensitive.

SPECIAL CONSIDERATION

Bacterial cultures should be considered in all hospitalized patients who develop sialadenitis, as they often have resistant organisms.

IMAGING TESTS

Much controversy exists regarding the routine use of imaging in the evaluation of salivary gland pathology. Some authors feel that if a discrete tumor is identified, then directly proceeding to surgical treatment and histopathologic diagnosis is indicated. Others routinely utilize imaging to better counsel the patient preoperatively and to better plan the definitive procedure. In the end, the decision comes down to the philosophy of the physician and patient.

PLAIN RADIOGRAPHY

Plain radiographs can be utilized to diagnose sialolithiasis.

PEARL... Approximately 90% of submandibular calculi are radiopaque, in contrast to only about 10% of parotid calculi.

Although inexpensive, the utility of plain radiographs is limited by the fact that they rarely change patient management.

SIALOGRAPHY

Sialography is performed to radiographically demonstrate the salivary ducts by instilling a radiopaque material through the main ductal system. This can be done with plain radiographs or with computed tomography. Although popular in the past for a wide array of pathology, the role for sialography is currently limited by its lack of specificity and cumbersome technique.

CONTROVERSY

Some authors still advocate sialography for evaluation of calculi, ductal obstruction, inflammatory disease, penetrating trauma, and mass lesions.

COMPUTED TOMOGRAPHY

The use of computed tomography (CT) scanning in the evaluation of salivary disease has increased over the last two decades. Indications for CT scanning include differentiation of abscess from sialadenitis, differentiation of diffuse sialadenosis from discrete tumor, and determination of extent of tumor or abscess prior to treatment. Traditionally superior for evaluation of bony anatomy, newer generation CT scanners have improved soft tissue definition. The addition of iodinated contrast further increases diagnostic accuracy for vascular, inflammatory, and neoplastic processes. CT scanning, however, lacks specificity for differentiating benign from malignant disease.

CONTROVERSY

Some authors feel that CT can be used to accurately determine malignancy. They point out that malignant tumors show irregular outlines, diffuse borders, and nodal metastasis.

CT scanning is helpful in differentiating deep lobe parotid tumors from tumors originating within the parapharyngeal space. CT demonstration of multiple thin-walled cysts in an HIV-infected patient is usually sufficient for the diagnosis of HIV-associated salivary gland disease. CT scanning is the imaging method of choice when evaluating bony anatomy. CT scanning is ten times more sensitive than plain radiographs for sialolithiasis, allowing for asymptomatic calculi to be visualized.

SPECIAL CONSIDERATION

Except in cases of gross bone destruction, CT is not sensitive or specific enough to definitively diagnose bone invasion by tumor.

ULTRASONOGRAPHY

Ultrasonography utilizes high-frequency sound waves for imaging. The main advantages are that it is inexpensive, noninvasive, and does not require radiation exposure. Its clinical use is limited to differentiating cystic from solid masses, and in the identification of calculi. Both of these functions can be more effectively accomplished with CT scanning.

RADIONUCLEOTIDE IMAGING

Radionucleotide imaging is based on the fact that technetium 99 is taken up by salivary tissue. The oncocytic component of adenolymphoma (Warthin's) and the oncocytoma readily and preferentially accumulate this radionucleotide, permitting their diagnosis. This test is occasionally clinically useful in elderly asymptomatic patients with a tail of parotid mass in whom parotidectomy is not warranted.

MAGNETIC RESONANCE IMAGING

The clinical role of magnetic resonance imaging (MRI) has increased over the past decade. The indications for MRI tend to overlap with those of CT scanning. MRI is the study of choice when evaluating vascular or neoplastic processes, whereas CT is more helpful in evaluating calculi and inflammatory disease. MRI is the best imaging technique available for definition of soft tissue. Utilization of MR angiography (MRA) and MR venography (MRV), as well as the addition of the paramagnetic contrast agent gadolinium-diethylenetriamine pentaacetic acid (DTPA), has further increased its ability to differentiate soft tissue pathology. Because MRI is limited in its ability to define bony anatomy, CT and MRI are often complementary when evaluating the extent of neoplastic processes.

PITFALL...
Despite its sensitivity in identifying soft tissue lesions, MRI still lacks specificity in differentiating benign from malignant neoplasms.

CONTROVERSY

Some authors feel that with proper interpretation, MRI can effectively and accurately differentiate benign from malignant tumors based on appearance.

The major disadvantages of MRI scanning are increased cost over other imaging technology, increased patient claustrophobia, and time required for the study. Its use is also contraindicated in patients with ferromagnetic implants.

HISTOPATHOLOGY TESTS

Pathology is currently the gold standard test for diagnosing salivary neoplasms and cysts. It is also extremely useful for certain inflammatory processes such as Sjögren's syndrome and sarcoidosis (Chapter 60).

FINE-NEEDLE ASPIRATION CYTOLOGY

Fine-needle aspiration (FNA) cytology is safe and effective and has increasingly aided diagnosis of salivary gland tumors not requiring excisional biopsy. The sensitivity has been reported to be between 66 and 100%. Sample error is the main limitation to improving sensitivity of this test. Image guided aspiration may decrease sample error and thus increase sensitivity. Specificity continues to improve as the familiarity of cytopathologists with salivary disease increases. Currently, it is estimated to be between 92 and 99% specific for neoplasm at institutions utilizing the technique frequently. Specificity decreases somewhat (70 to 80%) when attempts are made to differentiate benign from malignant neoplasms. FNA is indicated for poor surgical risk patients, patients with a history of malignancy, and patients in whom inflammatory disease has not yet been differentiated from neoplastic disease by imaging.

CONTROVERSY

Some authors recommend FNA cytology for all salivary tumors, to aid in preoperative planning and patient counseling.

FNA cytology, when performed with a 17-gauge needle, or smaller, is not associated with tumor seeding of the needle tract. The disadvantages of FNA cytology are occasional patient intolerance, problems of sample error, and need for an experienced cytopathologist.

FROZEN SECTION HISTOPATHOLOGY

Frozen section diagnosis of salivary tumors is generally quite good, with published accuracy rates of 96%. If, however, an attempt is made to specifically diagnose benign and malignant disease, the accuracy rates drop to 77% and 85%, respectively. Cellular pleomorphic adenoma, oncocytoma, mucoepidermoid carcinoma, and lymphoma can all present diagnostic difficulty on frozen section alone. The role for routine frozen section evaluation after excisional biopsy of salivary gland tumors remains controversial. A decision to do so should be based on a clear understanding of how the information may impact patient management, rather than as a "knee-jerk" response.

Incisional biopsy may be performed for frozen section diagnosis when malignancy is suspected preoperatively and confirmatory di-

agnosis is desired prior to performing radical or destructive surgery. As a general rule, radical or destructive surgery should not be performed on the basis of frozen section diagnosis alone but rather in combination with relevant history, physical exam, imaging, and/or FNA cytology information. When doubt exists, conservative surgical therapy with preservation of important structures should be undertaken, with a plan to await confirmatory diagnosis on permanent histopathologic evaluation.

CONTROVERSY

The role for frozen section analysis of margins, either soft tissue or neural, is controversial. Sample error and skip lesions complicate the effectiveness.

PERMANENT HISTOPATHOLOGY

Permanent histopathologic specimens may be obtained by large-needle, incisional, or excisional biopsy. Large needle biopsy often produces destruction of tissue architecture, making it extremely difficult to establish an accurate diagnosis. Additionally this type of biopsy can be associated with seeding of the needle tract and is recommended only in high-risk surgical patients in whom FNA is not diagnostic.

Incisional biopsy for permanent histopathologic evaluation is acceptable for minor salivary gland or sublingual gland tumors; however, excisional biopsy is still preferable for anticipated benign disease. Incisional biopsy for permanent histopathologic evaluation is contraindicated in tumors of the parotid or submandibular gland due to risk of tumor spillage and increased recurrence rates. Excisional biopsy through superficial or total parotidectomy, or submandibular gland removal, is indicated for tumors involving these glands. An exception may be in cases where lymphoma is suspected and definitive management would not include surgery. Tissue should be sent "fresh" in cases suspicious for lymphoma.

Incisional biopsy also has a role in the diagnosis of inflammatory diseases of the parotid gland. It should be performed only after labial minor salivary gland excisional biopsy has not proven diagnostic. The incisional biopsy should be taken in the direction of facial nerve fibers, from the tail of the parotid gland. Noncaseating granulomas suggest sarcoidosis. A focus of greater than 50 lymphocytes per 4 mm^2 is 95% specific for Sjögren's syndrome. (Other specific histopathologic findings are discussed in Chapter 60.)

Excisional biopsy is the gold standard diagnostic clinical test for salivary gland tumors. Many tumors can be diagnosed with standard hematoxylin and eosin (H&E) staining, but special stains may be necessary for others. Mucin and alcian blue stains are used to differentiate adenocarcinoma from mucoepidermoid carcinoma. Periodic acid-Schiff (PAS) is useful in differentiating acinic cell carcinoma, which stains positively and is diastase resistant, from clear cell carcinoma or metastatic renal cell carcinoma. Immunohistochemistry utilizes antibodies to differentiate tumors of different cell origins. Antibodies to S-100 protein identify neural tumors, adenoid cystic carcinoma, and melanoma. Melanoma is further identified with positive HMB45. Leukocyte common antigen (LCA) is positive in lymphoma. Cytokeratin is positive in squamous cell carcinoma, mucoepidermoid carcinoma, and carcinoma expleomorphic. These immunohistochemical techniques are extremely useful adjuncts to standard H&E staining, especially in poorly differentiated neoplasms.

In addition to diagnosis, permanent histopathologic evaluation can give information about local and regional metastatic involvement of nerves, vessels, lymph nodes, and adjacent soft or bony tissue. Margins may also be evaluated for adequacy of surgical resection and likelihood of residual disease.

SPECIAL CONSIDERATION

Abnormal DNA ploidy, a measure of frequency of aneuploid cells, has been associated with more aggressive tumors, but the clinical relevance remains uncertain.

FUNCTIONAL TESTS

Clinically relevant functional tests of the salivary system are limited to measurement of the salivary secretory flow rate (sialometry). Even this is burdensome and not routinely performed. Sialometry can be helpful to quantify salivary dysfunction, because drooling or xerostomia are only rarely associated with hypersalivation or hyposalivation, respectively (Chapter 59). Salivary flow rates can be measured in the stimulated or resting (unstimulated) state. Stimulated salivary flow can be achieved using 2% citric acid, chewing paraffin wax, or with pilocarpine. Saliva is collected over a period of 5 to 15 minutes in calibrated cylinders, from the oral cavity or from a specific salivary duct. Published normal total salivary flow rates are 0.3 to 0.5 mL/min for resting, and 1 to 2 mL/min for stimulated tests. Published normal unilateral parotid salivary flow rates are 0.02 to 0.17 mL/min for resting and 0.03 to 0.67 mL/min for stimulated tests.

Although the lacrimal gland is not part of the salivary system, it is an exocrine gland whose functional status can easily be measured. This is done in the workup of suspected autoimmune inflammatory diseases such as Sjögren's syndrome. Measurement of lacrimation is performed using a piece of litmus or filter paper placed under the lower eyelid. The distance moisture travels in 5 minutes is then measured (Schirmer's test). Values less than 5 mm are considered significant for hypofunction.

SUGGESTED READINGS

Brooks ML, Mayer DP. Imaging in salivary gland disorders. In: Granick MS, Hanna DC III, eds. *Management of Salivary Gland Lesions.* Baltimore: Williams & Wilkins; 1992:38–53.

Chan MK, McGuire LJ, King W, Li AK, Lee JC. Cytodiagnosis of 112 salivary gland lesions: correlation with histologic and frozen section diagnosis. *Acta Cytol* 1992;36:353–363.

Cohen MB, Britt-Marie E, Ljung MD, Boles R. Salivary gland tumors: fine-needle aspiration vs frozen-section diagnosis. *Arch Otolaryngol Head Neck Surg* 1986;112:867–869.

Coll J, Porta M, Rubies-Prat J, et al. Sjogren's syndrome: a stepwise approach to the use of diagnostic tests. *Ann Rheum Dis* 1992;51:607–610.

Cros DL, Gansler TS, Morris RC. Fine needle aspiration and frozen section of salivary gland lesions. *South Med J* 1990;83:283–286.

Gershon A. MUMPS. In: Fauci AS, Braunwald E, Isselbacher KJ, et al, eds. *Harrison's Principles of Internal Medicine.* 14th ed. New York: McGraw-Hill, 1998;1127–1128.

Gluckman JL, ed. Contemporary classification of salivary gland tumors. In: *Renewal of Certification Study Guide in Otolaryngology Head and Neck Surgery.* Dubuque, IA: AAO–Kendall/Hunt; 1998: 547–551.

Gluckman JL, ed. Sjogren's syndrome. In: *Renewal of Certification Study Guide in Otolaryngology Head and Neck Surgery.* Dubuque, IA: AAO–Kendall/Hunt; 1998:563–565.

Heller KS, Attie JN, Dubner S. Accuracy of frozen section evaluation of salivary tumors. *Am J Surg* 1993;116:424–427.

Moutsopoulos HM. Sjögren's syndrome. In: Fauci AS, Braunwald E, Isselbacher KJ, et al, eds. *Harrison's Principles of Internal Medicine.* 14th ed. New York: McGraw-Hill; 1998:1901–1903.

Rice DH. Diagnostic imaging. In: Cummings CW, Frederickson JM, Harker LA, et al, eds. *Otolaryngology Head and Neck Surgery.* Vol. 2. St. Louis: Mosby Year Book; 1998:1223–1233.

Seifert G, Miehlke J, Haubrich J, Chilla R. Methods of investigation. In: *Diseases of the Salivary Glands.* New York: Thieme; 1986:44–62.

Som PM. Salivary glands: In: Som PM, Bergion RT, eds. *Head and Neck Imaging.* 2nd ed. St. Louis: Mosby Year Book; 1991:277–348.

Chapter 58

CONGENITAL DISORDERS

David L. Steward and Thomas A. Tami

Congenital disorders of salivary glands are uncommon, with the majority being associated with the parotid gland. These congenital disorders can be categorized as being developmental anomalies of the branchial system, nonbranchial developmental anomalies, or neoplasms. This chapter reviews several of the more important of these.

FIRST BRANCHIAL ANOMALIES

Branchial anomalies may be cysts, sinuses, or fistuli. A cyst has no epidermal connection. A sinus connects to the epidermis or lumen of the foregut via an epithelial-lined tract. A fistula has communication between the epidermis and the lumen of the foregut via an epithelial-lined tract. Some authors further characterize branchial anomalies as being of cleft (ectoderm), arch (mesoderm), or pouch (endoderm) origin.

The first branchial cleft is the only cleft that persists in normal development. It invaginates to form the external auditory canal (EAC). First branchial anomalies tend to be duplication anomalies of the first branchial cleft. Work's classification of type I and II first branchial cleft anomalies has been widely accepted. He proposed that type I anomalies are of ectodermal origin and are considered a duplication of the membranous EAC. Type II anomalies are of ec-

todermal and mesodermal origin and are duplication anomalies of the membranous EAC and pinna (thus containing skin and cartilage). Both types may be intimately related to the parotid gland and the facial nerve. Tympanic cavity involvement is described but unusual. First branchial cleft cysts account for 8% of branchial anomalies, with type I occurring more frequently than type II.

Type I first branchial anomalies appear in the periauricular region (embedded within the parotid if preauricular) where they tend to be parallel to the EAC and lateral to the facial nerve. If a sinus or fistulous tract exists, it will open into the EAC (Fig. 58–1).

Type II first branchial anomalies appear posterior or inferior to the angle of the mandible and are intimately related to the parotid gland. They may lie lateral to, medial to, or between the branches of the facial nerve. Sinus or fistulous tracts, when present, connect to the EAC (Fig. 58–2).

> **PEARL...** Adequate and safe resection of these lesions (especially type II) requires identification and preservation of the facial nerve, often through a superficial parotidectomy approach. Branches of the nerve can occasionally be split by the sinus tract of the cyst.

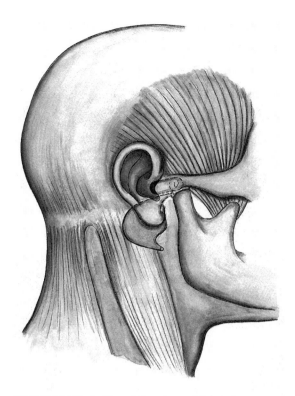

FIGURE 58-1 Type I first branchial defects.

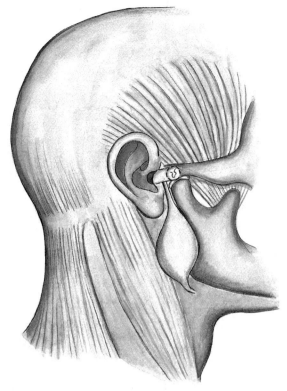

FIGURE 58-2 Type II first branchial defects.

SPECIAL CONSIDERATION

Branchial cleft anomalies cannot be differentiated from preauricular pits/sinuses. These lesions typically present as a pit or sinus tract arising from the skin overlying the crus of the helix. These congenital malformations arise from failed fusion of the hillocks during pinna development.

NONBRANCHIAL DEVELOPMENTAL ANOMALIES

Nonbranchial developmental anomalies encompass vascular and lymphatic malformations, pluripotential stem cell defects, as well as salivary glandular and ductal developmental anomalies.

HEMANGIOMAS

Hemangiomas are vascular developmental anomalies and are the most common congenital salivary gland tumor. Hemangiomas have been classified as capillary, cavernous, mixed, proliferative, and invasive. They may also have a lymphangiomatous component. They differ from other congenital vascular anomalies such as venous and arteriovenous malformations in that hemangiomas grow by cellular proliferation, whereas the latter two entities grow by dilatation of existing vessels.

Capillary hemangiomas predominantly involve the parotid gland, are more common in females (2:1), and usually occur on the left side (5:1). These tumors are generally contained within the capsule of the gland. Clinically, over 90% present within the first 6 months of life as a bluish mass over the parotid region that undergoes a rapid growth phase over a few months.

The head-hanging position or crying increases the size and bluish discoloration, and the mass may feel doughy to palpation. Many patients have other hemangiomas, which should be documented, as their resolution may provide prognostic information for the parotid lesion.

SPECIAL CONSIDERATION

Microscopically, mitotic figures may be demonstrated; however, this is not indicative of malignancy in this age group.

Slow resolution, over a period of 4 to 6 years, is the general rule for these lesions, and treatment should be reserved for functional impairment, hemorrhage, thrombocytopenia (Kasabach-Merritt syndrome), infection, or ulceration. Systemic steroids are capable of stopping growth and inducing resolution in some patients. The mechanism of action is unclear; however, the response is usually within days of initiation of treatment.

SPECIAL CONSIDERATION

Because of adrenal and immune suppression with steroid use, long-term therapy is not recommended in this age group.

The role for intralesional steroids is as yet undefined in this region. Low-dose and short-term cyclophosphamide has been used in conjunction with steroids in the medical management of hemangiomas and lymphangiomas. Interferon-2α is currently reserved for patients with the life-threatening coagulopathy associated with Kasabach-Merritt syndrome.

Surgical therapy can be accompanied by a significant risk of neurovascular injury and should not be undertaken lightly. Identification of and preservation of the facial nerve are mandatory. Superficial parotidectomy may not be curative as these lesions may involve the deep portion of the gland, and staged excision may be necessary. Preoperative embolization or external carotid artery ligation is often recommended.

Because sclerosing agents have proven ineffective, they cannot be recommended. Radiation therapy has been described but is associated with a risk of developing malignancy later in life and is rarely warranted in this age group.

LYMPHANGIOMAS

Lymphangiomas are lymphatic developmental anomalies that may occasionally occur within any of the major or minor salivary glands, or more commonly as an extension from jugulolymphatic sac defects to the parotid or submandibular glands. Lymphangiomas can be classified as capillary or cavernous or as cystic hygromas depending on the size of the lymphatic channels; however, all three histologic types may be present within the same lesion. Cavernous lymphangiomas predominantly involve the parotid gland, are more common in girls than boys (7:1), and have no side predilection.

Clinically, lymphangiomas present shortly after birth with 60% diagnosed within the first and 90% within the second year of life. They commonly present as asymptomatic, fluctuant masses. Local infection is speculated to result in rapid growth. Hemorrhage into a cystic component may also result in a rapid increase in size of these lesions.

Unlike hemangiomas, lymphangiomas do not usually involute. Intervention is therefore warranted; however, it may be prudent to delay therapy until the patient is 3 to 4 years old to allow the patient to grow if the mass is not enlarging. Recurrent infections, compressive symptoms, and a doubtful diagnosis may precipitate earlier intervention.

Surgical excision is the treatment of choice. Surgery should be conservative with preservation of important neurovascular structures as recurrence rates are low (5 to 10%) even when remnants of tumor are left behind.

Injection of sclerosing agents has not proven successful in managing these lesions. Radiation therapy is associated with an unacceptably high risk of malignancy later in life in this age group and should not be used.

DERMOIDS AND TERATOMAS

Dermoids and teratomas are developmental anomalies of pluripotential stem cells. They are classified as dermoid cysts (ectoderm and mesoderm), teratoid cysts (poorly differentiated ectoderm, mesoderm, and endoderm), teratomas (well-differentiated ectoderm, mesoderm, and endoderm), and epignathi (complete differentiation of organs and limbs). Neurogenic tissue is a common component of ectodermal origin within these lesions.

Teratomas usually present within the first year of life and are associated with maternal polyhydramnios in 18% of cases. Isolated cases of malignant teratomas have been documented in neonatal patients.

Surgical excision is the definitive therapeutic modality for these lesions. Identification and preservation of important neurovascular structures are paramount. Encapsulation is common, which facilitates complete and safe removal.

DEVELOPMENTAL SALIVARY ANOMALIES

Congenital ductal cysts occur primarily in the parotid, though they may also occur in the submandibular gland. True cysts differ from pseudocysts (such as a ranula) in that a true cyst contains an epithelial lining. The majority of true salivary cysts are acquired, however. No therapy is indicated for congenital ductal cysts in infancy, unless they become recurrently infected. Surgery is curative.

Heterotopic salivary glands have been reported to occur in the neck, usually with cervical lymph nodes. Treatment is surgical excision.

Agenesis of salivary glands has been reported. Imaging makes the diagnosis in a child with xerostomia of unknown etiology. Treatment is aimed at improving oral hygiene.

Imperforate submandibular ducts have been described. They present with retention cysts in infancy. Therapy is marsupialization of the submandibular duct.

Congenital sialectasia is thought to represent abnormal ductal development with progressive dilation and sacculation of the ductal system. The patient presents with diffuse enlargement of one salivary gland and may progress to recurrent or chronic sialadenitis. Initial therapy is conservative, with surgery reserved for recurrent or chronic infections.

NEOPLASMS

Other than the vasoformative tumors previously described (hemangioma and lymphangioma), congenital salivary gland neoplasms are extremely rare.

Sialoblastomas are congenital epithelial tumors (of basal cell type) of the parotid or submandibular gland. Treatment is surgical excision, though there have been cases of local recurrence. A malignant form has also been described.

Congenital parotid salivary gland carcinomas have been reported to be quite aggressive, with both reported cases requiring surgical excision followed by radiation and/or chemotherapy.

Neurofibromas have been described in both the parotid and submandibular glands of patients with neurofibromatosis (von Recklinghausen's disease), an autosomal-dominant disease with variable penetrance and an incidence of 1:3000 births. The diagnosis should be suspected in patients with a neurofibroma and café-au-lait spots or axillary freckling.

SPECIAL CONSIDERATION

Unlike schwannomas, neurofibromas are not encapsulated and often have nerve fibers running through them; therefore, surgical therapy almost always results in cranial nerve sacrifice.

Between 6 and 16% of neurofibromatosis patients have sarcomatous transformation of one of the neurofibromas.

SUGGESTED READINGS

Chitre VV, Premchandra DJ. Recurrent parotitis. *Arch Dis Child* 1997;77(4):359–363.

Donegan JO. Congenital neck masses. In: Cummings CW, Fredrickson JM, Harker LA, Krause CJ, Schuller DE, eds. *Otolaryngology—Head and Neck Surgery.* 2nd ed. St. Louis: Mosby Year Book; 1993:1554–1562.

Gluckman JG, Medina JE. Lymphangioma and hemangioma: evaluation and treatment. In: Gluckman JG, ed. *Renewal of Certification Study Guide in Otolaryngology—Head and Neck Surgery.* Dubuque: Kendall/Hunt, 1998:435–437.

Harris MD, McKeever P, Robertson JM. Congenital tumours of the salivary gland: a case report and review. *Histopathology* 1990;17(2): 155–157.

Hsueh C, Conzalez-Crussi F. Sialoblastoma: a case report and review of the literature on congenital epithelial tumors of salivary gland origin. *Pediatr Pathol* 1992;12(2):205–214.

Lack EE, Upton MP. Histopathologic review of salivary gland tumors in childhood. *Arch Otolaryngol Head Neck Surg* 1988;114:898–906.

Myer CM, Cotton RT. Salivary gland disease in children: a review. Part 2: congenital lesions and neoplastic disease. *Clin Pediatr* 1986;25 (7):353–357.

Pownell PH, Brown OE, Pransky SM, Manning SC. Congenital abnormalities of the submandibular duct. *Int J Pediatr Otorhinolaryngol* 1992;24(2):161–169.

Regauer S, Gogg-Kamerer M, Braun H, Beham A. Lateral neck cysts—the branchial theory revisisted. A critical review and clinicopathological study of 97 cases with special emphasis on cytokeratin expression. *APMIS* 1997; 105(8):623–630.

Schuller DE, McCabe BF. Salivary gland neoplasms in children. In: Work WP, Johns ME, eds. *The Otolaryngologic Clinics of North America—Symposium on Salivary Gland Diseases* 1977;10(2):399–412.

Seifert G, Donath K. The congenital basal cell adenoma of salivary glands. Contribution to the differential diagnosis of congenital salivary gland tumours. *Virchows Arch* 1997;430 (4):311–319.

Sevila A, Morell A, Navas J, Alfonso R, Silvestre JF, Ramon R. Orifices at the lower neck: heterotopic salivary glands. *Dermatology* 1997; 194(4):360–361.

Work WP. Cysts and congenital lesions of the parotid gland. In: Work WP, Johns ME, eds. *The Otolaryngologic Clinics of North America—Symposium on Salivary Gland Diseases* 1977; 10(2):339–343.

Chapter 59

FUNCTIONAL DISORDERS

David L. Steward and Thomas A. Tami

Functional disorders of salivary glands may be categorized as sialolithiasis, sialadenosis, sialectasia, hypersalivation, hyposalivation, and miscellaneous. This chapter reviews the important clinical entities within these categories. Inflammatory, neoplastic, and traumatic entities are discussed in Chapters 60 to 62.

> **PEARL···** Prior to making a diagnosis of a functional salivary gland disorder (e.g., sialadenosis), consideration should be given to chronic inflammatory etiologies (e.g., Sjögren's disease or sarcoidosis).

SIALOLITHIASIS

Sialolithiasis is defined as the presence of calculi or sialoliths within the ductal system of major or minor salivary glands. It is estimated that sialolithiasis is the most common dysfunction of salivary glands, with a slight female preponderance. The submandibular gland accounts for the majority of the cases (80 to 90%), compared to the parotid (8 to 19%) or the sublingual gland (1%). Although minor salivary gland calculi are unusual, they occur preferentially in the upper lip and buccal mucosa. In the majority of cases of sialolithiasis (75%) only one stone is

present, with multiglandular disease being unusual (3%).

Salivary calculi are usually composed of calcium phosphate and carbonate, along with other inorganic and organic salts and proteins. Calculi formation does not appear to be related to serum concentration of calcium or phosphorus levels. Despite having similar calcium concentrations, 90% of submandibular calculi are radiopaque, compared with only 10% of parotid calculi.

> **SPECIAL CONSIDERATION**
>
> Gout, the only systemic disease known to cause salivary calculi, produces stones composed of uric acid. In this situation, stone formation appears to be dependent on serum concentration.

Salivary stasis predisposes to calculi formation, often around a nidus of debris within the salivary duct. The submandibular gland is thought more vulnerable because the duct is longer, flows in an antigravity direction, and has a smaller-caliber lumen. Additionally, submandibular saliva is relatively more alkaline and has a higher mucus and calcium phosphate concentration than parotid saliva.

The most common presenting symptom is postprandial swelling and pain in the involved gland. Calculi may also be asymptomatic if located deep within the gland. Eventually, patients often present with acute or recurrent infection. Diagnosis is by history, palpation of the stone (especially in the submandibular duct), and possibly imaging studies. The diagnosis is often by history alone in the parotid gland as the calculi tend to be small, difficult to palpate, and radiolucent. Sialography may be helpful.

Treatment is aimed at removal of the calculus. Occasionally the calculus may respond to warm compresses, glandular massage, and fluids, but surgical removal is often required. This may be accomplished transorally when the stone is palpable via incision over the duct (Fig. 59–1). The parotid duct has a propensity to stenosis and

---

CONTROVERSY

Although sialography is occasionally used to direct therapy in cases of chronic inflammation and sialectasia, ultimate treatment most commonly is based on clinical presentation regardless of the radiographic findings.

---

should be stented. When the stone is contained within the gland or cannot be located within the duct, removal of the gland is necessary. For the parotid gland this may require a complete parotidectomy if the stone is within the deep portion of the gland. Secondary infection should be treated as bacterial sialadenitis (see Chapter 60).

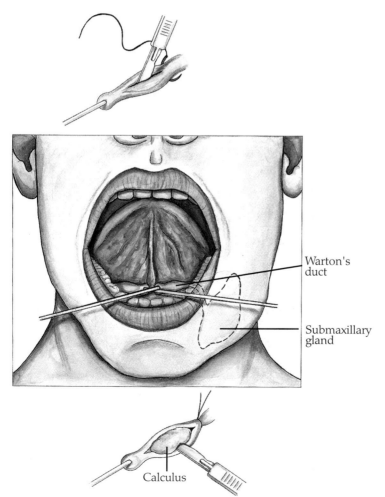

Warton's duct

Submaxillary gland

Calculus

FIGURE 59–1 Techniques for localization and retrieval of a submandibular duct calculus.

PEARL... Always palpate the ductal system intraorally at the end of the case to ensure a stone has not been forced into the duct during gland removal.

SIALADENOSIS

Sialadenosis is a noninflammatory, nonneo-plastic parenchymatous enlargement of salivary glands secondary to metabolic or secretory disorders of the glandular parenchyma. The parotid gland is principally affected as asymptomatic bilateral enlargement. However, due to the systemic nature of these disorders, any or all glands may be involved.

Sialadenosis may be classified by etiology into endocrine, metabolic, pharmacologic, or neurogenic groups (Table 59–1). There is evidence that sialadenosis results from changes in protein secretion from salivary gland acinar cells. Thus, all of these disorders may occur through aberrations in the autonomic nervous system, which regulates salivary flow and composition.

Endocrine abnormalities almost always result in some degree of sialadenosis, especially of the parotid gland. Diabetes mellitus is the most common, though the mechanism is not understood. Diabetes insipidus may affect salivary tissue through a decrease in fluid status. Thyroid disease, specifically hypothyroidism and myxedema, has been associated with sialadenosis.

SPECIAL CONSIDERATION

Salivary glands have an iodide concentrating mechanism similar to that of the thyroid, without the conjugation mechanism.

Other hypothalamic-pituitary axis causes of sialadenosis have been identified, including testicular or ovarian atrophy; menopause, lactation, and pregnancy; and Cushing's (adrenal hyperplasia) or Addison's (adrenal insufficiency) disease. An endocrine evaluation should be performed on a patient suspected of having sial-

TABLE 59–1 CAUSES OF SIALADENOSIS

Endocrine—diabetes, hypothyroidism, pregnancy, lactation, Cushing's, Addison's

Metabolic—malnutrition, vitamin deficiency, obesity, hyperlipidemia, cystic fibrosis

Pharmacologic—parasympathetic or sympathetic agonists or blockers, heavy metals, psychotropics

Neurogenic—dysautomia, Shy-Drager syndrome, diabetic autonomic neuropathy, phobia, depression

adenosis. Resolution of the underlying endocrine abnormality will usually return salivary gland size and function to normal.

Metabolic causes of sialadenosis are predominantly the result of nutritional deficiency. Alcoholic cirrhosis has long been associated with parotid gland enlargement (30 to 80% of patients), and this finding can be used to differentiate this type from other types of cirrhosis. The mechanism is mainly malnutrition. In fact, vitamin or protein deficiency or any disorder that affects absorption of nutrients can result in sialadenosis (Table 59–2). Other metabolic causes are uremia (through elevated ammonia levels), hypertension (possibly through sodium levels), hyperlipidemia, and obesity (through fatty deposition).

PITFALL... Prior to making a diagnosis of sialadenosis secondary to obesity, underlying endocrine etiologies must be evaluated and treated.

Cystic fibrosis warrants special mention as a cause of sialadenosis in children. This recessively inherited disease can result from genetic defects in multiple locations and can be diagnosed with a sweat chloride test. It predominantly affects the mucous-type glands (minor,

TABLE 59–2 NUTRITIONAL DEFICIENCY STATES ASSOCIATED WITH SIALADENOSIS

Malnutrition—alcoholism, anorexia, bulimia, celiac disease, Chagas disease, dysentary, esophageal cancer

Vitamin deficiencies—pellagra (niacin), beriberi (B_1, thiamine), scurvy (C), vitamin A and B_6 deficiencies sublingual, and submandibular glands, in decreasing order).

CONTROVERSY

Some authors believe the parotid glands are predominantly involved in cystic fibrosis, citing the association between pancreatic and parotid enzymatic digestion with amylase. This difference of opinion may result from studying different subsets of patients with cystic fibrosis. In fact, the predominant effect may be the result of malabsorption and malnutrition.

Treatment for metabolic sialadenosis is directed at reversing the underlying metabolic disorder.

SPECIAL CONSIDERATION

Because sialadenosis is commonly associated with the bulemia/anorexia syndrome, this potentially devastating condition, which frequently occurs in adolescent girls, must always be considered in this clinical setting.

Pharmacologic causes of sialadenosis could also be grouped under metabolic causes; however, separating the two is helpful in the clinical setting. Drugs may affect the salivary glands in different ways to produce sialadenosis and the mechanisms are often poorly understood. The majority act through parasympathetic or sympathetic stimulation or blockade (Table 59–3). Some act via changes in fluid states (diuretics). Others have direct toxic effects (heavy metals, iodine, mercury, bismuth, and arsenic) or cause hypersensitivity or allergic reactions (cornstarch), which result in salivary gland enlargement through an inflammatory response (see Chapter 60). Therapy for pharmacologic sialadenosis is drug cessation or change. With discon-

TABLE 59–3 DRUGS AFFECTING SALIVARY FUNCTION

Sympathomimetics—beta-agonists, decongestants, cocaine

Sympathetic antagonists—antihypertensives, beta-blockers

Parasympathomimetics—acetylcholinesterase inhibitors (neostigmine), cholinergic agonists (pilocarpine)

Parasympathetic antagonists—antihistimines, antiemetics, anticholinergics

Psychotropics—stimulants, sedatives, antiparkinsonian, anticonvulsants, antipsychotics, antidepressants

tinuance of the medication, symptoms generally resolve.

Neurogenic abnormalities of the autonomic nervous system (dysautonomia or autonomic neuropathy) will result in sialadenosis. Examples are Parkinson's disease and Shy-Drager syndrome, which both demonstrate atrophy of the autonomic nervous system and may represent a spectrum of the same disease. Autonomic neuropathy can also result from diabetes and alcoholism. Autonomic dysfunction usually results in hypofunction, but hyperfunction has also been described. Parotid hypertrophy has also been noted in individuals after strokes or resection of brain tumors.

SIALECTASIS

Sialectasis is defined as ductal dilatation within a salivary gland and has been classified as congenital (primary) or acquired (secondary). Sialectasia usually results from an obstructive process, such as sialolithiasis; ductal stricture, stenosis, or foreign body (seed); or chronic or recurrent infection. Additionally, it may result from Kussmaul's disease (sialodochitis fibrinosis), which occurs in dehydrated patients who develop mucous or fibrinous plugs within the ductal systems of salivary glands. Treatment is aimed at relieving the underlying obstruction. Hydration is helpful in sialolithiasis and Kussmaul's disease. Chronic sialectasia often results in salivary stasis and chronic or recurrent infection, which may necessitate gland removal (see Chapter 60).

Sialectasia can also occur in the setting of pneumoparotitis following increased intraoral pressure. This has been described in glass blowers, brass musicians, and patients undergoing a bag-mask airway.

HYPERSALIVATION

Hypersalivation (hyperptyalism) is almost always secondary to parasympathetic stimulation, which may be either physiologic or pharmacologic (acetylcholinesterase inhibitor, acetylcholine agonist). Transient hypersalivation is usually caused by psychogenic (food) or mechanical (acid from gastroesophageal reflux) stimulation of the parasympathetic system. Chronic hypersalivation (an increase in salivary flow) is uncommon and should be quantified to distinguish it from sialorrhea (drooling), which most often results from neuromuscular incoordination of swallowing a normal volume of saliva.

Sialometry is used to quantify salivary dysfunction. It involves measurement of resting (unstimulated) and stimulated salivary production by collection of saliva in 0.1-mL calibrated cylinders over a period of 6 minutes. The stimulated test utilizes chewing of paraffin wax or a 2% citric acid solution. Normal flow rates are 0.3 to 0.5 mL/min for resting, and 1 to 2 mL/min for stimulated tests.

Management of sialorrhea in the pediatric population initially involves behavioral therapy, physical therapy, and biofeedback techniques. As improving neuromuscular coordination may be difficult in some patients, medical and surgical therapies are often used to attempt to decrease the amount of salivary flow. Medical therapy is predominantly through the use of anticholinergic agents (glycopyrrolate), which have systemic side effects (tachycardia, urinary retention, and decreased gastrointestinal motility).

CONTROVERSY

Most pediatric otolaryngologists recommend surgical therapy over medical therapy for sialorrhea.

Surgical therapy usually involves bilateral submandibular gland excision and bilateral parotid duct ligation, with subsequent parotid gland atrophy.

PEARL••• Patients should be kept on low-dose antibiotics for at least 1 month postoperatively to prevent suppurative parotitis.

SPECIAL CONSIDERATION

Unlike the parotid gland, the submandibular gland does not undergo atrophy after duct ligation.

Sublingual gland excision is usually not necessary. Tympanic neurectomy, in conjunction with parotid duct ligation, or with chorda tympany section has been advocated by some authors. Because surgical therapy is aimed only at the major salivary glands and because the underlying neuromuscular disabilities persist, surgical therapy is not universally successful in the management of sialorrhea.

HYPOSALIVATION

Hyposalivation (hypoptyalism) is usually secondary to pharmacologic parasympathetic inhibition, autoimmune disease (see Chapter 60), or salivary gland destruction by radiation therapy. Chronic hyposalivation (a decrease in salivary flow) should be distinguished from xerostomia (a sensation of a dry mouth). Over 500 drugs have been linked to xerostomia; however, only a small number have been shown to significantly decrease salivation. Furosemide diuresis, for example, is associated with a high incidence of xerostomia; however, a controlled study found no significant change in salivary flow rate. The majority of drugs that do reduce salivary flow rate have direct anticholinergic properties (Table 59–3). The effect is usually reversed upon discontinuation of the medication. The reasons for xerostomia without hyposalivation are not well understood. Systemic and mucosal hydration as well as salivary composition has been postulated to play a role.

Hyposalivation is well described in transient psychogenic states such as fear, stress, hypnosis, and meditation. It has also been described in patients with depression.

Aging has long been associated with xerostomia; however, studies of salivary flow rate do not show significant decreases with age. This is despite histologic evidence of salivary gland atrophy with age.

Hyposalivation secondary to radiation therapy is well documented and becomes permanent when exposure exceeds 50 gray (Gy). Within 1 week of therapy (10 Gy), salivary function declines about 60%. After full-course therapy (60 to 70 Gy), salivary function is essentially absent unless the salivary glands were shielded. The mechanism is not entirely understood but involves salivary epithelial cell death. Treatment for patients with some residual functional salivary tissue is with the cholinergic agonist pilocarpine. For patients with complete absence of function, therapy is with salivary substitutes. Adherence to strict oral hygiene is mandatory to prevent dental carries in the absence of normal salivary function.

MISCELLANEOUS

Masseteric hypertrophy, usually secondary to bruxism, may simulate parotid enlargement. This may be differentiated clinically by having the patient bite down while palpating the masseter muscles. As chewing is known to stimulate salivary flow, it is possible that patients with masseteric hypertrophy could also have secondary sialadenosis.

Frey's syndrome (gustatory sweating) is seen clinically in 35 to 60% of postparotidectomy patients. It is speculated that all patients, if specifically tested using Minor's starch-iodine test, would demonstrate gustatory sweating. When it does present clinically, it usually occurs several months after surgery. The mechanism is cross-reinnervation of the normal fibers of the sympathetic supply to the sweat glands by the fibers of the parasympathetic supply to the parotid gland (see Chapter 57). Treatment is re-

served for patients who are symptomatic. Topical anticholinergic agents (glycopyrrolate, scopolamine) have proven simple and effective.

CONTROVERSY

Some authors recommend placement of tissue (fascia, dermis, alloplasts, or muscle flaps) between the skin flap and parotid bed at the time of surgery to prevent Frey's syndrome.

Additionally, some authors believe avoidance of injury to the auriculotemporal nerve during parotidectomy will prevent Frey's syndrome. Tympanic neurectomy has also been advocated to treat this syndrome but is not universally accepted as an effective therapeutic maneuver.

Cheilitis glandularis is an enlargement of the labial salivary glands, which secrete a clear thick sticky mucus. Lower lip eversion has been described secondary to this disorder. Vermilionectomy is recommended.

SUGGESTED READINGS

Batsakis JG. Salivary gland physiology. In: Cummings CW, Fredrickson JM, Harker LA, Krause CJ, Schuller DE, eds. *Otolaryngology—Head and Neck Surgery*. Vol. 2. 2nd ed. St. Louis: Mosby Year Book; 1993:986–996.

Fox PC. Acquired salivary dysfunction, drugs and radiation. *Ann NY Acad Sci* 1998;842:132–137.

Gill G. Metabolic and endocrine influences on the salivary glands. *Otolaryngol Clin North Am* 1977;10(2):363–369.

Guchelaar HJ, Vermes A, Meerwaldt JH. Radiation-induced xerostomia: pathophysiology, clinical course and supportive treatment. *Supportive Care Cancer* 1997;5(4):281–288.

Langlais RP, Benson BW, Branett DA. Salivary gland dysfunction. *Ear Nose Throat J* 1989;68:758.

Rice DH. Non-neoplastic diseases of the salivary glands. In: Paparella MM, Shumrick DA, Gluckman JL, Meyerhoff WL, eds. *Otolaryn-

gology Head and Neck. Vol. 3. 3rd ed. Philadelphia: WB Saunders, 1991.

Rice DH. Salivary gland physiology. *Otolaryngol Clin North Am* 1977;10(2):273–285.

Richardson EP Jr, Beal MF, Martin JB. Degenerative diseases of the nervous system. In: Braunwald E, Isselbacher KJ, Petersdorf RG, Wilson JD, Martin JB, Fauci AS, eds. *Harrison's Principles of Internal Medicine.* 11th ed. New York: McGraw Hill; 1989:2023–2024.

Ritter FN. Salivary gland involvement in systemic diseases. *Otolaryngol Clin North Am* 1977;10(2):371–377.

Screenby LM, Schwartz SS. A reference guide to drugs and dry mouth. *Gerontology* 1986;5:75–99.

Screenby LM, Valdini A. Xerostomia a neglected symptom. *Arch Intern Med* 1987;147:1333–1337.

Strome M. Nonneoplastic salivary gland diseases in children. *Otolaryngol Clin North Am* 1977;10(2):391–398.

Vissink A, Spijkervet FK, Van Vieuw Amerongen A. Aging and saliva: a review of the literature. *Special Care Dentistry* 1996;16(3):95–103.

Chapter 60

INFECTIOUS AND INFLAMMATORY DISORDERS

David L. Steward and Thomas A. Tami

Infectious or inflammatory disorders of salivary glands are defined as sialadenitis. These disorders are best classified according to the time course of the disease (acute, chronic, or recurrent) and by etiology (infectious, immunologic, allergic, or toxic). Successful management of sialadenitis is dependent on the recognition that inflammatory processes often have a multifactorial basis. Abnormalities of salivary gland anatomy can provide local predisposing factors to inflammation, whereas immune system abnormalities act as systemic predisposing factors.

ACUTE BACTERIAL SIALADENITIS

Acute suppurative sialadenitis is an ascending bacterial infection that affects the parotid gland more often than the submandibular gland. Primarily a disease of the aged and chronically ill, most cases occur in hospitalized patients. Reduced or absent salivary flow is the most important pathogenic factor, with changes in salivary composition playing a subordinate role.

The clinical picture demonstrates warm, tender swelling of the gland, often with overlying skin erythema. Leukocytosis and fever often accompany bacteremia. Purulent secretions may be expressed from the ductal orifice and should be cultured if present. *Staphylococcus aureus* is the most commonly identified organism, with *Streptococcus viridans* second.

PEARL... In the chronically ill, hospitalized patient, a mixed infection including gram-positive, gram-negative, and anaerobic flora should be assumed and empiric therapy instituted accordingly.

Treatment consists of hydration and empiric antibiotic therapy until specific therapy based on culture results can be employed. Additionally, reversal of underlying systemic disease and removal of anticholinergic medications will greatly expedite recovery. Glandular massage and sialogogues may also be helpful in restoring salivary flow.

Progression of the infection to abscess is common, especially in the parotid gland.

SPECIAL CONSIDERATION

Fluctuance is rarely present because of the dense fascia within and surrounding the parotid gland.

Surgical drainage is indicated when no improvement is seen within 48 hours of initiating intravenous antibiotic therapy, when purulent material is draining via Santorini's fissure into the external auditory canal, or when computed tomography (CT) scanning demonstrates abscess formation. Drainage is via a preauricular incision. Incisions parallel to the facial nerve should be made in the fascia overlying the gland. Dissection into the parenchyma should be done bluntly with a hemostat opened in a direction parallel to the branches of the nerve.

> **PITFALL•••** Failure to identify and open the multiple small abscesses within the separate lobules of the gland, or failure to identify and drain abscesses extending into the masseteric or parapharyngeal spaces, may result in deep neck space infection, sepsis, and death.

Preoperative CT scanning is useful to identify abscess location and direct surgical therapy.

> **PEARL•••** Blunt finger dissection into the parapharyngeal space at the time of surgery will identify a collection lurking there, if a CT scan is not obtained preoperatively.

Penrose drains should be left for several days, and the wound only loosely approximated.

Postoperative parotitis, although on the decline with improved intraoperative hydration, still complicates about 0.1% of major surgical procedures. Diagnosis and management are similar to suppurative parotitis.

> **CONTROVERSY**
>
> Given an increased incidence after abdominal procedures, some authors have proposed that an enzymatic autodigestive process similar to that seen in pancreatitis may be involved.

CHRONIC RECURRENT BACTERIAL SIALADENITIS

Chronic, recurrent sialadenitis continues to be a therapeutic challenge to the otolaryngologist. The disease is multifactorial with reduced salivary flow as a common initiator, ductal metaplasia as a common mediator, and chronic sialectasia as a common end stage. Acute exacerbations should be treated as acute suppurative sialadenitis. Conservative management involves optimizing salivary flow via hydration, sialagogues, and glandular massage, along with good oral hygiene. Identifying and treating any underlying etiology such as obstruction (stricture, stone), functional disorder (metabolic, medication), or autoimmune disease (Sjögren's, sarcoidosis) is critical to breaking the vicious cycle depicted in Figure 60–1.

When conservative therapy fails to relieve persistent symptoms of pain and swelling, surgical therapy is initiated. Excision of the gland is the recommended therapy for the chronically infected submandibular gland. Although cure rates approach 100% for near-total parotidectomy, this procedure should not be undertaken lightly. Facial nerve dissection is substantially more difficult in a chronically inflamed gland, resulting in higher complication rates. These risks should be weighed against the patient's age, health, and degree of symptoms.

> **CONTROVERSY**
>
> The facial nerve monitor, although not routinely used for parotidectomy, is highly recommended in the setting of chronic inflammation of the parotid gland.

A superficial parotidectomy may be therapeutic if an obstructive process is localized to the superficial portion of the gland and if performed early in the disease process.

> **PITFALL•••** Once the cycle of recurrent infection occurs, the entire gland undergoes inflammatory changes, which may result in inadequate treatment if only a superficial parotidectomy is performed.

Simple parotid duct ligation intraorally has a reported success rate of 60% in eliminating recurrent parotitis.

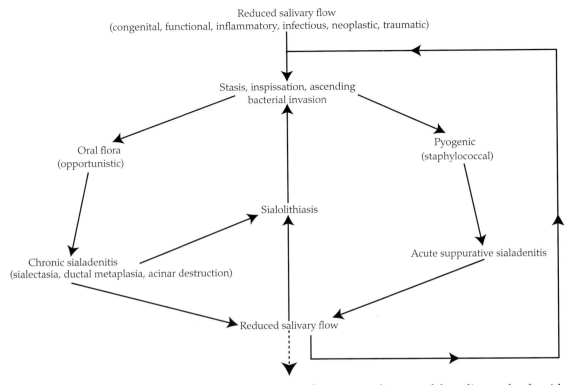

FIGURE 60–1 The relationship of acute and chronic inflammatory diseases of the salivary glands with resultant chronic recurrent sialadenitis.

Low-dose radiation therapy (600 rad) should be considered only for elderly debilitated patients as the beneficial effects are short lived and malignant transformation is a risk.

The prognosis is better for chronic recurrent parotitis in children, and therefore treatment differs from adults. This disease is more common in boys and may manifest as early as infancy. It will often resolve after puberty, with few cases persisting into adulthood. Therapy should be aimed at treatment of underlying factors, maximizing salivary flow, and antibiotic therapy for acute exacerbations until after puberty is reached.

Chronic, sclerosing sialadenitis of the submandibular gland was described by Kuttner in 1896. The hard, swollen submandibular gland is clinically difficult to distinguish from tumor. Histopathology demonstrates a chronic inflammatory process. This probably represents a common end stage of chronic, recurrent submandibular sialadenitis. At this late stage, surgical excision is curative.

ACUTE VIRAL SIALADENITIS

Acute viral sialadenitis is an inflammation of salivary gland tissue usually secondary to infection with a sialadenotropic virus such as mumps or cytomegalovirus. Less frequently, viral sialadenitis results from concomitant viral infection with Epstien-Barr virus (EBV), enterocytopathogenic human orphan virus (ECHO), coxsackievirus, measles, whooping cough, and encephalomyocarditis. After initial respiratory mucosal infection and replication, salivary gland infection is secondary to viremia with hematogenous spread. This is in contrast to ascending infection, as seen in bacterial sialadenitis. This difference is thought to be secondary to the antiviral efficacy of secretory immunoglobulin A (IgA) present in saliva. However, once viremia has occurred, viral secretion in saliva is common.

PEARL••• Many viruses are secreted in saliva and remain infectious without causing sialadenitis, for example, poliomyelitis, hepatitis, human immunodeficiency virus (HIV), rabies, rubella, and influenza.

Mumps is the most common cause of viral sialadenitis. The incidence has decreased markedly in the United States due to routine vaccination against the paramyxovirus causing the disease. It is predominantly a disease of childhood, with 85% of infections in children under 15 years of age. Clinically, the disease presents with unilateral or bilateral parotid swelling progressing from posterior to anterior, often with a general malaise. Submandibular involvement is less common. Inflammation of the pancreas, gonads, and meninges often follows but may be present without the salivary gland involvement. Orchitis during or after puberty occurs in about 10 to 30% of cases leading to sterility if both testes are involved. Meningoencephalitis is often subclinical but in rare cases may be fatal. A more common complication is unilateral deafness. Diagnosis can be made clinically or with mumps S and V antibodies. The virus may also be isolated from the urine within 2 weeks of infection. Treatment is generally supportive. Steroids and gamma globulin are reserved for treating encephalitis, pancreatitis, and orchitis. Childhood immunization is preventative and recommended.

Adult cytomegalovirus (CMV) sialadenitis is usually associated with immune suppression secondary to HIV, organ transplantation, or malignancy. The severity of the infection is usually dependent on the severity of the immune suppression.

Prenatal CMV infection is transmitted across the placenta and is 20 times more com-

---

CONTROVERSY

Some authors believe CMV infection in the immune-suppressed patient is secondary to latent CMV reactivation, possibly from salivary cells. In the immune-competent host, these infections are usually subclinical.

---

mon than perinatal infection, which is transmitted during birth or breast-feeding. A localized occult form of prenatal infection is also called salivary inclusion disease. The more severe, generalized CMV disease is characterized by cerebral, ophthalmologic, hematologic, and hepatic lesions. Typical nuclear inclusion bodies can be seen in salivary duct cells isolated from saliva.

Coxsackievirus sialadenitis is associated with gingivitis and herpangina. Other viral infections may produce concomitant sialadenitis. The diagnosis is usually made using serologic titers.

Human immunodeficiency virus sialadenitis is referred to as HIV-associated salivary gland disease and presents in a very different manner than the above mentioned entities. It predominantly involves the parotid gland, presenting with painless swelling during the early lymphadenopathy portion of the disease. It is bilateral 80% of the time. CT imaging reveals multiple thin-walled cystic masses. Histologically they resemble the lymphoepithelial lesion of Sjögren's syndrome but with a T4/T8 ratio less than 1. HIV testing along with the clinical picture and CT imaging is usually sufficient to make the diagnosis. Fine-needle aspiration (FNA) is reserved for cases where lymphoma is suspected. Occasionally, these cystic masses become secondarily infected and are easily treated with aspiration and appropriate antibiotic therapy. Parotidectomy is rarely indicated.

ACUTE ALLERGIC SIALADENITIS

Acute allergic sialadenitis is uncommon. It is seen after ingestion of foods or medications containing iodide. Patients sensitive to iodide demonstrate a rapid, simultaneous, painful enlargement of all salivary glands. The latency between ingestion and enlargement is usually minutes and represents a hypersensitivity reaction. Swelling generally resolves over a period of hours. Diagnosis is usually by history alone. Serum and salivary eosinophilia may be present. Treatment is supportive unless the patient has signs of anaphylaxis. Avoidance will prevent recurrence. Reactions to phenylbutazone and nitrofurantoin, as well as cornstarch, have also been documented in the literature.

ACUTE TOXIC SIALADENITIS

Radiation sialadenitis is dependent on dose and fractionation. The parotid gland is much more sensitive to radiation than the submandibular gland. This is due to the higher heavy metal content within secretory granules of the serous cells, which catalyze a lipid oxidation when exposed to radiation. This effect is potentiated by concomitant chemotherapy. Low-dose (1000 rad) radiation therapy results in acute and tender parotid gland swelling. Continued irradiation leads to complete destruction of serous acini and glandular atrophy.

Heavy metal ingestion is associated with toxic sialadenitis. Lead, copper, and bismuth are implicated.

CHRONIC SPECIFIC GRANULOMATOUS SIALADENITIS

Tuberculosis of the salivary glands is an infrequent infection by *Mycobacterium tuberculosis,* with a predisposition for the parotid gland. Usually unilateral, these infections most often represent secondary periparotid lymph node involvement often from a tonsil focus. Clinically, these infections present as tumors with a nontender mass present for many weeks. A draining fistula should raise suspicion for this entity. Usually pulmonary involvement is present and may be seen on chest X ray (CXR). Diagnosis is made by positive purified protein derivative (PPD) testing, sputum culture, and/or biopsy demonstrating caseating, necrotizing granulomas. Multiagent antituberculosis chemotherapy is usually therapeutic. Occasionally, surgical ex-

cision or curettage is indicated for persistent draining fistulae.

Atypical *Mycobacterium* infection is increasing in frequency and most commonly seen in children or immune-compromised hosts, manifesting as painful, periparotid lymph node infection with or without cervical lymphadenitis. PPD testing is usually negative or only weakly positive. Treatment can be effective using macrolide antibacterials. Surgical excision or curettage is reserved for persistent infection or draining fistulae.

Cat-scratch disease is a necrotizing, granulomatous lymph node infection caused by the gram-negative bacillus *Bartonella henselae,* which may be demonstrated on Warthin-Starry silver staining. The disease usually causes adenopathy in the region of the animal scratch and may involve periparotid lymph nodes with parenchymal involvement by direct extension. Serologic testing is positive in 70 to 90% of patients but is not currently commercially available. The disease is usually self-limited within 6 months and diagnosis is usually clinical. More symptomatic cases may be treated with doxycycline, fluoroquinolone, or macrolide antibiotic therapy, though this is of no proven benefit. Surgical excision or drainage of suppurative glands may be necessary and biopsy can confirm the diagnosis.

Actinomycosis of salivary glands predominantly involves minor salivary glands after dental manipulation; however, parotid and submandibular infections have been documented. In its chronic form, the disease resembles tuberculosis and may fistulize. Biopsy demonstrating sulfur granules or positive culture are diagnostic. Therapy is with long-term penicillin, and drainage of suppurative glands may be necessary.

> **PITFALL•••** Actinomycosis has been mistaken for malignancy, resulting in unnecessary disfiguring surgery.

Other specific diseases of the salivary glands are rare. Syphilis and gonorrhea have been described as presenting with bilateral painless parotid swelling. Histologically, these represent granulomatous infections. Diagnosis is by serology and culture. Directed antibiotic therapy is curative. Other unusual pathogens that cause cervical lymphadenitis may also present in periparotid lymph nodes (e.g., tularemia, toxoplasmosis). Biopsy and culture are diagnostic.

CHRONIC, NONSPECIFIC, GRANULOMATOUS SIALADENITIS (SARCOIDOSIS)

Chronic, nonspecific, granulomatous sialadenitis (epithelioid cell sialadenitis) is better known as sarcoidosis of the salivary glands. Sarcoidosis is a chronic, multisystem disorder of exaggerated T-helper lymphocyte immune response to as yet unidentified antigens and is characterized by noncaseating, epithelioid granulomas. It affects the parotid gland in about 6% of patients, often bilaterally. Approximately 9% of patients with chronic parotitis actually have sarcoidosis. In the United States the disease is seen more commonly in African Americans than in Caucasians (17:1), and slightly more commonly in females. In other parts of the world, this racial difference is not observed or is reversed. Clinically, patients often present with unilateral or bilateral painless swelling of the parotid gland. Xerostomia is uncommon but may be present. Parotid involvement may be nodal or parenchymal, and the gland may thus feel nodular to palpation. Submandibular and minor salivary gland involvement may be present subclinically in up to 60% of patients with parotid involvement. Definitive diagnosis is made by biopsy demonstrating noncaseating granulomas. As pulmonary involvement is most common, transbronchial biopsy is most often used to make the diagnosis. When this is negative but the diagnosis is still in question, then salivary gland biopsy is indicated.

> **PEARL...** Labial minor salivary gland biopsy may be performed easily in the office, reserving tail of parotid biopsy for negative results.

Elevated serum angiotensin-converting enzyme (ACE) levels and hilar adenopathy on CXR are suggestive of, but not specific for, sarcoidosis.

The triad of parotitis, anterior uveitis, and facial palsy often associated with fever is termed uveoparotid fever or Heerfordt's disease. Lacrimal gland involvement may cause xerophthalmia. Central nervous system involvement most commonly affects the facial nerve; however, other cranial and peripheral neuropathies may also be seen.

> **CONTROVERSY**
>
> Facial nerve involvement may be due to neurosarcoid and not primarily to parotid gland involvement.

Treatment is predominantly cellular immune suppression with steroids. Although the efficacy of cyclophosphamide and methotrexate has not yet been established in controlled studies, these agents are also often employed. As the disease is self-limited in about 50% of patients, treatment is reserved for active pulmonary, neurologic, or ophthalmologic involvement. Steroid therapy is reasonable for acute epithelioid sialadenitis; however, efficacy in reducing chronically swollen parotid glands has not been shown.

Granulomatous cheilitis is a nonspecific granulomatous disease affecting the minor salivary glands, predominantly of the upper lip. It occurs as part of the Melkersson syndrome (facial paralysis, labial edema, and tongue plication) but has also been seen in association with leprosy and more recently Crohn's disease. Interestingly, involvement in Crohn's may occur in the absence of gastrointestinal symptoms. Biopsy demonstrates epithelioid granulomas with inflammatory infiltrates.

CHRONIC, MYOEPITHELIAL SIALADENITIS (SJÖGREN'S SYNDROME)

Sjögren's syndrome is a chronic, slowly progressive autoimmune disease characterized by lymphocytic infiltration and destruction of the exocrine glands resulting in xerostomia and keratoconjunctivitis sicca. The autoimmune response involves lymphocytic T-cell infiltration and B-cell hyperactivity to an as yet undetermined antigenic initiator.

CONTROVERSY

Some authors believe a retrovirus may be the initiator.

Sjögren's syndrome is defined as primary when it occurs alone. In association with other autoimmune rheumatic diseases it is defined as secondary Sjögren's syndrome, which occurs in about half of the cases.

The incidence of Sjögren's syndrome is 0.5% in the general population, and middle-aged women are more commonly affected than are men (9:1). Sjögren's is the second most common autoimmune connective tissue disease behind rheumatoid arthritis, and approximately 25% of patients with rheumatoid arthritis have secondary Sjögren's syndrome.

Xerostomia is the most common symptom of the syndrome and manifests in soreness, altered taste sensation, dental caries, and difficulty chewing, swallowing, or speaking without a liquid bolus. Fissuring of the tongue may be present. Unilateral or bilateral salivary swelling, predominantly of the parotid glands, is present in 75% of primary and 40% of secondary cases of Sjögren's syndrome.

Ocular symptoms include burning, pain, photophobia, or persistent foreign body sensation. Slit-lamp examination after rose Bengal staining reveals superficial corneal erosions in about 25% of patients and is diagnostic of keratoconjunctivitis sicca. Schirmer's eye test (<5 mm in 5 minutes) is positive more frequently but is less specific.

Other symptoms relate to the involvement of exocrine glands throughout the aerodigestive and genitourinary tracts. Although involvement of other exocrine glands is common, this usually remains subclinical. When symptomatic, patients report dry nose and throat, chronic nonproductive cough, as well as dyspareunia secondary to dry genitalia.

About one third of patients with primary Sjögren's report systemic symptoms of fatigue, low-grade fever, myalgia, and arthralgia. The incidence of extraglandular manifestations in primary Sjögren's is summarized in Table 60–1. This extraglandular involvement is sometimes referred to as a lymphoproliferative disorder or as a pseudolymphoma.

SPECIAL CONSIDERATION

If extraglandular involvement includes an increase in monoclonal IgM, this may indicate Waldenström's macroglobulinemia. A sudden decline in the IgM level is considered a poor prognostic sign and may herald a transition to malignancy.

Patients with secondary Sjögren's syndrome have symptoms related to the associated autoimmune disorders (Table 60–2). Rheumatoid arthritis is the most common, presenting in about 50% of patients with secondary Sjögren's.

The risk of developing B-cell lymphoma with Sjögren's syndrome is 44 times greater than for the population at large. It is an additional 5 times greater when parotid swelling is part of the syndrome. Splenomegaly, lymphadenopathy, prior radiotherapy, and immune suppression are additional risk factors. CT scanning and vigilant surveillance for increased parotid swelling or lymphadenopathy are critical to the management of these patients. FNA should be performed, followed by biopsy, for any suspicious lesions.

TABLE 60–1 INCIDENCE OF EXTRAGLANDULAR MANIFESTATIONS IN PRIMARY SJÖGREN'S SYNDROME

Clinical Manifestation	Percent
Arthralgias/arthritis	60
Raynaud's phenomenon	37
Lymphadenopathy	14
Lung involvement	14
Vasculitis	11
Kidney involvement	9
Lymphoma	6
Liver involvement	6
Splenomegaly	3
Peripheral neuropathy	2

TABLE 60–2 AUTOIMMUNE DISEASES IN SECONDARY SJÖGREN'S SYNDROME

Rheumatoid arthritis
Systemic lupus erythematosus
Scleroderma
Vasculitis
Mixed connective tissue disease
Primary biliary cirrhosis
Chronic active hepatitis

Histology of involved parotid glands varies according to the duration of the disease process. Early, a T-cell lymphocytic infiltrate is seen. Later, ductal metaplasia and an increase in myoepithelial cells are noted. Late in the disease, islands of myoepithelial cells are surrounded by lymphocytes.

Minor salivary gland histology demonstrates a lymphocytic infiltrate. The presence of one focus of greater than 50 lymphocytes per 4 mm² (focus score >1) is 95% specific for Sjögren's syndrome. Confirmation of CD4 lymphocytes, versus CD8 lymphocytes as seen in HIV, is even more specific.

Serologic testing may be of benefit in some cases but lacks sensitivity and specificity. SS-A (Ro) and SS-B (La) are autoantibodies found in primary Sjögren's syndrome, 70% and 50% of the time, respectively. The frequency is lower for the secondary syndrome. Erythrocyte sedimentation rate (ESR) is elevated in 70% of all cases. Rheumatoid factor (RF) and antinuclear antibody (ANA) may also be positive, especially in the secondary syndrome.

Diagnosis is based on chronic (>3 month) signs and symptoms of xerostomia and keratoconjunctivitis sicca along with either positive histology or serology.

> **PITFALL•••** HIV must be excluded, in the absence of positive serology, as it may mimic Sjögren's clinically and histologically.

Treatment is primarily supportive and aimed at preventing complications from exocrine dysfunction. Artificial saliva and good oral hygiene to prevent caries are the mainstay for xerostomia. Methylcellulose eyedrops are effective in preventing corneal ulcerations. Severe cases may require closure of the lower lid puncta. Anticholinergic, sympathomimetic, antidepressant, and diuretic medications should be avoided when possible. Pilocarpine may be beneficial early in the disease to promote exocrine function before salivary and lacrimal gland atrophy occurs. Topical ophthalmic steroids are used for ocular complications. Systemic steroids or immune suppressants are reserved for extraglandular manifestations (Table 60–1). Suppurative sialadenitis is managed as described under bacterial infections. Parotidectomy is rarely indicated and should only be undertaken with great trepidation.

> **PITFALL•••** Sudden parotid swelling or lymphadenopathy in a patient with long-standing Sjögren's syndrome must be evaluated for lymphoma to avoid delay in diagnosis.

NECROTIZING SIALOMETAPLASIA

Necrotizing sialometaplasia is a salivary gland disease of uncertain etiology. Most commonly it involves a minor salivary gland of the palatal mucosa; however, it may occur in any salivary tissue.

> **CONTROVERSY**
>
> Some authors believe salivary infarct is the initiating event.

Histologically, mucosal ulceration with pseudoepitheliomatous hyperplasia, lobular necrosis, inflammatory response, and squamous metaplasia are seen. Mitotic figures may be present. The disease is self-limited with healing occurring over 1 to 3 months.

> **PITFALL•••** This disease may be mistaken for mucoepidermoid or squamous cell carcinoma with unnecessary therapy if the diagnosis is missed.

SUGGESTED READINGS

Crystal RG. Sarcoidosis. In: Fauci AS, Braunwald E, Isselbacher KJ, et al, eds. *Harrison's Principles of Internal Medicine.* 14th ed. New York: McGraw-Hill; 1998:1922–1928.

Deegan MJ. Immunologic diseases of the salivary glands. *Otolaryngol Clin North Am* 1977; 10(2):351–360.

Flexon PB, Baker AS. Infectious diseases of the salivary glands. In: Granick MS, Hanna DC, eds. *Management of Salivary Gland Lesions.* Baltimore: Williams & Wilkins; 1992:54–60.

Moutsopoulos HM. Sjogren's syndrome. In: Fauci AS, Braunwald E, Isselbacher KJ, et al, eds. *Harrison's Principles of Internal Medicine.* 14th ed. New York: McGraw-Hill; 1998:1901–1904.

Rice DH. Non-neoplastic diseases of the salivary glands. In: Paparella MM, Shumrick DA, Gluckman JL, Meyerhoff WL, eds. *Otolaryngology Head and Neck.* Vol. 3. 3rd ed. Philadelphia: WB Saunders; 1991:2089–2097.

Seifert G, Miehlke A, Haubrich J, Chilla R. Sialadenitis. In: Verlag GT, ed. *Diseases of the Salivary Glands.* New York: Thieme; 1986:110–163.

Solomon MP, Mandell BF. Salivary gland involvement in rheumatic disease. In: Granick MS, Hanna DC, eds. *Management of Salivary Gland Lesions.* Baltimore: Williams & Wilkins; 1992:61–65.

Travis LW, Hecht DW. Acute and chronic inflammatory diseases of the salivary glands: diagnosis and management. *Otolaryngol Clin North Am* 1977;10(2):329–338.

Weber MD, ed. Sjögren syndrome. In: Gluckman JL, ed. *Renewal of Certification Study Guide in Otolaryngology—Head and Neck Surgery.* Dubuque, IA: Kendall/Hunt; 1998:563–565.

Chapter 61

NEOPLASMS AND CYSTS

David L. Steward

Salivary gland neoplasms and cysts may be loosely referred to as salivary gland tumors. These tumors are best defined by location (parotid, submandibular, sublingual, or minor salivary gland), architecture (solid or cystic), metastatic potential (benign or malignant), and histogenesis (epithelial, mesenchymal, or metastatic). A modification of the World Health Organization classification is presented in Table 61–1. It should be noted that many tumor-like lesions of the salivary system are presented in the preceding chapters covering congenital, functional, and inflammatory disorders. This chapter reviews the more important salivary neoplasms and cysts.

SALIVARY GLAND CYSTS

Salivary gland cysts are lesions of the ductal system. These may be categorized as congenital cysts (Chapter 58), acquired epithelial lined cysts, mucoceles (pseudocysts), and cystic neoplasms. Nonneoplastic salivary gland cysts and pseudocysts represent about 5 to 15% of salivary gland tumors and are predominantly ex-

travasation mucoceles of the minor salivary glands (Table 61–2).

MUCOCELE

Mucoceles are created by granuloma formation around mucus extravasating from an injured salivary duct. They lack an epithelial lining and are thus called pseudocysts. They occur primarily around minor salivary glands of the lower lip where recurrent microtrauma from lip biting is a common etiology. Mucoceles may occur in or around any salivary gland. Treatment for minor salivary gland mucoceles, when required, is simple marsupialization. Minor salivary gland excision is rarely necessary.

RANULA

A ranula is a mucocele of the sublingual gland that usually produces swelling in the floor of mouth. The term *ranula* derives from the diminutive Latin term *rana,* for frog. It is named for the submental swelling that may occur if the extravasated mucus pierces the mylohyoid muscle (plunging ranula). As the etiology is a

TABLE 61–1 CLASSIFICATION SALIVARY GLAND TUMORS

Type of Tumor	Relative Incidence (%)
I. Salivary cysts and pseudocysts	14
II. Benign epithelial neoplasms	53
Pleomorphic adenoma	39
Monomorphic adenomas	
Adenolymphoma (Warthin's)	11
Duct adenoma	2
Basal cell adenoma	0.5
Oncocytoma	0.3
Sebaceous adenoma	
Clear cell adenoma	
Other adenomas	
III. Malignant epithelial neoplasms	19
Mucoepidermoid carcinoma	5
Carcinoma ex-pleomorphic adenoma	4.5
Adenoid cystic carcinoma	3
Acinic cell carcinoma	2
Squamous cell carcinoma	1.5
Undifferentiated carcinoma	1
Other carcinomas	2
IV. Benign mesenchymal neoplasms	3
Hemangioma	1
Lymphangioma	0.5
Lipoma	0.6
Neural	0.6
Others	
V. Malignant mesenchymal neoplasm	4.4
Lymphoma	4
Sarcomas	0.3
VI. Metastatic neoplasms	5.6
VII. Nonneoplastic tumor-like lesions	
Chronic sialadenitis	
Sialolithiasis	
Sialadenosis	
Sialectasia	
Lymphoepithelial lesion	
Parotid lymph node hyperplasia	
Oncocytosis	
HIV-associated salivary gland disease	
Necrotizing sialometaplasia	
Others	

TABLE 61–2 CLASSIFICATION OF SALIVARY CYSTS AND PSEUDOCYSTS

Cyst Type	Predominant Gland (Site)	Relative Frequency (%)
Mucoceles	Minor salivary glands (lower lip)	65
Duct cyst	Parotid, minor (oral cavity)	23
Lymphoepithelial cyst	Parotid, minor (floor of mouth)	6
Ranula	Sublingual	5

damaged sublingual ductal system, treatment is excision of the sublingual gland and marsupialization of the mucocele.

> **PITFALL•••** The lingual nerve and submandibular duct are easily injured if not identified and preserved during surgical treatment of a ranula.

Simple marsupialization or pseudocyst excision, without excision of the sublingual gland, often results in recurrence.

> **CONTROVERSY**
>
> A cervical approach for a plunging ranula may not be necessary if the sublingual gland is removed.

SALIVARY DUCT CYSTS

Salivary duct cysts (also called mucus retention cysts) occur predominantly within the parotid gland and the minor salivary glands of the oral cavity. These can be differentiated from mucoceles by the presence of an epithelial lining. Occasionally, small local mucoceles may form at the periphery due to leakage of mucus from the cyst. The etiology is ductal obstruction, either congenital (rare) or acquired. The acquired salivary duct cyst is often the result of sialithiasis, inspissated secretions, or chronic sialadenitis. Ductal cysts must be differentiated from cystic neoplasms (Warthin's tumor, adenoid cystic carcinoma, and mucoepidermoid carcinoma). Treatment for symptomatic patients is gland excision.

LYMPHOEPITHELIAL CYSTS

Lymphoepithelial cysts occur mainly in the parotid gland and minor salivary glands of the floor of the mouth. These cysts may be either single or multiple, unilocular or multilocular. They have a multilayered epithelial cyst wall surrounded by lymphoid stroma with lymphoid follicles.

The origin of lymphoepithelial cysts is controversial. Intraparotid lymph follicles with parenchymatous inclusions are relatively common within the parotid gland and may be responsible for lymphoepithelial cyst formation in this site. The same cannot be said for minor salivary gland lesions. Thus, chronic lymphoid inflammation with secondary epithelial proliferation has been proposed as etiologic in lymphoepithelial cyst formation in the minor salivary glands. Given the histologic similarity of these cysts to the lymphoepithelial lesions of Sjögren's syndrome and HIV-associated salivary gland disease, lymphoepithelial cysts may be part of a spectrum of lesions seen in chronic inflammatory salivary disease.

Diagnosis involves exclusion of cystic neoplasm, Sjögren's syndrome, and HIV-associated disease. Treatment is excision of the involved salivary gland.

SALIVARY NEOPLASMS

Salivary neoplasms may occur in any of the major or minor salivary glands. The majority of neoplasms (80%) occur in the parotid gland. Submandibular and minor salivary gland (mostly palatal) neoplasms each account for about 10% of the total, and the sublingual gland accounts for only 1%. The incidence of malignant neoplasms occurring at each site varies inversely with the total number of neoplasms. Although only 20% of parotid neoplasms and about 50% of submandibular and minor salivary gland neoplasms are malignant, nearly 90% of all sublingual gland neoplasms represent malignancy.

Of the 5% of salivary gland neoplasms that occur in children, most (85%) occur in the parotid gland and are benign (65%). Hemangiomas are the most common tumor type in the pediatric age group (see Chapter 58).

BENIGN EPITHELIAL NEOPLASMS

Pleomorphic Adenoma

Pleomorphic adenomas are the most common salivary neoplasm, and 85% occur in the parotid gland. The submandibular gland accounts for 8% of pleomorphic adenomas, and the minor salivary glands (mostly of the palate) account for 7%. These slow-growing parotid tumors present in the superficial lobe in 90% of cases, commonly during the fifth decade. Less often, pleomorphic adenomas may present in the parapharyngeal space, either as extensions of deep lobe tumors or from rests of minor salivary gland tissue.

Pleomorphic adenomas arise from intercalated and myoepithelial cells. Unless arising from minor salivary glands, these tumors are often encapsulated. Microscopic pseudopods of tumor are present and result in incomplete resection if enucleation is performed without a cuff of surrounding tissue.

The diagnosis can usually be made with fine-needle aspiration biopsy and treatment is by surgical excision of the gland.

> **PITFALL...** Incisional biopsies result in tumor spillage and possible seeding.

Recurrent Pleomorphic Adenoma

Since the widespread acceptance of superficial parotidectomy with facial nerve dissection, the incidence of recurrent pleomorphic adenoma (RPA) has decreased from 20 to 2%. However, it remains a very challenging problem when it occurs. Incomplete surgical excision secondary to pseudopod formation is the most likely mechanism for recurrence. Intraoperative tumor spillage has long been thought etiologic, however, a recent review with greater than 10-year follow-up did not support this. Risk factors for RPA include large tumors, deep lobe tumors, palatal tumors, tumors abutting the facial nerve, and young patients. Most cases of RPA are multifocal (70%), with 25% involving the deep lobe.

Malignant degeneration of pleomorphic adenomas may occur in 5 to 10% of cases and is more frequent in long-standing recurrent tumors. Diagnosis of RPA includes ruling out malignant transformation.

Treatment of RPA is based on patient age, patient symptoms, and previous treatment. Observation is recommended in the elderly patient without history of recent rapid tumor growth and without evidence of malignancy by fine needle aspiration (FNA). Young patients with a focal recurrence who previously underwent enucleation rather than parotidectomy are good candidates for successful surgical therapy with facial nerve preservation. Young patients with multifocal recurrence adjacent to or involving the facial nerve are difficult to cure with surgery alone. Additionally, surgery carries a risk for permanent facial paralysis, total or partial, in 10 to 30% of cases.

CONTROVERSY

Facial nerve monitoring may result in earlier identification and less facial nerve trauma in the surgical management of RPA.

Adjuvant external beam radiotherapy has proven effective in the management of microscopic disease left after revision surgery. The efficacy of radiation therapy is statistically worse in the presence of gross residual tumor, however.

PITFALL••• Radiation therapy, especially in young patients, may be associated with future malignancy induced by radiation.

Adenolymphoma (Warthin's Tumor)

Adenolymphoma, originally called papillary cystadenoma lymphomatosum by Warthin, is the most common of the monomorphic adenomas of the salivary glands. These tumors appear almost exclusively in the tail of the parotid gland, though submandibular and minor salivary gland involvement has been reported. They are more common in males than females (4:1) and can be bilateral (7 to 12%) and multifocal (4%).

CONTROVERSY

Histogenesis of adenolymphoma is related to proliferation of ductal epithelial inclusions within parotid or periparotid lymph nodes.

Diagnosis is by FNA or nuclear medicine study. The oncocytic component of these tumors allows visualization using technetium 99. Histology demonstrates a classic double layer of oncocytic cells. Malignancy is extremely rare; therefore, observation may be indicated in asymptomatic elderly patients. Surgical excision with a cuff of normal tissue and facial nerve preservation is curative. Recurrences are more likely the result of unidentified multifocal disease rather than residual tumor.

Basal Cell Adenoma

Basal cell adenomas are the second most common monomorphic adenomas of the salivary glands. These slow-growing tumors are usually located in minor salivary glands of the upper lip. Of the major salivary glands, the parotid is most often involved.

In making this diagnosis, adenoid cystic carcinoma, with which this tumor may be confused, must be ruled out. Treatment, as with all monomorphic adenomas, involves excision with a cuff of normal tissue and facial nerve preservation.

Oncocytoma

Oncocytomas are rare monomorphic adenomas composed of oncocytes. They are reported in the submandibular gland and minor salivary glands of the palate; however, they are seen most commonly in the parotid gland. These tumors show a slight female preponderance, present during the sixth decade, and may be bilateral.

Diagnosis is by characteristic histology demonstrating mitochondrially rich oncocytes without a lymphoid component as seen in adenolymphoma. Like adenolymphomas, they are well visualized with technetium 99 nuclear imaging. Malignancy is rare, though these tumors may be locally aggressive, especially in the minor salivary glands. Treatment is excision with a cuff of normal tissue.

BENIGN MESENCHYMAL NEOPLASMS

Nonepithelial tumors of the salivary glands arise from local mesenchymal structures including blood vessels, lymphatic vessels, neural tissue, connective tissue, and adipose tissue. These rare tumors make up about 5% of salivary tumors and are more common in children. The majority are angiomas. The parotid gland is involved about 90% of the time.

Hemangioma

Hemangiomas are the most common mesenchymal neoplasm of the salivary glands (40%) and are the most common salivary gland tumor in children (see Chapter 58). Hemangiomas presenting during adulthood are more likely cavernous than capillary in type.

Lymphangioma

Lymphangiomas are less common than hemangiomas and usually represent extension from cervical cystic hygromas (see Chapter 58).

Lipoma

Lipomas make up about 20% of mesenchymal salivary gland tumors, the great majority of which (95%) occur in the parotid gland. They are more common in men and may demonstrate extraglandular extension.

> **PEARL•••** Lipomas may be differentiated from lipomatosis (diffuse fatty infiltration) by the presence of a capsule. The distinction is important because lipomatosis is not treated surgically.

Despite the presence of the capsule, lipomas often have various intraglandular extensions and are more extensive than first appreciated. Diagnosis is by FNA and computed tomography (CT) scan. Surgical excision after identification and preservation of the facial nerve is curative.

Nerve Sheath Tumor

Neural tumors are rare salivary neoplasms occurring in middle age. They are more common in the parotid gland (85%) than in the submandibular gland. Histologically and clinically they do not differ from neural tumors in other sites.

Extratemporal facial nerve schwannomas are less common than intratemporal tumors. They are encapsulated and may cause slowly progressive facial nerve paresis through compression at the stylomastoid foramen.

Neurofibromas may be solitary or may occur as part of the neurofibromatosis of patients with von Recklinghausen's disease.

> **SPECIAL CONSIDERATION**
>
> Unlike schwannomas, neurofibromas arise from the nerve fibers and cannot usually be separated from the nerve of origin without sacrificing the nerve.

MALIGNANT EPITHELIAL NEOPLASMS

Salivary gland cancer is rare, with an incidence of 1 in 100,000 and representing about 1% of all head and neck tumors. The tumor, node, metastasis (TNM) staging of salivary gland malignancies is summarized in Table 61–3.

Prognosis of salivary gland malignancy is based on tumor histology (type and grade), tumor stage (size, local extension, nodes,

TABLE 61-3 STAGING SYSTEM FOR MAJOR SALIVARY GLAND CANCER

T_x	Primary tumor cannot be assessed			
T_0	No evidence of primary tumor			
T_1	Tumor ≤2 cm in greatest dimension			
T_2	Tumor >2 and ≤4 cm in greatest dimension			
T_3	Tumor >4 and ≤6 cm in greatest dimension			
T_4	Tumor >6 cm in greatest dimension			
	All categories are subdivided:	(a) no local extension		
		(b) local extension (skin, soft tissue, bone, nerve)		
N_x	Regional nodes cannot be assessed			
N_0	No regional lymph node metastases			
N_1	Single ipsilateral node <3 cm in diameter			
N_{2a}	Single ipsilateral node 3–6 cm in diameter			
N_{2b}	Multiple ipsilateral node, none >6 cm			
N_{2c}	Bilateral or contralateral nodes, none >6 cm			
N_3	Metastasis in a lymph node, >6 cm			
M_x	Presence of distant metastases cannot be assessed			
M_0	No distant metastases			
M_1	Distant metastases			
	Stage I	T_1	N_0	M_0
		T_2	N_0	M_0
	Stage II	T_3	N_0	M_0
	Stage III	T_1	N_1	M_0
		T_2	N_1	M_0
	Stage IV	T_4	N_0	M_0
		T_3	N_1	M_0
		T_4	N_1	M_0
		Any T	N_2	M_0
		Any T	N_3	M_0
		Any T	Any N	M_1

Source: *AJCC® Staging Handbook,* 5th ed. Philadelphia: Lippincott-Raven; 1998:57–60. Reprinted by permission of the American Joint Committee on Cancer [AJCC®], Chicago, IL.

metastasis), and tumor location (parotid, submandibular, or minor salivary gland). Of these, tumor stage and grade (low vs. high) are the most important. Overall, parotid malignancies have a better prognosis than minor salivary gland malignancies, with both having a better prognosis than submandibular gland malignancies. Prognosis is worse for minor salivary gland cancers outside the oral cavity and oropharynx, especially for laryngeal and sinonasal adenocarcinoma or adenoid cystic carcinoma.

Treatment is based on prognosis. In general stage I, low-grade malignancies are treated with surgery alone. Stage II, III, IV and all high-grade malignancies are treated with surgery and postoperative radiation therapy.

SPECIAL CONSIDERATION

Radical parotidectomy, with facial nerve sacrifice, should be performed only when the facial nerve is grossly invaded and not functioning preoperatively.

Neck dissection is definitely indicated for positive nodal disease.

SPECIAL CONSIDERATION

Elective neck dissection is reserved for high-grade mucoepidermoid and squamous cell carcinoma of the parotid gland, high-grade submandibular gland malignancies, and high-grade minor salivary gland malignancies of the tongue and anterior floor of the mouth.

Neutron beam therapy is associated with higher local and regional control rates than traditional photon radiotherapy but has not been shown to significantly alter survival. Additionally, it may be a useful tool for local recurrence after previous photon radiotherapy and surgery. The drawbacks of neutron beam therapy are increased complication rates and that it is not widely available.

PITFALL... Chemotherapy has not been promising and should be used for palliation or on study protocol only.

Mucoepidermoid Carcinoma

Mucoepidermoid carcinoma is a tumor with variable malignant potential. These tumors are classified as low-, intermediate-, or high-grade based on the ratio of mucoid to epidermoid components. High-grade tumors have very little mucoid cells and are distinguishable from undifferentiated and squamous cell carcinomas only with mucin stains on histology.

Mucoepidermoid carcinoma is the most common parotid malignancy, the second most common submandibular gland malignancy, and the most common malignancy of childhood. It is the most common type of salivary malignancy induced by radiation. Of minor salivary gland sites, the palate is the most frequently involved. Mucoepidermoid carcinoma is the most com-

mon oral cavity minor salivary gland malignancy.

Low-grade mucoepidermoid carcinomas have a 95% 5-year survival and are treated effectively with surgical excision. High-grade tumors have a <50% 5-year survival and have a significant incidence of regional (45%) and distant (10%) metastases. Treatment for the latter should include gland excision with neck dissection for N1–3 disease and postoperative radiation therapy. Given the high incidence of occult nodal metastases (16%) in clinically N0 necks, either empiric neck dissection or radiation therapy should be utilized to treat the N0 neck.

Adenoid Cystic Carcinoma

Adenoid cystic carcinoma is the most common submandibular gland malignancy and the most common minor salivary gland malignancy when all sites are considered. Perineural and perivascular invasion is the hallmark of this malignancy and skip lesions are often present. Histologically, it shows basaloid epithelium in cyclindric formations within a hyaline stroma (hence the term *cylindroma*). Histologic classifications (cribriform, solid, cylindromatous, and tubular) have not been reliably prognostic.

Adenoid cystic carcinomas have a high incidence (50%) of distant metastasis at the time of presentation but a very low incidence (5%) of nodal disease. Lung and bone are the most common sites of metastasis. Local recurrences are common because of neural involvement with skip lesions. Prognosis is poor, with 10 to 15% 15-year survival; however, the 5-year survival rates are 40 to 70%. Prognosis is worse in sinonasal and laryngeal sites.

Treatment is surgery followed by radiotherapy (photon or neutron). Neck dissection is indicated only for the rare case of grossly positive nodal disease.

Acinic Cell Carcinoma

Acinic cell carcinoma is a tumor of variable metastatic potential that occurs almost exclusively within the parotid gland. The predilection for the parotid gland is based on the serous cell origin of these tumors. Submandibular and minor salivary gland involvement is much less common. These tumors may be bilateral in 3% of cases, and are slightly more common in females. Acinic cell carcinomas have been classified as low-grade (Batsakis 1 and 2) or high-grade tumors (Batsakis 3 and 4). Low-grade tumors are more common (85%) and most closely resemble the normal salivary lobular architecture, whereas high-grade tumors are poorly differentiated and resemble the early phases of embryonic development of salivary acini.

Prognosis is initially good with 5-year survival rates of 70 to 90%; however, 10- and 15-year survival rates drop to 60% and 50%, respectively. Prognosis is worse for high-grade tumors, higher stage at presentation, age greater than 30 years, and submandibular site of involvement. Local failure occurs in about 30% of cases.

Treatment is parotidectomy with facial nerve preservation unless the nerve is grossly involved with tumor (indicating a high-grade tumor).

╔══════════════════════════════╗
║   **SPECIAL CONSIDERATION**   ║
║   ║
║ Data supporting the effectiveness of ra- ║
║ diotherapy are lacking; however, most ║
║ authors suggest adjunctive radiother- ║
║ apy (photon or neutron) for aggressive ║
║ tumors (high grade, high stage) and ║
║ patients with a poor prognosis (age ║
║ greater than 30 years, submandibular ║
║ gland involvement). ║
╚══════════════════════════════╝

Adenocarcinoma

Adenocarcinomas are located primarily within the parotid gland and minor salivary glands and less commonly in the submandibular and sub-

lingual glands. These generally behave as aggressive carcinomas with a high incidence of nodal (25 to 60%) and distant (30%) metastases at presentation, as well as a high incidence of local recurrence (50%).

Histologically, adenocarcinomas may be identified by a positive mucicarmine stain for mucus and a negative keratin stain. These tumors are graded by the degree of glandular formation. Polymorphous low-grade adenocarcinomas (PLGA) are a subset of minor salivary gland adenocarcinomas with a more benign course and better prognosis.

Prognosis is generally poor with 5-year survival rates of 25 to 70%. Treatment is surgical removal of the involved gland, preservation of the facial nerve, and adjunctive radiotherapy (photon or neutron).

Carcinoma Ex-Pleomorphic Adenoma

Carcinoma ex-pleomorphic adenoma is a malignancy arising within a preexisting benign neoplasm (pleomorphic adenoma). These tumors predominantly involve the parotid gland (80%), but may occur in the submandibular or minor salivary glands as well. The malignant portion and metastasis of the tumor are solely of epithelial origin.

╔══════════════════════════════╗
║   **SPECIAL CONSIDERATION**   ║
║   ║
║ This is in contrast to the much rarer ║
║ malignant mixed tumor, which con- ║
║ tains metastases of both epithelial and ║
║ mesenchymal components. ║
╚══════════════════════════════╝

The incidence of malignancy developing within a pleomorphic adenoma is estimated to be between 2 and 9%, with the higher percentage for tumors of greater than 5 years' duration (Fig. 61–1).

Clinically, these malignancies are associated with a rapid change in size of a previously stable salivary tumor. Histologic diagnosis may be difficult if the malignant portion has obliterated the preexisting pleomorphic adenoma.

Prognosis is poor for these aggressive tumors because of a high incidence of nodal (20 to

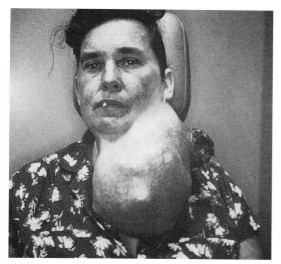

FIGURE 61–1 This otherwise benign pleomorphic adenoma was left unattended for 20 years before developing into a "carcinoma ex-pleomorphic adenoma."

70%) and distant (20%) metastases, as well as local recurrence (65%). Treatment is surgical excision with facial nerve preservation, neck dissection for nodal disease, and adjunctive radiotherapy (photon or neutron).

SPECIAL CONSIDERATION

Despite the high incidence of nodal metastasis, elective neck dissection for the N0 neck is not indicated because of the very low incidence of occult nodal disease and the need for radiotherapy to prevent loco-regional recurrence.

Squamous Cell Carcinoma

Primary squamous cell carcinoma of the salivary glands predominantly involves the parotid and submandibular glands and accounts for about 1% of salivary neoplasms and about 10% of salivary malignances.

Histologically, these tumors are indistinguishable from squamous cell carcinomas elsewhere in the body and stain positively for cytokeratin. Diagnosis includes exclusion of direct extension from a primary skin cancer, regional nodal metastasis from skin or mucosal primary,

distant metastasis, and other primary salivary carcinomas (high-grade mucoepidermoid, ex-pleomorphic).

PEARL... Thorough head and neck examination including the scalp, external auditory canal, and oropharyngeal mucosa is necessary to rule out regional metastatic disease.

Clinically, these cancers usually present in elderly males, often with facial paralysis (20%). Prognosis is poor because of a high incidence of nodal (40 to 70%) and distant metastases (15 to 20%), as well as local recurrence (40 to 70%).

Treatment for these aggressive tumors includes complete gland excision, with facial nerve sacrifice if grossly involved by tumor (preoperative paralysis), neck dissection, and postoperative radiotherapy.

SPECIAL CONSIDERATION

Elective neck dissection is indicated because of the high incidence (40%) of occult nodal disease.

Undifferentiated Carcinoma

Undifferentiated carcinomas of the salivary glands make up about 5% of salivary malignancies and are more common in the parotid gland. These highly aggressive tumors have high incidences of nodal (25%) and distant metastases (40%), as well as local recurrence (70%) and facial paralysis (25%). The prognosis is the worst of all salivary gland malignancies. Treatment is gland excision and postoperative radiotherapy in the absence of distant metastasis; otherwise, it is palliative only.

Other Carcinomas

A number of other salivary gland adenocarcinomas have been described. For each of the previously mentioned benign adenomas, a malignant form has been reported (basaloid, oncocytic, adenolymphomatous).

Other rare adenocarcinomas include the aggressive ductal carcinoma, the low-grade sclerosing clear cell carcinoma, endocrine small cell carcinoma (associated with carcinoid of the lung), and sebaceous carcinoma. Some authors designate these and other carcinomas as adenocarcinoma not otherwise specified (NOS).

An aggressive malignant lymphoepithelial lesion, also termed anaplastic carcinoma, has been reported primarily in the Eskimos and Chinese. Interestingly, it is not associated with the benign lymphoepithelial lesion of Sjögren's syndrome.

MALIGNANT MESENCHYMAL NEOPLASMS

Lymphoma

Malignant lymphomas of the salivary system are mostly non-Hogkin's lymphomas and occur primarily within the parotid gland (60%), and less commonly within the submandibular gland (35%). Salivary gland lymphomas have been classified as primary if they have no extrasalivary component. About 40% of lymphomas of the head and neck arise within the salivary glands.

Salivary gland lymphomas that arise within a lymphoepithelial lesion of myoepithelial sialadenitis (Sjögren's syndrome), are predominantly of plasma cell or B-cell origin. The risk of developing a lymphoma in a patient with Sjögren's syndrome is 40 times greater than the general population. Mean time to development of lymphoma is generally 10 years after onset of the syndrome.

SPECIAL CONSIDERATION

These patients require long-term follow-up because of the risk of developing lymphoma.

Prognosis is generally good and treatment is as for other lymphomas.

Sarcoma

Primary sarcomas of the salivary glands are rare, accounting for less than 1% of all salivary gland tumors. The majority of salivary gland sarcomas arise from adjacent structures. Malignant schwannomas, spindle cell sarcomas, fibrosarcomas, and malignant histiocytomas have been most frequently reported. Rhabdomyosarcomas are more common in the pediatric age group.

Prognosis for these aggressive tumors is poor. Treatment is generally with multimodality therapy.

Metastatic Salivary Gland Neoplasms

Metastatic lesions to the salivary glands predominantly involve the parotid and, less commonly, the submandibular gland. These should be classified as regional or distant metastases, with the former the more common.

Periparotid and intraparotid lymph nodes drain the skin in the periparotid area, including the auricle, external auditory canal, frontotemporal scalp, cheek, eyelids, upper lip, and nose (Fig. 61–2). Malignant melanoma (MM) and squamous cell carcinoma (SCCa) are the most frequent regional metastases to the parotid gland. Treatment includes management of the primary skin cancer, parotidectomy, neck dissection for positive nodes, and radiotherapy (SCCa) or chemotherapy (MM).

PEARL••• Elective superficial parotidectomy and neck dissection should be carried out for primary melanoma of intermediate depth (1.5–4 mm) located within the periparotid drainage area.

The submandibular lymph nodes drain the anterior oral cavity and lower lip. Regional metastases to nodes adjacent to the submandibular gland may involve the gland, and are predominantly SCCa. Treatment is neck dissection and radiotherapy.

Distant metastases to the salivary glands are very rare but when present generally involve the parotid gland. Lung and breast are the most

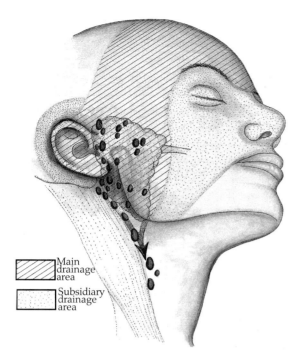

Main drainage area

Subsidiary drainage area

FIGURE 61-2 Drainage area of the periparotid and intraparotid lymph nodes.

likely primary carcinomas. Other carcinomas include papillary thyroid, renal cell, ovarian, colon, and melanoma.

SUGGESTED READINGS

Armstrong JG, Harrison LB, Spiro RH, Fas DE, Strong EW, Fuks ZY. Malignant tumors of major salivary gland origin. *Arch Otolaryngol Head Neck Surg* 1990;116:290–293.

Eisele DW, Johns ME. Salivary gland neoplasms. In: Johnson JT, Kohut RI, Pillsbury HA III, Tardy ME Jr, eds. *Head and Neck Surgery—Otolaryngology,* vol. 2. Philadelphia: JB Lippincott; 1993:1125–1147.

Goodman M, Pilch BZ. Salivary gland pathology: benign tumors. In: Granick MS, Hanna DC III, eds. *Management of Salivary Lesions.* Baltimore: Williams & Wilkins; 1992:66–111.

Goodman M, Pilch BZ. Salivary gland pathology: malignant tumors. In: Granick MS, Hanna DC III, eds. *Management of Salivary Lesions.* Baltimore: Williams & Wilkins; 1992:112–144.

Granick MS, Hanna DC III. Surgical management of salivary gland disease. In: Granick MS, Hanna DC III, eds. *Management of Salivary Lesions.* Baltimore: Williams & Wilkins; 1992:145–174.

Griffin TW, Pajak TF, Laramore GE, et al. Neutron versus photon irradiation of inoperable salivary gland tumors: results of an RTOG-MRC cooperative randomized study. *Int J Radiat Oncol Biol Phys* 1988;15:1085–1090.

Hoffman HT, Karnell LH, Robinson RA, Pinkston JA, Menck HR. National cancer database report on cancer of the head and neck: acinic cell carcinoma. *Head Neck* (July) 1999; 297–309.

Johns ME, Nachlas NE. Salivary gland tumors. In: Paparella MM, Shumrick DA, Gluckman JL, Meyerhoff WL, eds. *Otolaryngology,* 3rd ed. Philadelphia: WB Saunders; 1991:2099–2128.

Laramore GE, Krall JM, Griffin TW, et al. Neutron versus photon radiation for unresectable salivary gland tumors: final report of an RTOG-MRC randomized clinical trial. *Int J Radiat Oncol Biol Phys* 1993;27:235–240.

North CA, Lee DJ, Piantodaosi S, Zahurak M, Johns ME. Carcinoma of the major salivary glands treated by surgery or surgery plus postoperative radiation therapy. *Int J Radiat Oncol Biol Phys* 1990;18:1319–1326.

Olsen KD, Daube JR. Intraoperative monitoring of the facial nerve. *Laryngoscope* 1994;104: 229–232.

Seifert G, Miehlke A, Haubrich J, Chilla R. Lymph node diseases of the salivary gland. In: Verlag GT, ed. *Diseases of the Salivary Glands.* New York: Thieme; 1986:302–310.

Seifert G, Miehlke A, Haubrich J, Chilla R. Nonepithelial salivary tumors. In: Verlag GT, ed. *Diseases of the Salivary Glands.* New York: Thieme; 1986:286–297.

Seifert G, Miehlke A, Haubrich J, Chilla R. Salivary glands cysts. In: Verlag GT, ed. *Diseases of the Salivary Glands.* New York: Thieme; 1986: 90–91.

Seifert G, Miehlke A, Haubrich J, Chilla R. Salivary tumors of epithelial origin. In: Verlag GT, ed. *Diseases of the Salivary Glands.* New York: Thieme; 1986:171–281.

Shemen LJ. Salivary glands: benign and malignant disease. In: Lee KJ, ed. *Essential Otolaryngology.* 7th ed. Stamford, CT: Appleton and Lange; 1999:499–526.

Spiro RH. Salivary neoplasms: overview of a 35 year experience with 2807 patients. *Head Neck Surg* 1986;8:177–184.

Suen JY, Snyderman NL. Benign neoplasms of the salivary glands. In: Cummings CW, Fredrickson JM, Harker LA, Krause CJ, Schuller DE, eds. *Otolaryngology—Head and Neck Surgery,* 2nd ed. St. Louis: Mosby Year Book; 1993:1029–1104.

Suen JY, Snyderman NL. Malignant neoplasms. In: Cummings CW, Fredrickson JM, Harker LA, Krause CJ, Schuller DE, eds. *Otolaryngology—Head and Neck Surgery,* 2nd ed. St. Louis: Mosby Year Book, 1993:1043–1078.

Weber RS, Eisele DW, El-Naggar A, Poole M, Stringer S, Weinstein G. Management of salivary gland malignancies. In: Gluckman JG, ed. *Renewal of Certification Study Guide in Otolaryngology—Head and Neck Surgery.* Dubuque, IA: McGraw-Hill; 1998:555–559.

Weber RS, Eisele DW, El-Naggar A, Poole M, Stringer S, Weinstein G. Salivary glands—contemporary classification of salivary glands. In: Gluckman JG, ed. *Renewal of Certification Study Guide in Otolaryngology—Head and Neck Surgery.* Dubuque, IA: McGraw-Hill; 1998:544–545.

Weber RS, Eisele DW, El-Naggar A, Poole M, Stringer S, Weinstein G. Salivary glands—recurrent pleomorphic adenoma of the parotid gland. In: Gluckman JG, ed. *Renewal of Certification Study Guide in Otolaryngolgoy—Head and Neck Surgery.* Dubuque, IA: McGraw-Hill; 1998:552–554.

Chapter 62

TRAUMA

David L. Steward and Thomas A. Tami

Salivary gland trauma can be classified as either acute or chronic. Chronic trauma generally results in sialadenitis from obstructive and inflammatory processes and is discussed further in Chapter 60 (inflammatory). Radiation is a form of toxic injury discussed in Chapters 59 (functional) and 60 (inflammatory). This chapter reviews acute traumatic injury to the parotid and to the submandibular, parenchymal, and ductal systems. Additionally, associated acute traumatic extracranial facial nerve injury is reviewed.

SALIVARY DUCTAL INJURY

The majority of lacerations of a salivary duct involve the parotid. These must be identified and managed early to prevent sialocele, salivary fistula, or ductal stenosis. Parotid duct injury should be suspected in any facial laceration crossing a line drawn from the tragus to the upper lip and posterior to a line drawn perpendicularly from the lateral canthus (Fig. 62–1). Additionally, parotid duct injury should be suspected when the buccal branch of the facial nerve is injured, as it travels horizontally with and inferior to the duct. Arterial bleeding in a cheek wound should also arouse suspicion, as a small artery runs horizontal and superior to the duct. Fresh wounds in this area should be evaluated for ductal injury. This is best accomplished by intraoral retrograde probing of the parotid duct, using a lacrimal duct probe, and inspecting the wound for the probe.

> **PEARL•••** Avoid using size 00 probes, as the sharp tip will often penetrate the buccal mucosa without entering the parotid duct and give a false impression of injury.

A neglected parotid duct injury should be suspected in a patient with parotid swelling and upper lip weakness after primary closure of a cheek laceration.

Parotid duct lacerations should be repaired primarily over a Silastic stent. The stent should be removed in 10 to 14 days. Repeated dilation may be necessary to manage stenosis after stent removal. Distal duct laceration may alternatively be managed by transoral rerouting of the duct, with Silastic stenting to prevent orifice stenosis. The stent should be secured to the buccal mucosa to prevent extrusion.

Compression of the gland with resultant salivary flow into the wound will identify the proximal segment of the duct. In severely injured parotid ducts where primary anastomosis or transoral rerouting is not possible, proximal duct ligation with anticipated parotid gland

424 • SALIVARY GLANDS

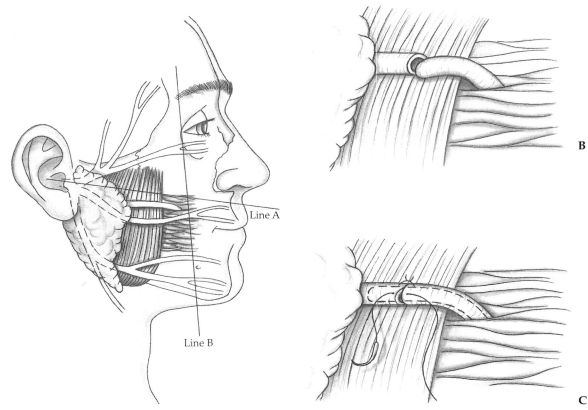

FIGURE 62-1 (A). Line *A*, marking the position of the parotid duct, extends from the tragus to the middle of the upper lip. The duct occupies the central third of this line. The buccal branch of the facial nerve runs inferior to the duct. Line *B* runs from the lateral canthus vertically to the mental foramen. Fibers of the facial nerve anterior to line *B* need not be repaired and they recover function if soft tissues are accurately approximated in layers. (B). Transected Stensen's duct. (C). Primary repair to the transected Stensen's duct by suturing over a Silastic catheter.

atrophy is possible. Alternatively, parotidectomy is effective in cases associated with facial nerve transection, where the nerve must be dissected for repair.

Chronic blunt trauma to the parotid, or less commonly the submandibular, duct can occur from dental abnormalities or poor-fitting dentures. Treatment of the underlying dental problem will usually resolve the problem. Occasionally, ductal orifice dilatation or sialodochoplasty may be necessary in severe cases.

SALIVARY PARENCHYMAL INJURY

Most salivary parenchymal injuries involve the parotid gland due to its location on the lateral face. After evaluation and appropriate manage-

ment of associated facial nerve and/or parotid duct injury, management of parenchymal injury can be undertaken. The rationale for acute treatment is to prevent sialocele and/or salivary fistula formation.

CONTROVERSY

Some authors recommend that the parotid fascia be closed primarily by placing sutures parallel to the fibers of the facial nerve at the time of primary skin closure, whereas other authors recommend only primary closure of the skin, with application of a pressure dressing.

Sialoceles and/or salivary fistulae may develop after either parenchymal or ductal injury. When ductal injury has occurred, exploration and repair as previously described should be undertaken, as conservative measures are rarely effective. Sialoceles should be aspirated. The diagnosis can be confirmed by an amylase concentration greater than 1000 units/mL. A pressure dressing should then be applied and replaced until the sialocele resolves. Attempts to decrease glandular secretion with the use of parasympatholytics have not proven effective. Some authors advocate tympanic neurectomy in refractory cases. Total gland excision is curative and is usually recommended for sublingual and submandibular glands, as well as difficult cases involving the parotid gland.

Salivary fistula is a frustrating problem that can result from either salivary ductal or parenchymal injury. When the main duct has been injured, exploration and repair as previously described are indicated. In the case of parenchymal injury, conservative therapy should be initiated with application of a pressure dressing. Parasympatholytics are often used but have no proven effectiveness. Tympanic neurectomy can also be considered in difficult cases. Total gland excision is often recommended for the submandibular gland and may be necessary in refractory cases involving the parotid. Fistulectomy and fistuloplasty have been described, but with poor reproducibility, and are not recommended.

EXTRACRANIAL FACIAL NERVE INJURY

Penetrating injury is the second most common cause of facial nerve injury, following temporal bone fracture. Facial lacerations, especially in the parotid region, should always be evaluated with special attention to facial nerve injury. Injuries anterior to a line drawn from the lateral canthus to the mental foramen (Fig. 62–1) rarely require repair because regeneration will often occur following meticulous closure of muscle and skin layers. However, injuries posterior to this line should be repaired immediately for best results. If repair cannot be performed within 48 hours, when a nerve stimulator can still be used to find the distal branches of the nerve, then tagging the ends for later repair is recommended.

PEARL... In unconscious patients, a Hilger nerve stimulator can be used transcutaneously to determine presence of facial nerve injury.

All facial nerve injuries should be repaired because even patients with severe closed head injuries often recover. The prognosis for delayed management is markedly worse.

Tension-free direct reanastomosis is recommended whenever possible. In cases where tension-free anastomosis is not possible, cable grafting, with the sural or great auricular nerve, is recommended.

PEARL... Using one or two fine (9-0) monofilament sutures is a simple and effective way to perform nerve anastomosis.

Delayed-onset facial paralysis from blunt trauma should be managed conservatively, often with systemic steroids. In cases of delayed presentation in penetrating trauma where no documentation of facial nerve function after injury is available, transection should be suspected and managed accordingly.

PITFALL... Watchful waiting is often rewarded with poor results in the management of traumatic facial paralysis with penetrating trauma.

SUGGESTED READINGS

Bailey BJ. Trauma. In: Cummings CW, Fredrickson JM, Harker LE, et al, eds. *Otolaryngology—Head and Neck Surgery*. Vol. 2. 2nd ed. St. Louis: Mosby Year Book; 1993:1018–1028.

Olson NR. Traumatic lesions of the salivary glands. *Otolaryngol Clin North Am* 1977;10(2): 345–350.

Seifert G, Miehlke A, Haulbrich J, et al. Salivary and branchial cleft fistulas. In: Verlag GT, ed. *Diseases of the Salivary Glands.* New York: Thieme; 1986:164–167.

Seifert G, Miehlke A, Haulbrich J, et al. Surgery of the salivary glands. In: Verlag GT, ed. *Diseases of the Salivary Glands.* New York: Thieme; 1986: 362–363.

SECTION X

MAXILLOFACIAL

Chapter 63

EMBRYOLOGY, ANATOMY, AND PHYSIOLOGY

Andrew C. Campbell and Kevin A. Shumrick

Embryologically, the formation of the facial anatomy is directly associated with the pharyngeal (branchial) arches. By the fourth week of gestation, four well-developed pairs of arches are easily seen, and a fifth arch lies buried beneath the surface. Other species with similar embryologic development have six pharyngeal arches, and therefore this fifth arch in humans is conventionally called the sixth arch for comparative purposes. Each arch contains an artery, nerve, cartilage, and muscle. Starting cranially, the cartilage of the first pharyngeal arch, also called Meckel's cartilage, ultimately becomes the mandible through the process of membranous bone formation. The malleus, incus, and maxilla are also formed from the first pharyngeal arch in a similar manner, though they are positioned more cranially. The second arch (Reichert's cartilage) becomes the stapes, the styloid process, and the lesser horn of the hyoid. The third arch cartilage forms the greater horn of the hyoid. The fourth and sixth arches form the cartilage of the airway.

The first arch gives rise to the mandibular division of the fifth cranial nerve (trigeminal nerve) and also the muscles that it innervates, the muscles of mastication (temporalis, masseter, medial, and lateral pterygoids), the mylohyoid, anterior digastric, tensor tympani, and tensor palatini. The second arch gives rise to the facial nerve and the muscles innervated by it, the stapedius, stylohyoid, posterior digastric, platysma, and the muscles of facial expression. The third arch gives rise to the glossopharyngeal nerve, which innervates the stylopharyngeus muscle and the superior and middle pharyngeal constrictors. The fourth arch gives rise to the superior vagus nerve, which provides sensation to the larynx and pharynx down to the level of the true vocal cords, and innervates the cricothyroid muscle. The sixth arch gives rise to the lower vagus nerve (recurrent), which provides sensation to the larynx, pharynx, and esophagus below the level of the true vocal cords, and innervates the intrinsic muscles of the larynx, inferior pharyngeal constrictor, and upper esophagus.

The arteries of the first and second arches ultimately involute, though a persistent dorsal artery of the second arch may be seen as the stapedial artery, passing through the crura of the stapes. The third arch artery becomes the proximal internal carotid artery. Later in development, the third arch forms the external carotid artery and provides a blood supply to its associated facial muscles. The fourth arch artery becomes the arch of the aorta. The sixth arch artery is the ductus arteriosis and normally is obliterated shortly after birth, becoming the ligamentum arteriosum.

Development of the middle third of the face is associated with the mesodermal tissues ventral to the overhanging forebrain. The midline mouth cavity or stomodeum is flanked on either side by the maxillary extensions of the first arch, caudally by Meckel's cartilage, and cranially by mesoderm and ectoderm overlying the forebrain. As the face develops, nasal pits arise near the frontonasal area. During fetal growth, the pits medialize as the orbits move to a frontal oblique position, primarily as the result of significant mesodermal development in the regions that ultimately form the parietal and squamous temporal bones. As the forebrain continues to enlarge, the cerebral hemispheres cause an elongation and enlargement of the forehead region. During this development, mesoderm forms a primitive connective tissue membrane. Ossification of this membrane then occurs as osteoblasts deposit bony matrix at multiple sites. This process continues until the sites coalesce into the facial bones with growth only at the suture lines. Fractured membranous bone heals by fibrous union.

In the adult, the malar eminence of the zygoma is the most prominent bone of the face and serves as a protective buttress. It is a very dense bone with four processes extending to articulations with the surrounding facial bones. Posteriorly, the thin zygomatic arch articulates with the temporal bone; superiorly, the zygoma articulates with the frontal bone; medially, it forms the lateral and inferior orbital walls and articulates with the maxilla at the infraorbital nerve; inferiorly, it forms a broad articulation again with the maxilla to form the zygomaticomaxillary buttress.

Other structurally important buttresses include the pyriform or nasofrontal buttress on either side of the nasal cavity and the pterygomaxillary buttress posteriorly. These buttresses provide tremendous strength in the vertical plane; however, they can be easily fractured by perpendicular forces. The significance of these buttresses will be discussed in greater detail in Chapter 69. Important muscles that attach to the zygoma include the masseter, the temporalis (passes medial to the zygomatic arch), and the zygomaticus major and minor.

The maxilla contains the antrum or maxillary sinus and forms the anterior midface and hard palate. It contributes to the majority of the orbital floor, articulates with the zygoma to form the zygomaticomaxillary buttress, establishes the posterior wall of the maxillary sinus/anterior wall of the pterygopalatine fossa, and extends to the hard palate where the upper dentition inserts.

The mandible is a dense **U**-shaped bone with the lower dentition inserting on its superior aspect. It is composed of dense cortical bone with a central spongy core in which the inferior alveolar nerve, artery, and vein travel. This neurovascular bundle exits the mandible at the mental foramen and provides sensation to the chin. The mandible is composed of a symphyseal region medially and parasymphyseal regions bilaterally in the paramedian position; there are also bilateral body, angle, and ramus regions. The ramus ends in two projections; anteriorly lies the coronoid to which the temporalis muscle attaches and posteriorly lies the condyle, which articulates with the temporomandibular joint.

The lateral pterygoid muscle attaches to the condyloid process and protracts and depresses the mandible. The medial pterygoid muscle attaches to the medial surface of the ramus and protracts, elevates, and pulls the mandible posteriorly. The masseter muscle attaches from the zygoma to the lateral portion of the mandibular angle and, with the temporalis muscle, elevates the mandible. Along the medial ramus, the inferior alveolar nerve enters the mandible at the mandibular foramen, just posterior to a bony prominence called the lingula spine.

PEARL... The entire lower teeth and chin can be anesthetized by injecting local anesthetic in the region of the lingula spine.

The temporomandibular joint is a synovial-lined, compound hinge and gliding joint. It is an unusual joint in that the articulating surfaces are covered not with hyaline cartilage but rather with fibrous connective tissue. A thin fibrous capsule surrounds the joint and is thickened laterally and posteriorly as the capsular ligament. This ligament helps prevent condylar dislocation. Within the capsule lies an articular disk or meniscus. This ovoid disk of avascular fibrous connective tissues lies between the mandibular condyle and the glenoid fossa and is attached to the inner surface of the joint capsule and to the tendon of the lateral pterygoid muscle. This disk divides the joint into separate upper and lower joint spaces. The temporomandibular joint lies just anterior to the external auditory meatus and can be easily palpated digitally at this site.

The facial mimetic musculature provides movement for facial expression and is described as having four layers. The most superficial two layers include the platysma, zygomatic major and minor, orbicularis oculi, and risorius. The third layer includes the orbicularis oris and levator labii superioris. Importantly, the facial nerve lies deep to the first three layers and thus inner-vates these muscles on their deep surface. Only the deepest layer of the buccinator, mentalis, and levator anguli oris is innervated at the superficial surface. These muscles are enveloped by the superficial cervical fascia, thus forming the superficial muscular aponeurotic system (SMAS). The SMAS invests the superficial facial muscles, and thus they function in concert to provide facial movement through the vertical fibrous septa (retinacula cutis) extending from the SMAS to the overlying dermis.

SUGGESTED READINGS

Anson BJ. The neck. In: Anson BJ, ed. *The Anatomy of the Head and Neck.* Vol. 1. 1st ed. Philadelphia: W.B. Saunders; 1956:67–94.

Beck AL. Deep neck infections. *Ann Otol Rhinol Laryngol* 1957;56:439–481.

Grodinsky M, Holyoke E. The fasciae and fascial spaces of the head, neck and adjacent regions. *Am J Anat* 1938;63:367–408.

Hollinshead WH. *Anatomy for Surgeons: The Head and Neck.* Vol. 1. 3rd ed. Philadelphia: Harper and Row; 1982:551.

Hollinshead WH. The neck. In: Hollinshead WH, ed. *Anatomy for Surgeons: The Head and Neck.* Vol. 1. 3rd ed. Philadelphia: Harper and Row; 1982:443–526.

Lang J. *Clinical Anatomy of the Nose, Nasal Cavity, and Paranasal Sinuses.* Vol. 1. 1st ed. New York: Thieme; 1989:144.

Paff GH. Introduction to the anatomy of the neck. In: Paff GH, ed. *Anatomy of the Head and Neck.* Vol. 1. 1st ed. Philadelphia: W.B. Saunders; 1973:1–9.

Tardy E. *Surgical Anatomy of the Nose.* 1st ed. New York: Raven Press; 1990:106.

Chapter 64

CLINICAL TESTS

Andrew C. Campbell and Kevin A. Shumrick

The major abnormalities affecting the maxillofacial region are trauma or various bony tumors. The primary means of evaluating the maxillofacial region are a thorough and knowledgeable physical examination and radiologic assessment.

The first test of the maxillofacial area should always be a thorough history and physical, including a complete cranial nerve exam. Clinically, one should examine for any lacerations or lesions of the skin or oral mucosa. Note should be made of any hematomas, crepitance, or ecchymosis of the soft tissue, any enophthalmos or exophthalmos, any numbness or weakness of the face, and any step-offs, depressions, or asymmetries of the facial skeleton. The patient's occlusion should be assessed as well as midface stability. Also, the extraocular muscles should be examined for signs of entrapment.

> **PEARL...** By performing a complete exam, one should be able to determine if any significant injury has occurred or any abnormality is present.

If significant injury or abnormality is suspected, further evaluation should be performed. For ocular abnormalities, a complete exam including slit-lamp and documented visual acuity should be done by an ophthalmologist. Computed tomography (CT) of the orbits is useful to assess the orbital contents and bony orbital walls. For soft tissue injury, damage to the facial nerve or parotid duct must be excluded. Once these structures are deemed intact, the wound should be thoroughly irrigated and meticulously reapproximated with fine suture. For soft tissue abnormalities (masses), magnetic resonance imaging (MRI) is the diagnostic tool of choice as it will delineate the facial planes and the depth of abnormality and often will be suggestive of a definitive diagnosis. For skeletal injury or abnormality, the test of choice is an axial and coronal CT with 5-mm cuts. Treatment of various midface and mandibular injuries is discussed in a later chapter in this section. If a mandibular injury is suspected, a Panorex is the test of choice to assess for fractures. The temporomandibular joint can be assessed by CT scan, MRI, or arthroscopy.

SUGGESTED READINGS

Lenz M. *Computed Tomography and Magnetic Resonance Imaging of Head and Neck Tumors: Methods, Guidelines, Differential Diagnoses and Clinical Results.* Vol. 1. 1st ed. Stuttgart: Georg Thieme Verlag; 1993:213.

Lufkin RB, Borges A, Nguyen KN, Anzai Y. *MRI of the Head and Neck.* Vol. 1. 2nd ed. Philadelphia: Lippincott, Williams and Wilkins; 2000:256.

Chapter 65

CONGENITAL DISORDERS

Andrew C. Campbell and Kevin A. Shumrick

A complete, in-depth discussion of maxillofacial congenital disorders is beyond the scope of this text. However, the more common syndromes are mentioned and highlighted.

Acrocephalosyndactyly, or Apert's syndrome, is characterized by acrocephaly and syndactyly of the hands and feet. Most cases are sporadic and are frequently associated with mental retardation. In affected individuals, the midface appears flattened due to an underdeveloped maxilla with a resulting apparent mandibular prognathism. A high arched palate, frequently with a posterior cleft, as well as malpositioned dentition is common. The cranium is brachycephalic with a very prominent forehead. Patients suffer from symmetric syndactyly, which varies in severity, and from hearing loss secondary to stapes fixation.

Craniofacial dysostosis, or Crouzon's syndrome, is characterized by premature craniosynostosis, midfacial hypoplasia, and bilateral proptosis. Inheritance is autosomal dominant with variable expression. Crouzon's is easily recognized by the marked proptosis resulting from shallow orbits, ocular hypertelorism, exotropia, and a hypoplastic maxilla. The proptosis can be severe enough to cause luxation of the globes and optic nerve damage. Patients have a short upper lip, a V-shaped palatal arch, dental malocclusion, a parrot-beaked nose, and frequently suffer from hearing loss, usually conductive. Brachycephaly with ridging of the sagittal suture due to premature synostosis can lead to mental retardation.

Cleidocranial dysplasia is characterized by short stature, a long neck, and narrow shoulders. The skull is brachycephalic, the clavicles aplastic or hypoplastic, and patients are noted to have supernumerary teeth and a hypoplastic maxilla. They also are noted to have a short midface with a broad-based nose and depressed nasal dorsum.

Mandibulofacial dysostosis, or Treacher Collins syndrome or Franceschetti-Zwahlen-Klein Syndrome, is characterized by down-sloping palpebral fissures with coloboma in the outer third of the lower lid, malar hypoplasia, deformed or atretic pinna and external auditory canals, mandibular hypoplasia with a large fishlike mouth, preauricular fistulas, conductive hearing loss, and frequent cleft palate and cleft lip. Inheritance is autosomal dominant with variable expressivity, and intelligence is normal. It is thought that an arrest in embryonic development at 6 to 8 weeks causes the characteristic abnormalities.

Oculomandibulodyscephaly with hypotrichosis, or Hallermann-Streiff-François syndrome, is characterized by a thin, pointed, parrot-like nose; mandibular hypoplasia with "double" chin; proportionate dwarfism; hypotrichosis, most commonly of the scalp, brows, and eyelashes; bilateral congenital cataracts with microphthalmia and nystagmus; and brachycephaly. Inheritance is unknown as there appears to be no genetic basis for this syndrome.

Craniometaphyseal dysplasia, or Pyle's disease, is characterized by bony overgrowth of the face and jaw, and altered metaphyses of the long bones. Inheritance is autosomal dominant, though it can be recessive. Patients have very broad, flat nasal bridges; ocular hypertelorism; late motor development; and marked thickening of the maxilla, mandible, and skull base. Due to bony overgrowth within the nasopharynx, patients frequently breathe with an open mouth. Ultimately, blindness may result from optic atrophy as bony overgrowth occurs in or near the optic canal.

Pyknodysostosis is characterized by short stature, osteopetrosis, frontal and occipital bulging, persistent fontanelles, agenesis of the angle of the mandible, and partial agenesis of the phalanges of the hands and feet. Patients consistently have absent frontal sinuses, and the other paranasal sinuses are hypoplastic. It is autosomal recessive.

Orofaciodigital syndrome type I is characterized by a pseudocleft in the median upper lip, hypoplastic nasal ala, asymmetric cleft palate, multilobulated tongue, multiple hyperplastic frenula, dystopia canthorum, various digital malformations, and mild mental retardation. Hamartomas between the lobes of the multilobulated tongue are common. It is X-linked recessive and is lethal in males. A similar syndrome, Mohr's syndrome (type II), is autosomal recessive.

Robin's sequence, or Pierre Robin syndrome, is characterized by a cleft palate, micrognathia, and glossoptosis. It can be a component of many syndromes, and many are thought to have Stickler's syndrome (hereditary arthro-ophthalmopathy). It is thought that the micrognathia allows the tongue to fall back over the epiglottis (glossoptosis), thus causing airway obstruction.

PEARL... The airway obstruction can be treated with a nasal trumpet airway; however, a tracheotomy is the definitive treatment in an unstable child.

Interestingly, the mandible grows to a normal size by age 4 to 6, and thus airway obstruction is a temporary problem. Other abnormalities include detached retina, glaucoma, low-set ears, and occasionally mental retardation. It is thought to be caused by an intrauterine insult at 4 months' gestation, or it may be genetically inherited.

Cleft lip-palate and *paramedian sinuses of the lower lip,* or van der Woude's syndrome, is characterized by bilateral, symmetrical fistulas or depressions at the vermilion border of the lower lip. These fistulas vary in size but most ultimately communicate through the orbicularis oris with underlying minor salivary glands. The pits can be associated with cleft lip and/or palate, and have been associated with orofaciodigital syndrome.

Congenital anomalies of the first and second branchial arches have multiple descriptions including hemifacial microsomia, craniofacial microsomia, unilateral and bilateral microsomia, oral-mandibular-auricular syndrome, hemignathia and microtia syndrome, unilateral facial agenesis, necrotic facial dysplasia, and intrauterine facial necrosis. The characteristics of the anomaly could include macrostomia, maldevelopment of the external and middle ear, mandibular hypoplasia, hemifacial hypoplasia, maldevelopment of the muscles of mastication, facial expression, and the tongue, and maldevelopment of the parotid gland. Commisural clefts can be closed primarily; however, often, multistaged procedures are required for treatment of severe cases.

Oculoauriculovertebral dysplasia, or Goldenhar's syndrome, may represent a variant of the first and second branchial arch syndromes and is characterized by varying degrees of craniofacial microsomia as well as epibulbar dermoids, ear tags, and abnormalities of the vertebral column. Mental retardation, heart abnormalities, and a mixed hearing loss have also been noted.

Multiple endocrine neoplasia (MEN) type 2B is characterized by multiple mucosal neuromas, pheochromocytoma, and medullary carcinoma of the thyroid. The mucosal neuromas usually involve the lip and tongue but can involve virtually any portion of the face. It has autosomal-dominant inheritance.

Gardner's syndrome is characterized by epidermoid inclusion cysts of the skin and polyposis of the colon. Frequently, fibromas and desmoid tumors of the skin occur as well as multiple osteomas of the skull and facial skeleton. It is autosomal dominant with variable penetrance.

Nevoid basal cell carcinoma syndrome, or basal cell nevoid syndrome or Gorlin's syndrome, is characterized by multiple basal cell carcinomas, cysts of the mandible, abnormal vertebra and ribs (bifid), calcification of the falx cerebri, and bilateral calcified ovarian fibromas. The mandible often has multiple destructive cysts, which frequently recur after surgical removal. The nevoid basal cell carcinomas occur frequently on the face and are excised as necessary. There is an association with medulloblastoma. It is autosomal dominant.

Osteogenesis imperfecta, or van der Hoeve's syndrome, has many clinical manifestations. Essentially all patients have abnormal osteoblastic activity and are prone to skeletal fractures. The severity ranges from slightly increased risk of long bone fractures to intrauterine death. Other associated findings include blue sclera, dentinogenesis imperfecta, otosclerosis, and capillary fragility. It is autosomal dominant with variable expressivity.

Craniofacial clefting, or facial clefting syndrome, is characterized by skeletal and soft tissue defects or clefts that occur in specific, common locations, categorized by Tessier. They frequently involve the mandible, maxilla, zygoma, orbits, and neurocranium, and severe ocular abnormalities are common. Clefts 0 to 4 involve the nasolacrimal apparatus, 5 to 8 involve the lower eyelid (6 is associated with Treacher Collins, 8 with Goldenhar's), 10 is usually caused by a frontal encephalocele, and 10 to 14 are associated with hypertelorism and ocular coloboma. These clefts are often inherited.

SUGGESTED READINGS

Gorlin RJ, Cohen MM, Levin LS. Syndromes of the head and neck. In: Motulsky AG, Bobrow M, Harper PS, Scriver C, eds. *Oxford Monographs of Medical Genetics.* Vol. 1. 3rd ed. New York: Oxford University Press, 1990.

Chapter 66

FUNCTIONAL DISORDERS

Andrew C. Campbell and Kevin A. Shumrick

Functional disorders of the maxillofacial region primarily involve the mandible and the temporomandibular joint. If the interrelationship of the maxillary and mandibular teeth during contact is not normal, the patient has malocclusion.

SPECIAL CONSIDERATION

A normal relationship occurs when the mesiobuccal cusp tip of the maxillary first molar is aligned with the buccal groove of the mandibular first molar. This is class I occlusion.

In class II occlusion, the mesiobuccal cusp of the maxillary first molar is positioned anterior to the buccal groove of the mandibular first molar, thus giving the maxilla a more prominent appearance. In class III occlusion, the mesiobuccal cusp of the maxillary first molar is positioned posterior to the buccal groove of the mandibular first molar, thus giving the mandible a more prominent appearance.

Pain in the region of the temporomandibular joint (TMJ) can arise from many areas, including the external or middle ear, muscles of mastication, referred pain from the pharynx, or from the joint itself. Nocturnal bruxism, malocclusion, or intrinsic abnormalities of the joint can all lead to temporomandibular joint dysfunction. A thorough history and physical including auscultation of the joint if the patient complains of popping, clicking, or grinding is necessary for an accurate diagnosis. Palpation of the muscles of mastication will help diagnose myofascial pain-dysfunction syndrome (muscle tenderness). Treatment includes nonsteroidal antiinflammatory drugs (NSAIDs), massage and heat, a soft diet, and an acrylic splint.

SPECIAL CONSIDERATION

For more severe cases, occlusal equilibration by removal of tooth substance, orthodontic therapy, or subcondylar osteotomy is done.

An internal abnormality of the disk space is treated with NSAIDs, splint therapy, meniscoplasty, meniscectomy, or subcondylar osteotomy. Degenerative joint disease of the TMJ is extremely common and is treated with NSAIDs, physical therapy, intraarticular steroid injections, or, in severe cases, reconstructive surgery.

Ankylosis of the TMJ refers to a true bony or fibrous fusion of the mandible to the glenoid fossa. If this occurs during facial development, significant deformity can occur. Treatment is surgical with vigorous postoperative physical therapy.

Because the TMJ is a sliding joint, it can become subluxed anteriorly during a wide opening of the mouth and become locked in place by the articular eminence. If the TMJ is anteriorly subluxed on one side, the chin deviates to the opposite side and an obvious "cross-bite" malocclusion is present. This is treated with manual reduction and a soft diet. In patients with recurrent subluxation and locking of the jaw, an eminectomy (excision of the articular eminence) is performed.

SUGGESTED READINGS

Auerbach SM, Laskin DM, Frantsve LM, Orr T. Depression, pain, exposure to stressful life events, and long-term outcomes in temporomandibular disorder patients. *J Oral Maxillofac Surg* 2001;59:628–33.

De Laat A. Temporomandibular disorders as a source of orofacial pain. *Acta Neurol Belg* 2001;101:26–31.

Glaros AG. Emotional factors in temporomandibular joint disorders. *J Indiana Dent Assoc* 2000;79:20–3.

Haley DP, Schiffman EL, Lindgren BR, Anderson Q, Andreasen K. The relationship between clinical and MRI findings in patients with unilateral temporomandibular joint pain. *J Am Dent Assoc* 2001;132:476–81.

Sonnesen L, Bakke M, Solow B. Temporomandibular disorders in relation to craniofacial dimensions: head posture and bite force in children selected for orthodontic treatment. *Eur J Orthod* 2001;23:179–92.

Sundqvist B, Magnusson T. Individual prediction of treatment outcome in patients with temporomandibular disorders. *Swed Dent J* 2001;25:1–11.

Chapter 67

INFECTIOUS AND INFLAMMATORY DISORDERS

Andrew C. Campbell and Kevin A. Shumrick

Infectious and inflammatory disorders covered here are also discussed in further detail under the sections on the nose and oral cavity.

BACTERIAL INFECTIONS

RHINOSCLEROMA

Definition

Respiratory scleroma (rhinoscleroma) is a chronic granulomatous infection produced by *Klebsiella rhinoscleromatis,* a gram-negative aerobic coccobacillus.

Clinical Presentation

This disease is endemic to Africa, Central and South America, south central and eastern Europe, the Middle East, and China. Sporadic cases have been reported in the United States, especially in persons who migrated from the aforementioned areas. The majority of cases affect the nose, but extension to the soft and hard palate, upper lip, and maxillary sinuses also is frequent. Typically the first area that is affected is the nose, with the onset of profuse rhinorrhea. Later crusting is a prominent symptom with eventual fibrosis and ulceration (Table 67–1). Other sites of involvement include the paranasal sinuses, orbit, larynx, tracheobronchial

tree, and middle ear. Acutely, the nose shows crusting with the infected mucosa being pale and showing diffuse nodular thickening.

Radiologic evaluation may provide a clearer picture of the extent of the disease process and possibly suggest the diagnosis. The main nasal and nasopharyngeal computed tomography (CT) findings are soft tissue masses of variable sizes. The lesions are characteristically homogeneous and nonenhancing, and have distinct edge definition; adjacent fascial planes are not invaded. In the subglottic area the lesions tend to form concentric irregular narrowing of the airway. In the trachea, crypt-like irregularities are considered diagnostic of scleroma in the appropriate clinical setting. Intraorbital, intracranial, and infratemporal parapharyngeal scleromatous masses have also been described. The hypertrophic stage of rhinoscleroma has characteristic mild to marked high signal intensity on both T1- and T2-weighted magnetic resonance imaging (MRI).

Pathology

A characteristic clinical picture may be suggestive of rhinoscleroma, but the diagnosis is made by histology. Cultures are of little benefit. Light microscopy shows a dense plasmacytic infiltrate, Mikulicz histiocytes (macrophages with

TABLE 67-1 STAGES OF RHINOSCLEROMA

Stage	Description
Catarrhal	Prolonged purulent rhinorrhea
Granuloma	Granulomatous nodules
Cicatricial (sclerotic)	Dense fibrotic reactions that stenose the nose, larynx, or tracheobronchial tree

clear foamy cytoplasm), and Russell bodies within the plasma cells.

> **PEARL•••** Warthin-Starry silver stain demonstrates the presence of the K. rhinoscleromatis, gram-negative bacteria within the macrophages.

Ultrastructural study reveals Mikulicz histiocytes, cytoplasmic vacuoles containing bacilli, and so-called A and B granules. Some authors favor the term *respiratory scleroma* for this lesion because it can affect not only the nose but also the upper and lower respiratory tracts as well as the mouth.

Treatment and Prognosis

Treatment of rhinoscleroma consists of local debridement and systemic antibiotics. Although a number of antibiotics have been found to be effective in this relapsing disorder, the lengthy duration of treatment can lead to problems with adverse effects and compliance. Patient compliance may be especially difficult with the traditional treatment modalities of streptomycin and tetracycline. A recent report describes a patient with extensive nasal rhinoscleroma who achieved pathologic and bacteriologic resolution during treatment with oral ciprofloxacin after failure of previous courses of tetracycline and trimethoprim-sulfamethoxazole. Ciprofloxacin may prove to be useful in the therapy of rhinoscleroma because it is convenient for oral administration, achieves good tissue levels, is concentrated in macrophages, and is generally well tolerated as long-term therapy. Rhinoscleroma must be distinguished from various inflammatory and neoplastic processes, including leprosy, paracoccidioidomycosis, sarcoidosis, basal cell carcinoma, and Wegener's granulomatosis.

ACTINOMYCOSIS

Definition and Description

Although the term *actinomycosis* seems to imply a fungal infection, actinomycosis is, in reality, a filamentous, branching, gram-positive anaerobic bacteria. Actinomycetes are normal saprophytic components of the oral flora. The most common species causing human disease is *Actinomyces israelii.*

Clinical Presentation

Infection with actinomycosis may present as either an acute, rapidly progressing infection or as a chronic, slowly spreading lesion that is associated with fibrosis. Actinomycosis may affect a number of different sites on the body (abdominal, thoracic, cutaneous, and genital), but greater than 50% of cases occur in the cervicofacial region.

> **SPECIAL CONSIDERATION**
>
> The suppurative reaction of actinomycosis infection may discharge large yellowish flecks that are visible. These flecks are composed of colonies of the bacteria and have been referred to as sulfur granules.

In the maxillofacial region the organism typically enters the tissue through an area of prior trauma, such as a tooth socket or mucosal tear. Actinomycosis infections do not travel along the typical fascial planes seen in other infections of the head and neck. Instead, the infection proceeds with direct extension through soft tissue. Classically, actinomycosis infections are described as having a firm woody feel that eventually forms a central abscess. This area of abscess formation will then typically track to either a mucosal or epidermal surface, forming a sinus, or if both surfaces are involved, a fistula.

Surprisingly, there is little pain associated with these infections despite their serious appearance. Additionally, it is rare for sensory or motor nerves to be compromised, and this may be a point of distinction when a malignancy may be in the differential.

Pathology and Microbiology

> **PITFALL...** The diagnosis of actinomycosis is ideally achieved by culture, but less than 50% of cases are positive due to the fastidious nature of the actinomycosis and its strict anaerobic culture requirements. Additionally, prior antibiotic treatment and overgrowth by contaminating organisms may obscure the actinomycosis.

Without a definitive culture for actinomycosis, a strong presumptive diagnosis can be made based on the typical clinical picture and supportive histologic findings. Consistent histologic findings would include chronically inflamed granulation tissue surrounding large collections of polymorphonuclear leukocytes and colonies of organisms. The actinomycosis colonies appear as club-shaped filaments that form a radiating rosette pattern. The organisms stain best with Gram and Gomori methenamine silver stains. Finally, fluorescein-conjugated antiserum can be used on the granules to specifically identify the *Actinomyces* species.

Treatment and Prognosis

The treatment of choice for actinomycosis in chronic fibrosing cases is prolonged high doses of antibiotics in conjunction with abscess drainage and excision of the sinus tracts. Penicillin is considered the antibiotic of choice. Patients who are allergic to penicillin can be treated with tetracycline. The prognosis is excellent with adequate treatment, which may require a 5- to 6-week course of penicillin.

LUDWIG'S ANGINA

Definition

Since Ludwig's original description, a variety of inflammatory conditions related to the floor of the mouth have been labeled Ludwig's angina, but in reality many would more appropriately be termed pseudoangina ludovici. These pseudo-Ludwig's are more limited infections that only involve the sublingual space, the submandibular lymph nodes, the submandibular gland, or the submental space, or are abscesses involving one or more of these spaces. There is a general consensus in the literature that to qualify as a true Ludwig's angina, the following features should be present: (1) a spreading cellulitis with no special tendency to form abscesses; (2) involvement of both submaxillary and sublingual spaces, and the angina is usually bilateral; (3) spread occurs by direct extension along fascial planes and not lymphatics; (4) involvement of muscle and fascia but not the submandibular gland or lymph nodes; and (5) origination in the region of the submaxillary space with progression to the sublingual space and floor of the mouth.

Clinical Presentation

Ludwig's angina occurs most commonly in young adults with periodontal disease. It is generally agreed that the most common cause of Ludwig's angina is an abscessed second or third molar tooth with penetration into the submaxillary space below the mylohyoid ridge and initiation of a cellulitis.

The clinical picture of Ludwig's angina is typically that of a young male with poor dentition who presents with a history of increasing oral or neck pain and swelling. Frequently, the patient's symptoms are unilateral, but soon progress to involve both sides. As the infection progresses, there is increasing edema and induration of both the external perimandibular region and the floor of the mouth. The soft tissues of the floor of the mouth become tremendously swollen and, as a result of the relatively unyielding superficial layer of the deep cervical fascia and mandible, the expansion progresses superiorly and posteriorly. This expansion has the effect of thrusting the tongue posteriorly and superiorly with approximation of the palatal vault. There is increasing neck rigidity, trismus, odynophagia, and, eventually, drooling. The temperature is typically elevated in the 100° to 102°F range, and 104° is not uncommon. As the swelling progresses there is increasing encroachment upon the airway and the patient assumes an erect posture with tachypnea. Dyspnea and stridor signal the imminent danger of airway obstruction. This is truly a desperate situation because visualization of the larynx by conventional techniques is impossible, and attempts at intubation may actually precipitate airway obstruction. Similarly, a tracheostomy is extremely difficult due to the inability of the patient to lie supine and the presence of significant neck edema. The point to stress is the rapidity with which this process may occur; many case reports detail the progression from onset of symptoms to respiratory obstruction within 12 to 24 hours.

Examination

The physical exam of a patient with Ludwig's angina typically finds fever, tachycardia, and variable degrees of respiratory obstruction, with dysphagia and drooling. The submandibular and submental regions are tense, swollen, and tender. The floor of the mouth is tense and indurated with massive mucosal swelling and pouting of soft tissue over the edges of the lower teeth; fluctuance is unusual. The tongue is pushed superiorly and there is marked trismus. Indirect examination of the larynx is, at best, difficult and usually impossible. Nasopharyngeal fiberoptic exam will reveal the presence of a greatly enlarged base of tongue pushing the epiglottis posteriorly, whereas the supraglottis and endolarynx are normal in appearance.

Microbiology

It is clear that these infections are, almost always, the result of mixed flora involving both aerobes and anaerobes. The most commonly reported aerobe is α-hemolytic streptococci followed by staphylococcus. As a rule, gram-negative organisms do not play a significant

role in Ludwig's angina, although *Haemophilus influenzae, Escherichia coli,* and *Pseudomonas* have all been reported.

Laboratory and Radiologic Findings

The diagnosis and treatment of Ludwig's angina are based on the clinical parameters outlined; laboratory and radiologic studies offer only supporting evidence. Typically, the white blood count (WBC) is moderately to markedly elevated in the range of 15,000 to 20,000 with a marked left shift. X rays show soft tissue edema, occasionally gas, and posterior displacement of the tongue with airway encroachment.

> **PEARL•••** Due to the fact that these infections are often of an odontogenic etiology, a Panorex may be helpful in determining the site of origin for the infection and aid in planning the treatment regimen.

Treatment and Prognosis

Treatment of Ludwig's angina depends on the disease stage when the patient presents. Ludwig's angina is a spectrum of conditions ranging from a periapical abscess and mild cellulitis, in its early stage, to massive sepsis with airway obstruction. Treatment may be tailored to the status of the individual patient with the understanding that this disease may progress very rapidly, and if initial steps are not successful, then more radical means must be employed.

In the early stages of Ludwig's angina with unilateral mild swelling and edema, simple intravenous antibiotics and supportive measures may be sufficient. They are often coupled with extraction of the inciting tooth, if this is identifiable.

Surgical treatment is directed at securing an airway and providing surgical drainage. The choice of airway management rests on the experience and availability of the treating personnel. Although airway management by nasotracheal intubation, with or without fiberoptic assistance, is well described in the literature, it should be borne in mind that airway manipulation may precipitate acute obstruction, and thus

SPECIAL CONSIDERATION

If the patient presents with more advanced disease or progresses to bilateral swelling, dysphagia with drooling, or any symptoms of airway compromise, then early airway intervention, in a controlled fashion, is advocated rather than waiting until emergency procedures are required.

a tracheostomy set should always be available. Due to the possibility of postoperative extubation, and the difficulty of reintubation, conversion to a tracheostomy is generally advocated for postoperative airway management. If intubation is not possible, then a tracheostomy under local anesthesia, often with the patient sitting upright, is required. This may be complicated by the presence of significant edema in the neck. Those cases with a rapidly deteriorating airway may require a cricothyrotomy. Once an airway is established, then surgical drainage is performed. Drainage consists of bilateral, wide surgical decompression of the suprahyoid region, with placement of multiple drains.

The choice of antibiotics must be tailored to the individual patient, but high-dose penicillin (12 to 16 million units per day) is considered the drug of choice. Chloramphenicol and clindamycin are alternate possibilities, especially in penicillin-allergic patients.

FUNGAL INFECTIONS

MUCORMYCOSIS

Definition and Description

Mucormycosis is an opportunistic, frequently fulminant, fungal infection that is caused by normally saprophytic organisms of the class Zygomycetes. These organisms are found throughout the world, growing on a variety of decaying organic materials. Numerous spores may be liberated into the air and inhaled by the human host. Mucormycosis may infect several different areas of the body, but the most frequently fatal is the rhinocerebral form. Mu-

cormycosis is classically noted to occur in poorly controlled (ketoacidotic) diabetics but may affect immunocompromised patients as well. It is extremely rare for mucormycosis to affect a healthy individual.

Clinical Presentation

Rhinocerebral mucormycosis may present in several ways, but a classic scenario is for a brittle diabetic to present in ketoacidosis with concomitant nasal obstruction, bloody nasal discharge, facial pain, and facial swelling. Often, these patients are comatose. With more advanced cases there may be gross proptosis.

> **PEARL...** A characteristic finding (some would say pathognomonic) is that of gross tissue necrosis with a black eschar of the lateral nasal wall and/or hemipalate.

This disease progresses rapidly with extension of tissue necrosis in a matter of hours. The disease progresses rapidly out of the nose and paranasal sinuses into the orbit and from there to the central nervous system via the orbital apex. Once in the central nervous system, death is the usual outcome.

Radiographically, mucormycosis is not distinctive, showing opacification of the affected sinuses and diffuse orbital swelling. Soft tissue air is not a typical feature.

Pathology and Microbiology

Histopathologically, there is noted to be massive soft tissue necrosis. This appears to be due to the tendency of the fungus to invade small blood vessels with resultant ischemic necrosis. The fungal elements may be observed in the soft tissue and appear as large, branching, nonseptate hyphae at the advancing edge of the infection. Culture will confirm the diagnosis but is of little help in an acute life-threatening infection of this nature. The diagnosis of mucormycosis is based on the clinical features and histologic picture. Due to the grave nature of this infection, definitive therapy must be instituted before culture results have been obtained.

Chapter 68

NEOPLASMS AND CYSTS

Andrew C. Campbell and Kevin A. Shumrick

BENIGN LESIONS

FIBROUS DYSPLASIA

Definition and Description

Fibrous dysplasia is an idiopathic, nonneoplastic bone disease in which normal medullary bone is replaced by structurally weak fibrous and osseous tissue.

Clinical Presentation

There are three variants of fibrous dysplasia: monostotic, polyostotic, and McCune-Albright syndrome.

MONOSTOTIC FIBROUS DYSPLASIA   A single osseous site is involved. Monostotic fibrous dysplasia accounts for 80 to 85% of cases of fibrous dysplasia. The jaws are the most commonly affected site. The disease is usually noted in the first or second decade of life, but milder forms of the disease may not be detected until later. Males and females are equally affected. The most common presenting symptom is that of a painless, hard mass. Not uncommonly attention is drawn to the mass as a result of trauma. However, there is no evidence that trauma incites fibrous dysplasia. Growth is generally slow, but there are cases where growth has been rapid.

The maxilla is involved more frequently than the mandible.

POLYOSTOTIC FIBROUS DYSPLASIA   By definition, polyostotic fibrous dysplasia involves more than one bone. It represents 15 to 20% of fibrous dysplasia cases. Although the skull and jaws may be affected with resultant facial asymmetry, the most notable feature of polyostotic fibrous dysplasia is typically its long bone involvement. It may be limited to a few bones in one anatomic region or may be diffuse, affecting virtually every bone in the skeleton. The bones of the head and neck are involved in up to 50% of the cases.

MCCUNE-ALBRIGHT SYNDROME   The McCune-Albright syndrome accounts for less than 5% of cases of fibrous dysplasia and refers to the following triad of findings:

1. Polyostotic fibrous dysplasia
2. Endocrine dysfunction, with sexual precocity among females the most dramatic manifestation
3. Areas of cutaneous hyperpigmentation similar to the café-au-lait spots noted in neurofibromatosis. However, the spots in patients with fibrous dysplasia have very irregular borders, whereas the spots of neurofibromatosis have smooth borders.

447

Regardless of the type of fibrous dysplasia, the majority of patients manifest the disease by the age of 30. There is no sex predilection. The most common presentation for fibrous dysplasia is that of a painless, asymmetric swelling. In some cases with polyostotic involvement there may be significant facial deformity. The teeth may be pushed and distorted by the process but are not usually loosened. Headaches, proptosis, nasal obstruction, and malocclusion may all be presenting symptoms, depending on the site of involvement. Routine laboratory studies (serum calcium and phosphorous levels) are normal.

> **PEARL...** Radiographically, the most notable feature is a fine "ground-glass" appearance, which results from superimposition of multiple poorly calcified bone trabeculae arranged in a disorganized matrix.

There is usually noted to be a poorly defined expansile mass with a thin, intact cortex. Usually there is no periosteal reaction unless there is an associated fracture. Lesions may vary with regard to the makeup of the bony versus the fibrous components. If predominantly fibrous, the lesions will appear radiolucent. If predominantly osseous, the lesions will appear radiodense. An equal mixture of the two will give the characteristic ground-glass appearance.

Pathology

Histopathologically, fibrous dysplasia shows irregularly shaped trabeculae of immature bone in a cellular fibrous stroma.

Differential Diagnosis

Fibrous dysplasia may be most easily confused with ossifying fibroma.

Treatment and Prognosis

The clinical presentation of fibrous dysplasia may range from an isolated fairly innocuous bony asymmetry that requires no treatment to massive distortion of the facial bones with severe cosmetic and functional disruptions. In many cases the disease tends to stabilize and stops progressing when skeletal maturation occurs. Thus treatment is best deferred until the mid- to late teens. Conservative surgical excision is the recommended treatment and is indicated only in patients with either functional or cosmetic concerns. Small lesions may be completely resected. However, larger lesions may be difficult to completely resect. In these cases just the functionally or cosmetically significant components should be removed.

> **SPECIAL CONSIDERATION**
>
> Recently, lesions impinging on the nasal airway and/or paranasal sinuses have been managed endoscopically.

The incidence of regrowth after surgery is difficult to ascertain, but it appears to occur to some degree in 30 to 40% of patients and is more common in younger patients. There is a low, but definite, rate of malignant transformation into osteosarcoma. For this reason radiation is generally felt to be contraindicated as a treatment modality for fibrous dysplasia.

OSSIFYING FIBROMA

Definition and Description

Ossifying fibroma is a sharply delineated neoplasm that is composed of fibrous tissue with varying amounts of calcified tissue suggestive of bone and/or cementum.

Clinical Presentation

Ossifying fibromas are distinctly more common in women than men. These tumors occur most commonly in the third and fourth decades of life. The most common site of occurrence is the third molar region of the mandible (upwards of 80 to 90%) followed by the maxilla. Ossifying fibromas generally present as an asymptomatic mass without pain or swelling or are discovered incidentally on an X ray. Larger tumors may displace teeth or change occlusion.

Radiographically, these lesions are sharply demarcated and unilocular. The degree of radiolucency is dependent on the amount of calcium contained in the tumor, which may vary with the maturity of the lesion (immature radiolucent; mature radiopaque).

Pathology

Most ossifying fibromas are not truly encapsulated but are microscopically and grossly separate from the surrounding bone. Microscopically these tumors are made up of fibrous tissue of varying degrees of cellularity and calcification. There may be some degree of bony trabeculae formation.

Differential Diagnosis

The most similar clinical entity to ossifying fibromas is fibrous dysplasia.

Treatment and Prognosis

Because ossifying fibromas are separate and discrete, they can usually be easily enucleated. However, if there has been considerable bone loss, bone grafting may be required. Tumor recurrence after removal is low and there is no evidence that ossifying fibromas undergo malignant transformation.

AMELOBLASTOMA

Definition

Ameloblastoma is the most common clinically significant odontogenic tumor. Ameloblastomas arise from odontogenic epithelium. They are slow-growing, locally invasive tumors, which usually pursue a benign course.

Clinical Presentation

There is no sex predilection and it may present at any age although it most commonly occurs in the third to fourth decades of life. Greater than 80% of ameloblastomas involve the mandible usually in the region of the third molar. Maxillary ameloblastomas most commonly occur in the molar region, with frequent involvement of the antrum and floor of the nose. The most common presenting symptom is that of a slow-growing, painless mass in the maxillary or mandibular region. Typically there is no disruption of motor or sensory nerves. Teeth may be displaced but are not loosened.

Radiographically, these tumors may have several presentations—either unilocular or multilocular radiolucent lesions. There may be significant thinning of cortical bone.

Pathology

Unencapsulated proliferating nests of odontogenic epithelial cells are found.

Differential Diagnosis

The differential diagnosis includes dentigerous cyst, odontogenic keratocyst, ameloblastic fibroma, and adenoid cystic carcinoma.

Treatment and Prognosis

PEARL... The conventional ameloblastoma tends to infiltrate between intact cancellous bone trabeculae at the periphery of the lesion before bone resorption is noted on radiographs. Thus, the margin of the tumor may extend beyond what would be expected on preoperative assessment.

SPECIAL CONSIDERATION

Simple curettage of these tumors leaves nests of cells behind with high rates of recurrence. En-bloc resection with 1-cm margins is advocated to ensure complete resection.

Ameloblastomas are generally considered radioresistant, and there are no accepted chemotherapy protocols. These tumors are locally invasive, and with recurrence or unchecked growth may involve significant portions of the facial skeleton and contiguous structures with resultant disfigurement, dysfunction, and even death.

Rarely, metastases may occur and do so in the setting of long-standing tumors, which have undergone multiple resections or have been treated with radiation. Typically, the metastatic lesions appear histologically benign. Ameloblastomas may undergo malignant transformation and are then referred to as ameloblastic carcinoma. Ameloblastic carcinomas look similar to squamous cell carcinoma and may metastasize to lungs, lymph nodes, and liver.

Pyogenic Granuloma

Definition

The pyogenic granuloma is a common tumor-like growth of the oral cavity. It is generally considered to be nonneoplastic. Despite its name it is not felt to be due to infectious agents. Also, it does not exhibit the typical histologic characteristics of a true granuloma.

Clinical Presentation

Pyogenic granulomas typically present as lobulated masses that have a narrower base than surface. The color is often quite red and the surface has a cobblestone appearance. Often, there is a history of bleeding with minor trauma. A history of trauma to the region is common but not universal. These lesions are more common in young adults and tend to occur on the gingiva. Pyogenic granuloma of the gingiva frequently develops in pregnant women and is sometimes referred to as "granuloma gravidarum."

Pathology

Pyogenic granulomas are notable for very vascular stroma that resembles granulation tissue with numerous endothelial-lined channels. There are scattered inflammatory cells. With time these lesions may take on a more fibrous appearance.

Differential Diagnosis

The distinctive clinical and histologic appearance is fairly straightforward. These lesions may be mistaken for other less common benign inflammatory lesions such as giant cell granuloma, ossifying fibroma, and fibrous histiocytoma.

Treatment and Prognosis

Treatment consists of conservative surgical excision. For lesions that develop during pregnancy, treatment should be held until after delivery when there is less chance of recurrence.

MALIGNANT LESIONS

MIDLINE MALIGNANT RETICULOSIS

Definition

This disease has many synonyms, such as lethal midline granuloma, Stewart's granuloma, polymorphic reticulosis, angiocentric lymphoproliferative lesion, and angiocentric T-cell malignant lymphoma. This is a rare disease that is characterized by aggressive, progressive ulceration of midline maxillofacial structures such as the palate, nasal septum, and nasal cavity. It is a lymphoproliferative disorder characterized by either polymorphous or monomorphous cellular infiltrate that causes necrosis and ulceration. There is angiocentricity and the lymphocytes are predominantly T cell.

Clinical Presentation

Midline malignant reticulosis affects males more than females and occurs most commonly in the fifth or sixth decades of life. The most commonly affected site is the nasal cavity or paranasal sinuses. Symptoms typically start with nasal crusting and ulceration with involvement of the septum and paranasal sinuses. Eventually, the palate is eroded. In late stages the orbits and cranial cavity may be affected.

Pathology

Histopathologic examination shows a mixed infiltrate of a variety of inflammatory cells, often arranged around blood vessels. There appears to be invasion and necrosis of surrounding normal tissue. Immunohistochemical evaluation shows a monoclonal T-lymphocyte predominance.

Differential Diagnosis

Other conditions with which this may be confused include Wegener's granulomatosis, histiocytosis X, non-Hodgkin's lymphoma, and un-differentiated carcinoma.

Treatment and Prognosis

Without treatment this condition is invariably fatal. Treatment is similar to T-cell lymphomas elsewhere—radiation therapy. Typically, at least 4500 cGy are given. Prognosis depends on the stage at diagnosis and treatment. If the disease is localized, radiation treatment may give 50% 5-year survival. Higher stages are in general rapidly fatal.

RHABDOMYOSARCOMA

Definition

Rhabdomyosarcomas are malignant tumors of skeletal muscle origin. They are the most common soft tissue sarcomas of children and occur most frequently in the head and neck.

Clinical Presentation

Rhabdomyosarcomas occur most commonly in the first decade but may also be seen in teenage and young adult patients. These tumors most commonly present as painless infiltrating masses that may exhibit a rapid increase in size. Other symptoms are related to the site of origin and include nasal obstruction, epistaxis, pain, refractory otitis media, otorrhea, temporofacial swelling or deformity, and neurologic deficits. There are no known associated etiologic factors.

SPECIAL CONSIDERATION

If an embryonal rhabdomyosarcoma arises within a cavity such as the nasopharynx it may demonstrate a distinctive growth pattern with an exophytic, polypoid appearance called *botryoid* (or grape-like).

Pathology

There are four histologic variants of rhabdomyosarcoma described:

Embryonal—the most common head and neck type; resembles various stages of the embryogenesis of skeletal muscle. Cross-striations are rarely seen.

Alveolar—aggregates of poorly differentiated round to oval cells separated by fibrous septa

Pleomorphic—least common histologic variant; predominantly occurs in adults; composed of spindle-shaped cells admixed with large, pleomorphic cells

Mixed—composed of two or more histologic types

Differential Diagnosis

Physically, rhabdomyosarcomas may be confused with nasal polyps, aural polyps, or other soft tissue tumors. Histologically, they may be confused with neuroblastomas, Ewing's sarcoma, malignant lymphoma, undifferentiated or poorly differentiated carcinoma, or any small round cell neoplasm.

Treatment and Prognosis

Prior to 1960, the prognosis for a patient with rhabdomyosarcoma was extremely poor, with more than 90% of patients dying. With multimodality therapy, including nonradical surgery, radiotherapy, plus multigene chemotherapy, the outlook for these patients has improved dramatically. For stage I disease the 5-year survival is over 80%. However, for stage IV disease the survival is less than 20%.

FIBROSARCOMA

Definition

Fibrosarcoma is a malignant tumor of fibroblasts.

Clinical Presentation

The most common site of occurrence for fibrosarcomas is the lower extremity. Only 10 to 15% of fibrosarcomas occur in the head and neck. Both sexes are affected equally. The most common head and neck sites are the paranasal sinuses, larynx, and neck. Symptoms vary with site and include nasal obstruction, epistaxis, pain, and dysphagia.

Pathology

These tumors show fasciculated growth patterns with spindle-shaped cells that have scanty cytoplasm and indistinct borders.

Differential Diagnosis

There are a number of entities that may be confused with fibrosarcoma: nodular fasciitis, fibromatosis, spindly cell carcinoma, malignant schwannoma, and spindle cell melanoma.

Treatment and Prognosis

Fibrosarcomas are generally not considered to be radiosensitive, and thus surgical excision with wide margins is considered the treatment of choice. Adjunctive radiotherapy may offer some benefit, but there is no conclusive evidence that it improves survival. At present, the efficacy of chemotherapy for soft tissue fibrosarcomas of the head and neck is not well established.

Lymph node metastasis is relatively rare and radical neck dissections are generally not felt to be necessary. If metastatic disease does occur, it is primarily to lung and bone. Recurrences are generally within 1 year but may recur many years following resection. Important prognostic features are tumor size, location, and histologic grade based on mitoses. Five-year survival varies with the histologic grade of the tumor, with grade I tumors having an 80% 5-year survival and grade IV a 25% 5-year survival.

OSTEOSARCOMA

Definition

Osteosarcoma is a malignant tumor of bone origin.

Clinical Presentation

Osteosarcomas are the most common type of primary malignant bone tumor. The distal femur and proximal tibia are the most frequent sites for this tumor; 6% of osteosarcomas occur in the head and neck. The most common sites of head and neck involvement are the mandible (in descending order, body, symphysis, angle, and ramus), maxilla, paranasal sinuses, and skull. Swelling and pain are the most common symptoms. Loosening of teeth, numbness, and nasal obstruction may be reported. Radiologically a number of findings may be noted, ranging from dense sclerosis to a mixed sclerotic and radiolucent lesion.

> **PEARL•••** A pathognomonic finding is that of a "sunburst" pattern created by formation of new spicules of bone within the tumor.

Pathology

Osteosarcomas display a sarcomatous stroma with the production of osteoid. Osteoid is the precursor to bone and appears as amorphous eosin staining material.

Differential Diagnosis

These tumors may be confused with benign lesions such as fracture callus, myositis ossificans, fibrous dysplasia, and aneurysmal bone cyst. They may be confused with several malignant lesions such as chondrosarcoma and fibrosarcoma.

Treatment and Prognosis

Complete surgical excision with postoperative radiation and adjuvant chemotherapy is generally recommended for osteosarcomas. Despite this, the prognosis remains relatively poor with a 30 to 50% 5-year survival.

SUGGESTED READINGS

Brodish BN, Morgan CE, Sillers MJ. Endoscopic resection of fibro-osseous lesions of the paranasal sinuses. *Am J Rhinol* 1999;13(2): 111–116.

Neville BW, Damm DD, Allen CM, Bouquot JE. Soft tissue tumors. In: Neville BW, Damm DD, Allen CM, Bouquot JE, eds. *Oral and Maxillofacial Pathology.* Vol 1. 1st ed. Philadelphia: WB Saunders; 1995:362–414.

Waldon CA. Bone pathology. In: Neville BW, Damm DD, Allen CM, Bouquot JE, eds. *Oral and Maxillofacial Pathology.* Vol. 1. 1st ed. Philadelphia: WB Saunders; 1995:443–492.

Chapter 69

TRAUMA

Andrew C. Campbell and Kevin A. Shumrick

Symptoms resulting from facial trauma are determined by the location and severity of the trauma inflicted. Symptoms of facial trauma range from those produced by simple abrasions to life-threatening airway obstruction or hemorrhage.

CLINICAL HISTORY

When evaluating a patient with facial trauma it is important to obtain as accurate and complete a history as possible regarding the traumatic event and subsequent course. Optimally, this should come from the patient. If the patient is not capable of supplying accurate information secondary to intoxication or altered mental status, then an attempt should be made to interview anyone else who may be familiar with the specifics of the case.

The *history of a traumatic event* should answer the following questions:

What was the mechanism of injury?

Was the patient mobile, restrained, or stationary?

Was the impacting object mobile or stationary?

Was the injury the result of blunt or penetrating trauma, or both?

Was the degree of energy transfer high or low?

Were there coincident fatalities?

Are there associated thermal or chemical injuries?

REVIEW OF SYSTEMS

As a general rule, one should never assume an isolated injury exists until all other systems have been cleared such as orthopedic, gastrointestinal, chest, etc. Specifically, the treating physician should screen the patient for potentially life-threatening symptoms distant from the head and neck:

Is chest pain present (this may be the only symptom of a subacute aortic transection)?

Does it hurt to breathe (a prominent symptom of rib fractures)?

Is the patient experiencing dyspnea or shortness of breath (indicating possible pneumothorax or hemothorax)?

Are abdominal symptoms such as cramping, pain, or nausea present?

Are extremity symptoms present, such as pain on motion, numbness, weakness, or paralysis?

Neurologic Symptoms

Of specific concern to physicians managing patients with facial trauma is the possibility of associated neurologic injuries. Before eliciting symptoms confined to the head and neck (extracranial), the examining physician should perform a screening neurologic trauma history. This should inlude, but not be limited to, the following issues:

> Was there a loss of consciousness? Was it witnessed?
>
> Has amnesia—anterograde vs. retrograde—been documented?
>
> Has there been a lucid interval bracketed by decreased levels of consciousness?
>
> Is there a documented change in the senses of vision, smell, or hearing?
>
> Is there a sensory, movement, or speech deficit?

Upper Aerodigestive Symptoms

After symptoms of neurologic injuries have been ruled out, the treating physician should address specific symptoms related to head and neck trauma. The symptoms indicative of a significant upper aerodigestive tract injury include dyspnea, cough, hemoptysis, drooling, dysphagia, and odynophagia. It should also be noted that an occult esophageal injury may produce constitutional ills such as fever, chills, and chest pain as the result of an evolving mediastinitis.

General Symptoms of Maxillofacial Soft Tissue and Bony Injuries

Injury to the facial soft tissue and bones often produces symptom constellations that can be conceptually organized according to four anatomic structures: the orbits and visual axis, nasal airway, dental occlusion, and the distributed neurovascular support. Patients will rarely be able to volunteer specific symptoms but note should be made of visual disturbance such as blurred vision or double vision. Additionally disturbances of dental occlusion are often noted by patients and they will frequently volunteer this observation. Nasal airway obstruction is also often noted. A thorough discussion of injury-specific symptoms is reserved for the relevant sections later in this section.

Physical Examination and Management

Facial injuries tend not to be life threatening. However, the clinician must be mindful of associated injuries and never assume an injury is isolated until all appropriate systems have been cleared.

Primary Survey and Cardiorespiratory Resuscitation

Initial cardiorespiratory stabilization is managed per established resuscitation protocols. This primary survey and emergent management is followed by a neurologic trauma assessment.

Neurologic Assessment

Associated intracranial injuries are the most common cause of death for head and neck trauma patients. Teasdale and Jennett (1974) described the Glasgow Coma Scale in an attempt to quantify a patient's mental status and establish an initial reference point against which future changes could be compared (Table 69–1). The scale uses three parameters: eye opening, best motor response, and best verbal response. With severe head injury the scale usually reads between 0 and 8; moderate head injury, 9 to 12; and with mild injury, 13 to 15. This scoring system permits cautious prognostication of expected outcome.

SPECIAL CONSIDERATION

An assessment and documentation of the level of consciousness (LOC), using the Glasgow Coma Scale (GCS), should be noted on the initial exam of every patient with more than minor trauma.

TABLE 69–1 GLASGOW COMA SCALE

Eye opening
    4—Opens eyes spontaneously
    3—Opens eyes to voice
    2—Opens eyes to pain
    1—No eye opening
Best motor response
    6—Obeys commands
    5—Localizes to pain
    4—Withdraws to pain
    3—Abnormal flexor response
    2—Abnormal extensor response
    1—No movement
Best verbal response
    5—Appropriate and oriented
    4—Confused conversation
    3—Inappropriate words
    2—Incomprehensible sounds
    1—No sounds

Source: Teasdale G, Jennett B. Assessment of coma and impaired consciousness. A practical scale. *Lancet* 1974;2: 81–84. Reprinted by permission of the publishers.

Early, frequent, and accurate documentation may flag the progressive and often subtle deterioration of mental status that accompanies intracranial bleeding. If no initial reference point is documented, the mental decline of a patient may not be appreciated by medical staff as the patient is processed through the emergency room system.

UPPER AERODIGESTIVE ASSESSMENT

After initial stabilization and neurologic assessment, the remainder of the secondary survey is completed including a thorough evaluation of the head and neck. Following neurologic injury, the second major cause of death in head and neck trauma patients is airway obstruction. Trauma severe enough to involve the airway is usually the result of a high-speed deceleration mechanism. Airway embarrassment may be acute or insidious in onset. Acute airway obstruction is addressed during the initial stabilization.

PEARL... If a patient with slowly evolving airway compromise is misdiagnosed or mistreated, this, too, may prove fatal. Therefore, patients with significant facial or neck trauma should have their laryngotracheal anatomy assessed thoroughly.

Valuable information regarding airway status may be gained from careful observation of the patient. Which position does the patient assume to facilitate respiration? Can the patient lie flat or must he or she sit up? Respiratory distress and/or stridor are serious signs that may not be present initially but develop as edema and/or hematoma progress. If present, these signs suggest moderately severe airway trauma and are indicative of a 60 to 70% compromise in the airway diameter. Such patients should never be left unattended, and plans should be made to secure the airway expeditiously. Hemoptysis, too, is present only in moderately severe injuries.

Examination of the oral cavity and oral pharynx should be undertaken to determine whether the following potential upper airway insults are present:

1. Blood, loose teeth, dentures, or foreign body
2. Edema of tongue, soft palate, or pharyngeal walls
3. Stable or expanding hematoma of pharyngeal walls
4. Disrupted integrity of mandibular arch with tongue prolapse

If there is concern over the possibility of an injury to the larynx, then the most reliable and accurate exam is with a flexible nasopharyngoscope looking for:

1. Presence of ecchymosis, edema, or expanding hematomas
2. Mucosal lacerations, hemorrhage, and exposed cartilage
3. Position and motion of the vocal cords
4. Position and motions of the arytenoids

The other essential component of the upper aerodigestive tract is the hypopharynx and esophageal conduit. Hematomas usually indicate a fracture of the hyoid or esophageal contusion. On occasion, an actual laceration of the mucosa of the hypopharynx or esophagus may be present. In advanced aerodigestive injuries, imaging studies (usually a contrast swallow), in conjunction with formal bronchoscopy and esophagoscopy, should document the exact nature of the insult and set the stage for definitive repair.

ASSESSMENT AND TREATMENT OF NASAL AND MAXILLOFACIAL INJURIES

After possible life-threatening situations or serious aerodigestive injuries have been ruled out, the physician may turn to the maxillofacial injuries. Maxillofacial injuries are very common. Consequently, in what follows, a point has been made to supplement general assessment of these injuries with some practical treatment guidelines. Classically, these injuries have been divided into soft tissue disruptions and bony fracture-dislocations.

There are a number of possible types of soft tissue injuries, including contusions and avulsions, but the most common soft tissue injuries are lacerations. Lacerations may range from simple, superficial wounds, easily repaired, to injuries that penetrate to involve deeper structures including muscles, nerves, and ducts. Major lacerations, improperly treated, can leave dysfunctional and deforming sequelae.

> **PEARL•••** The single most important factor in managing any injury is proper initial evaluation and assessment, so that relevant concerns are identified and a comprehensive treatment plan formulated.

Chart documentation is an integral part of medical care for both medical follow-up and medicolegal concerns. The following specifics of soft tissue injury should be noted and documented:

1. *Laceration shape:* Is the wound a straight laceration with clean margins? If so, it can probably be closed primarily with an acceptable result. Is the wound stellate with multiple trifurcations? It should be noted if the wound margins are very irregular or have adjacent devitalized tissue, as this may have implications for treatment and outcome. Although a simple clean laceration may be repaired primarily, a complicated wound with devitalized tissue may require resources not available in the emergency room.

2. *Surrounding soft tissue injury–associated contusion:* Contusions often result in a very irregular disruption of the skin with surrounding devitalized tissue. These wounds should be documented and managed conservatively. The patient should be informed that these injuries often result in depressed scars, which benefit from scar revision when mature.

3. *Loss of soft tissue coverage and/or lining:* Fortunately, actual loss of soft tissue is uncommon, but when it occurs it has significant implications for wound management and eventual outcome. These injuries should be carefully documented and the patient informed accordingly.

4. *Injury to structural margins or borders:* Soft tissue injuries involving the eyelid, nasal alar rims, auricular helical rims, and the oral stoma must be carefully examined and noted. Full-thickness injuries involving these structures have significant cosmetic and functional implications. The specifics of repairing these structures are discussed in Chapter 70.

5. *Penetrating soft tissue injuries:* Penetrating wounds are dangerous because although the exterior entrance point may seem relatively benign, the possibility of deeper structures being involved must be considered, and a thorough physical examination should be performed to rule out the possibility of injury to a significant structure such as a branch of

the facial nerve, the parotid duct, or the lacrimal apparatus. Timely identification of such an injury is important because delay in repairing these structures can significantly decrease the chances of a successful outcome.

Management of Facial Fractures

Facial fractures are a common finding in patients suffering facial trauma and can range from a simple closed nasal fracture to a panfacial injury where virtually every bone in the face is fractured. The type of trauma will often dictate the nature of the facial fracture. A single isolated blow (as from a fist) will usually result in an isolated discrete fracture, whereas a high-speed motor vehicle accident causes widespread comminution of the facial bones. A detailed description of management for each type of facial fracture is beyond the scope of this chapter; however, the application of the general principles set forth herein will permit the treating surgeon to assess a patient, order a radiologic workup, and formulate a general treatment plan regarding fractures of the midface and nose. Mandibular fractures are an extensive topic in their own right and the reader is referred to Chapter 19 as well as standard texts on this subject.

General Features of Nasal Fractures

Due to the fact that the nose is the most prominent facial feature, it is often involved in traumatic events. Not only are the nasal bones the most commonly fractured facial bones, they are the most commonly fractured bones of the body. The nasal bones are thin laterally and thicken centrally and superiorly. Additionally, they have relatively weak attachments to the frontal bone and maxilla.

The type of nasal fracture is determined mainly by the direction of the traumatic force. With mild, lateral nasal trauma, just the ipsilateral nasal bone fractures, moving medially by fracturing at the transition of thin to thick bone and at the suture with the ipsilateral maxilla and contralateral nasal bone. The deformity resulting from just an isolated nasal bone fracture consists of depression of the ipsilateral nasal wall. With more substantial trauma the ipsilateral nasal bone (which is fractured) pushes the contralateral nasal bone laterally. This gives rise to the C-shaped deformity of the nose commonly associated with nasal trauma. Note that the nose has greater resistance to fracturing from frontal trauma than lateral trauma due to the midline support of the septum. However, when fractures from frontal trauma do occur, they tend to splay the nasal bones laterally with buckling of the underlying nasal septum.

With more substantial nasal trauma, the maxilla may become involved, with fractures of the ascending maxilla as well as the medial orbital rims. However, these are no longer isolated nasal fractures and are now moving into the realm of nasoethmoidal fractures.

SPECIAL CONSIDERATION

A common, and often overlooked, coincident injury with nasal fractures is avulsion of the ipsilateral upper lateral cartilage from the nasal bone.

This will leave a residual depression of the side of the nose even after reduction of the fracture. For complete correction, cartilage grafting may be required. An additional injury that may be overlooked is a fracture of the septum, which may be associated with a septal hematoma. It is important to rule out a coincident septal hematoma because, if left untreated, the hematoma may result in pressure necrosis of the septal cartilage with an eventual saddle-nose deformity.

General Features of Zygomatic Complex Fractures

A separate category of midface fractures is the so-called zygoma fracture or tripod fracture. Both these terms are in popular usage and are inaccurate. They are probably best avoided for the following reasons. First, the zygoma itself rarely actually fractures. Instead, the fractures occur at the articulation of the zygoma with its surrounding bones. Second, because the zygoma articulates with four bones (the sphenoid, temporal bone, frontal bone, and maxilla), not three, the term *tripod fracture* is inaccurate. Several authors have suggested that the term *zygomatic complex fracture* (ZCF) be adopted as a substitute. The difficulty with this term comes when one is trying to describe such a fracture. Nonetheless, it appears that the term is becoming popular, and it is a more accurate description of the condition than previous terminology.

Although the most commonly fractured facial bones are the nasal bones, ZCFs are the next most frequent (excluding mandibles). Approximately 85% of all zygomatic fractures occur in males and 15% in females. Most ZCFs (80%) occur in patients between the ages of 18 and 45 years.

The history in a ZCF patient is usually one of laterally centered trauma without loss of consciousness. Common mechanisms include being punched or being struck by a baseball. Because the zygoma is a strong, dense bone, the traumatic force is transmitted throughout the entire bone and the fractures occur at the weakest points, which happen to be at the sutures of the zygoma's articulations. Thus, with a ZCF the entire zygoma is displaced in a direction determined by the vector of the traumatic force.

A history of unilateral epistaxis is not uncommon. Epistaxis results from the zygoma rotating medially into the maxillary sinus with bleeding from the sinus mucosa. Because the medial portion of the fracture passes through or very close to the infraorbital foramen, ipsilateral upper lip numbness is very common.

By definition a ZCF involves a portion of the lateral orbital rim and floor. This orbital involvement can have several features that may be apparent on physical examination. A very common finding is inferior displacement of the lateral canthus due to the fact that the lateral canthal tendon attaches to the lateral orbital rim (which is the superior extension of the zygoma) and is pulled inferiorly with the rest of the zygoma. Additionally, the orbital floor component of the fracture may cause enophthalmos, exophthalmos, or diplopia secondary to orbital content entrapment, most commonly the inferior rectus muscle in the fracture line. Trismus due to the temporalis muscle being trapped between the body of the zygoma laterally and the coronoid

process medially is also a common finding. Many of these physical findings may be obscured by edema and by pain that limits patient cooperation. Precise assessment of the fracture and treatment planning, therefore, require coronal and axial computed tomography (CT) images.

There have been several attempts to classify ZCFs based on the amount and direction of the zygoma's displacement, in the hope that this would help direct treatment. For the most part we have not found these classifications helpful. Instead, the recommended approach emphasizes accurate clinical and radiologic assessment with determination of the type and degree of fracture dislocation prior to surgically attempting anatomic reduction. With an accurate understanding of each individual fracture, the surgeon may focus on the key components of the fracture and tailor the surgical reduction and fixation to address the major areas of concern.

SPECIAL CONSIDERATION

Over the last decade it has become increasingly apparent that the key structure that needs to be accurately realigned in virtually every ZCF fracture (except for isolated arch fractures) is the zygomaticomaxillary buttress.

It is this buttress that determines the position of the body of the zygoma, which, in turn, determines the position of the malar eminence. The most common type of ZCF fracture is a simple rotation of the body of the zygoma into the maxillary sinus, with minimal displacement of the zygomaticofrontal suture; additionally, the orbital floor and rim are displaced but not comminuted.

A separate type of zygoma fracture is the zygomatic arch fracture. Arch fractures result from direct, lateral trauma, which causes a buckling of the midportion of the zygomatic arch, leaving a depressed central segment. In an isolated arch fracture the remaining anterior zygoma is not disturbed, so that all physical findings and symptoms are located laterally. The major physical finding is an externally visible depression overlying the arch, and the major symptom is trismus secondary to impingement of the fracture segments on the temporalis muscle and coronoid process of the mandible.

General Features of LeFort Fractures

To understand midface fractures, it is helpful to consider the organization of the facial skeleton. Basically, the facial skeleton consists of multiple cavities filled with either air (nose and paranasal sinuses) or soft tissue (orbits). These cavities are surrounded, for the most part, by thin cortical bones that are connected to each other and the skull by a series of thicker bones referred to as buttresses. Several teleologic explanations have been offered for this arrangement of facial bones. First, it allows the skull to be significantly lighter than if the face were composed of solid bone. Second, the arrangement of air-filled spaces with intersecting struts of thicker bone allows the midface to act as a shock absorber for the cranium. With significant trauma the facial skeleton crumples, much as a car bumper would, absorbing the kinetic energy of the traumatic event and sparing the more critical central nervous system. Given this arrangement of struts of strong bone juxtaposed to thin bone, facial fractures tend to occur along predictable patterns. Renee LeFort first described the patterns of midface fractures when he subjected cadavers to various blows to the face and then dissected off the soft tissue. He discovered that midface fractures tended to occur along lines that run perpendicular to the buttresses of the midface. LeFort noted that there were three common fracture patterns, and these fractures have been named after him based on their level of the midface.

> **PEARL...** A common feature of all true LeFort fractures is that they pass through the pterygoid plates and disrupt the position of the maxilla resulting in malocclusion.

The LeFort I (Guerin type) pattern consists of a fracture across the lower nasal septum, the lower portion of the piriform apertures, the canine fossae, and the two zygomaticomaxillary

buttresses. The fracture then passes above the maxillary tuberosity to and through the pterygoid plates. The LeFort II (pyramidal type) fracture starts at the nasofrontal junction and then passes across the medial orbits and medial orbital rim. It then passes laterally through the zygomatico-maxillary buttresses and posteriorly through the posterior wall of the maxillary sinus and then through the pterygoid plates. The LeFort III (also called craniofacial separation), basically separates the facial bones from the skull with the skull base as the line of separation. The fracture starts medially at the nasofrontal suture, and extends across the orbit at the medial wall, floor, and lateral wall. It continues through the zygomatic-frontal suture and across the zygomatic arch. More posteriorly the fracture line extends across the back of the maxilla and through the pterygoid plates.

Note that this separation of midface fractures into pure LeFort I, II, and III fractures is somewhat artificial because panfacial injuries often produce a combination of LeFort fracture patterns.

Physical Examination for Signs of Facial Fractures

Following the general exam for facial trauma, the patient should be examined specifically for the possibility of a facial fracture keeping the following specific points in mind.

General Appearance

A considerable amount of force is generally required to cause a fracture of a facial bone, and there is almost always associated edema and ecchymosis. This edema may make it difficult to appreciate changes in facial contour secondary to a facial fracture. Often, palpation is a more accurate means of assessing the underlying skeleton. The most important points of palpation are along the inferior and lateral orbital rims plus the zygomatic arches. Note should be made of tenderness, crepitance, and, most importantly, any step-offs or discontinuity.

Ocular Status

Considerable information regarding the presence of midface fractures may be gained by examining the eyes. The initial concern when considering a possible periorbital fracture should be to rule out injury to the globe or optic nerve. At the very least, a visual acuity and pupillary response to light should be obtained and recorded. It is also important to note a possible hyphema and to perform a fundal exam to look for occult papilledema. Assessment of the globes should include noting their position and movement:

> Are they positioned at the same height?
>
> Is there evidence of enophthalmos or exophthalmos?
>
> Are the extraocular movements present and full?
>
> Is there evidence of entrapment?

Entrapment occurs when the orbital floor is fractured and orbital contents (fat and ocular muscles) are pushed into the fracture line. If just orbital fat is caught, then the major symptom is enophthalmos secondary to loss of orbital volume. However, if the fracture impinges upon an ocular muscle, then the globe will have a decreased range of motion. The most commonly entrapped muscle is the inferior rectus (by virtue of the fact that it is closest to the floor). However, the medial rectus may also be entrapped with medial wall fractures. In cases of ocular muscle entrapment (inferior rectus), the eye will be positioned slightly more inferiorly than the contralateral eye, but with a straight-ahead gaze there will be no diplopia because the contralateral eye will focus on what the entrapped eye is focusing on. Symptoms arise when the patient tries to look around without moving the head. The entrapped muscle restricts the range of motion of the affected eye and causes diplopia. The diplopia is most prominent on upward gaze. It is important to perform forced duction testing to distinguish true entrapment of orbital contents causing diplopia from diplopia secondary to muscle dysfunction from edema or nerve injury.

Nasal Airway Status

An intranasal examination should be performed on all midface trauma patients. The nasal airway should be carefully assessed bilaterally. Is there bony or cartilaginous fracture-dislocation causing nasal obstruction? Is there a septal hematoma? If so, this must be drained in a timely fashion.

Dental Status

An almost universal consequence of both mandibular and LeFort fractures is some disruption or alteration of occlusion. Patients should be questioned about how their teeth are fitting together and asked to compare this fit with their pretrauma status. Additionally, patients should be questioned about prior dental history and if there were known occlusal abnormalities such as overbites, cross-bites, etc. If a question arises regarding a change in occlusion, it can be very helpful to obtain pretrauma dental records.

Facial Sensation

Several branches of the trigeminal nerve gain access to the facial soft tissues by exiting the facial skeleton through canals and foramina. Note that the supraorbital, infraorbital, and mental nerves penetrate the facial skeleton in approximately the same sagittal plane bilaterally.

SPECIAL CONSIDERATION

A diagnostic test of muscle entrapment is the forced duction test, which is performed by grasping the insertion of the inferior rectus muscle on the sclera with fine forceps and comparing the ease of moving the globes through a range of motion. The entrapped globe will have a restricted range of motion.

PEARL... A classic finding for LeFort fractures is the so-called open bite, which results from the teeth-bearing maxillary segment being pushed posteriorly and inferiorly. This results in retruded maxillary teeth (class III), with the maxillary molars striking the mandibular molars early and causing the open bite.

Thus, fractures of the orbital floor and zygoma commonly present with numbness of the ipsilateral upper lip, and mandibular fractures at the symphysis or body frequently have ipsilateral lower lip numbness. Any deficit of sensation of either the upper or lower lip should be clearly noted in the preoperative documentation to distinguish it from a possible operative complication.

Radiologic Evaluation of Facial Fractures

Following a thorough history and physical exam, an attempt should be made to document a fracture and delineate its extent. In the past, plain films of the face were used for evaluating facial fractures. However, plain films rarely give the detailed information needed to manage these patients without operative exploration of the various fracture sites. A good example of this is with the ZCF, where it is known that, by definition, a fracture will involve the orbital floor. Unfortunately, conventional X rays (even tomograms) give little accurate data regarding the orbital floor. Consequently, it has become standard practice, as mentioned earlier, to use coronal and axial CT scans of the facial bones. Optimally, these images should be separated by a maximum of 1.5-cm intervals for sufficient resolution.

Although their role has diminished, plain films have not been completely abandoned. They may be used to document a nasal fracture or demonstrate an isolated zygomatic arch fracture. These specific injuries are largely assessed clinically, however, with little emphasis on radiograms for operative management.

For assessing the status of the mandible, a Panorex or panoramic technique gives the best visualization of the entire mandible.

Management of Facial Fractures

The two major concerns associated with the management of facial fractures are function and cosmesis. The three major functional considerations are ocular function, nasal airway function, and occlusion/mastication. With regard to cosmesis, the external facial features are heavily dependent on the underlying bony structure and position. Even minor shifts of the nasal bones can dramatically alter an individual's appearance and nasal functioning. Similarly, if the orbital component of a zygomatic fracture is inadequately reduced, it may result not only in cosmetically apparent enophthalmos but also in functionally significant diplopia. Therefore, the dual issues of cosmesis and function actually go hand in hand, and, if the fracture is accurately repaired, the result should be satisfactory on both counts.

To achieve the most accurate possible repair of a facial fracture requires a precise and comprehensive diagnosis of the fracture's extent. To accurately diagnose most facial fractures requires the use of high-resolution coronal and axial CT scans as mentioned earlier. Simple nasal fractures can usually be assessed with an accurate physical exam and plain films of the nasal bones.

Once the site and extent of the fracture(s) have been determined, a method of fracture reduction and fixation of the fractured segments must be chosen. Previously, the management of facial fractures involved a balancing act in which the surgeon attempted to make the smallest possible external incision to expose the fracture site, yet at the same time had to ensure that the incision was long enough to provide adequate exposure for fracture reduction and fixation. Once the fracture was exposed by the limited external incision, it was reduced by approximating the two ends of the bone visible in the incision and stabilizing it with interfragment wires.

Significant improvement in the management of facial fractures has resulted from two new developments: (1) the introduction of plates and screws, which provide rigid internal fixation of fractures; and (2) the development of extended access/internal approaches to the facial skeleton, which are performed with internal or camouflaged incisions that provide maximum exposure of the facial skeleton while minimizing external scars. These extended access approaches are performed in a subperiosteal plane and are under muscles, nerves, and blood vessels, thereby avoiding these possible sites of morbidity.

Rigid Fixation of Facial Fractures

For most of the 19th century, facial fractures were stabilized with interfragmentary wiring, which provides support to a fracture but is not truly rigid for several reasons. First, the wire only contacts that portion of the drill hole closest to the fracture leaving the remaining 350 degrees or more without support. This allows the fracture to pivot around the wire. Moreover, interfragment wires do not provide support beyond the two drill holes on either side of the fracture. The recently introduced plating systems provide substantially greater stability than interfragment wiring, and this improved stability or fixation has been referred to as "rigid" fixation. Because the plates are placed underneath the facial soft tissues, this method of fixation has been termed "internal." Hence the term *rigid internal fixation* is applied to the use of plates and screws to distinguish it from other methods of fracture fixation (e.g., wires, external pins, splints, etc.).

The introduction of plates and screws to provide rigid internal fixation of facial fractures has been a significant advance over the use of simple interfragment wiring. Modern-day plates and screws also provide a means of spanning or bridging areas of bony loss or comminution. Note that the screw contacts 360 degrees of the drill hole and it consequently provides a much stronger grip than a wire, which contacts only a small portion of the drill hole.

The first plates used for rigid internal fixation of the facial skeleton were mandibular plates made of stainless steel with screw diameters of 2.7 mm and combined plate-screw profiles approaching 3.0 mm. Since that time, there has been steady advancement in the engineering of plates with the introduction of superior metals, such as titanium and Vitallium, and the progressive miniaturization of the systems such that there are now microplating systems with profiles and screw diameters of less than 1 mm. Complications were relatively common with the initial mandibular plating systems probably due to the fact that they were made of stainless steel and that many surgeons were relatively inexperienced with their application. However, with improvement in the design of plating systems and the routine teaching of plating techniques in surgical residencies, the incidence of complications has steadily decreased.

Closed Reduction of Nasal Fractures

As mentioned, the majority of nasal fractures consist of shifting the nasal pyramid to the side opposite the trauma force. Repositioning the nasal bones can often be accomplished through a closed reduction by elevating the depressed ipsilateral nasal bone and moving the contralateral nasal bone back to the midline. To accomplish this, a blunt elevator is inserted under the depressed nasal bone to elevate it, and digital pressure is placed on the out-fractured bone to move it medially.

> **PEARL...** Many surgeons feel that a closed reduction of a nasal fracture is most expediently accomplished in conjunction with some form of general anesthetic.

> **PITFALL...** Attempts at closed reduction with regional anesthesia are often disappointing for the surgeon and quite painful for the patient.

A key point is to thoroughly decongest the nasal mucosa, particularly at the superior nasal vault. After suitable anesthesia and decongestion have been achieved, a blunt elevator is placed into the nasal cavity on the depressed side of the fracture. Two points regarding placement of this elevator are critical to the success of a closed reduction. First, the tip of the elevator must not be placed any further internally than the posterior edge of the fracture.

PITFALL••• A common mistake is to place the tip of the elevator under solid bone, which not only restricts the ability to perform the closed reduction but also causes bleeding.

The second crucial point to be made regarding placement of the elevator is that it must be positioned as superiorly in the nasal vault as possible. Failure to position the elevator at the apex of the nasal vault will cause it to impact the middle turbinate, resulting in an ineffective reduction and troublesome bleeding.

Once the elevator is in place, the surgeon (standing on the contralateral side of the fracture) wraps the fingers of the most superior hand around the patient's forehead (to provide countertraction) and places the thumb over the laterally displaced nasal bone. The inferior hand grasps the elevator with the thumb on the medial side. The fracture is then reduced with a simultaneous motion of pushing the elevated bone medially (with the thumb) and the depressed bone laterally (with the elevator). Often there is a distinct click, signifying a successful reduction. If the elevated nasal bone does not feel stable, the nose can be packed for several days. Externally, the nose is taped and a loose metal splint applied.

Zygomatic Complex Fractures

The treatment of zygomatic complex fractures is determined by the degree of rotation and displacement of the fracture and whether or not there is significant orbital involvement. For a simple rotated zygomatic complex fracture, a sublabial approach with realignment and fixation of the zygomaticomaxillary buttress is all that is required. If the orbital rim is comminuted or the orbital floor needs to be addressed, then a tarsoconjunctival approach is employed with rim realignment and, if necessary, orbital floor augmentation. If there is severe displacement of the arch or body of the zygoma, then a hemicoronal approach is used to expose the arch and lateral orbital rim in conjunction with a transconjunctival and sublabial approach for the other fractured sites.

For isolated zygomatic arch fractures, an attempt at closed reduction is first made. A closed reduction may be accomplished through either a temporal approach (Gilles) or a sublabial approach. In each case an elevator is placed medial to the arch, and it is elevated with a firm lateral motion. If the elevated arch appears stable, the procedure is terminated. However, if the reduction is incomplete or unstable, then the arch is approached through a hemi-coronal incision and the arch rigidly fixated with 1.00-mm or 1.3-mm plates.

LeFort Fractures

LeFort fractures are complex injuries that can result in severe cosmetic and functional sequelae if improperly managed, and it is the surgeon's responsibility to be properly trained in their management. Although this chapter is not intended to provide a complete overview of midface trauma management, the following are some of the major points to consider.

The single most important step in managing midface trauma is an accurate assessment of the fracture's extent so that proper preoperative planning may be accomplished. An accurate assessment requires a careful physical exam and radiologic survey (coronal and axial CT scans). Once the fractures are identified, an operative plan is formulated to expose the area of concern using the appropriate extended access approach. The fracture is then accurately reduced and rigidly fixated.

As mentioned, by definition any true LeFort fracture will disturb the occlusal relationships. Therefore, the first step in repair of a LeFort fracture is to place arch bars on the teeth, reestablish the occlusion, and place intermaxillary fixation wires to maintain the occlusion. Once the occlusion is reestablished, attention is turned to exposing, reducing, and fixating the involved facial buttresses as follows:

LeFort I: The major buttresses disrupted are the zygomaticomaxillary and, to a lesser extent, the nasomaxillary buttresses running along the piriform aperture. These buttresses are approached through bilateral sublabial incisions exposing virtually the entire maxilla. The buttresses are then rigidly fixated with 1.5- or 2.0-mm-diameter plates and screws.

LeFort II: A LeFort II fracture passes across the nasal bridge and medial orbital rims before crossing the zygomatic (ZM) buttresses and extending through the pterygoid plates. In most instances the nasal and medial orbital rim components can be reduced with a closed technique, and the ZM buttresses managed similarly to the LeFort I.

LeFort III: A LeFort III implies significant trauma affecting virtually all the major bones of the midface. In a complicated case such as this, it is preferable to initially expose all the fractures and then sequentially reduce and fixate them, moving from areas of stability to less stable areas. A decision as to whether or not an orbital approach and repair will be required is made separately for each orbit, based on preoperative physical exam and X-ray information. A typical reduction for a LeFort III would involve a coronal approach for exposure of the zygomatic arches, Z-frontal suture, and nasofrontal suture; a transconjunctival approach for one or both orbital rims and floors; and bilateral sublabial approaches for exposure of the maxilla. In addition, 1.5- and 2.0-mm plates are used for the maxilla and lower profile, and 1.0- or 1.3-mm plates are used in the upper facial skeleton.

For all LeFort fractures, if a successful reduction has been achieved with rigid internal fixation, then the intermaxillary fixation is released at the end of surgery. The patient is then kept on a soft diet for 3 weeks to avoid unduly stressing the fracture reduction.

SUGGESTED READINGS

Gruss JS. Complex maxillary fractures: role of buttress reconstruction and immediate bone grafts. *Plast Reconstr Surg* 1986;78:9–22.

Gruss JS. The importance of the zygomatic arch in complex midfacial fracture repair and correction of post traumatic orbitozygomatic deformities. *Plast Reconstr Surg* 1990;6:878–890.

LeFort R. Etude experimentale sur les fractures de la machoire inferieure, parts I, II, III. *Rev Chir Paris* 1901;23:208,360,479.

Raveh J, Vuillemin T, Ladrach K, Roux M, Sutter F. Plate osteosynthesis of 367 mandibular fractures: the unrestricted indication for intraoral approach. *J Craniomaxillofac Surg* 1987;15:244–253.

Shumrick K, Kersten R, Kulwin D, Sinha P, Smith T. Extended access/internal approaches for the management of facial trauma. *Arch Otolaryngol Head Neck Surg* 1992;118:1105–1112.

Teasdale G, Jennett B. Assessment of coma and impaired consciousness. A practical scale. *Lancet* 1974;2:81–84.

Zingg M, Chowdhury K, Ladrach K, et al. Treatment of 813 zygoma-lateral orbital complex fractures. *Arch Otolaryngol Head Neck Surg* 1991;117:611–620.

Chapter 70

SPECIAL CONSIDERATIONS IN MAXILLOFACIAL TRAUMA

Andrew C. Campbell and Kevin A. Shumrick

CLINICAL EVALUATION

In the initial evaluation of all facial trauma patients, but particularly those with penetrating trauma, it is important to assess the status of the facial nerve, the parotid duct, and the lacrimal apparatus and to look for the possibility of retained foreign bodies.

FACIAL NERVE

The status of the facial nerve and all its branches should be noted and recorded on the initial evaluation of all facial trauma patients. It is not uncommon for a facial nerve deficit to be noted in a delayed fashion. The question then arises as to whether the deficit occurred immediately (implying a severance of the nerve requiring repair or decompression) or later, secondary to tissue edema (implying a contusion of the nerve, which will recover spontaneously).

> **PITFALL•••** When using local anesthesia on a facial laceration, it may be noted that there is a facial nerve deficit. If the status of the nerve has not been established initially, it becomes unclear whether the palsy is secondary to initial injury, anesthesia-induced (transient), or iatrogenic.

It is important to establish early on if there has been a transection of the nerve or one of its branches because an early and accurate repair maximizes the chances of functional regeneration. Note also the fact that the distal portion of the nerve can be stimulated for up to 72 hours following injury. This greatly facilitates accurate identification of the distal end of the nerve for coaptation and repair.

PAROTID DUCT

Injury to the parotid (or Stensen's) duct should always be considered with any deep cheek laceration or penetrating injury. Although an injury or transection of the duct is relatively uncommon, the morbidity of an unrecognized, and unrepaired, ductal injury is high and can be avoided with timely surgical intervention. The parotid duct exits the parotid gland at approximately the posterior border of the masseter muscle and then travels across the lateral border of the masseter. At the anterior border of the masseter the duct turns medially and enters the oral cavity just lateral to the second upper molar.

> **PEARL•••** It should be remembered that the facial nerve lies just lateral to the duct and there is almost always an associated injury to the buccal branch of the facial nerve with any parotid duct injury.

The most common sign of a ductal injury is saliva draining from the wound. The most direct way to confirm a ductal injury is to cannulate the duct intraorally with a lacrimal probe and use the probe to check the integrity of the duct in the depths of the wound. If a laceration or transection is discovered, it should be repaired with fine nylon suture (8-0 or 9-0) using magnification. Some authors advocate leaving a Silastic stent in place for 7 to 10 days after repair.

> **PITFALL•••** If a ductal injury is unrecognized, the patient will return with a sialocele that is often infected. Repair of the duct after formation of a sialocele or fistula is very difficult because of the maceration and friability of the tissues. Treatment at this point usually consists of pressure dressings and anticholinergics to suppress saliva production, with the hope that the gland will atrophy or the ductal injury seal itself. If the fistula persists, a superficial parotidectomy may be required.

LACRIMAL APPARATUS

There should be a high index of suspicion for injury to the lacrimal drainage apparatus with any laceration involving the medial portion of the upper or lower eyelid in the region of the medial canthus. The major sequela of a lacrimal canalicular laceration is epiphora, but this may not be obvious in the acute setting due to associated pain and edema. If there is a question of a canalicular laceration or lacrimal duct laceration, the lacrimal punctum and duct should be cannulated with a lacrimal probe and the wound examined to see if the probe appear in the wound. If a ductal laceration is identified, it should be repaired over Silastic stents under magnification with fine (8-0) sutures.

RETAINED FOREIGN BODY

The treating physician should always consider the possibility of a retained foreign body in penetrating injuries involving glass or wood or resulting from striking the ground. Special mention should be made of the phenomenon of "debris tattooing," resulting from particulate matter being embedded in the dermis and not

appropriately removed. The epidermis will then heal over this retained material, which will be visible externally. Once this healing has occurred, the debris is virtually impossible to remove short of excising the affected area.

> ## SPECIAL CONSIDERATION
>
> It is important to identify wounds with the potential for debris tattooing because the optimum time to treat this condition is at the time of injury, when the epidermis is still open and the foreign material can be removed by scrubbing, irrigation, and/or dermabrasion.

REPAIR OF SUPERFICIAL SOFT TISSUE INJURIES

After ruling out injuries to associated deep structures, attention may be turned to repair of the superficial soft tissue injury. Generally speaking, the treating physician should always take the time to meticulously remove all foreign bodies from the wound. If the wound appears grossly contaminated, it should be irrigated with copious quantities of saline under mild pressure. With regard to debridement of tissue in acute wounds, conservative removal only of obviously devitalized tissue should be performed. The specific method of wound repair depends primarily on the laceration morphology and those other relevant factors noted during the prior wound evaluation.

In the following discussion, technical pointers are emphasized for the repair of a clean, simple laceration. Additional guidelines are provided for management of complicating factors and those cosmetically challenging injuries involving margins and borders.

When repairing a straightforward uncomplicated laceration, the aim should be to provide an anatomically accurate, secure repair. This is best accomplished with complete anesthesia, fine instruments, excellent lighting, and comfortable working conditions for the surgeon. Often these conditions are not met in the usual emergency room setting and the surgeon has a duty to the patient to ensure that the proper conditions and resources are available before beginning a repair. This may mean taking the patient to the operating room, particularly if the patient is a child or has high aesthetic standards.

ANESTHESIA

Most uncomplicated facial lacerations can be repaired with infiltration of local anesthetics. The standard preparation is 1% Xylocaine with 1:100,000 epinephrine. A useful adjunct to diminish the pain of soft tissue infiltration (which is due primarily to the low pH of the anesthetic solution) is the addition of sodium bicarbonate to the Xylocaine. By mixing 1 cc of 8% sodium bicarbonate with 9 cc of Xylocaine, the pH will be brought up from roughly 3.0 to 7.0. It has been noted, however, that this pH adjustment also decreases the duration of action of the anesthetic effect. It is the responsibility of the treating physician to be aware of the safe dosage of any drug being administered.

> **PEARL...** As a rough rule of thumb, 40 cc of 1% Xylocaine per hour is considered the upper limit of appropriate local anesthesia use in the average 70-kg adult.

Although the vascular supply of the facial skin is probably the best of the entire body, necessitating the addition of the vasoconstrictor to the Xylocaine, there may be situations where the use of a vasoconstrictor is inappropriate. In particular, vasoconstrictors should probably be avoided in situations where there is clearly a limited pedicle type blood supply. Examples of this type of limited blood supply would include the tip of the nose or ear or an avulsion type injury where a pedicled flap of skin has been raised. In these types of injuries consideration should be given to using plain anesthetic without epinephrine or performing the repair under regional or general anesthesia.

INSTRUMENTATION AND SUTURE

To perform an atraumatic and accurate repair of a facial laceration, it is necessary to have a set of instruments available that allow the surgeon to work with a high degree of accuracy. With regard to suture, the least amount of the finest suture that will hold the tissues together should be used. The wound should be closed in layers, with identification and approximation of those anatomic structures that can support a suture under some tension. Fascia and dermis can withstand a tensile force. Fat and muscle, without fascia, are not strong enough to support a suture repair. When placing subcutaneous sutures, 5-0 or 6-0 absorbable polyglycolic acid is preferred. For skin repair, a 6-0 or 7-0 monofilament is used and the sutures are removed in 3 to 5 days.

REPAIR OF COMPLICATED SOFT TISSUE WOUNDS

CONTUSIONS

Blunt trauma often presents with an associated stellate laceration resulting from the skin being caught between the striking object externally and the facial skeleton internally. In these situations the skin is actually ripped rather than cut and this gives rise to widespread surrounding tissue disruption. These wounds often do poorly from an aesthetic standpoint even with the most meticulous repair. The scars are irregular and often widen and become depressed. Initial treatment should be directed at obtaining as accurate a repair as possible.

> **SPECIAL CONSIDERATION**
>
> As a general rule, extensive debridement should not be performed at the time of primary repair because of the difficulty in assessing what tissue will be important for the final outcome.

When the wound has fully matured (a minimum of 6 months to 1 year), a scar revision may be considered.

AVULSIONS

Actual loss of soft tissue represents one of the most difficult wound management situations. If the soft tissue is available, it is not unreasonable to reattach it as a full-thickness graft. Some authors feel hyperbaric oxygen may facilitate the survival of these grafts. Adjunctive treatment might include some form of anticoagulation or platelet inhibition. If it is a large portion of tissue with identifiable blood vessels that has been avulsed, such as a scalp or ear, then a microvascular reattachment with microvascular anastomosis may be considered. If the reattached portion survives long enough to develop venous stasis, surgical leeches have been used with some success.

If the avulsed tissue is not available, then the surgeon must manage the wound in its absence. If the defect is not too wide, an attempt at primary closure with undermining can be considered. However, if there is going to be excessive tension on the wound, then it is probably best to allow the wound to granulate on its own and revise it secondarily. No matter how tempting, there is almost no situation (except perhaps with massive tissue loss) where split- or full-thickness skin grafting is indicated.

PITFALL••• Placement of skin grafts in situations where soft tissue has been avulsed stops the wound contraction of secondary healing (which can be very helpful in closing a wound) and almost always provides a poor tissue match. This is particularly true where full-thickness skin and subcutaneous tissue have been lost.

For these situations placement of a skin graft, even a full-thickness one, will not only have a poor tissue match but will also leave a contour deformity. It is usually best to allow the wound to stabilize and plan a local or regional flap repair with facial skin that matches the skin surrounding the wound.

LACERATIONS INVOLVING A MARGIN OR BORDER

Special consideration should be given to any laceration that extends through an anatomic margin or border because of the aesthetic and functional importance of these junctional structures. From an aesthetic consideration, the eye is attracted to discrepancies in facial lines and contours and a misaligned margin or border will immediately be noticed. Technically these structures are somewhat more demanding because they have an external and internal surface that may be lacerated. If an optimal repair is to be performed, all three layers (internal, middle, and external) must be completely and accurately realigned. If the internal surface laceration is not repaired, the wound contraction associated with secondary wound healing may cause distortion of the external surface. The sites that merit particular attention are discussed in the following subsections.

Vermilion Border of the Lip

This smooth line of transition between the pale cutaneous lip skin and the red mucosa is a critical facial landmark and any malalignment, even as much as a millimeter, will be quite noticeable. With any lip repair the vermilion border should be accurately aligned first with a temporary suture to place the rest of the lip structures in their correct anatomic position. The lip should then be repaired in layers with the inner mucosa closed loosely with 4-0 plain gut sutures, the muscular layer with 6-0 polyglycolic acid, and the external skin and mucosa with a fine monofilament.

Nostril Margin

Lacerations involving the margin of the nostril need to be accurately repaired to ensure that unsightly notching does not occur. Additionally, it must be remembered that in the medial portion of the nostril and superior columella, the lower lateral cartilage is quite close to the margin and relatively superficial. If a laceration of the lower lateral cartilage is not recognized and repaired, there is a high likelihood that the nose will shift and twist as the forces of healing put stress on the ipsilateral nose, and the ends of the lower lateral cartilage slip over one another. If the inner mucosa is not repaired, the contraction resulting from secondary wound healing may cause superior retraction of the nostril margin. Because the nose has such a high aesthetic importance and secondary repair of the complications discussed herein is so difficult, lacerations of the nostril margin are often best repaired in the operating room. The principle of a three-layer closure is followed, with the exception that a laceration of the lower lateral cartilage is identified and repaired with 5-0 or 6-0 clear monofilament nylon to impart some permanent strength to the wound.

Auricular Helical Rim

Lacerations of the helical rim traverse skin and cartilage and require a three-layer repair with accurate reapproximation of the auricular cartilage, as in the nose, to avoid notching. Again, the perichondrium of the cartilage is reapproximated with 5-0 or 6-0 clear nylon and the skin with 6-0 nylon.

Eyelids

Management of eyelid lacerations could well take up an entire chapter on its own, but a few brief remarks are in order. Although laceration of the globe is a primary concern (this should be ruled out with appropriate ophthalmologic consultation/examination), there are several structures that may be involved with eyelid trauma that must also be considered. With upper eyelid lacerations, the surgeon should also consider the possibility of injury to the levator palpebrae, which could cause ptosis of the upper lid if not repaired.

> **PITFALL•••** The lacrimal gland may be involved with lacerations of the lateral portion of the upper lid and may be mistaken for orbital fat.

There are reports of the lacrimal gland being excised under the mistaken assumption that orbital fat was being debrided. In the lower eyelid, the possibility of a laceration to the lacrimal sys-

tem should always be considered with any medial lid laceration. In both the upper and lower eyelids, special concern should be given to lacerations that involve the lid margin. As in lacerations that involve margins elsewhere on the face, if this is improperly repaired, unsightly notching may occur. Briefly, repair of a lid margin laceration involves a three-layer closure with a fine, 6-0 or 7-0 plain gut suture on the conjunctival side (to avoid irritation of the scleral conjunctiva), a fine absorbable suture in the tarsal plate, and a fine monofilament on the external surface.

SUGGESTED READINGS

Bucci MN, Hoff JT. Neurologic evaluation and management. In: Fonseca RJ, Walker RV, eds. *Oral and Maxillofacial Trauma.* Vol. 1. 1st ed. Philadelphia: W.B. Saunders; 1991:137–156.

Heymans O, Nelissen X, Medot M, Fissette J. Microsurgical repair of Stensen's duct using an interposition vein graft. *J Reconstr Microsurg* 1999;15:105–8.

Lentrodt J. Maxillofacial injuries—statistics and causes of accidents. In: Kruger E, Schilli W, eds. *Oral and Maxillofacial Traumatology.* Vol. 1. 1st ed. Chicago: Quintessence Publishing Co.; 1982:43–47.

Levine CL, Berger RJ, Lazow SK. Parotid salivary fistula secondary to external pin fixation: case report. *J Cranio-Maxfac Trauma* 1996;2:20–23.

Parekh D, Glezerson G, Stewart M, et al. Posttraumatic parotid fistulae and sialoceles. A prospective study of conservative management in 51 cases. *Ann Surg* 1989;209:105.

Shumrick K, Kersten R, Kulwin D, Sinha P, Smith T. Extended access/internal approaches for the management of facial trauma. *Arch Otolaryngol Head Neck Surg* 1992;118:1105–1112.

Tachmes L, Woloszyn T, Marini C, et al. Parotid gland and facial nerve trauma: A retrospective review. *J Trauma* 1990;30:1395–1398.

SECTION XI

NECK

ANATOMY AND PHYSIOLOGY

Louis G. Portugal, Tapan A. Padhya, and Jack L. Gluckman

TRIANGLES OF THE NECK

For the purposes of description, the neck is traditionally divided into triangles. The sternocleidomastoid muscle divides each side of the neck into anterior and posterior triangles (Fig. 71–1).

The anterior triangle is bounded by the midline of the neck, the sternocleidomastoid muscle, and the lower border of the mandible. The anterior triangle is further subdivided by the digastric and omohyoid muscles into smaller triangular units. The submandibular triangle is bounded by the anterior and posterior bellies of the digastric muscle and the lower border of the mandible. The submental triangle is bounded by both anterior bellies of the digastrics and the hyoid bone inferiorly. The remaining portion of the anterior triangle is divided by the omohyoid into the carotid triangle superiorly and the muscular triangle inferiorly.

The posterior triangle is bounded by the sternocleidomastoid, the anterior border of the trapezius, and the middle third of the clavicle. This triangle is further subdivided by the omohyoid into a smaller subclavian triangle inferiorly and a larger occipital triangle superiorly.

FASCIAL LAYERS OF THE NECK

The cervical fascia represents a condensation of connective tissue that extends between anatomic structures. This fascia is divided into a su-

perficial and deep layer, with the deep layer dividing further into the superficial, middle, and deep layers of the deep cervical fascia (Figs. 71–2 and 71–3).

SUPERFICIAL FASCIA

The superficial fascia lies just below the dermis. It is an indistinct layer that blends with the continuous sheet of subcutaneous fat extending throughout the body. In the head and neck, the deep portions of this layer encase the platysma muscle as well as the voluntary muscles of the face and scalp.

SUPERFICIAL LAYER OF THE DEEP CERVICAL FASCIA

The superficial or investing layer of the deep cervical fascia begins posteriorly from the vertebral spinous processes and splits to enclose the trapezius. At the anterior border of the trapezius, the two layers unite to form a single layer until it reaches the posterior border of the sternocleidomastoid muscle, where it splits to invest this muscle as well as the strap muscles anteriorly.

Superiorly, this fascia is attached to the occipital protuberance and the superior nuchal lines at the back of the skull. At this level, the layer envelops the parotid and submandibular

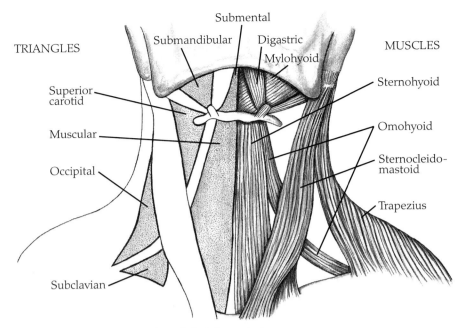

TRIANGLES

MUSCLES

Submental

Submandibular   Digastric

Mylohyoid

Superior
carotid

Sternohyoid

Muscular

Omohyoid

Sternocleido-
mastoid

Occipital

Trapezius

Subclavian

FIGURE 71-1 Triangles of the neck and their boundaries.

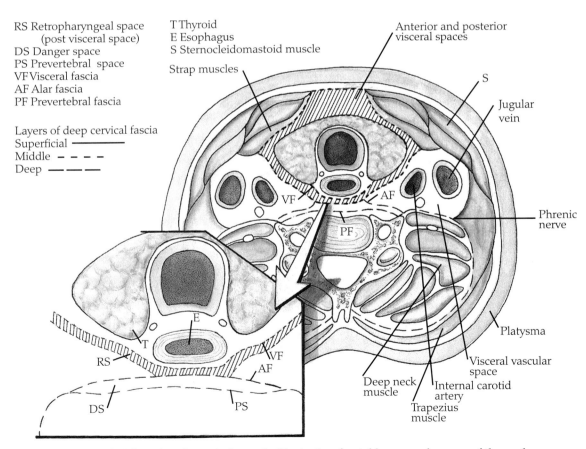

RS Retropharyngeal space
    (post visceral space)
DS Danger space
PS Prevertebral space
VF Visceral fascia
AF Alar fascia
PF Prevertebral fascia

Layers of deep cervical fascia
Superficial ———————
Middle – – – –
Deep — — —

T Thyroid
E Esophagus
S Sternocleidomastoid muscle

Strap muscles

Anterior and posterior
visceral spaces

S

Jugular
vein

VF

AF

PF

Phrenic
nerve

E

T

RS

VF

AF

Platysma

DS

PS

Deep neck
muscle

Internal carotid
artery

Trapezius
muscle

Visceral vascular
space

FIGURE 71-2 Axial section through the neck, illustrating fascial layers and spaces of the neck.

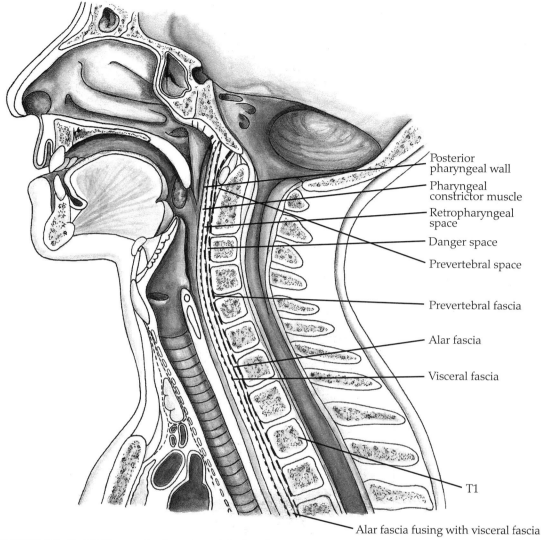

Posterior
pharyngeal wall

Pharyngeal
constrictor muscle

Retropharyngeal
space

Danger space

Prevertebral space

Prevertebral fascia

Alar fascia

Visceral fascia

T1

Alar fascia fusing with visceral fascia

FIGURE 71–3 Midline sagittal section of the head and neck, illustrating fascial layers and spaces of the neck.

glands, the mandible posterior to the mental foramen, and the pterygoid musculature. The lateral component, enveloping the parotid, attaches superiorly to the zygomatic arch. The medial component extends along the base of the sphenoid from the mastoid tip toward the opening of the carotid canal where it merges with the fascia of the internal carotid artery. Between the parotid and submandibular glands, the two layers rejoin to form the stylomandibular ligament.

In the midline inferiorly, the fascia between the sternocleidomastoid muscles splits just be-

fore attaching to the anterior and posterior surfaces of the sternum. The small space created by these two layers is referred to as the suprasternal space of Burns.

MIDDLE LAYER OF THE DEEP CERVICAL FASCIA

The middle or visceral layer of the deep cervical fascia encloses the thyroid gland, trachea, pharyngeal constrictor muscles, and esophagus.

Anteriorly, it extends from the hyoid bone down to sternal attachments and is continuous with the fibrous pericardium. The portion overlying the anterior trachea is particularly well developed and is referred to as the pretracheal fascia. The posterior portion of this layer behind the esophagus and pharynx extends all the way to the skull base.

DEEP LAYER OF DEEP CERVICAL FASCIA

The deep layer of the deep cervical fascia, also referred to as the prevertebral fascia, lies immediately anterior to the vertebral bodies, extending laterally to the tips of the transverse processes (Figs. 71–2 and 71–3). It extends over the deep muscles of the neck and attaches to the vertebral spines posteriorly. Superiorly this layer continues to the skull base and inferiorly to the coccyx. The deep layer of the deep cervical fascia is composed of a prevertebral and alar layer. This alar fascia lies immediately anterior to the prevertebral layer of the deep cervical fascia, extending across the midline from transverse process to transverse process. The superior extent is the same as the prevertebral layer but inferiorly it ends about the level of the first thoracic vertebra, where it fuses anteriorly with the visceral fascia.

SPECIAL CONSIDERATION

A potential space is created between the alar and prevertebral fascias that is referred to as the "danger space," because it communicates directly with the mediastinum.

The prevertebral space lies between the prevertebral fascia and vertebral bodies, and the retropharyngeal space lies between the alar and the visceral fascia.

TISSUE SPACES OF THE NECK (SEE ALSO CHAPTER 75)

Between cervical fascia exist potential spaces. Knowledge of these spaces is critical in understanding the spread of infection and disease in the neck.

PEARL... Because superficial and deep layers of the deep cervical fascia fuse at the hyoid bone, infection in the spaces above the hyoid does not spread directly to spaces below the hyoid.

Communication along the entire length of the neck occurs posteriorly along the retropharyngeal and prevertebral spaces (Figs. 71–2 and 71–3).

The *submandibular space* is located between the outer surface of the mylohyoid muscle and more superficial structures within the submandibular triangle. Along the posterior free edge of the mylohyoid muscle, this space is continuous with the sublingual space in the floor of the mouth. It is also continuous with the submental space within the submental triangle. Although typically infection in this space will not spread in the infrahyoid direction, infection can spread from one submandibular space across the neck to affect the contralateral space.

The spaces surrounding the pharynx in the suprahyoid region can be divided into an intrapharyngeal space and a parapharyngeal space. The *intrapharyngeal space* lies between the inner surface of the superior constrictor muscle and the pharyngeal mucosa. This space is commonly known as the peritonsillar or paratonsillar space and is the site of peritonsillar abscesses. The *parapharyngeal space,* which is bounded medially by the superior constrictor and laterally by the pterygoid muscles and fascia of the parotid gland, is limited inferiorly by the fascial attachment to the hyoid. However, posteromedially, this space communicates with the retropharyngeal space providing a route through which infection entering the parapharyngeal space can spread dangerously down into the mediastinum. Odontogenic or peritonsillar infections therefore have the potential to follow this route.

The *retropharyngeal space* is the first of three posteriorly located spaces involving the entire length of the neck. This space lies between the visceral fascia behind the pharynx and the alar fascia posteriorly. It extends from the skull base down to about the level of T1, where this space is believed to end with the fusion of the alar fascia anteriorly to the visceral fascia. The "danger space" describes the potential space between the alar fascia anteriorly and the prevertebral fascia posteriorly. Infection from the retropharyngeal space can enter the danger space, providing direct access to the mediastinum. The *prevertebral space* lies between the prevertebral fascia anteriorly and the vertebral column posteriorly extending from the skull base to the lower thoracic area.

ARTERIES OF THE NECK (FIG. 71–4)

COMMON CAROTID ARTERY

The common carotid artery lies beneath the sternocleidomastoid muscle arising on the right from the brachiocephalic artery and on the left directly from the aortic arch. As it ascends in the

neck, the common carotid is crossed superfically by the superior belly of the omohyoid muscle and the superior and middle thyroid veins. The common carotid artery terminates, bifurcating into the internal and external carotid arteries about the level of the thyroid notch.

INTERNAL CAROTID ARTERY

The internal carotid artery extends from the bifurcation toward the skull base without branching. It is crossed laterally by the hypoglossal nerve, the occipital artery, and the posterior belly of the digastric muscle. The digastric muscle serves as an important surgical landmark as all structures within the carotid sheath lie deep to this muscle. Near the skull base, the internal carotid artery is crossed laterally by the glossopharyngeal nerve, the stylohyoid, stylopha-

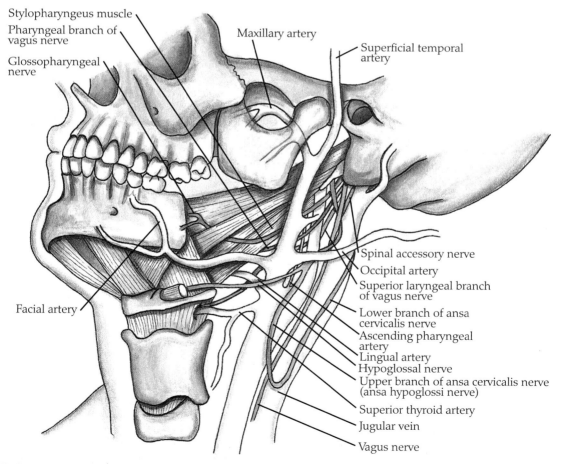

Stylopharyngeus muscle
Pharyngeal branch of vagus nerve
Glossopharyngeal nerve
Maxillary artery
Superficial temporal artery
Spinal accessory nerve
Occipital artery
Superior laryngeal branch of vagus nerve
Lower branch of ansa cervicalis nerve
Ascending pharyngeal artery
Lingual artery
Hypoglossal nerve
Upper branch of ansa cervicalis nerve (ansa hypoglossi nerve)
Superior thyroid artery
Jugular vein
Vagus nerve
Facial artery

FIGURE 71–4 Arteries and nerves of the neck.

ryngeus, and styloglossus muscles, as well as the styloid process.

EXTERNAL CAROTID ARTERY AND BRANCHES

After leaving the bifurcation, the external carotid artery passes behind the posterior belly of the digastric muscle, crossing superficially to the styloglossus and stylopharyngeus muscles. Its terminal branches continue behind the condylar process of the mandible passing into the parotid gland. The external carotid artery has eight branches.

The *superior thyroid artery* is the first anterior branch of the external carotid supplying the upper part of the thyroid gland as well as parts of the sternocleidomastoid muscle and the larynx. It arises just below the greater horn of the hyoid bone and runs directly inferiorly on the surface of the inferior constrictor muscle to the superior pole of the thyroid gland.

The *ascending pharyngeal artery* is the smallest branch of the external carotid, arising posteriorly at about the same level as the superior thyroid artery. It passes vertically to supply the muscles of the pharynx and palate, the tonsil, the middle ear, and the meninges.

The *lingual artery* arises just above the superior thyroid artery. It runs anterior and superior along the surface of the middle constrictor as the hypoglossal nerve passes superficial to it. The artery then passes beneath the hyoglossus muscle to enter the tongue. Ligation of the lingual artery can be accomplished by an approach through Lesser's triangle, which is bordered by the posterior belly of the digastric muscle posteriorly, the anterior belly of the digastric anteriorly, and the hypoglossal nerve superiorly. The artery can be found just deep to the hyoglossus muscle in the posterior portion of the triangle.

The *facial artery* arises on the anterior surface of the external carotid passing anteriorly and superiorly, deep to the digastric muscle. It passes through the submandibular gland, crosses the inferior border of the mandible over the antegonial notch of the mandible, and rises into the face at the anterior edge of the mas-

seter muscle. Branches of the facial artery in the neck include the ascending palatine artery, the tonsillar artery, branches to the submandibular gland, and the submental artery to the suprahyoid muscles.

The *occipital artery* arises from the posterior surface of the external carotid at about the same level as the facial artery. As it runs posteriorly across the carotid sheath, the hypoglossal nerve hooks around it. It supplies the suboccipital region of the scalp as well as the sternocleidomastoid, digastric, and stylohyoid muscles.

The *posterior auricular artery* also arises posteriorly at about the level of the upper border of the digastric muscle. It passes between the ear and the mastoid process, giving branches to the parotid gland, auricle, and scalp.

The *superficial temporal* and *maxillary arteries* are the terminal branches of the external carotid artery. The superficial temporal artery passes upward toward the scalp after it emerges from the superior surface of the parotid gland. The internal maxillary artery passes into the infratemporal fossa, entering the pterygopalatine fossa via the pterygopalatine fissure.

THYROCERVICAL TRUNK AND BRANCHES

The thyrocervical trunk provides two major branches important in the lower portion of the neck: the *transverse cervical artery* and the *inferior thyroid artery.* The trunk arises from the first part of the subclavian artery just anterior to the scalenus anterior muscle at the root of the neck. The transverse cervical artery runs posteriorly along the lower portion of the posterior triangle just superficial to the scalenus anterior muscle and sends branches to the sternocleidomastoid and trapezius muscles.

The inferior thyroid artery ascends from the trunk in a course deep to the carotid sheath passing medially to supply the inferior part of the thyroid gland, the superior and inferior parathyroid glands, and a portion of the larynx and trachea. The inferior thyroid artery runs along the same plane as the more superficial middle thyroid vein. Both vessels enter the thyroid gland at about the level of the cricoid.

VEINS OF THE NECK

Most of the veins in the neck eventually drain into either the internal or external jugular vein.

INTERNAL JUGULAR VEIN

The internal jugular vein lies within the carotid sheath along with the carotid artery and vagus nerve. As a continuation of the sigmoid sinus, it extends from the skull base down to thoracic inlet, where it joins the subclavian vein and forms the brachiocephalic vein. In its descent from the skull base, several major tributaries join it. In the uppermost part of the internal jugular vein in the region of the jugular bulb, the inferior petrosal sinus joins the internal jugular vein. At the level of the greater horn of the hyoid, the internal jugular vein is joined by the prominent common facial vein, which is formed by the facial vein and the anterior branch of the retromandibular vein. The facial and the common facial veins take a more superficial course than the facial artery passing laterally to the submandibular gland, digastric muscle, hypoglossal nerve, and carotid vessels. Below the common facial vein, the smaller lingual veins drain into the internal jugular vein. The lingual vein is formed from the dorsal lingual vein, which drains the dorsum of the tongue, and the deep lingual vein, which is visible beneath the mucosa of the ventral surface of the tongue. The latter may drain directly into the internal jugular vein. The superior thyroid vein accompanies the superior thyroid artery and drains the thyroid gland and portions of the larynx. The prominent middle thyroid vein drains directly into the internal jugular vein and runs along the same plane as the deeper inferior thyroid artery.

EXTERNAL JUGULAR VEIN

The external jugular vein arises near the tail of the parotid gland by a confluence of the posterior branch of the retromandibular vein and the posterior auricular vein. The external jugular vein passes inferiorly in a plane deep to the platysma but superficial to the sternocleidomastoid, terminating in the subclavian vein in the posterior triangle of the neck. The external jugular vein is joined at its midpoint by the posterior external jugular vein, which drains the posterior portions of the upper neck. Sometimes a communicating vessel with the internal jugular vein may be seen superiorly at its origin.

ANTERIOR JUGULAR VEIN

The anterior jugular vein arises from a confluence of veins in the submandibular region. Above the sternal notch, the anterior jugular veins communicate via the jugular arch. The anterior jugular veins then pass beneath the sternocleidomastoid muscle to drain into the external jugular or subclavian vein.

NERVES OF THE NECK (FIG. 71–4)

GLOSSOPHARYNGEAL NERVE

The glossopharyngeal nerve enters the neck through the jugular foramen with cranial nerves X and XI. The nerve contains sensory, motor, and parasympathetic components and has a superior and inferior ganglion in the region of the jugular foramen. Cell bodies for afferent fibers are primarily in the inferior ganglion with some somatosensory cell bodies in the superior ganglion. Immediately below the foramen, the glossopharyngeal nerve is located anterior to the vagus and accessory nerves. It runs anterior to the internal and then deep to the external carotid arteries. Following the stylopharyngeus muscle, it passes between the superior and middle constrictor muscles of the pharynx to innervate the tonsil, pharynx, and tongue. As one follows the course of the glossopharyngeal nerves, specific branches are identified in the neck.

The *tympanic nerve* arises from the inferior ganglion. It passes upward through the tympanic canaliculus to enter the middle ear as Jacobson's nerve and contributes to the tympanic plexus. From here it provides sensory fibers to the middle ear, eustachian tube, and mastoid cavity.

The *lesser petrosal nerve* contains preganglionic parasympathetic fibers that pass from the tympanic plexus through the anterior wall of the tympanic cavity and onto the floor of the middle cranial fossa. It then emerges from the foramen ovale to join the otic ganglion in the infratemporal fossa. Within this ganglion, the nerve synapses with postganglionic parasympathetic fibers that supply the parotid gland.

The *carotid branch* arises from the glossopharyngeal nerve just below the skull base. This nerve descends to unite with the carotid branch of the vagus nerve and carries sensory information back from the carotid body and carotid sinus.

The *pharyngeal branches* of the glossopharyngeal nerve form the pharyngeal plexus on the middle constrictor muscle with branches from the vagus nerve and sympathetic trunk. Through the plexus the pharyngeal branches of the glossopharyngeal nerve provide sensory innervation of the pharynx.

The *stylopharyngeus branch* supplies the stylopharyngeus muscle and represents the only motor branch of the glossopharyngeal nerve.

The *tonsillar branches* form a plexus with the lesser palatine nerve. Branches from this plexus are distributed to the tonsil and soft palate.

The *lingual branches* of the glossopharyngeal nerve supply both taste and general sensation to the posterior one-third of the tongue.

VAGUS NERVE

The vagus nerve contains sensory, motor, and parasympathetic fibers and, like the glossopharyngeal nerve, has both a superior and an inferior ganglion in the region of the jugular foramen. The vagus nerve exits the brainstem through the jugular foramen, taking a position between the internal jugular vein and carotid artery and passing downward within the carotid sheath. As one follows the course of the vagus nerve, specific branches are identified in the neck.

The *meningeal branches* arise from the superior ganglion and supply sensory innervation to the dura of the posterior cranial fossa.

The *auricular branch* also arises from the superior ganglion. It takes a course through the temporal bone to eventually provide sensory innervation to the pinna, external auditory canal (Arnold's nerve), and tympanic membrane.

The *pharyngeal branch* runs from the inferior ganglion of the vagus to the pharyngeal plexus lying on the middle constrictor muscle. Through the plexus, the vagus nerve provides motor innervation to the muscles of the pharynx and palate.

The *superior laryngeal nerve* also arises from the inferior ganglion of the vagus passing deep to both carotid arteries on its way to the larynx and dividing into internal and external branches. The internal branch passes between the middle and inferior constrictor muscles to supply sensation to the larynx. The external branch runs with the superior thyroid artery to supply the cricothyroid muscle of the larynx.

The *right recurrent laryngeal nerve* arises from the vagus in front of the subclavian artery, looping below and behind the artery and then rising in the tracheoesophageal groove toward the larynx. In a similar manner, the left recurrent laryngeal nerve leaves the left vagus nerve in front of the aortic arch, passing below and then behind the arch to ascend in the tracheoesophageal groove. The recurrent nerves pass beneath the inferior borders of the inferior constrictor muscles at the cricothyroid joint to supply all the intrinsic muscles of the larynx except the cricothyroid muscle.

ACCESSORY NERVE

The accessory nerve has both cranial and spinal components. The cranial component is primarily sensory, arising from the medulla oblongata and joining the vagus as it exits the jugular foramen. These fibers appear to be responsible for the vagal contributions to the pharyngeal plexus. The spinal component of the accessory nerve is primarily motor, originating from segments C2 through C4 of the spinal cord. Soon after leaving the jugular foramen, the accessory nerve heads toward the posterior triangle of the neck. It crosses laterally or on occasion medially to the internal jugular vein. The nerve remains anterior and inferior to the palpable transverse process of the atlas before entering the anterior portion of the sternocleidomastoid at the apex of the carotid triangle. The nerve emerges on the posterior border of the muscle at 1 cm above

Erb's point (see Cervical Plexus, below) passing through the posterior triangle to innervate the trapezius muscle.

HYPOGLOSSAL NERVE

The hypoglossal nerve exits the cranial cavity through the hypoglossal canal of the occipital bone passing downward under the posterior belly of the digastric muscle to emerge between the internal jugular vein and internal carotid artery. After looping around the occipital artery, it continues anteriorly across the internal and external carotid arteries and then deep to the submandibular gland and posterior belly of the diagastric muscle onto the surface of the hyoglossus muscle. From here, the nerve is distributed to the intrinsic muscles of the tongue and styloglossus, hyoglossus, and genioglossus muscles. Branches of the hypoglossal nerve also include contributions to the ansa cervicalis.

ANSA CERVICALIS

The ansa cervicalis provides motor innervation to the strap muscles. Contributions to the ansa cervicalis include upper and lower branches. The upper branch, sometimes referred to as the ansa hypoglossi, arises from the hypoglossal nerve as it loops around the occipital artery. Lower branches of the ansa cervicalis are derived from C2 and C3 fibers from the cervical plexus.

CERVICAL SYMPATHETIC TRUNK

Sympathetic innervation to the neck is derived primarily from preganglionic sympathetic fibers from the thoracic spinal cord. These fibers ascend via the sympathetic trunk and synapse at one of three major sympathetic cervical ganglia.

The *superior cervical ganglion* is the largest of these ganglia and is located at the level of the second and third cervical vertebrae behind the carotid sheath. Arising from the superior ganglion is the internal carotid nerve, which passes into the carotid canal to form the internal carotid plexus around the internal carotid artery.

This plexus sends sympathetic branches that communicate with different cranial nerves.

The *middle cervical ganglion,* the smallest cervical ganglion, is usually situated at the level of the sixth cervical vertebra close to the inferior thyroid artery just before it enters the gland.

The *inferior cervical ganglion* is located in the root of the neck just posterior to the vertebral artery.

CERVICAL PLEXUS

The cervical plexus is formed by fibers from C1 through C4 segments of the spinal cord and contains both motor and sensory nerves. The phrenic nerve is the motor branch of the plexus arising from C3 and C4 as well as C5. The phrenic nerve lies on the anterior scalene muscle deep to the prevertebral fascia entering the chest behind the subclavian artery, eventually supplying the diaphragm. The sensory branches of the plexus emerge as a bundle at an area along the posterior border of the sternocleidomastoid muscle referred to as Erb's point. There are four major sensory nerves: the lesser occipital nerve; the great auricular nerve; the anterior cutaneous nerve, also referred to as the transverse cervical nerve; and the supraclavicular nerve, which provides the lateral, intermediate, and medial supraclavicular nerves.

LYMPHATICS OF THE NECK

Anatomically, the cervical nodes are divided into superficial and deep groups. The superficial groups consist of the submental nodes, submandibular nodes, anterior cervical nodes, and superficial cervical nodes. These nodes are in direct communication with the superficial nodes of the face and scalp, which include the occipital nodes, retroauricular nodes, parotid nodes, and buccal nodes. Most of the deep cervical nodes are closely associated with the internal jugular vein. Other groups of deep cervical nodes include the pretracheal, perithyroid, paratracheal, and retropharyngeal nodes. To provide standardization in terminology, the lymphatics are classified into levels.

Level I The submental and submandibular triangles are bounded by the posterior belly of the digastric muscle, the hyoid bone inferiorly, and the body of the mandible superiorly.

Level II The upper jugular lymph node group lies along the course of the upper one-third of the internal jugular vein and the proximal portion of the spinal accessory nerve. This level extends from the base of the skull downward to the carotid bifurcation (surgical landmark) or hyoid bone (clinical landmark). The posterior border is the posterior edge of the sternocleidomastoid muscle, and the anterior border is the lateral edge of the sternohyoid muscle.

Level III The middle jugular group of lymph nodes lies along the middle one-third of the internal jugular vein from the carotid bifurcation to the omohyoid muscle (surgical landmark) or cricothyroid notch (clinical landmark). The anterior and posterior boundaries are the same as in level II.

Level IV The lower jugular group lies along the inferior one-third of the internal jugular vein from the omohyoid muscle superiorly to the clavicle inferiorly.

Level V The lymph nodes in the posterior triangle are bounded by the anterior border of the trapezius posteriorly, the posterior border of the sternocleidomastoid muscle anteriorly, and the clavicle inferiorly. Level V may be further subdivided into upper, middle, and lower levels corresponding to the superior and inferior planes that define levels II, III, and IV.

Level VI The anterior compartment group is composed of the lymph nodes surrounding the midline visceral structures of the neck from the hyoid bone to the sternal notch. The lateral border is the carotid sheath. This group of lymph nodes includes the paratracheal nodes, perithyroid nodes, precricoid nodes (Delphian nodes), and nodes lying along the recurrent laryngeal nerves.

Level VII The upper mediastinal lymph nodes are inferior to the suprasternal notch.

NODAL ANATOMY

Anterior Group

The anterior group is subdivided into the anterior jugular chain and the juxtavisceral chain. The *anterior jugular chain* runs along the anterior jugular vein superficial to the strap muscles. These nodes draining the anterior cervical skin and muscles ultimately drain into the lower internal jugular chain. The *juxtavisceral chain* consists of prelaryngeal, prethyroid, pretracheal, and paratracheal nodes. The prelaryngeal nodes are located over the thyrohyoid membrane. The upper nodes of this group drain the supraglottis, whereas the lower nodes or prethyroid nodes drain the infraglottic larynx, thyroid isthmus, and anteromedial thyroid lobes. The *Delphian node* is usually a solitary node that lies immediately superficial to the cricothyroid membrane. The pretracheal nodal group lies over the trachea extending from the thyroid isthmus to the innominate vein. The number of nodes in this group can vary from 2 to 12, and they drain the thyroid gland and trachea. The paratracheal nodes are in close proximity to the recurrent nerve and drain the lateral aspect of the thyroid and parathyroid glands, the postcricoid larynx, the trachea, and the esophagus.

All nodes from the anterior cervical group communicate with the superior mediastinal nodes, as well as the lower jugular nodes.

Lateral Group

The lateral cervical nodes consist of a superficial and deep chain. The superficial group is closely related to the external jugular vein and drains into the transverse cervical nodes of the deep group. The deep group consists of the spinal accessory chain, the transverse cervical chain, and the internal jugular chain.

All of these nodal groups form a triangle, with the base formed by the transverse cervical group, the posterior limb by the spinal accessory group, and the anterior limb by the internal jugular group. The *spinal accessory chain* follows the route of the spinal accessory nerve and can consist of up to 20 nodes. These nodes are interconnected with other nodal groups, especially the upper internal jugular chain nodes. The transverse cervical group follows the transverse cervical vessels and may number 12 nodes. The medial nodes lie on top of the scalene muscles and their drainage area overlaps that of the lower internal jugular nodes. The *internal jugular chain* consists of a large system of nodes covering the anterior and lateral aspects of the internal jugular vein extending from the digastric muscle superiorly to the junction of the internal jugular vein and the subclavian vein inferiorly. These nodes, which can number as many as 30, are classified as upper, middle, and lower groups. On the left, the internal jugular chain drains into the thoracic duct, subsequently emptying into the left subclavian vein. On the right, it drains into the right lymphatic duct emptying at the junction of the right internal jugular and subclavian veins.

SPECIAL CONSIDERATION

The internal jugular chain, although interconnected with other nodal groups, can receive direct drainage from the entire upper aerodigestive tract, major salivary glands, and thyroid and parathyroid glands.

The lateral group remains the most significant group of nodes that drain the upper aerodigestive tract and therefore need to be carefully dissected during neck dissections.

Submandibular Nodes

The submandibular nodes are classified into five subgroups: (1) preglandular, (2) postglandular, (3) prevascular, (4) postvascular, and (5) intra-

capsular. The preglandular and postglandular lie anterior and posterior to the submandibular gland, respectively. Likewise, the prevascular and postvascular groups lie anterior and posterior to the facial artery. An occasional node can be located within the capsule of the submandibular gland. The submandibular nodal group drains the ipsilateral upper and lower lip, cheek skin, nose, nasal vestibule mucosa, medial canthus, anterior alveolus, anterior tonsillar pillar, soft palate, and anterior two-thirds of the tongue and submandibular salivary gland. The nodes drain into the upper internal jugular chain nodes. There is an accessory lymphatic channel from the submandibular group to the nodes along the posterior aspect of the omohyoid muscle, therefore accounting for multilevel involvement with infections of the anterior oral cavity.

Submental Nodes

These nodes can vary in number from 2 to 8. They are located in the soft tissue between the anterior bellies of the digastric, mylohyoid, and platysma muscles. These nodes drain the mentum, the midportion of the lower lip, the anterior alveolus, and the anterior one-third of the tongue. The nodes subsequently drain into the ipsilateral and contralateral preglandular or prevascular submandibular nodes or into the internal jugular chain via lymph channels traveling along the hypoglossal nerve.

Sublingual Nodes

The sublingual nodes are located along the collecting trunk of the tongue and sublingual gland. These nodes drain the anterior floor of the mouth and the ventral surface of the tongue. They connect either to the submandibular group or to the upper internal jugular chain nodes at various levels.

Parotid Nodes

The parotid nodes are divided into an extraglandular and intraglandular group. The extraglandular group is further subdivided into preauricular and infrauricular nodal groups. They drain the lateral and frontal aspects of the scalp as well as the anterior auricle, external auditory canal, skin of the lateral face, and buccal mucosa. The intraglandular nodes drain the same sites and are interconnected with the extraglandular group. Embryologically, these nodes were trapped as the gland formed. Both groups drain into both the internal and external jugular chains and can number as many as 20 nodes. Infections of the anterior scalp, temporal bone, and buccal mucosa may require a Blair/parotidectomy incision with facial nerve preservation to drain these nodes and any abscess collection.

Retropharyngeal Nodes

The retropharyngeal nodes are classified into a lateral and medial group, both of which are located between the pharyngeal wall and the prevertebral fascia. The lateral group usually consists of one to three nodes, which are located at the level of the atlas (C1) next to the internal carotid artery. The medial group is located in the midline and located more inferiorly. There may be multiple nodes in this group extending all the way to the level of the cricoid. They primarily drain the nasal cavity, sphenoid sinus, ethmoid sinus, hard and soft palate, nasopharynx, and posterior pharyngeal wall to the level of the cricoid. These nodes drain into the upper internal jugular group. This space is commonly involved in children and in infections that connect to the lateral parapharyngeal space.

SPECIAL CONSIDERATION

The retropharyngeal space can be accessed by rotating the pharynx medially and opening the infected tissue between the pharynx and the cervical spine.

Occipital Nodes

The occipital nodes are divided into a superficial and a deep group. The superficial group consists of 2 to 5 nodes that are located between the sternocleidomastoid and trapezius muscles at the apex of the posterior triangle. They are superficial to the splenius muscle and just deep to the superficial investing fascia. The deep group

of 1 to 3 nodes is located deep to the splenius muscle and is situated along the course of the occipital artery. The superficial group drains the occipital scalp and the posterior cervical skin and subsequently drains into the deep group and upper spinal accessory nodes. The deep group also drains the deep musculature of the neck in the occipital region.

Postauricular Nodes

The postauricular nodes can vary in number from 1 to 4 and are located over the dense fibrous insertion of the sternocleidomastoid onto the mastoid tip. They drain the posterior parietal scalp as well as the skin overlying the mastoid and postauricular area. These nodes subsequently drain into the infraauricular parotid nodes and also into the internal jugular and spinal accessory nodes.

THORACIC DUCT

The thoracic duct is an important lymphatic structure that can be encountered in the root of the neck during a neck dissection. The thoracic duct passes up through the mediastinum to enter into the left root of the neck posterior to the carotid sheath and medial to the anterior scalene muscle. It empties often through multiple branches into the lowest portion of the internal jugular vein, the subclavian vein, or both. The main duct may extend as high as 5 cm above the clavicle and may on rare instances terminate on the right side of the neck rather than on the left.

SUGGESTED READINGS

Hollingshead WH. *Anatomy for Surgeons: Volume I, The Head and Neck.* 3rd ed. Philadelphia: Harper and Row; 1982.

Jones KR. Anatomy of the neck. In: Shockley WW, Pillsbury HC III, eds. *The Neck: Diagnosis and Surgery.* St. Louis: CV Mosby; 1994.

Robbins KT, Medina JE, Wolfe GT, et al. Neck dissection classification and TNM staging of head and neck cancer. In: Robbins KT, ed. *Pocket Guide to Neck Dissection Classification and TNM Staging of Head and Neck Cancer.* Alexandria, VA: American Academy of Otolaryngology; 1991.

Chapter 72

CONGENITAL DISORDERS

Greg R. Licameli and Louis G. Portugal

Neck masses in the pediatric population are common, with the majority of lesions arising from inflammatory causes. The embryonic development of the head and neck is a complicated series of events, and any defect in this developmental progression can lead to the formation of a mass in this region. Although present at birth, masses may not become clinically apparent until childhood or even adulthood. Knowledge of the embryology of this area allows one to formulate a differential diagnosis and plan treatment accordingly.

Congenital head and neck masses include anomalies of the branchial system, thyroid gland, dermoid and teratoid masses, and vascular anomalies. Age of presentation, location of the mass, and associated symptoms help to narrow the differential diagnosis. Management of these masses is usually surgical, with the timing of surgery dictated by the severity of the symptoms.

THYROGLOSSAL DUCT CYSTS

The most common congenital neck mass is a thyroglossal duct cyst. Although the majority of these lesions present before age 12, they may present in early and middle adulthood. Males and females are affected equally. Knowledge of the embryology of the thyroid gland predicts the possible locations of this anomaly.

The normal thyroid gland develops from a small epithelial rest on the floor of the pharynx. The descent of this tissue caudally begins in the third week of life and is complete by the eighth week.

SPECIAL CONSIDERATION

As the gland descends, it is intimately associated with the hyoid bone, which is in the process of fusing in the midline.

The gland remains attached to the pharynx at the foramen cecum of the tongue by the thyroglossal duct, and it is the failure of this duct to involute that causes thyroglossal duct cysts.

PEARL••• The majority of thyroglossal duct cysts (Fig. 72–1) present at or below the level of the hyoid in the midline neck, with less common presentations occurring at any point along its descent.

An arrest in the normal descent of the thyroid gland leads to ectopic thyroid tissue. Complete arrest presents as a mass in the base of the tongue known as a lingual thyroid, and when present is

487

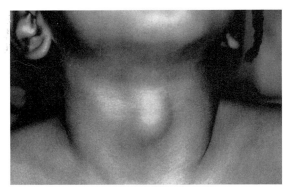

FIGURE 72–1 Thyroglossal duct cysts.

usually the only functional thyroid tissue in the patient. Thyroid tissue has also been found as far inferiorly as the superior mediastinum.

On physical exam thyroglossal duct cysts are smooth and nontender and do not trans-illuminate. With swallowing, the cyst may rise owing to its close association with the hyoid and also with tongue protrusion due to its at-tachment to the foramen cecum. Infection of the cystic material is common and is associated with an acute increase in size, overlying skin erythema, tenderness, and occasionally sponta-neous drainage through a sinus tract.

PEARL••• Because of the connection of the thyroglossal duct to the pharynx via the foramen cecum, infections are often polymicrobial, and antibiotic therapy is directed to the most common oral pathogens.

Radiologic evaluation is necessary to estab-lish the presence of normal thyroid gland tissue. In the past computed tomography and radionu-clide thyroid scanning were employed. However, B-mode ultrasonography has now emerged as the preferred diagnostic modality secondary to a lack of radiation exposure, ease of examination, the ability to discern the composition of the mass, and the identification of normal thyroid gland tissue.

Early removal of the cyst is advocated to pre-vent potential complications from repeated in-fection, including an increased difficulty in surgi-cal exploration and formation of fistulas. Sistrunk described the preferred method of excision in

PITFALL••• Determination of the location of normal thyroid tissue is essential prior to the excision of any suspected thyroglossal duct cyst or ectopic thyroid. Although ultrasound is the preferred mode of imaging, an uncooperative child or a very dense cyst may give a false-positive result. In these instances a thyroid-scan should be considered.

1920. It involves the complete removal of the cyst, the middle portion of the hyoid bone, and all remnants of the duct inferior to the cyst and superiorly up to the foramen cecum. An initial transverse incision is made over the cyst, which is usually sufficient to follow the course of the tract in its entirety. On occasion, additional smaller transverse incisions are made to facilitate expo-sure, particularly when the tract extends inferi-orly. When faced with an acute infection, antibi-otic therapy should be instituted prior to surgery. Recurrence rate following this technique is re-ported to be less than 10%. Although rare, malig-nancy may be found within the excised duct and is usually papillary adenocarcinoma.

PITFALL••• Recurrence after excision is often due to failure to remove the midportion of the hyoid, failure to remove an en-bloc section of tissue in the tongue around the tract, and rupture of the cyst during surgery. Recurrence is also higher for repeat surgical explorations.

DERMOIDS AND TERATOMAS

Teratomas and dermoid cysts are uncommon causes of head and neck masses in children, presenting at or shortly after birth. Felt to be true developmental neoplasms, they arise from pluripotent cells at anatomic sites where they are not normally found. Dermoids are composed of ectoderm and mesoderm, and teratomas are composed of all three germ layers. Dermoids are lined by epidermis and may contain hair follicles and sebaceous glands. In contrast, teratomas can display a wide range of differentiation, from dis-organized teratoid cysts to true teratomas. *Epig-nathi* is the term given to the best-differentiated teratomas, demonstrating hair, teeth, and primitive limbs.

Dermoids are commonly found as smooth, nontender masses in the submental region (Fig. 72–2). Teratomas are usually found in the cervical region and are firm, mobile, and may be both cystic and solid in composition (Fig. 72–3). Surgical removal is the procedure of choice for both dermoids and teratomas.

SPECIAL CONSIDERATION

Although both dermoid cysts and thyroglossal duct cysts usually present as midline cervical masses, the former is removed traditionally with a simple excision, and the latter is excised with the more extensive Sistrunk procedure. It may be possible to differentiate between the two with needle aspiration or incisional biopsy and intraoperative pathologic interpretation, but the risk of cyst content spillage, incomplete resection, or erroneous intraoperative pathologic diagnosis leads some surgeons to remove all midline cervical cysts below the strap muscles via the Sistrunk procedure.

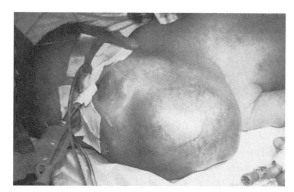

FIGURE 72–3 Massive teratoma (intubated at birth).

BRANCHIAL ARCH ANOMALIES

Branchial sinuses, fistulas, and cysts result from abnormalities in the normal development of the branchial apparatus. As with thyroglossal duct cysts, they are present at birth but may not become clinically apparent until early childhood into adulthood. The branchial apparatus consists of six pairs of arches separated by four paired grooves externally and by four paired pouches internally. The fifth arch is not apparent in the fetus and is not clinically significant. Each branchial arch is composed of mesodermal condensations in the pharynx with a surface covering of ectoderm around the fourth week. Cartilage and muscles that subsequently develop in each arch are associated with specific cranial nerves and arteries (Table 72–1). Development of this region occurs during the third to seventh embryonic week. Branchial pouches are lined with endoderm, and branchial grooves with ectoderm.

FIRST ARCH

The first branchial arch cartilage is also known as Meckel's cartilage. This gives rise to the maxilla, malleus, incus, mandible, and the sphenomandibular ligament. Muscle derivatives include the mylohyoid, anterior belly of the digastric, tensor tympani, and tensor veli palatini, as well as the muscles of mastication: the masseter, temporalis, and medial and lateral pterygoids. The associated nerve is the trigeminal or fifth cranial nerve. The artery is the first aortic arch artery, which forms the maxillary artery.

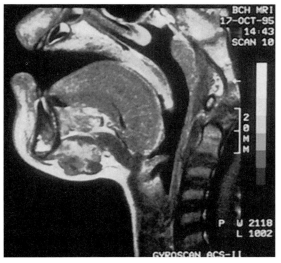

FIGURE 72–2 Dermoid on floor of mouth.

TABLE 72-1 THE BRANCHIAL APPARATUS AND THE HEAD AND NECK: STRUCTURES DERIVED FROM BRANCHIAL ARCH COMPONENTS AND INNERVATION OF THE BRANCHIAL ARCHES

Arch	Nerve	Muscles	Skeletal Structures	Ligaments
First mandibular	Trigeminal (V)	Muscles of mastication Mylohyoid and anterior belly of digastric Tensor tympani Tensor veli palatini	Malleus Incus Mandible	Anterior ligament of malleus Sphenomandibular ligament
Second hyoid	Facial (VII)	Muscles of facial expressions Stapedius Stylohyoid Posterior belly of digastric	Stapes Styloid process Lesser cornu of hyoid Upper part of body of the hyoid bone	Stylohyoid ligament
Third	Glossopharyngeal (IX)	Stylopharyngeus Constrictors	Greater cornu of hyoid Lower part of body of the hyoid bone	
Fourth and sixth	Superior laryngeal branch of vagus (X) Recurrent laryngeal (branch of vagus) (X)	Cricothyroid Levator veli palatini Constrictors of pharynx Intrinsic muscles of larynx	Thyroid cartilage Cricoid cartilage Arytenoid cartilage Corniculate cartilage Cuneiform cartilage	

SECOND ARCH

Cartilage of the second arch is known as Reichert's cartilage and develops into the lesser cornu and upper body of the hyoid bone, the stylohyoid ligament, the styloid process, and the stapes except for the footplate. Its muscles are the muscles of facial expression, the platysma, the stylohyoid, the posterior belly of the digastric, and the stapedius muscles. The nerve of the second arch is the facial or seventh cranial nerve. A portion of the second aortic arch artery may persist as the stapedial artery.

THIRD ARCH

The cartilage of the third arch develops into the greater cornu and lower portion of the body of the hyoid. The muscles of the third arch are the stylopharyngeus and superior and middle constrictors of the pharynx, which are innervated by the nerve of the third arch, the glossopharyngeal, or ninth cranial nerve. The third aortic arch artery persists as part of the internal carotid artery.

FOURTH AND SIXTH ARCH

The fourth arch cartilage develops into the thyroid cartilage. The muscle of the fourth arch is the cricothyroid muscle, which is innervated by the vagus or tenth cranial nerve. Both the sensory and motor component of the vagus develops within this arch. The fourth arch artery becomes the arch of the aorta. The sixth arch cartilage becomes the cricoid and arytenoid cartilages as well as the cuneiform and corniculate cartilages of the larynx. The nerve of the sixth arch is the recurrent laryngeal branch of the vagus, which supplies the inferior constrictor muscles. The sixth arch artery persists as the ductus arteriosus and obliterates in the postnatal period.

PHARYNGEAL POUCHES

Each of the five arches has an intervening pouch and groove. The first pouch forms the eustachian tube and middle ear cleft and the first groove forms the external auditory meatus. The pouch and groove are separated by mesoderm and form the three-layered tympanic membrane.

The palatine tonsil arises from the second pouch. The third pouch forms the inferior parathyroid gland and the thymic duct. The fourth pouch forms the superior parathyroid gland. The sixth pouch forms the ultimobranchial body, which subsequently becomes infiltrated by cells of neurocrest origin and develops into the C cells of the thyroid gland. The remaining grooves of the branchial apparatus are obliterated by the caudal overgrowth of the second branchial arch.

SPECIAL CONSIDERATION

A cyst is a collection of fluid in an epithelium-lined sac. A cyst arising from a branchial groove is lined with squamous epithelium. A cyst arising from a branchial pouch is lined with respiratory epithelium. However, this respiratory epithelium may undergo squamous metaplasia with recurrent infections. A sinus is a tract leading from the epithelial surface into deeper tissues and is often associated with a cystic mass. A fistula is a tract between the skin externally to the pharynx or larynx internally.

BRANCHIAL CLEFT ANOMALIES

Branchial fistulas or sinuses usually become clinically apparent at birth or shortly thereafter. Small openings along the anterior border of the sternocleidomastoid may remain asymptomatic for many years. Recurrent mucoid discharge often associated with upper respiratory tract infections brings these lesions to the attention of the parents and physician. These fistulas may be elucidated with contrast material injected through a small catheter placed within the tract (Fig. 72–4). A complete fistula is uncommon, with most ending before the pharynx is reached.

Branchial cleft cysts are often unnoticed until they become infected, with a subsequent increase in size and tenderness. These masses may present in the neck as a discrete fullness along the anterior border of the sternocleidomastoid. Cysts are more common than fistulas or sinuses. The majority of branchial cleft cysts arise from the second branchial cleft, with the remainder arising from the first branchial cleft. Third and fourth branchial cleft anomalies are very rare.

The usual course of branchial cleft apparatus anomalies is recurrent infection. Surgical excision is performed early rather than later to better ensure that excision is complete. In cases of recurrence a preoperative fistulogram or intraoperative injection of methylene blue into the sinus tract may aid in removal. However, extravasation of contrast material into the surrounding tissues can hinder subsequent removal.

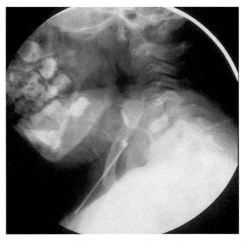

FIGURE 72–4 Contrast study outlining tract of second branchial arch sinus.

FIRST BRANCHIAL CLEFT ANOMALIES

Anomalies of the first branchial cleft are uncommon and fall into two categories. In the first category, absent or abnormal development of the cleft leads to an absent external auditory canal or an aplastic/stenotic canal. The second category is referred to as duplication anomalies and has been characterized by Work (Fig. 72–5). Type I anomalies are duplications of the membranous external auditory canal and are of ectodermal origin. A tract forms that parallels the external auditory canal and may open into the medial canal or middle ear space. Type II first branchial anomalies are considered duplications of both the membranous and bony external auditory canal and are composed of both ectoderm and mesoderm. These lesions are commonly found at the angle of the mandible. If present, a fistula or sinus tract opens into the external auditory canal at the bony cartilaginous junction (Fig. 72–6). Both type I and type II branchial cleft cysts may course above or below the facial nerve, and previous infections can make excision difficult.

> **PEARL•••** Drainage may occur from the external auditory canal with palpation of a preauricular or angle-of-mandible mass. Expression of this material from the ear helps to confirm the embryologic origin of the lesion.

> **PITFALL•••** A common mistake is the failure to recognize a mass in the periparotid region with an opening anterior to the sternocleidomastoid as a potential first branchial cleft cyst. Often a simple incision and drainage are performed, with the surgeon believing this is to be a simple cyst or node, with subsequent recurrence and persistent drainage.

SPECIAL CONSIDERATION

Congenital preauricular sinuses are often confused with first branchial cleft anomalies. However, they are considered a malformation of the six hillocks (from the first and second arches) that form the auricle. The most common lesion is the preauricular sinus or cyst with its opening anterior to the root of the helix. Excision is performed for recurrent infections and drainage.

SECOND BRANCHIAL CLEFT ANOMALIES

Second branchial cleft anomalies are the most common of the branchial defects. If present, fistulous tracts open externally in the lower half of the neck along the anterior border of the sterno-

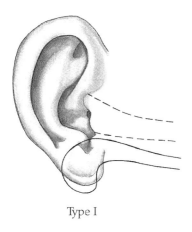
Type I

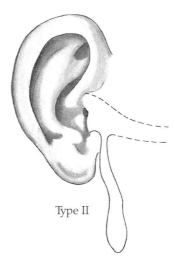
Type II

FIGURE 72–5 First branchial cleft anomalies (type I and type II).

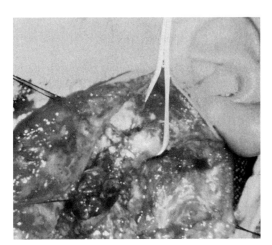

FIGURE 72–6 First branchial cleft cyst (type I) loop at cartilage. See Color Plate 72–6.

cleidomastoid. Cystic dilatations may be seen along the course of the tract. Internal openings, if present, are found in the region of the tonsillar fossa. Surgical removal is typically performed through stepladder incisions. If a sinus tract ex-

ists, an ellipse of skin surrounding the opening is included in the incision.

> **PEARL...** First branchial sinuses open anterior to the sternocleidomastoid muscle above the hyoid, and second branchial sinuses open anterior to the sternocleidomastoid below the thyroid.

Knowledge of the structures associated with each arch is critical in the successful removal of these lesions. The tract of the fistula or sinus will be lateral to the structures found in the lower arches. Following this logic a second branchial arch sinus tract runs externally from the skin through the platysma muscle and deep to the sternocleidomastoid muscle. The tract runs between the internal and external carotid arteries and passes lateral to the hypoglossal and glossopharyngeal nerves (nerves of the third and fourth arch) and continues inferior to the posterior belly of the digastric, opening into the region of the tonsillar fossa (Fig. 72–7).

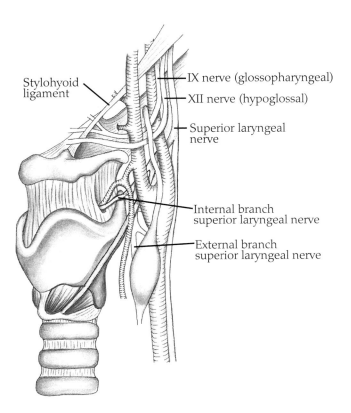

Stylohyoid ligament

IX nerve (glossopharyngeal)

XII nerve (hypoglossal)

Superior laryngeal nerve

Internal branch superior laryngeal nerve

External branch superior laryngeal nerve

FIGURE 72–7 Second branchial cleft anomalies.

THIRD BRANCHIAL CLEFT CYSTS

Third branchial cleft cysts are very rare and present similarly to their second branchial arch counterparts. Anatomically the tract courses posterior and lateral to the internal carotid artery and hypoglossal nerve, terminating its course in the pharynx at the level of the piriform sinus (Fig. 72–8).

LYMPHANGIOMAS (CYSTIC HYGROMA)

Lymphangiomas, also known as cystic hygromas, are uncommon congenital masses. They arise from abnormal lymphatic development along the jugular lymphatic sacs; 50% of these lesions present by 1 year of age, and 90% present by age 2. There is no gender predilection.

Embryologically, this malformation occurs in the sixth week of embryonic development. Narrow outpouchings composed of thin-walled endothelial-lined cysts infiltrate into the surrounding tissues. Arrested development leads to sequestration of tissue, which does not communicate with the rest of the lymphatic system.

Lymphangiomas can be classified into three groups: lymphangioma simplex, consisting of thin-walled lymphatic channels; cavernous lymphangiomas, which are composed of larger lymphatic channels; and cystic hygromas, which con-

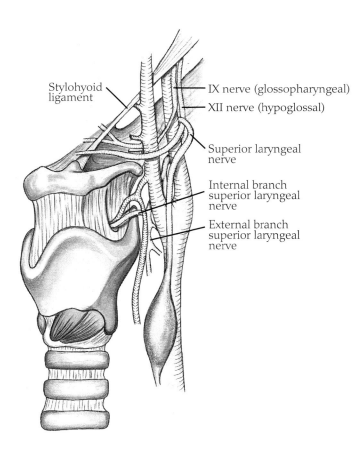

Stylohyoid ligament

IX nerve (glossopharyngeal)

XII nerve (hypoglossal)

Superior laryngeal nerve

Internal branch superior laryngeal nerve

External branch superior laryngeal nerve

FIGURE 72–8 Third branchial cleft anomalies.

tain large lymphatic dilatations. Practically, most lesions on histologic examination are composed of all three types and subclassification does not have diagnostic significance. Clinically, these lesions present most often in the posterior cervical triangle of the neck and are soft, nontender, poorly defined masses that transilluminate.

Acute enlargement is often temporally related to a concurrent upper respiratory tract infection. Evaluation is performed with a combination of computed tomography scanning and endoscopy. Involvement of the oral cavity, hypopharynx, and larynx poses the most immediate risk to the patient and may necessitate tracheostomy for airway protection. On endoscopy, thin-walled cystic lesions are seen submucosally. Imaging of both the neck and thorax is required to evaluate the extent of the lesion. Multiloculated cystic masses in radiologic imaging are pathognomonic for this condition (Fig. 72–9).

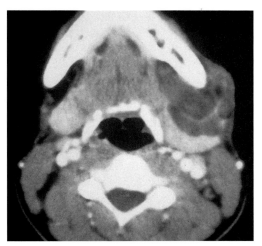

FIGURE 72–9 Computed tomography of cystic hygroma.

CONTROVERSY

Surgical excision is the treatment of choice; however, the timing of surgery is dependent on the surgeon's personal philosophy. Those advocating early excision point to the possibility of infection, rapid growth, and potential airway compromise. Others recommend waiting until the child is 3 to 4 years of age because of the possibility of involution and the relative technical ease of operating on an older child.

The main principle of lymphangioma removal is preservation of all vital structures. Because of the infiltrating nature of this lesion, portions of the lesion are left behind at the time of surgical resection. Partial staged resections are often required, especially in large suprahyoid lesions. Use of the CO_2 laser aids in the treatment of pharyngeal and laryngeal lesions. Therapies such as radiation therapy and sclerosing agents have been tried without success and cause significant fibrosis, which hinders subsequent surgical dissection. A lower than expected recurrence rate of 10 to 15% may be due to postoperative scarring limiting further growth.

HEMANGIOMAS

Hemangiomas are the most common benign tumors of infancy, with a majority of lesions recognized by 6 months of age. They are the result of defective embryonic development of the peripheral blood vessels. Angiocysts form interconnected endothelial blood lakes, which then coalesce into capillary networks with distinct arteries and veins. Arrested development at the endothelial stage gives rise to these subcutaneous vascular masses. They are classified histologically as capillary, cavernous, and juvenile.

Hemangiomas in the head and neck appear as soft, compressible, nonpulsatile bluish masses. Involvement may include the parotid, neck, tongue, and skin. They may enlarge with crying or staining. Growth can be rapid in the neonatal period, but spontaneous involution may occur in 50% of children by age 5, and 70% by age 7. Lesions that do not involve critical structures, such as the airway or the orbit, are usually observed as the cosmetic result after involution is better than after surgical resection.

Radiologic evaluation includes computed tomography, which will outline the limits of the lesion but is not specific for this type of tumor. Angiography is useful for both diagnosis and embolization prior to resection. Embolization alone does not retard the growth of the lesion. Lesions that are symptomatic may be treated with a course of corticosteroids. In addition, interferon-α_{2a} has been used in patients with massive lesions with some success.

CONTROVERSY

The use of radiation therapy is controversial, with complications including skin atrophy, fibrosis of underlying tissues, potential arrest of growth, and risk of malignancy seen as potentially unacceptable side affects. However, its use is reported in the literature with low complication rates, and this likely reflects the type of radiation schedule and dosing used.

Surgical excision is performed on lesions involving critical areas, and those exhibiting spontaneous bleeding, recurrent infection, or the presence of consumption coagulopathies.

FIBROMATOSIS COLLI

Fibromatosis colli is a congenital tumor of the sternocleidomastoid. The mass is often detected 2 to 3 weeks after birth in an otherwise healthy child. The mass is firm, nontender, and intimately involved with the underlying muscle. Torticollis may be a part of the presenting symptoms, and physical therapy has been advocated to prevent any long-term difficulties. Although its origin is unknown, it has been associated with difficult vaginal deliveries and subsequent traction on the head and neck during delivery. These masses usually resolve by 18 months of age. The diagnosis can be confirmed by the clinical appearance and by ultrasound demonstrating the intimate nature of the lesion with the underlying sternocleidomastoid muscle. Surgery is indicated for lesions that do not resolve after 18 months or in children with persistent torticollis.

SUGGESTED READINGS

Cunningham MJ. The management of congenital neck masses. *Am J Otolaryngol* 1992;13(2): 78–92.

Guarisco JL. Congenital head and neck masses in infants and children. *Ear Nose Throat* 1991; 70(1,2):75–82.

May M. Neck masses in children: diagnosis and treatment. *Pediatr Ann* 1976;5(8):518–535.

Myers E, Cunningham M. Inflammatory presentations of congenital head and neck masses. *Pediatr Infect Dis J* 1988;7:S162–S168.

Rood S, Johnson J, Myers E, et al. Congenital masses of the head and neck. *J Postgrad Med* 1982;72:141–149.

Sonnino RE, Spigland N, Laberge JM, Desjardins J, Guttman FM. Unusual patterns of congenital neck masses in children. *J Pediatr Surg* 1999;24(10):966–996.

Torsiglieri AJ, Tom LW, Ross AJ III, Wetmore RF, Handler SD, Potsic WP. Pediatric neck masses: guidelines for evaluation. *Int J Pediatr Otorhinolaryngol* 1988;16:199–210.

Chapter 73

INFECTIOUS AND INFLAMMATORY DISORDERS

Tapan A. Padhya and Jack L. Gluckman

LYMPHATIC INFECTIONS

The lymphatic tissue in the neck accounts for one-third of all nodal tissue in the entire body. Most cervical lymph nodes are located in the anterior triangle traversing along the carotid sheath from the skull base to the thoracic inlet (Fig. 73–1). In general, the pattern of nodal involvement from cutaneous, dental, and mucosal upper aerodigestive tract infections occurs in a predictable and sequential manner. Extracapsular extension of infection from the involved nodes occupies the potential neck space in which they are located. Once one neck space is involved, adjacent spaces can also become involved by the infectious process. In general there is a continuum from isolated lymphadenitis to frank neck abscess.

Nodal groups should be defined by their specific anatomic location; however, most surgeons now refer to nodal levels in describing nodal groups involved by infectious and malignant disease (see Chapter 71).

CERVICAL LYMPHADENITIS

Infectious involvement of cervical lymph nodes is most often implicated in bacterial and viral infections of the upper aerodigestive tract. Clinically palpable, tender, and possibly fluctuant nodes are common in the pediatric population.

PEARL... Viral infections usually affect bilateral nodal groups and may accompany systemic symptoms. Bacterial infections are usually unilateral and have a higher propensity for suppuration.

Acute bacterial lymphadenitis is most commonly caused by group A β-hemolytic streptococcus or *Staphylococcus aureus*. Viral involvement, cat-scratch disease, mycobacterium tuberculosis, atypical mycobacterium, and toxoplasmosis account for a more chronic form of lymphadenitis.

A thorough history should be the starting point in evaluating cervical lymphadenitis. The patient's age, duration of symptoms, possible infectious contacts, animal exposure, recent travel, consumption of poorly handled foods, and coexisting conditions are very important in establishing a differential diagnosis. Physical inspection includes site, size, and inflammatory characteristics of the involved node(s). Looking for coexisting head and neck disease and systemic disease is imperative.

Diagnostic tests include needle aspiration, excisional biopsy, and incision and drainage for acute suppuration. All obtained fluid or tissue should be submitted for Gram stain, acid-fast bacterial stain, and cultures for aerobic and anaerobic bacteria. Additional special stains can be

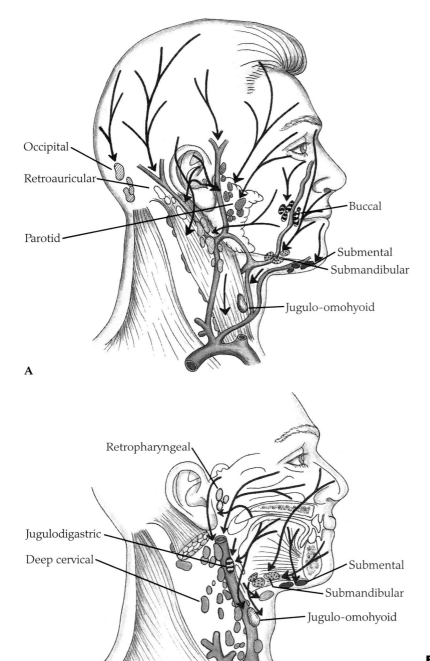

Occipital

Retroauricular

Parotid

Buccal

Submental

Submandibular

Jugulo-omohyoid

A

Retropharyngeal

Jugulodigastric

Deep cervical

Submental

Submandibular

Jugulo-omohyoid

B

FIGURE 73–1 Superficial (A) and deep drainage (B) of the neck.

utilized for viral, fungal, and unusual bacterial organisms.

Serology may include a white blood cell count with differential, sedimentation rate, and serum immunoglobin titers. Tuberculin skin test-

ing is very important in patients suspected of having a mycobacterium infection. Imaging such as a lateral neck X ray or a chest X ray may be indicated for possible coexisting sources of infection. An axial computed tomography (CT) scan with intravenous contrast, except in acutely toxic patients, is usually reserved until primary therapy proves unresponsive.

Treatment for suppurative lymphadenitis is oral or intravenous broad-spectrum antibiotics with surgery reserved for refractory cases. Antibiotic choices may include penicillin, first- and second-generation cephalosporins, and clindamycin. Treatment for most viral infections with lymphadenitis is usually supportive including analgesics and antipyretics. Occasionally, a warm compress on the affected nodes will ease the associated discomfort and will possibly hasten abscess formation.

Viral infection remains the most common cause of cervical lymphadenitis. Common viral pathogens include respiratory syncytial virus, parainfluenza, adenovirus, enterovirus, herpes simplex virus, Epstein-Barr virus, cytomegalovirus, and human immunodeficiency virus. Viral infections are commonly associated with generalized lymphadenopathy and occasional exanthems. Lymphadenitis present for more than 1 week is highly suggestive of a viral or granulomatous origin.

Group A β-hemolytic streptococcus and *S. aureus* account for the vast majority of unilateral cervical lymphadenitis. These organisms should be suspected especially if suppuration is present. Lymphadenitis present for 1 to 3 days again points to a bacterial origin. The nodes most often affected include the submandibular triangle (level I) and upper jugulodigastric nodes (level II). Treatment with oral antibiotics should be considered as a first-line treatment.

Cat-scratch disease presents in late fall and most of winter. Greater than 90% of patients have a history of cat exposure and/or cat scratch. The offending organism is the bacteria *Bartonella henselae,* which first causes axillary adenopathy followed by cervical adenopathy. A skin lesion occurs 7 to 14 days at the site of inoculation. One to two weeks later, tender lymphadenitis occurs. These nodes can remain enlarged for up to 4 months. Treatment for cat-scratch is usually observation unless the patient exhibits toxic symptoms, in which case azithromycin may be helpful. Needle aspiration may relieve acute pain and discomfort. Incision and drainage should be avoided.

Mycobacterium species (*Mycobacterium tuberculosis* and atypical mycobacterium) account for the most cases of chronic, unilateral, suppurative cervical lymphadenitis. Other species of note include *M. avium-intracellulare, M. scrofulceum,* and *M. malmoense.* A positive tuberculin skin test will differentiate *M. tuberculosis* from atypical mycobacterium. Involved nodes may undergo spontaneous rupture with purulent drainage and are minimally tender.

SPECIAL CONSIDERATION

M. tuberculosis has a high association with concomitant pulmonary disease, whereas atypical mycobacterium is rarely associated with pulmonary involvement.

Treatment for lymphadenitis due to *M. tuberculosis* is medical therapy using rifampin, isoniazid, and pyrazinamide, instituted for 6 months. Treatment for atypical mycobacterium is usually surgical excision in conjunction with oral clarithromycin.

Toxoplasma gondii is a protozoan that uses the cat as a host and is excreted in cat feces as oocytes. Infection via undercooked meats and unpasteurized milk can cause mononucleosis-like viral illness in immunocompetent patients. In immunocompromised patients, such as those with human immunodeficiency virus (HIV), the central nervous system is targeted as well as other major organ systems.

Dental caries and gingivitis implicate anaerobic species and actinomyces as possible sources of cervical lymphadenitis. Fungal oral candidiasis may have cervical node involvement in immunosuppressed patients. Herpes simplex and enterovirus are implicated in gingivostomatitis.

Kawasaki disease is an inflammatory condition that is diagnosed with five hallmark features: (1) fever, (2) rash, (3) nonpurulent conjunctivitis, (4) mucositis, and (5) cervical lymphadenopathy. The pediatric population is most commonly affected, especially those under 4 years of age. A toxin of *S. aureus* had been implicated as a possible etiology.

FASCIAL SPACE INFECTIONS

The fascial spaces of the neck are potential spaces (see also Chapter 71). Intimate knowledge of the interrelationship of these spaces is especially important when dealing with neck infections but is of less significance in surgery for cervical metastases.

The submandibular space is bounded superiorly by the mucosa of the floor of the mouth and inferiorly by the hyoid bone, extending from the lower border of the mandible anteriorly to the tongue musculature posteriorly. The mylohyoid muscle subdivides the space into the sublingual and submaxillary spaces. The submandibular gland traverses both subspaces, but the hypoglossal nerve, lingual nerve, sublingual gland, and submandibular duct are all located solely within the sublingual space. The submental space, which is continuous with the submandibular space, is located between the two anterior bellies of the digastric muscle and the symphysis of the mandible.

The peritonsillar space is a potential space located between the fibrous capsule of the palatine tonsil and the pharyngeal fascia/superior constrictor musculature.

The masticator space contains the pterygoid muscles, temporalis muscle, and masseter muscle, all of which are enveloped by the superficial layer of the deep cervical fascia. The parotid space, which contains the parotid gland and intraparotid nodes, abuts the lateral aspect of the masticator space and can connect to the parapharyngeal space. Numerous septa perforate the gland, and so parotid space infections are often loculated.

DEEP NECK SPACES

The parapharyngeal space extends from the skull base to the hyoid bone. It is bounded medially by the pharyngeal constrictors and laterally by the mandible, pterygoid musculature, and parotid gland. The styloid process separates the space into an anterior prestyloid compartment and a posterior postyloid compartment. The prestyloid compartment contains fat, the parotid gland, the internal maxillary artery, the lingual nerve, and the inferior alveolar nerve. The poststyloid compartment includes the internal ca-

rotid artery; the internal jugular vein; cranial nerves IX, X, XI, and XII; the cervical sympathetic chain; and lymph nodes. The parapharyngeal space communicates with the submandibular space (anteriorly), the parotid space (posterolaterally), the masticator spaces (laterally), the carotid sheath (posteriorly), and the retropharyngeal space (posteromedially). Because of this, the parapharyngeal space is commonly involved in deep cervical space infections.

The retropharyngeal space is between the midline pharyngeal mucosa and the alar or prevertebral fascia and contains connective tissue and lymph nodes. This space extends from the skull base to the tracheal bifurcation. Infection of this space can therefore extend inferiorly into the mediastinum and into the parapharyngeal space. Deep to the alar or prevertebral fascia lies the true prevertebral space (danger space), which extends along the entire length of the spinal column.

PATHOPHYSIOLOGY OF NECK SPACE INFECTIONS

The medical literature cites the most common sources of neck space infections as dental followed by the oropharyngeal sites. In the preantibiotic era, the tonsils and pharynx were responsible for 70% and the dentition for 20% of infections. In the antibiotic era, tonsils and pharynx account for 30%, a dental etiology for 30%, followed by cervical adenitis, trauma, and most recently intravenous drug use especially in larger urban areas.

The bacteriology of neck space infections usually exhibits a mixed flora with anaerobic abscesses predominating over aerobic abscesses. Anaerobic species include *Peptostreptococcus*, *Bacteroides*, anaerobic *Staphylococcus*. Aerobic organisms include *S. aureus*, *Streptococcus* species, *Haemophilus influenzae*, *Escherichia coli*, and *Klebsiella*.

MANAGEMENT OF NECK SPACE INFECTIONS

Patient evaluation begins with a complete history, which includes recent dental work, dental pain, intravenous drug abuse, a recent upper respiratory tract infection, recent surgery, and trauma. The history will help to localize nodes and spaces at risk. Next, a thorough physical should be performed including inspection of the dentition and palpation of the soft tissue of the head and neck. A patient's vital signs such as temperature, pulse, respiratory rate, and blood pressure may all indicate a more serious evolving process.

Radiography can be a useful tool in determining an overall treatment plan. A lateral neck film may show widening of the long neck spaces, especially the retropharyngeal space, which is commonly involved in children.

> **PEARL...** The lateral neck film may show increased prevertebral width (>7 mm at C2, >20 mm at C6).

The presence of gas on plain film is an indication for surgical drainage. A chest roentograph must always be performed to assess possible mediastinal involvement.

Fluctuance is the exception rather than the rule in deep neck spaces, and an axial CT scan with intravenous contrast is very beneficial in these cases. The CT scan will enhance frank abscess pockets and give valuable information regarding proximity to vital structures like the carotid sheath.

> **SPECIAL CONSIDERATION**
>
> In patients who are initially managed with intravenous antibiotics, a CT scan should be used only when the patient is not progressing as expected.

Serology tests such as a white blood cell count with differential, sedimentation rate, and electrolyte profile will give additional insight as to the patient's current status. Wound cultures via needle aspiration are not routinely obtained unless the patient is immunocompromised or the infection is unresponsive or life-threatening.

In cases where there is a question of cellulitis versus abscess, 12 to 24 hours of antibiotics will usually decide the issue. Failure to improve after 24 hours of antibiotics is an indication for surgery.

> **SPECIAL CONSIDERATION**
>
> Airway control is the first priority when the submandibular, parapharyngeal space, and retropharyngeal spaces are involved.

When a patient has severe trismus or Ludwig's angina, a tracheotomy should be performed. In patient's with a retropharyngeal abscess, there is a potential risk of rupture and subsequent aspiration during intubation. If the surgeon opts for intubation, Trendelenburg positioning with frequent suctioning may be an option.

Antimicrobial coverage for deep neck space infections includes clindamycin as a first-line choice. Alternative choices may include ampicillin/sulbactam, cefuroxime plus Flagyl, and amoxicillin/clavulanate.

Surgical drainage of a neck space abscess includes wide exposure, vascular identification and control, drainage of all septated pockets of pus, copious irrigation, and finally the placement of drains. Blunt dissection is accomplished with a hemostat. Most surgeons prefer to leave the drains in place for a duration of 3 to 5 days. Intraoperative wound cultures should be obtained for a more organism-directed use of antibiotics.

Drainage of the canine and sublingual spaces can be achieved intraorally with frequent suctioning. The buccal space can be drained via an intraoral or extraoral approach. The masticator, submandibular, and submental spaces should be drained through an incision below and parallel to the lower border of the mandible (Fig. 73–2). The peritonsillar space can be aspirated and/or incised transorally in adults but general anesthesia may be required in children. The parapharyngeal space, although contiguous with many other spaces, must be accessed through a transcervical incision. This incision is placed two finger breadths below the mandible horizontally or can extend along the anterior

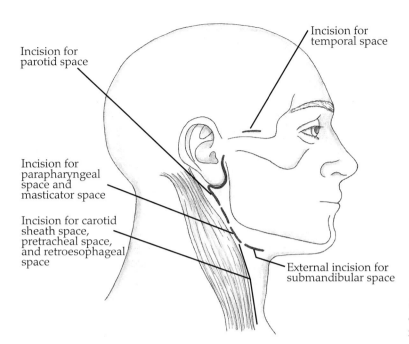

Incision for temporal space

Incision for parotid space

Incision for parapharyngeal space and masticator space

Incision for carotid sheath space, pretracheal space, and retroesophageal space

External incision for submandibular space

FIGURE 73–2 Incisions for draining the fascial spaces in the neck.

border of the sternocleidomastoid muscle. Identifying and isolating the carotid sheath is imperative before any further dissection or drainage procedure is performed. The retropharyngeal space can be drained transorally; however, any possibility of aspiration or extension into the parapharyngeal space should make one access the abscess through a transcervical approach. The parotid space should be drained through a standard Blair/parotidectomy incision.

Intravenous antibiotics should be used liberally and rearranged once culture results return. Frequent wound dressing changes and wound surveillance is imperative. Should the patient not improve, repeat CT imaging followed by repeat surgical drainage may be required.

NECROTIZING FASCIITIS

Necrotizing fasciitis is extremely rare in the head and neck, with fewer that 70 cases reported in the literature. One must keep a strong index of suspicion, especially if an infection progresses rapidly or is unresponsive to standard management principles. Necrotizing fasciitis usually occurs in the extremities, trunk, and perineum. Etiologies include dental abscesses, blunt or penetrating trauma, peritonsillar abscess, osteoradionecrosis, insect bites, burns,

lacerations, and needle punctures. Dental abscesses account for most cervical infections, whereas trauma usually affects the midface and lower face. In most of the cases reported, patients possess some predisposition to infection, such as diabetes mellitus, peripheral vascular disease, cirrhosis, previous malignancy, immunosuppression, or alcoholism. At least 50% of patients with cervicofacial necrotizing fasciitis have at least one predisposing factor.

The infectious process may arise over a few hours or a few days after the initial insulting event and progress rapidly. Usually there is a central zone of necrosis, surrounded by a tender purplish area, which is encircled by a wide peripheral zone of erythema. Probing of the central necrosis will allow the surgeon to palpate down to the fascia. Also of note is the lack of frank purulence and the presence of thin gray "dishwater" exudate emanating from the necrotic area. Subcutaneous emphysema may be a hallmark feature of rapidly progressing disease. The patient usually presents in a toxic state with hyperpyrexia, tachypnea, tachycardia, and progressive lethargy.

Treatment involves correction of any electrolyte imbalance, anemia, and hypovolemia. Immediate wide surgical debridement is the keystone to treatment. The patient usually is treated concurrently with broad-spectrum antibiotics. Postoperative care includes aggressive bedside dressing changes and frequent debridements under general anesthesia. The benefit of hyperbaric oxygen should be considered but should not replace aggressive surgical treatment.

SUGGESTED READINGS

Fairbanks DNF. *Antimicrobial Therapy in Otolaryngology–Head and Neck Surgery.* 9th ed. Alexandria, VA: American Academy of Otolaryngology–Head and Neck Surgery Foundation; 1999.

Har-El G, Aroesty JH, Shaha A, Lucente FE. Changing trends in deep neck abscess. A retrospective study of 110 patients. *Oral Surg Oral Med Oral Pathol* 1994;77:446.

Hollinshead WH. *Anatomy for Surgeons–The Head and Neck.* 3rd ed. Philadelphia: Lippincott; 1982.

Johnson JT. Abscesses and deep space infections of the head and neck. *Infect Dis Clin North Am* 1992;6:705.

Moloy PJ. *Diagnosis of Inflammatory Disease in Cervical Lymph Nodes.* Alexandria, VA: American Academy of Otolaryngology–Head and Neck Surgery Foundation; 1987.

Moore KL. *Clinically Oriented Anatomy.* 4th. Philadelphia: Lippincott; 1999.

Rabuzzi DD, Johnson JT, Weissman JL. *Diagnosis and Management of Deep Neck Infections.* 3rd ed. Alexandria, VA: American Academy of Otolaryngology–Head and Neck Surgery Foundation; 1993.

Chapter 74

Neoplasms and Cysts

Jack L. Gluckman

This chapter describes tumors arising in the soft tissues of the neck that are nonlymphatic in origin, that is, excluding lymph node metastases and lymphoma and those from salivary glands and thyroid. These tumors are quite rare but need to be considered in the evaluation of a patient with a mass in the neck.

TUMORS OF NEUROGENIC ORIGIN

Peripheral nerves are surrounded by Schwann cells (neural crest origin) and fibroblasts (mesenchymal origin), both of which can be the precursor of neurogenic tumors. Although there are a host of obscure tumors that can be included in the differential diagnosis, only the commonly occurring tumors will be discussed.

NEUROMA

This is not a true neoplasm but rather a regenerative process secondary to trauma—usually iatrogenic. It consists of a mass of Schwann cells, endoneural and perineural connective tissue, and axons that present as a small subcutaneous mass usually in a previously operated neck.

> **PEARL•••** Pressure on the mass causes a shock-like sensation, which is diagnostic.

Treatment, if indicated at all, is surgical excision.

SCHWANNOMA

Schwannomas arise from the nerve sheath and are solitary, discrete, and well encapsulated. The axons of the nerve of origin are displaced by the tumor. The histologic appearance is classical, consisting of varying elements of Antoni–A tissue (palisading pattern of Schwann cell nuclei surrounding a central mass of cytoplasm known as Verocay bodies) and Antoni–B tissue (loose textured with no distinct pattern). Immunohistochemically the tumor stains positively for S-100 protein.

The neck is a common site for these tumors. Although it is often difficult to identify the nerve of origin, the tumor may arise from cranial nerves IX, X, XI, or XII, the brachial plexus, or the cervical plexus. It is usually asymptomatic and slow growing, but occasionally is associated with neuralgic-like pain. Malignant degeneration is rare.

The imaging findings, particularly on magnetic resonance imaging (MRI), are quite characteristic, consisting of a fusiform mass with central cystic areas, which may be misinterpreted as malignant degeneration. The mass is hypovascular but shows up brightly on T2-weighted imaging. Treatment consists of surgical excision by means of subcapsular dissection. This technique frequently permits preservation of nerve function. Malignant schwannoma is treated with wide resection and radiation with or without chemotherapy, with a 50 to 75% 5-year survival rate.

NEUROFIBROMA

These tumors can be solitary but usually are multiple in patients with von Recklinghausen's disease (multiple neurofibromatosis). This is an autosomal-dominant disorder characterized by café-au-lait spots and multiple subcutaneous nodules. In this syndrome the neurofibromas may present as solitary or multiple encapsulated masses or as plexiform neurofibromas with characteristic fusiform multilobular enlargement ("bag of worms"). They may arise from peripheral nerves or cranial nerves.

> **SPECIAL CONSIDERATION**
>
> Unlike schwannomas, the axons are present within the tumor, and hence nerve function cannot be preserved during surgical excision.

Solitary neurofibromas can easily be removed. However, in plexiform neurofibromatosis, surgery should only be considered if a malignancy is suspected or there is pressure on surrounding vital structures. Malignant degeneration is associated with a poor prognosis. Clinical features suggestive of malignancy include rapid growth, nerve dysfunction, and pain. Treatment of a malignant neurofibroma is surgery, radiation, and chemotherapy, with a poor 15 to 30% 5-year survival rate.

PARAGANGLIOMA

Extraadrenal paragangliomas are derived from neural-crest–derived cells, which are related to the arterial vasculature, cranial nerves, and sympathetic ganglia. The most common head and neck sites for paragangliomas are the carotid body (carotid body tumor), the jugulotympanic

area (glomus jugulare and glomus tympanicum), and intravagal (glomus vagale). Less commonly, they may arise in the orbit and larynx.

The inheritance pattern is autosomal dominant modified by genomic imprinting.

> **SPECIAL CONSIDERATION**
>
> Children of female carriers will never develop tumors but will carry the gene in 50% of cases. Children of male carriers will have a 50% incidence of developing tumors.

In general, paragangliomas are very slow growing with only the carotid body tumor and vagal paraganglioma presenting as a neck mass. They may be multicentric, 2 to 10% in sporadic cases and 25 to 50% if familial; they are rarely malignant and very occasionally secrete catecholamines. Manifestations of catecholamine secretion include episodic or sustained hypertension, headache, palpitations, and excessive sweating. Malignancy usually manifests as metastases to nodes, lung, liver, and bone. It occurs in under 1% of cases.

CAROTID BODY TUMOR

This is the most common head and neck paraganglioma. It arises from the carotid body, presenting as a slowly increasing neck mass. It usually is asymptomatic, although cranial nerve palsies in large lesions have been described, particularly vagal and hypoglossal palsy.

> **PEARL...** Clinically it is firm to palpation and is characterized as being freely mobile from side to side but not in a vertical direction.

Carotid bruit may be present if the lesion is large enough to compress the artery.

Although the diagnosis is easily apparent on magnetic resonance angiography (MRA) and angiography, these tests are not essential to confirming the diagnosis. Biopsy is not neces-

> **PEARL•••** Diagnosis is confirmed by the finding on imaging of a vascular tumor, splaying the internal and external carotid arteries apart. This is well demonstrated on both MRI and computed tomography (CT) scan.

sary and is discouraged. MRI is useful in identifying multicentric disease. Similarly, an octreotide study can be used to rule out other paragangliomas elsewhere. Angiography is particularly useful for larger lesions in determining ipsilateral and contralateral cerebral blood flow and identification of vessels for preoperative embolization.

The mainstay of treatment is surgical, although observation for very early lesions or patients ineligible for surgery is a consideration given the tumor's slow rate of growth. Radiation can be considered in lesions that are thought to warrant treatment but are not surgical candidates for any reason. The main concern regarding surgical resection is the risk of carotid injury and cranial nerve deficit, particularly in the larger lesions. This should always be a consideration in deciding how best to manage an individual patient.

Preoperative embolization is only indicated for large lesions. Small tumors are easily dissected free of the carotid system once a suitable subadventitial plane has been obtained. Larger lesions and lesions that are firmly adherent to the carotid system may necessitate carotid resection and replacement.

VAGAL PARAGANGLIOMA (GLOMUS VAGALE)

These tumors arise from paraganglionic tissue within the perineurium of the vagus just below or at the ganglion nodosum. These tumors usually present as a slow-growing neck mass but may extend intracranially through the skull base. They may manifest as a parapharyngeal mass.

Diagnostic workup includes CT scan, MRI and/or MRA, and usually angiography to determine tumor extent, skull base involvement, and possible intracranial extension. Angiography may display feeder vessels that can be embolized preoperatively.

Treatment consists of surgical excision, which necessitates sacrifice of the vagus nerve.

> **PEARL•••** The patient should clearly understand the functional consequences of this and rehabilitative steps necessary postoperatively.

Radiation has been used for those patients not deemed suitable for surgery with reportedly good results.

TUMORS OF VASCULAR ORIGIN

ANGIOSARCOMA

The most common sites for angiosarcoma are the scalp and the soft tissues of the neck. This tumor arises from vascular endothelial cells and is therefore very vascular.

> **PITFALL•••** Angiosarcoma presents in the neck as a cutaneous or subcutaneous ill-defined mass and is often mistaken for a bruise or hemangioma, thereby delaying diagnosis.

It infiltrates the surrounding tissues and may spread to regional nodes or more commonly distantly by hematogenous spread.

Treatment consists of wide resection followed by postoperative radiation with an overall poor 5-year survival of 12 to 33%.

HEMANGIOPERICYTOMA

These uncommon tumors arise from the pericytes of Zimmermann that surround capillaries; 15 to 25% arise in the head and neck area, although rarely primarily in the neck itself. In the neck they present as fairly rapidly growing masses. They are extremely vascular and tend to infiltrate the surrounding tissues. The behavior of these tumors is highly unpredictable, with a high local recurrence rate and propensity for distant metastases even many years later.

Treatment consists of wide local excision, but local recurrence is common because of inadequate excision. Postoperative radiation is usually recommended.

TUMORS OF ADIPOSE ORIGIN

LIPOMA

This is the most common tumor of mesenchymal origin, with approximately 13% occurring in the head and neck. It presents as an asymptomatic subcutaneous mass, which is soft to palpation. Treatment consists of local excision. Hibernomas are tumors of immature (brown) fat that likewise present as a subcutaneous mass indistinguishable grossly from regular lipomas.

Benign symmetric lipomatosis (Madelung disease) is characterized by the presence of nonencapsulated fat in the neck and shoulder area. It commonly affects middle-aged men of Mediterranean descent. It may cause cosmetic deformity, impaired range of motion, and even airway obstruction due to compression. Conservative resection for cosmetic and functional reasons is appropriate.

LIPOSARCOMA

This is the second most common soft tissue sarcoma after fibrous histiocytoma in adults; however, it rarely occurs primarily in the neck. It has a propensity to local infiltration and distant metastases. The well-differentiated and myxoid types have a good prognosis, whereas the round cell and pleomorphic variants have a poor 5-year survival. Distant metastases and local re-

currence are the common cause of failure. Treatment consists of local excision with postoperative radiation.

TUMORS OF FIBROUS ORIGIN

COLLAGENOUS FIBROMA (DESMOPLASTIC FIBROMA)

This is a benign, well-circumscribed, fibrous tumor. Histologically it is hypocellular, consisting of spindle and stellate-shaped cells that are arranged haphazardly and separated by bundles of collagen and fibromyxoid stroma. Treatment consists of local excision.

AGGRESSIVE FIBROMATOSIS (DESMOID FIBROMATOSIS)

Also known as extraabdominal desmoid tumors, fibromatosis is seen more commonly in females. It may arise anywhere in the neck, invading and surrounding vital structures. It usually presents as a painless mass that is nondiscrete. Histologically it characteristically consists of an infiltrating mass of mature fibrous tissue, that is, mature fibroblasts, lacking mitotic figures, arranged in interlacing fascicles surrounded by a dense collagen matrix.

Preoperative MRI or CT scan is useful in delineating the lesion.

Treatment consists of wide resection and postoperative radiation. Intraoperatively it is difficult to discern the extent of the tumor.

Local recurrence is a common phenomenon.

FIBROSARCOMA

Improvement in pathologic diagnostic techniques resulted in the differentiation of many similar-appearing lesions such as aggressive fibromatosis. Fibrosarcomas can be divided into low- and high-grade types with good correlation between the degree of differentiation and prognosis. Treatment consists of wide local excision with postoperative radiotherapy with or without various chemotherapy regimes. Local recurrence is a common cause of failure, as are distant metastases.

FIBROSING CERVICITIS

This is not a true neoplasm, but it is important to consider in the differential diagnosis of tumors of fibrous origin. It is similar to other idiopathic fibrosing syndromes, including Riedel's thyroiditis, sclerosing cholangitis, and retroperitoneal fibrosis. It causes obstructive symptoms by gradually encompassing vital structures in the neck. A trial of steroids may be useful, but surgical excision is probably the treatment of choice.

TUMORS OF SKELETAL MUSCLE ORIGIN

RHABDOMYOMA

Adult rhabdomyoma is rare and occurs almost exclusively in the head and neck, with 25% arising in the soft tissue of the neck. Patients present with a gradually increasing neck mass. Histologically, it is characterized by the presence of large cells with abundant glycogen and granular eosinophilic cytoplasm. Treatment consists of surgical excision.

RHABDOMYOMASARCOMA

This is the most common soft tissue sarcoma in children and can occur anywhere in the head and neck, but rarely is the neck itself the site of origin. Traditionally, there are four histologic types: embryonal, botryoid, alveolar, and pleomorphic. It usually presents with a neck mass infiltrating into surrounding structures. Distant metastases need to be excluded. Prognosis has improved dramatically with multimodal therapy combining surgery, radiation, and multiagent chemotherapy.

CONTROVERSY

The exact role of surgery remains controversial, with some surgeons proposing wide resection, others debulking, and yet others only recommending surgery for salvage.

SUGGESTED READINGS

Biller HF, Lawson W, Som P. Glomus vagale tumors. *Ann Otol Rhinol Laryngol* 1989;98:21–26.

Evans HL, Soule EH, Winklemann RK. Atypical lipoma, atypical intramuscular lipoma and well-differentiated retroperitoneal liposarcoma: a reappraisal of 30 cases formerly classified as well-differentiated liposarcoma. *Cancer* 1979;43:574–584.

Kwekkeboom DJ, Van Urk H, Pauw B. Octreotide scintigraphy for the detection of paragangliomas. *J Nucl Med* 1993;34:873–878.

Lydiatt WM, Shaha AR, Shah J. Angiosarcoma of the head and neck. *Am J Surg* 1994;168: 451–454.

Mark RJ, Tran LM, Secarz J. Angiosarcoma of the head and neck: the UCLA experience 1955 through 1990. *Arch Otolaryngol Head Neck Surg* 1993;119:973–978.

McCaffrey TV, Meyer FB, Michaels VV. Familial paragangliomas of the head and neck. *Arch Otolaryngol Head Neck Surg* 1996;120:1211–1216.

Nielsen G, O'Connell J, Dickersin G. Collagenous fibroma (desmoplastic fibroblastoma): a report of seven cases. *Mod Pathol* 1996;9:781–785.

Olsen KD, DeSanto LW, Wold LE, Weiland LH. Tumefactive fibro-inflammatory lesions of the head and neck. *Laryngoscope* 1986;96: 940–944.

Staples JJ, Robinson RA, Wen BC. Hemangiopericytoma—the role of radiotherapy.

Int J Radiat Oncol Biol Phys 1990;19:445–449.

Toriumi D, Atiuch R, Murad T. Extracranial neurogenic tumors of the head and neck. *Otolaryngol Clin North Am* 1986;19:609.

Valdagni R, Amichetti M. Radiation therapy of carotid body tumors. *Am J Clin Oncol* 1990;13:45–48.

Van der May AG, Friyns JH. Does intervention improve the natural course of glomus tumors? A series of patients seen in a 32-year period. *Ann Otol Rhinol Laryngol* 1992;101:635–642.

Walike JW, Bailey BJ. Head and neck hemangiopericytomas. *Arch Otolaryngol Head Neck Surg* 1971;93:345–348.

Chapter 75

TRAUMA

Tapan A. Padhya and Jack L. Gluckman

BLUNT TRAUMA

The incidence of blunt trauma in the United States has been drastically reduced with the advent of mandatory seat-belt legislation in most states. However, blunt neck trauma still occurs in unrestrained car passengers and people involved in violent altercations. The anterior neck is fairly well shielded by the anterior mandible and the clavicle. When blunt trauma to the neck does occur, the laryngotracheal tree is the most vulnerable to injury. (For a more detailed discussion, see Chapter 39.) Major vessel injury due to blunt trauma is an extremely rare phenomenon but must be considered when dealing with a patient with an expanding hematoma, carotid bruit, or neurologic findings. A perforation or tear of the pharynx, hypopharynx, or esophagus must be viewed with strong suspicion whenever a patient presents with subcutaneous air (crepitance), dysphagia, or odynophagia.

PENETRATING TRAUMA

Management of penetrating neck trauma presents a diagnostic challenge in light of the number of vital structures that traverse this relatively small area. No one single algorithm or approach has been universally accepted. Both mandatory exploration and selective exploration carry low morbidity and mortality rates. Until World War II,

penetrating injuries resulted in an overall 15% mortality rate. With advancements in anesthesia, blood replacement, antibiotics, and resuscitation techniques, mortality today approaches 1 to 2% regardless of the philosophical approach to exploration.

Most penetrating trauma results from stab wounds, handgun injuries, and shotgun injuries. The male to female ratio is 5:1. Most injuries occur in the anterior triangle of the neck because it represents the most surface area of the neck. The type of injury depends on the type of object, size of the object, and the area of the head and neck injured. Stab wounds are usually less severe than small handgun wounds. The firearm's muzzle velocity (v) is the most important factor in the kinetic energy (KE) of the moving object (KE = $\frac{1}{2}$ mv^2). Therefore, a high-power rifle has 60 times more energy than a handgun.

ANATOMIC CLASSIFICATION (FIGS. 75–1 AND 75–2)

The neck is surrounded by investing fascia commonly divided into a superficial and deep layer. The superficial layer envelopes the platysma muscle, and the deep layer is further subdivided into superficial, middle, and deep layers. Because of these tight fascial layers, exsanguination is limited but airway compression is a real life-threatening problem.

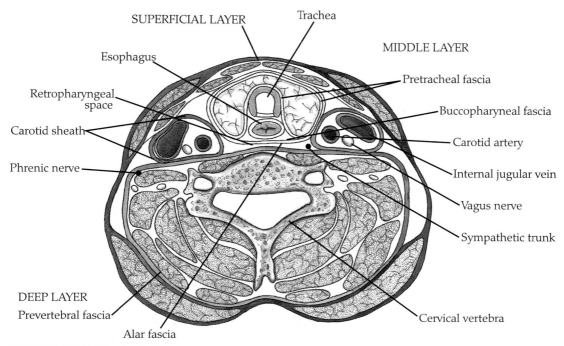

SUPERFICIAL LAYER
Trachea
MIDDLE LAYER
Esophagus
Pretracheal fascia
Retropharyngeal space
Buccopharyneal fascia
Carotid sheath
Carotid artery
Internal jugular vein
Phrenic nerve
Vagus nerve
Sympathetic trunk
DEEP LAYER
Prevertebral fascia
Cervical vertebra
Alar fascia

FIGURE 75-1 The fascial layers.

The platysma, which extends from the lower facial muscles to the clavicle, remains the key anatomic landmark when dealing with penetrating neck trauma. Old surgical doctrine regarded penetration of the platysma as an indication for mandatory neck exploration. With today's sophisticated imaging techniques, a more selective neck exploration approach is in place at most trauma centers. The neck has been subdivided vertically into three distinct zones:

Zone I is the area of the neck between the clavicle and the cricoid cartilage, containing the proximal common carotid artery, vertebral artery, subclavian artery, upper mediastinal vasculature, lung apices, trachea, esophagus, and thoracic duct.

> ## SPECIAL CONSIDERATION
>
> It is difficult to gain emergent proximal control of hemorrhage and it is difficult to expose intrathoracic neurovascular structures.

Zone II is the area of the neck extending between the cricoid cartilage and the angle of the mandible, containing the carotid bifurcation, vertebral artery, internal jugular vein, larynx, trachea, esophagus, vagus/recurrent laryngeal nerves, and spinal cord.

Zone III is the area of the neck from the angle of the mandible to the base of the skull, containing the distal external carotid artery branches, vertebral artery, salivary glands, pharynx, spinal cord, and cranial nerves VII, IX, X, XI, and XII.

> ## SPECIAL CONSIDERATION
>
> It is difficult to gain emergent distal control of hemorrhage and it is difficult to expose skull base neurovascular structures.

EVALUATION

When evaluating a neck trauma patient, the primary survey should always assess the ABC (airway, breathing, and circulation) of trauma as out-

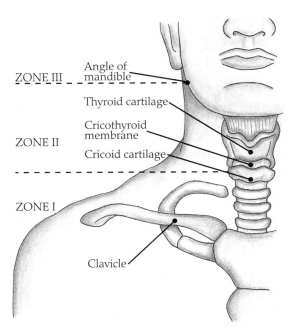

ZONE III

Angle of
mandible

ZONE II

Thyroid cartilage

Cricothyroid
membrane

Cricoid cartilage

ZONE I

Clavicle

FIGURE 75–2 Anatomic zones of the neck.

lined in the advanced trauma life support (ATLS) protocol. Early airway intervention in the emergency room is paramount, especially in the face of an expanding hematoma. Whether the patient is awake or unconscious, a quick survey of the patient's airway status must be made. A cricothyrotomy or vertical tracheotomy is the preferred airway of choice compared to oral or nasal intubation in a patient with overt respiratory distress.

PITFALL... Endotracheal intubation may be considered in select situations, but it may further exacerbate bleeding, pharyngeal perforations, or laryngotracheal injuries.

SPECIAL CONSIDERATION

One must assume a cervical spine injury until further testing can be done. This is especially important whenever one is establishing a surgical airway.

Concurrently, the patient's circulatory status must be assessed rapidly. Any frank bleeding must be controlled with direct pressure only.

PITFALL... Any use of clamping instruments should be condemned.

Establishment of large-bore intravenous access will facilitate rapid fluid resuscitation in light of large blood loss or hemodynamic instability. Indications for immediate surgical management include life-threatening hemorrhage, hemodynamic instability, or expanding hematomas. The operating room is the only place where a wound is explored or probed or a foreign body is removed. An anesthesia team and ancillary staff should be present to facilitate continued resuscitation.

Secondary survey and definitive management can be done in a system-by-system fashion once the airway has been addressed and the patient is hemodynamically stable. Vascular trauma can be present in 25% of patients with penetrating neck trauma. Mortality can reach 66% with any major vessel injury. Inspection, palpation, and auscultation of the head, neck, upper extremities, and thorax is of extreme importance. Obvious signs of hypovolemic shock, frank brisk bleeding, expanding hematoma, decreased breath sounds (hemothorax), decreased radial pulse, and carotid bruits should alert the trauma surgeon to a possible vascular injury.

Respiratory tract injury accounts for 10% of penetrating neck trauma. Sites that are affected include the oropharynx, hypopharynx, larynx, trachea, and lung apices. The patient may exhibit cyanosis, air per wound, subcutaneous emphysema, hemoptysis, dysphonia, hoarseness, and decreased breath sounds.

PITFALL... An initial respiratory tract injury may appear stable but may rapidly decompensate, requiring emergent surgical airway intervention.

The digestive tract is involved in 5% of all penetrating neck trauma. This area accounts for the most frequently missed injury due to its occult nature. Findings like dysphagia, odynophagia, hematemesis, crepitus, and free air on imaging all suggest a possible perforation or tear. Early intervention is to exteriorize the leak to prevent the more devastating complication of mediastinitis.

The nervous system can involve a range of injuries. Cranial nerve, phrenic nerve, and brachial plexus injury can all result depending on the missile trajectory. Complete or incomplete spinal cord transection should be considered if localizing or lateralizing deficits are found. Carotid or vertebral artery injury can cause an interruption of blood flow, resulting in a global neurologic defect or hemiplegia.

Soft tissue injury may include glandular or ductal injury. This includes parotid gland, submandibular gland, or thoracic duct injury. Saliva exiting the wound or associated facial or hypoglossal nerve injury may point to a gland/duct injury. Repair of the duct over a stent is required as well as drainage of the glandular bed. Right-sided penetrating neck trauma in zone III can also injure the thoracic duct. Treatment usually involves a high index of suspicion, isolation, and ligation of the duct.

Management

Biffl et al (1997), in their review, based treatment on the level of zone penetration and whether the patient was symptomatic or not.

Symptomatic

Zone I—arteriography with or without esophageal studies

Zone II—to operating room if hemoptysis, dysphonia, crepitus, hematemesis, dysphagia, or nerve deficit is present

Zone III—arteriography with or without embolization

Asymptomatic

Zone I—arteriography with or without esophageal studies

Zone II—observe

Zone III—with or without arteriography for possible occult vascular injury (all patients admitted for overnight observation)

CONTROVERSY

Surgical exploration of zone II still remains an area of great controversy.

The concept of mandatory exploration of all wounds with platysmal penetration dates back to the military campaigns of this century. Military surgeons were able to effectively reduce mortality using this approach. This concept was carried over to the civilian population, where it did reduce overall mortality but it also resulted in >50% negative exploration rate. More selective approaches have emerged resulting in lower costs, shorter hospital stays, and fewer negative explorations. With the advent of today's advanced imaging techniques, a more selective approach has been adopted by many centers.

Emergent exploration in the operating room is indicated in times of overt vascular injury and hemodynamic instability. Diagnostic procedures such as arteriography, esophagography, computed tomography (CT) imaging, and flexible laryngoscopy will give important information and allow the surgeon to manage the patient in a more selective fashion. Arteriography in the hemodynamically stable and asymptomatic patient is indicated for zone I and III injuries and will detect any occult vascular injury while providing excellent intravascular control. Esophagography by itself has a 90% sensitivity in detecting occult pharyngoesophageal leaks and tears. CT imaging, again used only in the asymptomatic and stable patient, provides excellent detail of the laryngotracheal complex, subcutaneous air, and the bony cervical spine. Flexible laryngoscopy is to be used in the awake patient with a stable airway. Mucosal tears, edema, and laryngeal derangements may cause the surgeon to surgically manage the airway and explore the larynx. The above tests can be used alone or in combination depending on the zone of injury and the patient's stability. A positive finding on any of the above tests usually requires open exploration of the neck.

When taking a stable patient to the operating room, flexible laryngoscopy will provide adequate information as to the status of the larynx.

SPECIAL CONSIDERATION

All attempts should be made to clear the cervical spine prior to any operative manipulation.

Any oropharyngeal or laryngotracheal trauma may preclude endotracheal intubation and an awake tracheostomy must be considered. Once the airway is controlled, a rigid endoscopic evaluation that includes rigid laryngoscopy, rigid bronchoscopy, and rigid esophagoscopy should be performed. Prior to neck exploration, one must give parenteral antibiotics and a tetanus toxoid booster for all penetrating injuries.

Occult vascular injuries in zone III may often be managed with endovascular embolization techniques but on rare occasion a lateral swing mandibulotomy may be required for actual surgical repair. Zone II vascular injuries can be directly accessed via a transcervical approach.

PEARL... The anesthesia team should have packed red blood cells on hand in the event of an acute hemorrhage.

Simple lacerations of the carotid or the internal jugular vein can be primarily repaired. If the arterial vessel wall is too damaged, one must consider either ligation or saphenous vein interposition. Exploration for zone I vascular injuries

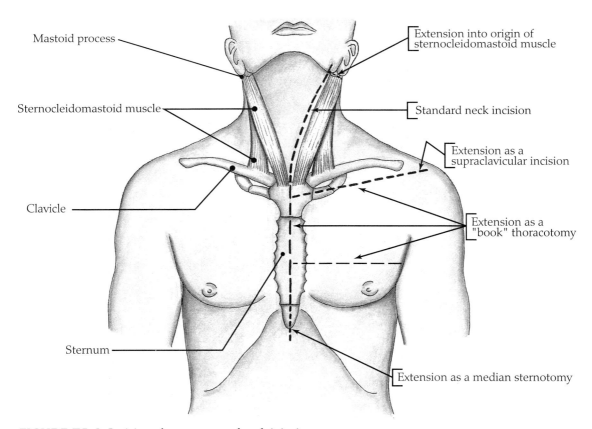

FIGURE 75–3 Incisions for exposure of neck injuries.

may require a supraclavicular incision with a possible median sternotomy or "book" thoracotomy (Fig. 75–3). Repair can be facilitated with primary closure or a polytetrafluoroethylene (PTFE) graft. In general, all arterial vessels should be repaired, and venous injuries can be ligated.

Pharyngoesophageal injuries as documented by esophagography or rigid esophagoscopy should be explored, debrided, and closed primarily in one or two layers. An additional tissue buttress using strap muscles or the sternocleidomastoid should be considered for larger tears. These wounds must be drained with either a closed suction or a Penrose drain. Prior to closure and under direct vision, one should place a nasogastric tube for initiation of enteral feeds while the wound heals. In esophageal perforations with delay in diagnosis (>12 hours) the wound should be drained due to the higher risk of wound contamination and mediastinitis.

Penetrating laryngotracheal injuries follow the same principles outlined for blunt laryngotracheal trauma. Most important is airway management. If the patient presents with airway instability, the safest and most expedient way to intervene is through a cricothyrotomy or tracheotomy in the emergency room. In stable patients, flexible laryngoscopy with or without CT imaging of the larynx will allow the surgeon to decide about the patient's airway status. Any suggestion of potential respiratory compromise should make the surgeon intervene early with a surgical airway. Once the airway is addressed, cervical exploration can be done in conjunction with laryngeal exploration. Inspection of the carotid sheath, esophagus, and cartilaginous framework can be accomplished. Further repair of the endolarynx can be accomplished via a laryngofissure. Thyroid cartilage fractures can be reapproximated with suture, wire, or microtita-nium plating. Tracheal lacerations can be sutured or used for the tracheotomy site.

CONCLUSION

Whether one subscribes to the mandatory or selective approach to penetrating trauma, one must always follow a systematic and stepwise approach to patient management. A system-by-system checklist will facilitate complete evaluation and treatment of the cervical trauma patient.

SUGGESTED READINGS

Biffl WL, Moore EE, Rehse DH, Offner PJ, Franciose RJ, Burch JM. Selective management of penetrating neck trauma on cervical level of injury. *Am J Surg* 1997;174:678–682.

Brennan JA, Meyers AD, Jafek BW. Penetrating neck trauma: a 5-year review of the literature (1983–1988). *Am J Otolaryngol* 1990;11:191–197.

Demetriades D, Asensio JA, Velmahos G, Thal E. Complex problems in penetrating neck trauma. *Surg Clin North Am* 1996;76(4):661–682.

Hollinshead WH. *Anatomy for Surgeons—The Head and Neck.* 3rd ed. Philadelphia: Lippincott; 1982.

Kendall JL, Anglin D, Demetriades D. Penetrating neck trauma. *Emerg Med Clin North Am* 1998;16(1):85–105.

Meyer JP, Barrett JA, Schuler JJ, Flanigan P. Mandatory vs selective exploration for penetrating neck trauma. *Arch Surg* 1987;122:592–597.

Miller RH, Duplechain JK. Penetrating wounds of the neck. *Otolaryngol Clin North Am* 1991;24(1):15–28.

SECTION XII

THYROID GLAND

Chapter 76

ANATOMY AND PHYSIOLOGY

Jack L. Gluckman

ANATOMY

The thyroid gland is a bi-lobed gland connected by an isthmus lying over the second and third tracheal rings (Fig. 76–1). A pyramidal lobe arising from the isthmus is present in 40 to 50% of cases. In adults, the average weight is 20 to 30 g. Histologically the gland consists of follicles lined by a single layer of cuboidal epithelium. The colloid in the follicles is glycoprotein (thyroglobulin). The follicles are surrounded by a vascular stroma. The gland itself has a true connective tissue capsule separate from the fibrous fascia (derived from the pretracheal fascia) that envelops it.

The blood supply of the gland is as follows: The superior thyroid artery runs with the superior laryngeal nerve before entering the thyroid.

> **PEARL···** It is important to ligate the superior thyroid artery close to the gland to avoid injury to the nerve during thyroidectomy.

It divides into anterior and posterior branches just before it enters the gland, with these branches anastomosing with the contralateral vessels and ipsilateral inferior thyroid artery. The inferior thyroid artery arises from the thyrocervical trunk and enters the gland at the mid-

lobe after crossing the recurrent laryngeal nerve and divides into two branches. It may be absent in up to 6% of cases. The thyroidea ima artery arises directly from the aorta, innominate artery, or right common carotid artery, and enters the isthmus. It is present in up to 12% of cases.

The superior thyroid veins run with the superior thyroid artery and drain the upper pole into the internal jugular or common facial vein. The inferior thyroid veins usually form two trunks or a plexus draining directly into the innominate vein or lower internal jugular vein. The middle thyroid veins may be single, multiple, or occasionally absent in 50% of cases. They drain directly into the internal jugular vein.

The lymphatics accompany the veins and drain into the paratracheal nodes and then to the superior mediastinum. They may also drain to the middle deep cervical nodes and into the lateral neck.

In performing thyroidectomy, intimate knowledge of the relationship between the inferior thyroid artery and the recurrent laryngeal nerve is imperative to avoid damaging this important nerve.

EMBRYOLOGY

The thyroid anlage develops as a median endodermal derivative that migrates from the tongue base (foramen cecum). The distal portion of this

519

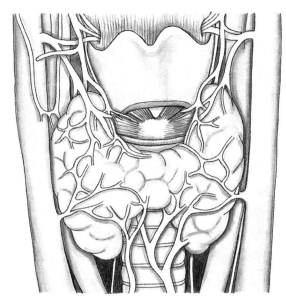

FIGURE 76-1 Anatomy of the thyroid gland.

thyroglossal duct forms the thyroid gland and reaches its normal position by the seventh week. The rest of the thyroglossal duct obliterates by the tenth week.

SPECIAL CONSIDERATION

The thyroglossal duct may remain patent to varying degrees, resulting in ectopic tissue or cysts along its course.

PHYSIOLOGY

The purpose of the thyroid gland is to concentrate iodine; 20 to 30% is stored in the thyroid and only a small percentage is carried in thyroid hormones and nonthyroid tissue. The iodide is trapped in the follicular cells, then oxidized to iodine. Iodine is attached to tyrosine to form monoiodinated tyrosine (MIT) and di-iodinated tyrosine (DIT). Two DIT molecules couple to form thyroxine (T_4), or MIT and DIT can couple to form tri-iodothyronine (T_3). All tyrosine compounds are bound to thyroglobulin and stored in thyroid follicles as colloid.

Thyrotropin-releasing hormone (TRH) is released from the hypothalamus, which stimulates the anterior pituitary gland to secrete thyroid-stimulating hormone (TSH). This in turn stimulates the thyroid to synthesize and release thyroid hormone. TSH release is inhibited by elevated thyroid hormone levels. When released from thyroglobulin, the thyroid hormone enters the circulation, where over 90% is bound to protein molecules. The unbound thyroid hormone is responsible for influencing metabolism.

SUGGESTED READINGS

Hansen JT. Embryology and surgical anatomy of the lower neck and superior mediastinum. In: Falk SA, ed. *Thyroid Disease.* Philadelphia: Lippincott-Raven; 1997:15–28.

Johnson JT. Applied anatomy of the thyroid and related structures. In: Johnson JT, Gluckman JL, eds. *Carcinoma of the Thyroid.* Oxford: Isis Medical Media; 1999:7–12.

Johnson JT. Applied physiology of the thyroid gland. In: Johnson JT, Gluckman JL, eds. *Carcinoma of the Thyroid.* Oxford: Isis Medical Media; 1999:13–14.

LoPresti JS, Singer PA. Physiology of thyroid hormone synthesis, secretion, and transport. In: Falk SA, ed. *Thyroid Disease.* Philadelphia: Lippincott-Raven; 1997:29–40.

Moosman DA, DeWeese MS. The external laryngeal nerve as related to thyroidectomy. *Surg Gynecol Obstet* 1968;127:1011–1016.

Singer PA. Clinical approach to thyroid function testing. In: Falk SA, ed. *Thyroid Disease.* Philadelphia: Lippincott-Raven; 1997:41–52.

Chapter 77

CONGENITAL DISORDERS

Jack L. Gluckman

THYROGLOSSAL DUCT ANOMALIES

This duct extends from the foramen cecum to the pyramidal lobe. Seven percent of the population has remnants of the thyroglossal duct. Persistent tissue and failure to obliterate or descend result in anomalies of the thyroglossal duct.

THYROGLOSSAL DUCT CYST

This cyst can be found anywhere along the length of the duct (60% infrahyoid, 24% suprahyoid, 1% intralingual). Fifty percent present before the age of 20. It usually manifests as a 1- to 2-cm cystic mass that is mobile on swallowing and protruding of the tongue. Occasionally, it may swell with acute infection. In rare cases, malignancy may develop in the cyst. The cyst contains mucus-like clear fluid, and in addition 60% of these cysts also contain thyroid tissue. Imaging, including radioactive scanning, has been advocated as routine to determine whether the thyroid with the cyst is the only functioning thyroid, but probably this is unnecessary, as the cyst will need to be removed anyway if it is symptomatic. Excision is by the Sistrunk operation, which includes the whole tract to the foramen cecum and includes the body of hyoid bone.

PITFALL... Surgeons should never be tempted to excise only the cyst; the whole tract, including the body of the hyoid, should always be excised.

LINGUAL THYROID

Lingual thyroid results from failure of the thyroglossal duct to descend. It presents as a mass at the foramen cecum. It may be asymptomatic or present with airway obstruction due to the mass. It may represent the only thyroid tissue, and after excision, hypothyroidism may result.

ECTOPIC THYROID TISSUE

Ectopic thyroid tissue may occur anywhere along the migratory route of the thyroid. Rarely, thyroid tissue may migrate to the superior mediastinum. It has also been identified in the larynx, trachea, pericardium, and esophagus.

CONGENITAL INTRATHYROID CYSTS

These cysts present in children. They are possibly derived from persistent ultimobranchial bodies or an intrathyroidal thyroglossal duct cyst.

SUGGESTED READINGS

Myer CM III, Cotton RT. Congenital thyroid cysts and ectopic thyroid. In: Falk SA ed. *Thyroid Disease.* Philadelphia: Lippincott-Raven; 1997:467–474.

Pinczowler E, Crockett DM, Atkinson JB, Kun S. Preoperative thyroid scanning in presumed thyroglossal duct cysts. *Arch Otolaryngol Head Neck Surg* 1992;118:985–988.

Taylor WE, Myer CM III, Hays LL, Cotton RT. Acute suppurative thyroiditis in children. *Laryngoscope* 1982;92:1269–1273.

Topf P, Fried MP, Strome M. Vagaries of thyroglossal duct cysts. *Laryngoscope* 1988;98: 740–742.

Chapter 78

INFECTIOUS AND INFLAMMATORY DISORDERS

Jack L. Gluckman

ACUTE SUPPURATIVE THYROIDITIS

This uncommon form of thyroiditis has an equal male to female incidence. It is usually preceded by an upper respiratory tract infection, with *Staphylococcus* being the most frequent organism. Clinically it is characterized by a painful enlargement of the gland, fever, and fluctuance if an abscess should develop. Treatment consists of antibiotics and drainage if abscess formation should occur.

PAINLESS THYROIDITIS

There are two forms of painless thyroiditis: sporadic and postpartum. The etiology is unknown, but thought to be possibly autoimmune, that is, a variant of Hashimoto's thyroiditis. The sporadic form can occur at any age and is more common in females. Clinically, it is characterized by diffuse thyroid enlargement without pain or tenderness, and temporary hyperthyroidism early in the course of the disease. Fifty percent of patients become hypothyroid, which spontaneously resolves in 6 months.

Postpartum thyroiditis has a similar history to the sporadic variant except that the initial hyperthyroidism is mild. Histologically there is lymphocytic infiltration and thyroid follicle disruption. As the disease is self-limiting, treatment is rarely necessary; however, steroids may be of value.

SUBACUTE THYROIDITIS (DE QUERVAIN'S THYROIDITIS)

This form can occur at all ages; however, it is most common in the fifth decade. Females are more commonly affected than males. The etiology is unknown but is thought to be possibly viral. It is a painful thyroiditis, with diffuse thyroid enlargement that is tender to palpation. There is associated malaise and fever, and the patient is usually thyrotoxic. In general there are four distinct phases related to endocrine function: hyperthyroid (1–3 months); euthyroid (1–3 weeks); hypothyroid (2–6 months); and recovery, which is usually complete. Histologically there is lymphocyte, monocyte, and giant cell infiltration. Treatment consists of analgesics, steroids, and antiinflammatory agents.

HASHIMOTO'S THYROIDITIS

This is extremely common, affecting 2% of the population; 95% of cases occur in females, most commonly between 30 and 50 years of age. The etiology is thought to be autoimmune with a strong genetic predisposition.

The gland may be diffusely enlarged with a fine nodularity or multinodular. It is firm to palpation. The patient is usually left with residual hypothyroidism.

Histologically, disrupted follicles and infiltration with lymphocytes and plasma cells are found with variable fibrosis.

> **PEARL•••** A thyroid scan demonstrates a "salt and pepper" pattern.

Antithyroglobulin antibodies are present in 55 to 90% of patients; however, antibodies to thyroid microsomes are noted in a higher percentage. Fine-needle aspiration biopsy can be diagnostic. Not only may patients develop other autoimmune conditions, but they are at increased risk for developing B-cell lymphoma in the gland.

RIEDEL'S THYROIDITIS

This uncommon condition affects females more commonly than males, and usually occurs in older patients. It may be associated with mediastinal and retroperitoneal fibrosis. It is characterized by a fixed, rock-hard thyroid enlargement, which may involve the strap muscles and surrounding structures. Histologically the gland is replaced by fibrosis. Obstructive symptoms are uncommon but can be significant, for example, airway obstruction and dysphagia. Treatment consists of palliative surgery to relieve obstruction.

HYPERTHYROIDISM

GRAVES' DISEASE

This condition usually presents in the third to fourth decade, with females seven times more likely than males to be affected. The autoimmune etiology occurs with development of abnormal immunoglobulins that fix on the thyroid-stimulating hormone (TSH) receptor of the thyroid epithelial cell. Autonomous hypertrophy and function result. Clinically there is a diffuse toxic goiter with ophthalmopathy occurring in 55% of cases and dermopathy in 5% of cases. Nervousness, sweating, hypersensitivity to heat, palpitation, and fatigue are prominent symptoms. The ophthalmopathy is characterized by a stare, lid lag, eyelid retraction with secondary chemosis, and conjunctival irritation.

Increased serum triiodothyronine (T_3) and thyroxine (T_4) levels and radioactive iodine uptake are noted, confirming the diagnosis. Drug therapy includes thionamides, sympathetic blockers, and iodine. Radioactive iodine is generally accepted as the treatment of choice.

> **SPECIAL CONSIDERATION**
>
> Pregnant women should not be treated with this modality.

Eighty to ninety percent are cured after a single treatment, with the majority of persistent cases cured after a second or third treatment.

Surgery is indicated for those patients who refuse radioactive iodine or those with thyroid nodules suspicious for malignancy. Patients should be rendered euthyroid prior to surgery.

> **CONTROVERSY**
>
> Subtotal thyroidectomy leaving 7 to 8 g of nodule-free tissue is recommended; however, total thyroidectomy is proposed by many.

TOXIC MULTINODULAR GOITER

This goiter usually is found in older patients and differs from Graves' disease in that there is usually no ophthalmopathy or dermopathy. Surgery, consisting of total thyroidectomy, is the preferred treatment. It can be treated with radioactive iodine but not as successfully as surgery.

TOXIC ADENOMA

This is a rare condition usually found in younger patients. The nodule is usually quite large (2.5–3.0 cm). Surgical excision is the treatment of choice.

SMOOTH DIFFUSE AND MULTINODULAR NONTOXIC GOITER

This goiter is usually a compensatory response occurring most commonly in females. The diffuse goiter usually evolves into a multinodular goiter. Although it is physiologic, occurring in adolescence and pregnancy, it may be secondary to dietary deficiency.

It usually manifests with pressure symptoms and signs.

SPECIAL CONSIDERATION

A small percentage (1–2%) of multinodular goiters may harbor a malignancy.

Treatment consists of thyroid suppression, with the indications for surgery being cosmetic deformity, pressure symptoms and signs refractory to suppression, fear of malignancy, and the development of toxicity.

SUGGESTED READINGS

Berger SA, Zonszein J, Villamena P, Mittman N. Infectious diseases of the thyroid gland. *Rev Infect Dis* 1983;5:108–122.

Burch HB, Wartofsky L. Graves' ophthalmopathy: current concepts regarding pathogenesis and management. *Endocr Rev* 1993;14:747–793.

Falk SA. Hyperthyroidism: a surgeon's perspective. In: English GM, ed. *Otolaryngology.* Philadelphia: Harper & Row; 1985:4–70.

Hamburger JI. The various presentations of thyroiditis: diagnostic considerations. *Ann Intern Med* 1986;104:219–224.

Woolf PD. Thyroiditis. In: Falk SA, ed. *Thyroid Disease.* Philadelphia: Lippincott-Raven; 1997: 393–410.

Chapter 79

NEOPLASMS AND CYSTS

Jack L. Gluckman

INCIDENCE

Thyroid cancer is not uncommon. The American Cancer Society estimated 13,900 new cases with 1,120 deaths occurring in the United States in 1995. The vast majority occur in females.

PATHOLOGY

All benign and malignant thyroid cancers are listed in Table 79–1.

BENIGN

Adenoma

An adenoma is an encapsulated tumor composed of glandular epithelium with varying degrees of intratumoral degenerative changes, for example, hemorrhage, fibrosis, and calcification. Histologically, adenomas can be differentiated into follicular, colloid, embryonal, fetal, and Hürthle variants. These, with the possible exception of Hürthle adenomas, are all benign in behavior.

CONTROVERSY

Some pathologists question the existence of Hürthle cell adenomas and regard all as well-differentiated carcinomas.

Follicular adenomas may demonstrate unusual cellularity, numerous mitoses, and spontaneous necrosis but are benign in behavior. Adenomas may rarely cause thyrotoxicosis and may undergo malignant transformation.

MALIGNANT

Papillary Carcinoma (60–65%)

Most commonly seen in the third to fifth decades, papillary carcinoma can present at any age. The female to male ratio is 2:1. Generally these carcinomas tend to be biologically indolent, with an overall excellent prognosis. The etiology is obscure. They may arise from a benign adenoma. There is some evidence to suggest a relationship with Hashimoto's thyroiditis, but this may be purely coincidental. Low-dose and high-dose external radiation is probably a causative factor in their development.

Macroscopically, these tumors can be divided into *occult* (under 1.5 cm in size), *intrathyroidal* (confined to the thyroid gland), and *extrathyroidal* (spread beyond the confines of the thyroid gland). Occult cancers have been coincidently noted in 35.6% of autopsies. Intrathyroidal tumors compose approximately 70% of papillary cancers. Extrathyroidal tumors may infiltrate the surrounding structures, particularly the larynx, trachea, strap muscles, and great vessels. Microscopically, most are purely

TABLE 79-1 Classification of Thyroid Tumors

Benign
  Adenoma (follicular, colloid, embryonal, fetal, Hürthle)
  Other (thymoma, paraganglioma, teratoma, hemangioma)
Malignant
  Papillary adenocarcinoma
  Follicular adenocarcinoma
  Hürthle cell carcinoma
  Medullary carcinoma
  Anaplastic
    Small cell
    Giant cell
  Sarcoma
  Lymphoma
  Squamous cell carcinoma
  Mucoepidermoid carcinoma
  Clear cell tumors
  Plasma cell tumors
  Metastases

papillary but some may have areas of follicular carcinoma.

SPECIAL CONSIDERATION

The propensity for invasion of the intraglandular lymphatics results in a high incidence of multicentricity and nodal metastases. Neither the multicentricity nor the presence of regional metastases has any prognostic significance, hence the lack of value of the clinical staging system.

Venous invasion is seen in 10% of cases. Dedifferentiation in a tumor is common with an unclear prognostic significance; however, anaplastic transformation, although rare, has an ominous prognosis. Negative prognostic indicators include advanced age at the time of presentation, male gender, extrathyroidal extension, and distant metastases. Dedifferentiation, vascular invasion, and atypical variants, such as tall cell, follicular, columnar cell, and sclerosing, may also have negative prognostic significance.

Follicular Carcinoma (15%)

These tumors have a propensity for vascular invasion, with metastases to bone, brain, and liver. Lymph node metastases are rare. Anaplastic transformation is more common than in papillary carcinomas. Pathologically there are two variants: the *overtly invasive carcinoma*, which overtly infiltrates the thyroid and surrounding structures, and the *minimally invasive tumor*, which resembles an adenoma histologically and grossly appears well encapsulated; however, microscopically it has capsule invasion.

PEARL... Definitive diagnosis of a minimally invasive cancer can often be established only on permanent section and may be missed on frozen section.

The overtly invasive variant has a high incidence of metastases and a 20 to 50% mortality rate, whereas the minimally invasive tumor has a mortality rate of under 5%. Poor prognostic indicators in follicular carcinoma include advanced age at the time of presentation, male gender, extrathyroidal extension, and distant metastases. Vascular invasion, anaplastic transformation, and trabecular growth pattern have negative prognostic implications.

Hürthle Cell Carcinomas (5%)

PEARL... Not all nodules containing Hürthle cells are neoplastic. The vast majority are Hürthle cell changes in benign follicular adenomatous nodules or thyroiditis.

Hürthle cell tumors should be regarded as a variant of follicular tumors and as such can be divided into the overtly invasive and minimally invasive groups. The former has a much higher mortality rate with a higher incidence of cervical lymphatic metastases.

Medullary Carcinoma (3–5%)

The vast majority of medullary carcinomas are sporadic in origin, with only 10 to 20% of cases being familial, that is, associated with Sipple's syndrome (multiple endocrine neoplasia [MEN] type 2A), which entails medullary thyroid cancer, C-cell hyperplasia, adrenal pheochromocytoma, adrenal medullary hyperplasia, and parathyroid hyperplasia, or with MEN type 2B, which, in addition, entails mucosal neuromas, gastrointestinal ganglioneuromas, and musculoskeletal abnormalities. Most sporadic cases present at around 50 years of age, but familial cases may present in childhood. The tumor is usually located in the area of the highest C-cell concentration, that is, the lateral upper two-thirds of the gland, and may be multicentric. The tumor may be well circumscribed and encapsulated or more diffusely infiltrative. Commonly intrathyroid lymphatics and veins are invaded. Fifty percent have nodal metastases and 15 to 25% have distant metastases at presentation. Poor prognostic indicators include MEN type 2B, nodal and distant metastases, and extrathyroidal extension. Small cell tumors, pleomorphism, poor calcitonin staining, and high carcinoembryonic antigen (CEA) staining are also poor prognostic indicators.

Anaplastic Carcinoma (1–5%)

This rare tumor is thought to arise in well-differentiated cancers, usually in older women. It usually presents at an advanced stage with diffuse thyroid enlargement or as a large nodule. Surrounding structures are infiltrated early. There are two histologic variants: small cell and giant cell. The prognosis is extremely poor.

Lymphoma (1–3.5%)

Lymphoma may arise primarily in the thyroid or as part of systemic disease. It commonly arises in a gland with Hashimoto's thyroiditis. It usually affects elderly women, and it may present as a diffusely enlarged gland or a single nodule. Hypothyroidism may result from infiltration by the malignancy or preexisting thyroiditis. The most common histologic type is a large cell diffuse malignant lymphoma. The prognosis for thyroid lymphoma is good in 50 to 77% of cases.

Miscellaneous

Rare tumors such as sarcomas, mucoepidermoid carcinomas, and squamous cell carcinomas may occur. Cancer may also involve the thyroid by direct extension, for example, from the larynx or pharynx, or by retrograde lymphatic spread and by hematogenous spread. Carcinoma of the kidney and colon and melanoma are the most common distant sites. Cancer may arise in aberrant thyroid tissue, such as the lingual thyroid, thyroglossal duct, and intratracheal, intralaryngeal, and mediastinal thyroid tissue.

CLINICAL PRESENTATION

A neoplasm of the thyroid may present with one or a combination of the following clinical features:

1. *Thyroid enlargement (goiter)* Thyroid enlargement may be smooth and diffuse or nodular. A nodular goiter may consist of a single nodule or multiple nodules.

SPECIAL CONSIDERATION

A smooth, diffuse enlargement is usually a sign of benign thyroid disease; however, rarely an anaplastic carcinoma or lymphoma may present this way.

The most common is the multinodular goiter, which usually represents the end stage of benign disease. In this case, the nodules consist of areas of colloid storage, degeneration, hyperplasia, cyst formation, and inflammation. Occasionally, however, a multinodular goiter may harbor a neoplasm (10–15% of cases). Of these, 90% are benign and 10% malignant. Therefore, the overall incidence of malignancy in a multinodular goiter is only 1 to 2%.

PEARL... A true single nodule is far more likely to be a neoplasm and the chances of this being malignant are 5 to 10%. Therefore, a true single nodule should be regarded with a higher index of suspicion than a dominant nodule in a multinodular goiter.

---

2. *Symptoms and signs of pressure on adjacent structures* The sheer mass of an enlarged thyroid gland may cause pressure on adjacent structures. Pressure on the esophagus results in dysphagia, which is usually discomfort on swallowing. As the pressure increases, the dysphagia will gradually become obstructive. Pressure on the trachea results in mild to moderate stridor, although in long-standing tumors, chondromalacia of the tracheal rings may cause significant airway obstruction. Hoarsness is usually due to vocal cord edema. Very rarely a recurrent nerve palsy may result from pressure on the nerve alone. Retrosternal extension may cause tracheal deviation and superior mediastinal syndrome with facial edema and venous engorgement of the neck.

3. *Symptoms and signs of infiltration* A rapidly increasing mass, particularly if painful and associated with tethering of the overlying skin, is suggestive of malignancy. Stridor and even hemoptysis is due to direct infiltration into the laryngotracheal complex. Unilateral vocal cord paralysis or even bilateral paralysis, for practical purposes, indicates malignancy due to infiltration of the recurrent laryngeal nerve. Infiltration of the esophagus causes obstructive dysphagia and odynophagia. Lateral extension may result in the cervical sympathetics and even the brachial plexus being infiltrated.

4. *Evidence of regional and distant metastases* Regional lymphatic spread to the lateral neck and superior mediastinum or distant metastases may be the only obvious clinical evidence of thyroid cancer. Papillary cancer has a propensity for nodal metastases, of which 20% may be cystic. Follicular carcinoma, on the other hand, tends toward hematogenous spread to bone, lung, and elsewhere, although Hürthle cell cancer can spread to regional nodes. Medullary and anaplastic nodal metastases have a tendency toward extracapsular spread.

5. *Evidence of endocrine dysfunction* Most patients with thyroid tumors are euthyroid; however, rarely secreting benign adenoma or even carcinoma may result in hyperthyroidism. Occasionally, the tumor may have destroyed enough of the surrounding gland to cause hypothyroidism. Medullary cancer may have symptoms related to calcitonin, or rarely, adrenocorticotropic hormone (ACTH) or prostaglandin secretion.

EVALUATION OF A THYROID MASS

A thorough clinical evaluation usually enables the clinician to establish a working differential diagnosis and determine the role of special investigations. The following tests of the thyroid may be of value.

X-RAY OF THE NECK

Patchy calcification is present in any long-standing benign thyroid disease, well-differentiated cancers, and medullary cancer. Therefore, X-ray of the neck is of little practical value diagnostically.

X-RAY OF THE CHEST

Retrosternal extension, tracheal deviation, superior mediastinal nodal involvement, and even pulmonary metastases may be apparent, and therefore a chest X-ray should always be obtained.

ESOPHAGRAM

This investigation is helpful in differentiating thyroid from nonthyroid causes of dysphagia and whether the dysphagia is due to pressure or malignant infiltration of the esophagus. Therefore, an esophagram should be ordered if the patient complains of significant dysphagia.

RADIONUCLIDE SCAN

Radionuclide studies used to represent the cornerstone of thyroid imaging but are no longer commonly used as a first-line imaging study in the routine evaluation of thyroid nodules. These studies, however, are able to differentiate a diffusely enlarged gland from nodular enlargement and a true single nodule from a multinodular goiter, and to determine the functional status of the nodules, that is, hot versus cold.

The following agents are available for scanning: technetium 99m (Tc-99m); radioactive iodine (^{131}I, ^{125}I, ^{123}I), and thallium 201 chloride. Tc-99m is popular because of its low cost, ready availability, short half-life, and optimal imaging capabilities. It is only trapped by the thyroid and not organified, therefore, a "hot" nodule identifies only that the drug is being trapped and not necessarily that the nodule is functional. Radioactive iodine is the only agent that is trapped and organified and therefore is able to determine function. ^{123}I is the best of these compounds but is expensive and has a short shelf-life, and thus is not very practical. Thallium 201 is taken up by well-perfused cellular lesions and has been advocated for detection of lymph node metastases, retrosternal extension, recurrent cancer, and functioning nodules within a suppressed normal thyroid gland, but it is not commonly ordered.

SPECIAL CONSIDERATION

Octreotide scintigraphy is particularly useful for detecting metastatic medullary carcinoma, although it has been shown to detect metastatic Hürthle cell carcinoma as well.

ULTRASONOGRAPHY

Ultrasonography is a highly sophisticated imaging modality that is ideal for evaluating thyroid disease. High-resolution, real-time ultrasonography enables the radiologist to detect thyroid nodules as small as 3 mm in diameter and has a wide variety of uses in evaluating thyroid disease:

1. Screening high-risk patients, for example, patients with a past history of radiation, for nodules
2. Differentiating a true single nodule from a dominant nodule in a multinodular goiter
3. Evaluating the status of the nodule, whether cystic or solid, and if solid, demonstrating whether it is well circumscribed or has infiltration into surrounding structures
4. Facilitating the performance of fine-needle aspiration biopsy for the smaller and deeper nonpalpable thyroid nodules
5. Permitting objective monitoring of the status of medically treated nodules
6. Evaluating the clinically negative neck for metastases
7. Detecting recurrent cancer after thyroidectomy

COMPUTED TOMOGRAPHY (CT) AND MAGNETIC RESONANCE IMAGING (MRI)

Both these sophisticated imaging modalities demonstrate the thyroid gland well. The high iodine content allows the gland to be highlighted on CT scan, and MRI is particularly useful in both T1- and T2-weighted images. Both CT and MRI are able to demonstrate any extrathyroidal extension of the tumor, particularly where airway infiltration is suspected; to determine the presence of retrosternal involvement; and to detect metastatic disease, either locally or regionally.

SPECIAL CONSIDERATION

These modalities are unnecessary in the evaluation of a routine thyroid mass.

METASTATIC WORKUP

Where advanced medullary carcinoma, anaplastic carcinoma, or well-differentiated cancer is suspected, a metastatic workup is indicated. The sophistication of the workup depends on the philosophy and index of suspicion of the clinician. It should include a bone scan and CT scan of the abdomen and chest if there is a high level of concern. An octreotide study is particularly sensitive for metastatic medullary carcinoma.

Blood Tests

As a routine, thyroxine (T_4), tri-iodothyronine (T_3), and thyroid-stimulating hormone (TSH) levels should be assessed. Thyroid antibodies for Hashimoto's thyroiditis may also be indicated if appropriate. If a well-differentiated cancer is suspected, a serum thyroglobulin can be obtained, although it is not essential.

> **PITFALL•••** These levels may increase after fine-needle aspiration biopsy (FNAB); therefore, this test should be performed prior to FNAB.

The levels are also raised in subacute thyroiditis, but usually return to normal following steroid therapy. It is most useful as a marker in follow-up after treatment of well-differentiated thyroid cancer.

> **PEARL•••** Postoperative serum thyroglobulin levels under 10 ng/mL in patients on thyroid supression are indicative of cancer control.

A serum calcitonin level should be obtained if a medullary carcinoma is suspected, particularly if there is a family history.

Fine-Needle Aspiration Biopsy

FNAB has become an essential part of the evaluation of the thyroid mass. There are three aspects to this procedure that influence its successful use:

1. The ability to obtain a satisfactory specimen from the nodule. Ultransonography-guided biopsy may enhance this technique.

> **PEARL•••** The best results are not necessarily obtained from the center of the nodule (where central necrosis may be present) but from the periphery. One aspirate of a nodule is rarely sufficient and multiple aspirates are frequently necessary.

2. The ability of the cytopathologist to accurately interpret the specimen. The diagnostic accuracy is excellent for papillary, anaplastic, and medullary cancer, but is of no value in microinvasive follicular neoplasms where malignancy is defined by capsule invasion.

3. The clinician's ability to correlate the biopsy results with the clinical findings. If the report of the cytopathologist is either malignant or benign, the subsequent approach is simple. If it is suspicious (usually dealing with a Hürthle cell or follicular neoplasm), the patient should probably proceed to surgery, as the diagnosis of malignancy can only be established histologically. If the specimen is inadequate, the aspirate should be repeated. If the specimen is again inadequate, other factors will have to be taken into consideration before proceeding to surgery.

> **PEARL•••** A negative fine-needle aspiration should never preclude surgical exploration in a patient with a clinically suspicious lesion.

Large-Bore Needle Biopsy

This technique, which yields a true surgical specimen, has an advantage over fine-needle aspiration in that a portion of the capsule and surrounding tissue can be included and evidence of capsule invasion detected. But given the accuracy of FNAB today, it is rarely indicated.

Surgical Exploration

Open surgical exploration and excisional biopsy of the nodule remains the ultimate diagnostic technique. Indications for this vary from institution to institution and from clinician to clinician based on the personal experience of the physician, the sophistication and reliability of the ancillary tests, and the individual needs of the patient. The indications for open exploration are divided into two groups:

1. Obvious malignancy:
   a. Clinical or radiographic evidence of infiltration
   b. Clinical or radiographic evidence of regional or distant metastases
   c. Fine-needle aspiration positive for malignancy (papillary, medullary, anaplastic)
   d. Thyroid mass with raised serum level of calcitonin

2. Suspicion of malignancy:
   a. Suspicious fine-needle aspiration
   b. Nodule refractory to suppression
   c. Solitary thyroid nodule with raised serum thyroglobulin level
   d. Recurrent cyst refractory to two aspirations and thyroid suppression
   e. Nodule "going wrong," for example, a solitary nodule increasing in size and associated with pain
   f. True single nodule in males, elderly women, children, or in any patient with a history of prior radiation treatment.

CONTROVERSY

Some believe that all of these criteria should indicate the need for thyroidectomy, whereas others believe that careful follow-up with scans and fine-needle aspiration allows these patients to be treated conservatively. All, however, agree that there is a higher incidence of malignancy in this group and if there is concern, open exploration should be performed.

MANAGEMENT OF THYROID TUMORS

In general, the treatment of thyroid tumors is surgical excision. Every patient undergoing a thyroid exploration should sign a very specfic, detailed, and informed consent that should include the possibility of performing subtotal or total thyroidectomy and nodal dissection as indicated. Potential complications, such as recurrent and superior laryngeal nerve injury, hypoparathyroidism, hemorrhage, and infection, should be mentioned.

PEARL... The patient should also be aware that the tumor may be misdiagnosed as benign and may require a second surgery (completion thyroidectomy) at a later date.

Once the thyroid is exposed, an excisional biopsy of the nodule is performed usually consisting of lobectomy and isthmusectomy. In very advanced disease or certain types of cancer where aggressive surgery is not considered, for example, anaplastic carcinoma and lymphoma, an incisional biopsy alone will suffice. A frozen-section analysis is then obtained and further surgery performed depending on the intraoperative findings, the histologic type, and the philosophy and experience of the surgeon. If a diagnosis of a benign tumor is made, the operation is terminated with the understanding that the pathologist may reverse the diagnosis after permanent section analysis, and completion thyroidectomy may subsequently be necessary.

Total vs. Subtotal Thyroidectomy

If malignancy within the thyroid gland is diagnosed, the approach is as follows. The first decision to be made is whether a total or subtotal thyroidectomy should be performed. A total thyroidectomy consists of removal of the whole gland, preserving the parathyroid glands at least on the contralateral side, and bilaterally if feasible. A subtotal thyroidectomy is anything less then a total thyroidectomy and may vary from removal of a lobe (a lobectomy) to removal of most of the gland, leaving a rim of thyroid tissue on the contralateral side to protect the parathyroids and recurrent laryngeal nerve.

The advantages of total thyroidectomy are the following:

1. It is a better oncologic operation. Papillary and medullary tumors may appear well circumscribed but usually are not encapsulated, and delineation of the extent of the tumor is difficult. Follicular carcinoma may have extracapsular extension, and tumor extent is difficult to determine intraoperatively. Papillary and medullary carcinoma are frequently multicentric, and therefore total thyroidectomy is the best technique to encompass these lesions.

2. Although leaving residual well-differentiated tumor in the contralateral lobe may statistically have no impact on the survival of the patient, probably because of the use of postoperative thyroid suppression, anaplastic transformation of residual well-differentiated tumor is well documented and this is reason enough to ensure removal of all tumor, no matter how minuscule.

3. The incidence of recurrent and superior laryngeal nerve injury and hypoparathyroidism can be kept extremely low following total thyroidectomy provided good technique is used.

4. Removal of all thyroid tissue facilitates the use of postoperative diagnostic scans necessary to rule out recurrence or metastases. If residual thyroid is left, this will need to be ablated prior to effective scanning or treatment with radioactive iodine.

5. Serial postoperative thyroglobulin levels will be more valid if total thyroidectomy has been performed.

The advantages of subtotal thyroidectomy are the following:

1. It is a far simpler and less time-consuming procedure.

2. The morbidity is significantly lower, that is, there is less damage to the recurrent and

superior laryngeal nerves and parathyroids, particularly in the occasional surgeon's hands.

3. The prognosis in well-differentiated tumors is not affected by performing the lesser procedure.

> **PITFALL...** Herein lies the most compelling argument for performing a subtotal thyroidectomy. Unfortunately, there is no means of predicting which well-differentiated tumor, if inadequately excised, will exhibit aggressive behavior or even undergo anaplastic transformation.

The above agruments need to be weighed and a decision made by the surgeon as to the type of thyroidectomy to be performed. When performing a thyroidectomy for medullary carcinoma, all four parathyroids should be carefully identified and examined because of the associated incidence of parathyroid hyperplasia and adenomas.

MANAGEMENT OF EXTRATHYROID EXTENSION OF CANCER

Although extension beyond the thyroid gland into local and regional structures is common with anaplastic carcinoma, it rarely (9–16%) occurs in well-differentiated thyroid tumors. Structures most frequently involved are the recurrent laryngeal nerves, trachea, pharynx, esophagus, larynx, and overlying strap muscles. The structures can be involved by direct extension or from a metastatic lymph node. The optimal therapy for the patient will depend on the histology of the tumor, the extent of the extrathyroidal extension, the patient's physical status, the patient's expectations, and the surgeon's own philosophy. To this end, careful preoperative patient evaluation and counseling as to the various possibilities are imperative.

If the patient has advanced anaplastic cancer, radical resection should not be attempted, but rather the tumor should be biopsied and a tracheostomy inserted and the patient treated with external radiation. Likewise, lymphoma usually requires biopsy and, if necessary, tracheostomy.

Well-differentiated tumors with extrathyroidal extension are treated surgically and then followed with radioactive iodine and/or external radiation. The dilemma is whether to just "shave" the tumor off the vital structures or complete an "en bloc" resection, including the structure involved. In general, if the tumor can be shaved leaving no gross tumor, this is preferable and survival rates are comparable to wide-field resection. On the other hand, if gross tumor would be left using the shaving technique, wide-field resection should be performed.

RECURRENT LARYNGEAL NERVES

If a nerve is enveloped by tumor and paralyzed, it should be sacrificed. If, however, the nerve is functioning, particularly if it is the *only* functioning nerve, and tumor can be dissected off, this should be done.

TRACHEA

Superficial invasion can be shaved, but direct extension into the lumen should be treated by sleeve or wedge resection and primary anastomosis.

LARYNX

If the thyroid cartilage is superficially involved, a shave resection is possible. If the hemilarynx is involved, a vertical partial laryngectomy will suffice. If the anterior larynx is involved, the tumor may be resected and the larynx reconstructed using an epiglottic pull-down procedure. If the cricoid is extensively involved or the larynx is bilaterally involved, total laryngectomy will be necessary.

PHARYNX AND ESOPHAGUS

If only a small segment of the hypopharynx is involved, partial pharyngectomy may suffice. Often the pharynx and cervical esophagus involvement is associated with laryngeal involvement, and a total laryngopharyngectomy and cervical esophagectomy is needed, which en-

tails reconstruction using free jejunal graft, gastric pull-up, and so on.

> **PEARL•••** In all such cases, aggressive use of postoperative radioactive iodine and even external beam radiation is indicated and may be successful in treating microscopic residua.

MANAGEMENT OF REGIONAL LYMPH NODES

Attention is now directed to all the regional lymph nodes, including the pre- and paratracheal, superior mediastinal, and lateral neck nodal groups. In all patients, the pericapsular and paratracheal nodes need to be routinely removed with the thyroidectomy. If there are overt nodal metastases in these groups, the superior mediastinum and lateral neck need to be explored and, if necessary, nodal dissection performed. Usually the superior mediastinum can be dissected bluntly without sternotomy. The management of the lateral neck depends on the type of tumor, whether any metastases are identified, and the philosophy of the surgeon. In general, the more extensive the paratracheal nodal involvement, the greater the likelihood of lateral neck involvement.

PAPILLARY CARCINOMA

Only 20 to 25% of patients with papillary carcinoma present with clinical evidence of nodal metastases; however, the incidence of metastases determined pathologically is far higher, varying from 30 to 79%. The significance of this knowledge is obscure, as the presence of metastases appears to have no adverse effect on the prognosis of these patients.

Types of neck dissection include node plucking, limited anterior compartment dissection, or a full functional neck dissection, with each type of dissection having its proponents and detractors. Extracapsular extension does not appear to have an ominous prognosis. The surgeon's experience and philosophy will ultimately dictate the type of neck dissection performed.

CONTROVERSY

As the ability to accurately establish the presence of nodal metastases intraoperatively is extremely poor, and patient survival does not seem to be affected whether a neck dissection is done at all, let alone what type of neck dissection is performed, it is little wonder that the management of nodal metastases in this cancer is so controversial.

FOLLICULAR CARCINOMA

Lymph node metastases in follicular carcinoma are very rare, being detected in under 10% of patients clinically and 20% on pathologic evaluation, and have little prognostic significance. Therefore, neck dissections are performed only for overt metastases, with the philosophy being similar to that for papillary cancer.

HÜRTHLE CELL CARCINOMA

Hürthle cell carcinomas have a higher incidence (30%) of lymphatic metastases than does follicular carcinoma. Therefore, a higher index of suspicion for nodal metastases should exist, and functional neck dissections should be performed when disease is encountered.

MEDULLARY CARCINOMA

CONTROVERSY

Because of the high incidence of cervical metastases (50–63%), some authors advocate prophylactic paratracheal, superior mediastinal, and lateral neck dissections on a routine basis. Others feel that paratracheal and central compartment dissection only are necessary, and only if positive nodes are identified in the superior mediastinum and lateral neck, should these areas be dissected.

If a neck dissection is to be performed, a modified radical neck dissection preserving the accessory nerve should be recommended because of the propensity for extracapsular extension.

ANAPLASTIC CARCINOMA

In anaplastic carcinoma the neck is usually not surgically treated even with overt metastases, as the primary is almost never amenable to surgical excision.

FOLLOW-UP

A reversal of the frozen section diagnosis of benign follicular neoplasm with a permanent-section diagnosis of microinvasive cancer is an occasional development. If the surgeon is of the philosophy that a total thyroidectomy is the treatment of choice for microinvasive follicular cancer, then the patient will require completion thyroidectomy, usually performed within the first postoperative week. On the other hand, if subtotal thyroidectomy is considered adequate, no further treatment is indicated.

WELL-DIFFERENTIATED TUMORS

The patient is rendered hypothyroid and at 4 to 6 weeks a diagnostic radioiodine scan is performed. If any significant residual thyroid tissue is present, it will need to be ablated using radioactive iodine. There is no conclusive evidence that radioactive iodine is of benefit as an adjunct in all patients with well-differentiated cancer, but in patients with distant metastases or overt local or regional residual cancer it should be used. Further scans should be performed at 6 months, 1 year, and then every 2 years as indicated. Serum thyroglobulin levels are drawn every 6 months.

MEDULLARY CARCINOMA

Following definitive resection of the disease, calcitonin levels are drawn. For the first year, calcitonin levels are obtained every three months, then every six months thereafter.

If the calcitonin level remains high, this invariably means undetected recurrent or metastatic disease. The determination of the site of this residual disease necessitates a full metastatic workup and CT or MRI of the neck or an octreotide scan. If no overt disease is apparent, some authorities recommend open exploration of the neck and prophylactic neck dissections if these have not already been performed, whereas others recommend external radiation to the neck.

ROLE OF POSTOPERATIVE EXTERNAL RADIATION

The main indication for external beam radiation in well-differentiated and medullary cancers is residual, inoperable cancer or cancer that has undergone anaplastic transformation. At least 50 Gy should be administered, with the results being better for microscopic residua but rarely for macroscopic tumor as well. External radiation appears more effective than radioactive iodine in treating local recurrence in well-differentiated cancer, whereas radioactive iodine is better for managing distant metastases. Radiation is the treatment of choice for anaplastic carcinoma, often combined with chemotherapy.

ROLE OF CHEMOTHERAPY

In advanced, well-differentiated cancers and medullary carcinomas that have proved to be refractory to conventional therapy, a wide variety of chemotherapeutic drugs have been used, but results have been most disappointing; likewise for anaplastic cancer, with predictably poor results.

ROLE OF POSTOPERATIVE THYROID HORMONE ADMINISTRATION

Thyroid hormone replacement in patients who have unergone ablation of all thyroid tissue either by surgery or radiation is necessary. It is in addition most useful in controlling any microscopic residual well-differentiated thyroid cancer that may have been left locally, regionally, or distantly.

CONTROVERSY

The role of thyroid suppression in patients who have undergone subtotal thyroidectomy is more controversial, with some believing that it is of value in improving survival by suppressing any residual cancer.

PROGNOSIS

Overall, patients with well-differentiated cancer do extremely well with excellent long-term survival. In low-risk patients (the vast majority), the mortality rate is 1 to 2%. In high-risk patients (those with adverse prognostic indicators), the mortality rate is 40 to 50%. Patients with medullary carcinoma, detected by screening at an early stage, have an excellent prognosis. Hereditary and sporadic medullary cancers have similar survivals (82% at 5 years and 43% at 20 years). Anaplastic cancer has a dismal survival rate and is usually incurable by the time the patient presents.

SUGGESTED READINGS

Friedman M, Toriumi D, Maffee M. Diagnostic imaging in thyroid cancer. *Am J Surg* 1988;155:215.

Goepert H, Callender G. Differentiated thyroid cancer—papillary and follicular carcinoma. *Am J Otolaryngol* 1994;15:167–179.

Schroder DM, Chambers A, France CJ. Operative strategy for thyroid cancer. Is total thyroidectomy worth the price? *Cancer* 1986;58:2320–2328.

Shah JP, Loree T, Dharker D. Prognostic factors in differentiated carcinoma of the thyroid gland. *Am J Surg* 1992;164:658–661.

Simpson WJ, Panzarella T, Carruthers JS. Papillary and follicular thyroid cancer: impact of treatment in 1,578 patients. *Int J Radiat Oncol Biol Phys* 1988;83:679–688.

Singer PA. Clinical approach to thyroid function testing. In: Falk SA, ed. *Thyroid Disease*. 2nd ed. Philadelphia: Lippincott-Raven; 1977.

Chapter 80

SPECIAL CONSIDERATIONS: PARATHYROID GLANDS

Jack L. Gluckman

ANATOMY

There are usually four parathyroid glands. However, in 2 to 5% of the population, five or more may be present. The gross appearance is bean-like, with a pink color that changes to reddish-brown when manipulated. The glands are small (average dimension 5 × 3 × 2 mm) and weigh 30 to 50 mg. Histologically they are well encapsulated, with the parenchyma consisting of chief and oxyphilic cells and fibrous stroma with fat cells. The blood supply to the parathyroids is from the inferior thyroid artery (the superior gland is supplied by a branch from this artery or occasionally from the superior thyroid artery).

EMBRYOLOGY

The superior glands arise from the fourth branchial pouch (they share their origin with the ultimobranchial complex, which gives rise to calcitonin-secreting C cells of the thyroid). They descend to the posterior aspect of the thyroid gland. Rarely, they may overdescend into the upper posterior mediastinum. If they fail to descend, they may be found close to the larynx.

The inferior glands arise from the third branchial pouch (together with the thymus). They are usually found related to the lower pole of the thyroid. If they overdescend, they may be found in the anterior mediastinum or tracheo-esophageal groove. The supernumerary glands may be found almost anywhere in the neck and upper mediastinum.

PHYSIOLOGY

Ninety-nine percent of the total body calcium is present in the skeleton and only a small percentage is in extracellular and intracellular fluid. In the blood, 50% of the calcium is protein bound, whereas 45% is ionized and 5% complexed to phosphate and citrate. Only the ionized calcium is active. Patients with hypoalbuminemia will therefore have elevated ionized calcium levels.

Calcium homeostasis is controlled by the interaction of parathyroid hormone, vitamin A metabolism, and calcitonin on bone, kidney, and gastrointestinal mucosa. Ingested calcium is absorbed by the gastrointestinal mucosa and this is affected by vitamin D and parathyroid hormone. Non–protein-bound calcium is excreted via the kidney, being initially filtered and then being 95% resorbed. Calcium is actively transported between bone and extracellular fluid, influenced by parathyroid hormone, calcitonin, and vitamin D. Secretion of parathyroid hormone is inversely related to the concentration of calcium in the blood. It has a direct effect on bone and kidney and an indirect effect on the gastrointestinal mucosa. In severe magnesium deficiency, parathyroid hormone secretion

TABLE 80–1 CAUSES OF HYPERCALCEMIA

Primary hyperparathyroidism
Malignancy
   Skeletal metastases
   Humoral hypercalcemia of malignancy
Granulomas
Hyperthyroidism
Adrenal insufficiency
Drugs
   Thiazide diuretics
   Lithium
   Estrogens/antiestrogens
   Milk-alkali syndrome
   Vitamin A and D toxicity
Immobilization
Acute and chronic renal disease
Benign familial hypocalciuric hypercalcemia

is blunted. Causes of hypercalcemia are listed in Table 80–1).

PRIMARY HYPERPARATHYROIDISM

The female to male ratio is 2:1 particularly in the over 60 age group. A large percentage have only biochemical evidence of hyperthyroidism, and many others have only vague nonspecific manifestations, such as malaise and myalgias. Classic features of hyperparathyroidism are noted in Table 80–2.

TABLE 80–2 CLINICAL FEATURES OF HYPERPARATHYROIDISM

Constitutional	Fatigue, anorexia, weight loss
Musculoskeletal	Bone and joint pain, weakness
Renal	Calculi, renal failure, hematuria, polyuria
Gastrointestinal	Constipation, peptic ulcer, pancreatitis
Neurologic	Headache, memory loss, insomnia, hallucinations, depression, apathy
Cardiovascular	Arrythmias, hypertension
Skin	Pruritus

PEARL... Eighty to ninety percent of cases are due to an adenoma; rarely double adenomas can occur. Ten to twenty percent are due to diffuse parathyroid hyperplasia.

Those patients with multiple endocrine neoplasia (MEN) syndromes 1 and 2A have hyperplasia. One percent is due to parathyroid carcinoma.

An adenoma presents as a solitary mass that is usually solid and rarely cystic. It is almost never clinically palpable. Histologically a rim of normal tissue is useful in distinguishing it from hyperplasia. Usually the chief cell is predominant with marked pleomorphism.

Hyperplasia may be either chief cell hyperplasia or clear cell hyperplasia; 25 to 35% of chief cell hyperplasia patients have MEN syndrome. The glands may be enlarged unequally. Clear cell hyperplasia is more likely to have large glands with the superior frequently larger than the inferior glands.

Parathyroid carcinoma is rare, with the average age of presentation being the fifth decade. There is a male to female ratio of 1:1. It usually presents with elevated calcium. It may infiltrate locally or spread to lungs, liver, and bones. Usually, however, it has an indolent course, with a 50% 5-year survival.

SECONDARY HYPERPARATHYROIDISM

This is due to increased parathyroid hormone secretion secondary to chronic hypocalcemia and is associated with parathyroid gland hyperplasia. Chronic renal failure is the most common cause. Features include all the manifestations of hypercalcemia.

SPECIAL CONSIDERATION

Rarely in chronic renal failure, the parathyroids develop autonomous unregulated secretion of parathormone (tertiary hyperparathyroidism).

FAMILIAL HYPERPARATHYROIDISM

WERNER'S SYNDROME—MEN TYPE I

This syndrome is characterized by parathyroid hyperplasia (occasionally adenoma), pituitary tumors, and pancreatic tumors. Occasionally carcinoid, ovarian, differentiated thyroid tumors, and melanoma may be associated.

SIPPLE'S SYNDROME

This syndrome is divided into two types: Type 2A consists of parathyroid hyperplasia or adenoma, medullary thyroid cancer, and phaeochromocytoma. Type 2B consists of features of type 2A plus mucosal neuromas and marfanoid habitus, but there is no hyperparathyroidism.

PATIENT EVALUATION

Careful history regarding family, drug usage, and renal symptoms is essential. The parathyroids are usually not palpable. There may be manifestations of MEN syndrome on clinical examination.

Biochemically, the serum calcium should be elevated on at least three separate samples (ionized calcium). Serum protein levels are needed if total serum calcium levels are measured. Alkaline phosphatase is usually elevated and serum phosphorus is usually low. Renal function is assessed with blood urea nitrogen (BUN) and serum creatinine. Parathyroid hormone assays can differentiate hypercalcemia of parathyroid and nonparathyroid origin.

LOCALIZATION STUDIES

Some clinicians believe that no localization studies are needed prior to the initial surgical exploration and these tests should be confined to those cases that have failed surgical exploration. Most surgeons however perform localization studies of some sort. Computed tomography (CT) scan is of little value except in detecting mediastinal adenomas. Ultrasonography has an accuracy rate of 90%, but it may be difficult to differentiate thyroid nodules from parathyroid adenomas, and ultrasonography may fail to localize parathyroid disease in the presence of

large nodular goiters. Magnetic resonance imaging (MRI) has a high sensitivity and accuracy but is quite expensive. It is, however, readily available and is the modality of choice for many physicians. Thallium-technetium subtraction studies have an over 90% accuracy rate reported in experienced hands and are the least expensive. Sestamibi-technetium scintigraphy is the most accurate of all tests but is not readily available in some centers. Angiography and selective venous catheterization for parathormone should be reserved for the patient who has failed exploration. It is labor intensive, expensive, and difficult to perform.

SURGICAL MANAGEMENT OF HYPERPARATHYROIDISM

The ideal patient for surgery is a healthy individual with symptomatic hyperparathyroidism and serum calcium levels 1 mg above normal limits. As most patients are postmenopausal women, early surgery is indicated to decrease the incidence of osteoporosis. If an adenoma is encountered, it should be removed and sent for frozen section. The other glands should be inspected and one other gland can be carefully biopsied to compare histology to that of the removed adenoma if necessary. Because of the possibility of double adenoma, it is recommended to routinely explore both sides. If hyperplasia is encountered, 3½ glands should be removed. One can also remove all four glands and autotransplant one gland into a muscle bed (usually forearm). Autotransplantation provides normocalcemia in 80% of patients.

If neck exploration is negative, the thyroid gland should be carefully inspected for intrathyroidal tissue (2–5% of patients). If negative, then a systematic exploration of the neck, particularly the tracheoesophageal groove, paratracheal fat, and thymus, should be undertaken.

> **PEARL...** Before reexploration for persistent hyperparathyroidism, every attempt should be made to localize the adenoma preoperatively using techniques already described.

SUGGESTED READINGS

Davidson J, Noyek AM, Gottesman I, et al. The parathyroid adenoma: an imaging/surgical perspective. *J Otolaryngol* 1988;17:282–287.

Hindie E, Melliere D, Simon D. Primary hyperparathyroidism: is technetium 99 sestamibi iodine 123 scanning the best procedure to locate enlarged glands before surgery? *J Clin Endocrinol Metab* 1995;80:302–307.

Petti G. Hyperparathyroidism: a study of 100 cases. *Otolaryngol Head Neck Surg* 1982;90:413–417.

Ralston S, Gallacher S, Patel U. Cancer associated hypercalcemia: morbidity and mortality. Clinical experience with 126 patients. *Ann Intern Med* 1990;112:499–506.

Thompson NW. The history of hyperparathyroidism. *Acta Chir Scand* 1990;156:5.

SECTION XIII

SKULL BASE

Chapter 81

ANATOMY AND PHYSIOLOGY

Myles L. Pensak

An intimate and detailed knowledge of the architecture of the bony skull base along with neural and vascular structures is requisite for any surgeon performing contemporary otorhinolaryngologic surgery (Figs. 81–1 to 81–7).

The irregular and complex bone structure of the skull base makes it one of the most difficult regions to navigate surgically. Compounding this is the fact that vital neural and vascular structures traverse a number of fissures, foramina, and septations in the skull base. To conceptually understand this region, the skull base has been anatomically divided into three cavities. This chapter describes the related regional architecture, recognizing that this anatomic compartmentalization simplifies understanding but does not reflect functional divisions in the purest sense.

ANATOMY AND DEVELOPMENTAL EMBRYOLOGY

THE SKULL

The embryologic development of the skull results from mesenchyme developing around the forming brain. The neurocranium is the protective cover found encasing the brain, and the viscerocranium is the skeleton covering the jaw. The skull base takes origin from the chondrocranium (fused cartilage), which later undergoes enchondral ossification.

There are two principal fusion plates. The parachordal cartilage fuses about the cranial end of the notochord, subsequently fusing with the sclerotome regions of the occipital somites. The growth of this cartilaginous mass forms the base of the occipital bone. Further growth forms the boundaries of the foramen magnum. Anteriorly, the hypophyseal cartilages fuse about the developing pituitary gland, and upon fusion form the progenitor for the sphenoid bone. The trabeculae crani form the ethmoid bone, the ala orbitalis forms the lesser wing of the sphenoid, and finally the petrous and mastoid portions of the temporal bone form the otic capsule while the nasal capsule helps form the ethmoid bones.

During fetal life and infancy, the flat bones of the skull are separated by dense connective tissue membranes called sutures. Six large fibrous areas are present called fontanelles. Developmental molding of the skull during rapid growth periods is accommodated by these soft fontenelles.

SPECIAL CONSIDERATION

The skull at birth is round, and the bones are thin. The cranium and skull are large in proportion to the rest of the skeleton and in particular to the face.

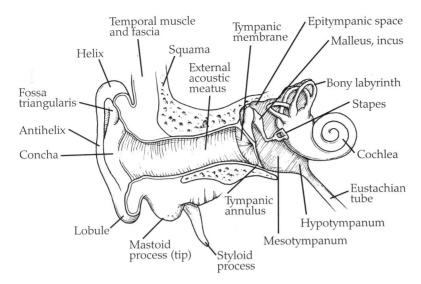

FIGURE 81–1 Embryologically, the auricle, the middle ear complex, and the inner ear develop from disparate sources. Natural pathways and fissures as well as neural and vascular channels invite unimpeded extension of both infectious processes and tumors progressing along the bony skull base.

The face is small due to the small size of the jaw and the absence of paranasal air sinuses. Maturation of the viscerocranium reflects the development of the cartilaginous skeleton of the first three branchial arches: (1) Meckel's cartilage, (2) Reichert's cartilage, and (3) third arch cartilage.

Intramembranous ossification occurs within the maxillary process of the first branchial arch and forms the premaxilla, maxilla, zygomatic, and squamous portions of the temporal bone. The mesenchyme of the mandibular process condenses around the first arch cartilage, undergoes intramembranous ossification, and forms the mandible.

There is an intimate relationship between the developing foregut and the developing central nervous system. The notochord lies between the roof of the foregut and the nervous system in a bed of mesoderm. Rathke's pouch pri-

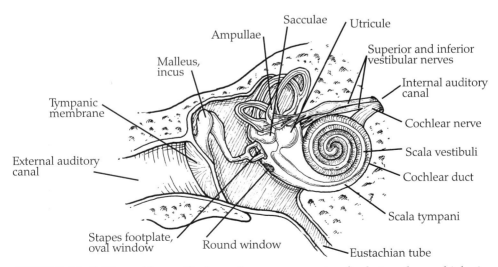

FIGURE 81–2 The cochleovestibular end-organ represents a finely tuned neurobiologic receptor and transducer. Enclosed within this, the hardest bone in the body, the fluids and neural elements contained within the scala tympani, vestibuli, and cochlear duct account for auditory signal processing as well as balance.

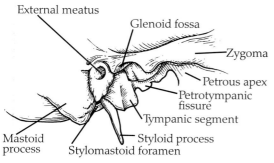

FIGURE 81–3 As the tympanic ring expands and the mastoid process descends, the stylomastoid foramen and facial nerve come to occupy a fixed location in the adult. The intimate juxtaposition of the facial nerve at this junction with the skull base needs to be addressed when dealing with tumors, in particular glomus jugulare lesions.

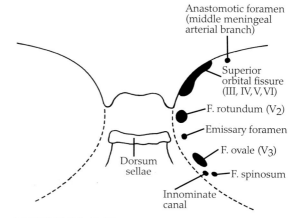

FIGURE 81–5 The cavernous sinus contains not only venous structures but also neural and arterial elements. F., foramen.

mordium for the anterior pituitary lies ventral to the anterior buccal pharyngeal membrane, developing from the dorsal ectoderm of the stomodeum or mouth. This is important as the notochord is thought to terminate anteriorly in the body of the basisphenoid immediately posterior to the sella turcica.

VASCULAR STRUCTURES

The skull base vascular embryology is complex. In the 4- to 6-mm crown rump length embryo, the aortic arch noted in the first three pharyngeal bars forms the basis for the common and internal carotid arteries. Capillaries drain into a superfi-

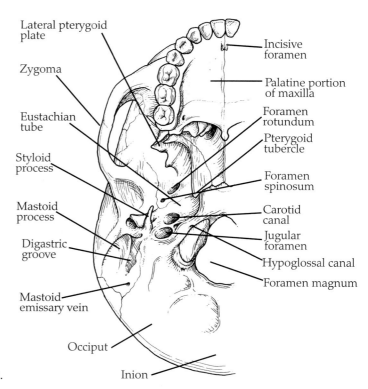

FIGURE 81–4 The bony skull base is perforated by numerous named (and unnamed) fissures and foramina.

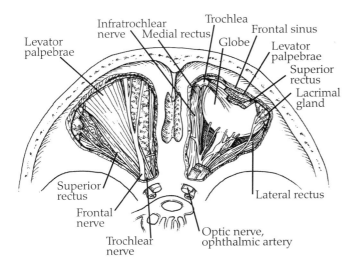

FIGURE 81–6 The orbital contents are intimately aligned such that violation by infection, tumor, or trauma may have devastating consequences.

cial venous plexus, which subserves the dural layer dorsal and lateral to the developing neural tube. A plexus of tributaries pools and drains into a ventrally located primary head sinus.

The primary head sinus in continuity with the anterior cardinal vein gives rise to the inter-nal jugular vein. At this early stage, the primitive lingulofacial vein (future common facial vein) is noted to feed into the future internal jugular vein. Immediately adjacent to this venous plexus lies the ventral pharyngeal artery, which will soon form the external carotid artery.

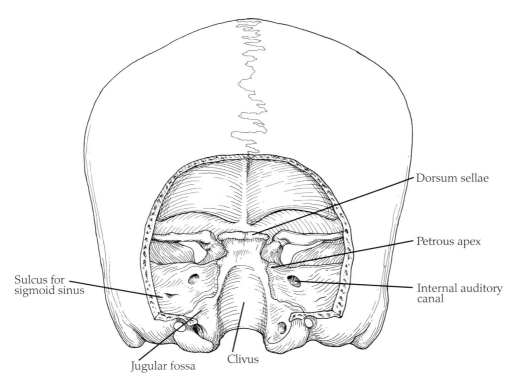

FIGURE 81–7 The clivus lies at the central portion of the bony skull base and is quite difficult to approach, although numerous routes are currently described.

An independent arteriovenous plexus noted about the optic vesicle in the developing maxillary process can be seen.

Finally, it is noted that the anterior cardinal vein (from the head) joins the posterior cardinal vein (from the trunk) to form the common cardinal vein (the duct of Cuvier) entering the primitive heart.

In the 6-mm embryo, the primitive maxillary vein is noted to drain the ventral caudal optic vessel and the olfactory region above and Rathke's pouch below. Ultimately, this vessel becomes the drainage port for all ophthalmic and orbital veins in the adult.

SPECIAL CONSIDERATION

As the embryonic brain matures, dural venous channels migrate laterally, whereas neural ganglion remain medially placed.

During the 7- to 12-mm embryonic stage, the expansion of the frontal and maxillary regions is significant, whereas the mandibular and hyoid bars develop slowly. Concomitantly, the basilar and vertebral arteries mature as the auricular hillocks elevate and the glossopharyngeal bar is overgrown by the cervical sinus.

As the head sinus migrates laterally, there is simultaneous caudal migration of the posterior dural root, which will join the primitive jugular vein, becoming the caudal end of the sigmoid sinus. This venous ring lies lateral to cranial nerve X and dorsocranially to fibers of cranial nerve XI. The proximal pia arachnoid vein forms the inferior petrosal sinus juxtaposing the roots of cranial nerves X and XI.

During the 12- to 14-mm stage the chondrocranium overlying the future skull base is noted. Condensations of mesenchyme radiate from separate cartilages surrounding the noted dorsal venous tributaries. During this period the ventral jugular vein completes its migration to the lateral side of the cranial nerve XII primordium. Fibers of the second and third cervical nerves join cranial nerve XII to form the ansi hypoglossae.

At the 16- to 18-mm stage the head sinus is noted more laterally than dorsally to the optic capsule. The head sinus is now being replaced by secondary anastomoses that drain the sigmoid sinus. At this time the cephalically positioned primitive transverse sinus is noted. Inferiorly, the facial region is drained cranially by the proximal ophthalmic vein and maxillary tributaries of the head sinus, whereas caudal drainage is through the lingulofacial vein.

SPECIAL CONSIDERATION

This bidirectional flow of blood circumscribing the developing facial architecture is important because this is the first time that a definitive extracranial venous system is appreciated.

During this period the maxillary vein once confined to the maxillary process with the maxillary division of cranial nerve V redistributes cranially and caudally, encompassing the territory of the ophthalmic and mandibular divisions of the trigeminal nerve.

During the 16- to 18-mm embryo growth stage, the plexiform vertebral vein and companion artery are noted. The early vertebral vein empties into the internal jugular vein or primitive subclavian vein.

During the 18- to 21-mm stage the external jugular system is noted, followed shortly by the establishment of the external carotid system. The head sinus has almost disappeared except for a short segment, the lateral portion of the future cavernous sinus. The caudodorsal end of the parotic sinus forms the adult superior petrosal sinus. The anterior and middle branches develop into a tentorial plexus.

By the 22-mm stage, the chondrocranium is prominent at the base of the brain and surrounds the roots of the cranial nerves especially in the basi-occipital and temporo-occipital region. As this development occurs, the newly formed inferior petrosal sinus and cavernous sinuses allow direct caudal blood flow into the internal jugular vein.

Arterial development of the skull base centers around the growth and arborization of four vessels: (1) the dorsal ophthalmic artery, (2) the stapedial artery, (3) the trigeminal artery, and (4) the primitive maxillary artery. The dorsal ophthalmic artery is responsible for supplying the optic nerve and the globe itself after entering the orbit through the superior orbital fissure, initially noted in primitive mesenchymal tissue. While regressing by the time of birth, its proximal remnant is often described as the resultant inferior lateral trunk, the second most prominent branch of the intracavernous internal carotid artery.

The stapedial artery may be followed in the cephalic direction entering the floor of the temporal fossa through a small unnamed foramen on the upper surface of the petrous bone. Ultimately it will contribute to the development of the middle meningeal artery and the maxillary mandibular artery, which eventually leaves the cranial cavity through the foramen spinosum as the future maxillary artery. The adult trigeminal artery, which is noted to remain patent with an incidence of 0.1 to 0.5%, takes origin from the basilar system and is noted to run medially to the trigeminal nerve following the ophthalmic division as it enters the cavernous sinus.

Finally, the primitive maxillary artery, taking origin from the carotid siphon, supplies the posterior portion of the pituitary anastomoses with its counterpart from the contralateral side.

NEURAL STRUCTURES

The relationship of the carotid artery to the venous vasculature, neural elements, and osteomeningeal interfaces is central to the concern with which surgeons approach lesions of the skull base. The proximal intracranial portion of the carotid artery is relatively fixed lying within the carotid canal, ensheathed by a variable thickness fibrous membrane at the level of the gasserian ganglion. By contrast, the intracavernous carotid artery is free and unencumbered by either a fibrocartilaginous or osseus sheath.

Intrapetrous (subtemporal or middle fossa) dissection with an intact cochleovestibular end organ via either Glasscock's triangle or Kawase's triangle demonstrates the variable thickness of the intrapetrous carotid canal. Access to the petrous internal carotid artery shows fibers of the sympathetic plexus in this region before branches join cranial nerve VI. In general, this portion of the internal carotid artery is referred to as the posterior loop, and the tensor tympani and eustachian tube can be noted to lie lateral to this structure. As the carotid passes above the foramen lacerum toward the posterior clinoid process, it then turns anteriorly as its horizontal component passes upward at the level of the anterior clinoid process. In a significant majority of cases the internal carotid is exposed under the trigeminal nerve, whereas in a lesser number the bone is quite thin. Before reaching the fibrocartilage of the foramen lacerum, an interperiosteal venous plexus is noted. In a small number of cases, there is continuity of the venous plexus about the middle meningeal artery at the foramen spinosum. However, in the vast majority, the pericarotid venous plexus represents an extension of the posterior lateral cavernous sinus plexus or connects directly to the superior petrosal sinus.

Once fully matured, the carotid relationship with the petrous otic capsule structure is well defined. The cochlea may be found at a variable depth from the transition zone between the vertical and horizontal carotid canal, averaging approximately 2.5 mm in the posterior or posterior/superior direction. Variable pneumatization patterns are expected and account for the variability of distances. Furthermore, the cochlea intimately effacing the lateral portion of the internal carotid artery is quite close to the facial nerve, averaging 0.7 mm from the geniculate ganglion. After passing through the region of the foramen lacerum, the intracavernous carotid artery is defined with two main segments noted after passing between the petrous apex and the sphenoid base. The medial and anterior roots are noted to be free, whereas the posterior and lateral roots are not only confined by the carotid canal but are also fixed by the banding of the gasserian ganglion.

In the developed skull base, the anterior fossa supports the frontal lobes. The boundaries of the anterior fossa are represented anteriorly by the inner table of the frontal bone and a midline attachment for the falx cerebri. Posteriorly, the lesser wing of the sphenoid articulates laterally with the frontal bone and juxtaposes the inferoanterior angle of the parietal bone or pterion. The tentorium cerebelli is attached to the lesser sphenoid wing at the anterior clinoid process. The cribriform plate of the ethmoid bone is noted medially with an osseous projection representing an upward projection of the ethmoid bone medially in the midline wherein the falx cerebri is attached. The foramen cecum is noted opening for the transmission of a nasal mucosal vein. The anterior ethmoid nerve transverses a bone in the cribriform plate, whereas the olfactory bulb passes through small perforations in the plate before joining to form the olfactory nerve.

The middle cranial fossa houses the temporal lobes. Anteriorly it is effaced by the lesser wings of the sphenoid and posteriorly by the superior border of the petrous ridge. Laterally, the squamous portions of the temporal lobe and greater wings of the sphenoid join with the parietal bones to form its boundaries. Lying between the greater and lesser wings of the sphenoid the superior orbital fissure transmits cranial nerves III, IV, and VI along with the superior ophthalmic vein. The optic canal anteriorly transmits both the ophthalmic artery and the optic nerve. Along the floor, immediately behind and medial to the superior orbital fissure perforation of the greater wing of the sphenoid is the foramen rotundum through which the maxillary division of the trigeminal nerve passes. Posterior to this lies the foramen ovale through which the lesser petrosal nerve and the sensory root and small motor roots of the trigeminal nerve pass to the infratemporal fossa. Just posterior to the foramen ovale lies the foramen spinosum for the transmission of the middle meningeal artery. At the apex of the petrous ridge, the trigeminal ganglion is located. Along the anterior surface of the petrous ridge, both the greater and lesser petrosal nerves can be identified. Medial to the trigeminal ganglion in Dorello's canal, the abducens nerve is noted to pass across the apex of the petrous bone before entering the lateral wall of the cavernous sinus.

The cerebellum, pons, and medulla can be noted to be contained within the posterior fossa cavity. Anteriorly, it is bordered by the superior walls of the petrous pyramid and posteriorly by the internal surfaces of both the squamosa portion of the temporal bone and the occipital bones. Lying anterior and lateral to the margins of the foramen magnum, the hypoglossal canal is responsible for transmission of cranial nerve XII. Juxtaposed between the occipital bone and the lower portion of the petrous temporal bone, the jugular foramen is identified. The anterior compartment contains the inferior petrosal sinus and cranial nerves IX, X, and XI. The posterior component houses the terminus of the sigmoid sinus as it passes through the bony skull base to form the internal jugular vein. Cephalic to the jugular foramen lies the porous acousticus for the transmission of both cranial nerves VII and VIII as they pass through the cerebellopontine angle. Upon entrance into the internal auditory canal, the nerves are compartmentalized with the facial nerve occupying the anterior-superior quadrant of the canal, the cochlear nerve occupying the anterior-inferior portion, and the two vestibular nerves located posteriorly. At the fundal region of the canal, the crista falciformis divides the superior from inferior compartment, whereas Bill's bar is noted to demarcate the posterior from anterior compartment superiorly.

ANATOMY: THE TEMPORAL BONE

The temporal bone is situated as a pyramidal structure at the center of the skull base. Superiorly, the tegmen separates it from the middle fossa; posteriorly is the posterior fossa; and anteriorly are the parotid and temporomandibular joint. Inferiorly, the infratemporal fossa is noted, whereas at the temporal bone's apex the anterior-most segment of the bone is attached to the clivus by the petroclival ligament. Along the floor of the temporal bone, passing from a posterior to anterior position, lie the stylomastoid foramen, the jugular bulb, and the carotid canal.

On the temporal bone's posterior surface the endolymphatic sac impression is noted. Just medially, the porous acousticus is appreciated.

Passing from their respective root entry zones from the brainstem, the seventh and eighth nerves traverse the cerebellopontine angle to enter the internal auditory canal (IAC) at the porous acousticus. Within the IAC, the posterior fossa dura covers the nerves until it thins out at the Obersteiner-Redlich zone. The facial nerve comes to occupy the anterior-superior compartment; the cochlear nerve, the anterior-inferior compartment; and the vestibular divisions superior and inferior, the posterior field of the IAC. At the lateral end of the canal a horizontal shelf of bone separates the superior from inferior compartments and the crista falciformis vertical wedge of bone separates the facial and superior vestibular nerves in the superior compartment of the fundal region of the IAC. This bone is called Bill's bar, named for William House, M.D.

The internal auditory artery travels within an arachnoid plane between the anterior and posterior compartments. The anterior-inferior cerebellar artery is found to curl within the IAC in upward of 40% of specimens studied.

Leaving the fundal area of the IAC, the facial nerve can be found within a narrow bony channel between the cochlea anteriorly and the superior canal posteriorly. At the level of the geniculate ganglion, the greater superficial petrosal nerve is given off, exits the facial hiatus, and is directed anteriorly, providing preganglionic parasympathetic fibers to the parotid gland.

At the geniculate ganglion the nerve is directed posteriorly at its first genu and passes into the middle ear directed just above the cochleariformis process. At the horizontal canal the nerve turns inferiorly and is directed within the mastoid compartment to the stylomastoid foramen. Within the vertical segment it gives off two branches: the chordae tympani, which supplies taste to the ipsilateral tongue, and the branch that innervates the stapedius muscle.

At the stylomastoid foramen the nerve passes through a fibrocartilaginous channel before it enters the belly of the parotid gland, where it divides into major constituent branches that innervate the mimetic muscles of facial expression.

At the petrous apex the carotid artery can be seen to lie just below the eustachian tube. Entering the floor of the petrous bone, it travels superiorly, intimately effacing the cochlea until the level of the protympanum, where it turns in an anterior direction and is directed cephalically. Viewed from the middle fossa it sits medial to the greater superficial petrosal nerve and the trigeminal nerve. The artery is noted to pass through the foramen lacerum, a cartilaginous covering just before the anterior clinoid process, where it breaches the dura. The branches of the trigeminal nerve can be seen to pass forward, directed to the superior orbital fissure (V_1), foramen ovale (V_2), and the foramen rotundum (V_3). The middle meningeal artery passes through the foramen spinosum.

The venous anatomy that encompasses the temporal bone is made up of the superior and inferior petrosal sinuses. The latter, upon entering the jugular bulb, is noted to have several points of entry. The sigmoid sinus receives substantial blood flow from the transverse sinus. The sigmoid is directed in an anterior-inferior direction toward the variably placed jugular bulb. A high jugular bulb may sit just under the annular margin well within the middle ear space.

Cranial nerves IX, X, and XI are noted to lie in the pars nervosa of the jugular foramen. Nerve VI lies in a small channel referred to as Dorello's canal at the petrous apex and can be followed along the lateral tentorial edge until it passes into the cavernous sinus.

SUGGESTED READINGS

Grant JCB, ed. *Grant's Atlas of Anatomy.* 6th ed. Baltimore: Williams & Wilkins; 1972.

Hollinshead WH, ed. *Anatomy for Surgeons.* Vol. 1. 2nd ed. New York: Harper & Row, 1968.

Jackler RK, ed. *Skull Base Surgery.* St. Louis: CV Mosby; 1996:121–162.

Pensak ML. *The Cavernous Sinus: An Anatomic Study with Clinical Implication.* Triologic thesis, The Triologic Society, 1992.

Schuknecht HF, ed. *Pathology of the Ear.* Philadelphia: Lea & Febiger; 1993.

Chapter 82

CLINICAL TESTS

Myles L. Pensak

In the extirpation of skull base lesions, the surgeon endeavors to remove the tumor with optimal preservation of neurologic and vascular structures. Although the complete excision of neuromas most often requires the sacrifice of the principal nerve and in cases of malignancy may mandate the elective sacrifice of neighboring neural structures, utilization of intraoperative monitoring techniques have enhanced our ability to accomplish this goal with the greatest element of safety. Moreover, evoked potential feedback increases operative safety by immediately reporting that brainstem function may be threatened by a given surgical maneuver.

INTRAOPERATIVE MONITORING OF OCULAR AND EXTRAOCULAR MOTOR FUNCTION

Tumors of the skull base including those that arise from the pituitary or extend from the clivus and ultimately invade the cavernous sinus may compromise oculomotor function. Furthermore, extensive dissections that require the manipulation of the extraocular muscles or nerves may lead to visual dysfunction and so monitoring during surgery is extremely important.

EXTRAOCULAR ANATOMY

Cranial Nerve III— The Oculomotor Nerve

The nucleus of the third nerve lies within the midbrain at the level of the superior calliculus. As fibers pass ventrally through the red nucleus, they are directed below the floor of the third ventricle and the Edinger-Westphal nucleus. The fibers exit the brainstem between the cerebral peduncles juxtaposing the posterior and superior cerebellar arteries. Posterolaterally, the nerve enters the lateral wall of the cavernous sinus through which it is directed anteriorly. Enveloped in a dural sheath, it passes through the superior orbital fissure wherein it divides into superior and inferior branches to innervate four of the six ocular muscles, including the medial and inferior recti, inferior oblique, superior recti, and levator palpebrae superiori.

Cranial Nerve IV— The Trochlear Nerve

At the level of the inferior colliculus the nucleus of the fourth nerve can be noted within the tegmentum of the midbrain. The trochlear nucleus is noted to indent the medial longitudinal fasciculus with axons passing caudally in the periaqueductal gray matter about the cerebral aqueduct and the fourth ventricle. The nerve exits the brainstem dorsally, passing anteriorly and ventrally around the basis pedunculi to enter the lateral wall of the cavernous sinus ventral to the third nerve. It decussates into three divisions within the superior orbital fissure and innervates the superior oblique muscle.

Cranial Nerve VI— The Abducens Nerve

The nucleus of the sixth nerve lies within the tegmental portion of the caudal pons, ventral to the floor of the fourth ventricle, and intimately related to the internal genu of the facial nerve, forming the facial caliculus. The fibers pass directly to the ventral surface of the pons, exiting at the pontomedullary junction. Coursing laterally and rostrally, the nerve passes through Dorello's canal at the apex of the petrous ridge. The nerve passes through a dural sheath and runs with the internal carotid artery medially within the cavernous sinus until it exits the superior orbital fissure to innervate the lateral rectus muscle.

TECHNIQUE OF INTRAOPERATIVE MONITORING

There are a number of devices currently on the market that directly monitor the extraocular motor nerves during surgery. At the University of Cincinnati, we currently employ the Xomed-Treace NIM-II Nerve Integrity Monitor. This device facilitates simultaneous monitoring and has the added advantage of providing both visual and auditory feedback. The device also includes a muting system that automatically eliminates electrical artifact during the procedure.

> **PEARL•••** No muscle relaxant or neuromuscular blockade should be employed by the anesthesiologist.

Kartush and Bouchard (1992) have advocated the complete elimination of muscle relaxant or neuromuscular blocking agents during cases that are monitored to avoid the camouflaging of even

small amplitude responses that may result from mechanical manipulation. Short-acting, reversible paralytic agents, however, may be employed during intubation (Fig. 82–1).

The choice of electrode array is important. Surface electrodes require a paste interface with the skin. During the procedure the electrodes may shift. Furthermore, because of variable skin thickness or debris, there may be increased artifact or resistance, thus distorting the quality and character of the generated evoked potential. By comparison, needle electrodes allow for a fixed reference point and are generally quite stable once affixed in place with a sticky tape or drape (Fig. 82–2).

In monitoring cranial nerves III, IV, and VI, electrodes are placed in or near the inferior rectus, superior oblique, and lateral recti muscles respectfully.

> **PITFALL•••** Be specific regarding anatomic field being monitored. Nerve "cross-talk" is very common.

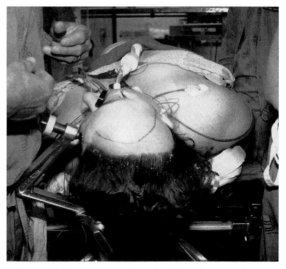

FIGURE 82–1 Immediately following intubation and positioning of the patient, the electrode array for intraoperative monitoring is set. Often with multiple nerves being concomitantly followed, the neurophysiologist monitoring the patient must set the wires and electrodes in a fashion so as not to be caught by drapes, anesthesia equipment, or field equipment. See Color Plate 82–1.

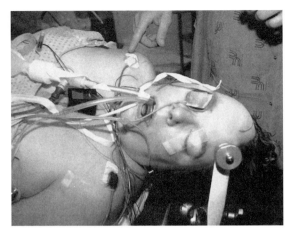

FIGURE 82-2 The choice of electrode array is important. Needle electrodes allow for a fixed reference point and are quite stable. See Color Plate 82–2.

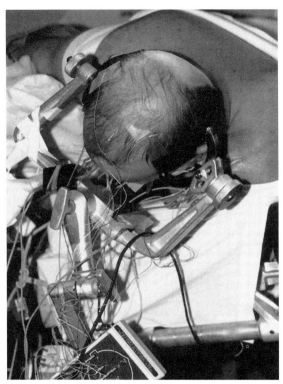

FIGURE 82-3 With electrodes set, only one reference electrode is employed despite the number of nerves being assessed. Impedance is checked relative to both interelectrode and field impedance before proceding. See Color Plate 82–3.

It is important that when monitoring nerve VI along with VII, the electrodes be intimately applied within the anatomic field of nerve VI to avoid cross-field stimulation from the orbicularis oculi muscle. Once set, a ground electrode is placed and a reference electrode is set to the contralateral side. However, it does not matter which nerve is isolated, as no more than one reference electrode is employed despite the number of nerves being assessed. With the electrode array set, impedance is checked and established to be less than 1000 ohm (interelectrode) and less than 5000 ohm (field impedance) to reduce field or operating room environmental electromagnetic interference (Fig. 82–3).

Irrespective of the monitoring array employed, a monopolar or bipolar stimulus may be utilized. Monopolar stimulators are thinner and do not become ineffective if blood or cerebrospinal fluid (CSF) passes between the probe tips and target nerve. However, bipolar stimulation is more selective and does not result in artifact due to current spread. The unit employed for stimulation should be adjustable for variable current delivery. Clearly, the lower the amperage (0.05 mA), the more sensitive the response.

The generated EMG may be a burst or a repetitive response. The former is usually transmitted and results from mechanical stimulation,

SPECIAL CONSIDERATION

Stimulus response may result from a number of electromechanical phenomena. Dissection with mechanical manipulation of the nerve either directly or through transmitted stimulation as the tumor is manipulated will result in a generated wave response. Furthermore, cold water irrigation or thermal transfer from bipolar cautery, ultrasonic aspiration, or laser manipulation may all result in neural stimulation.

whereas the latter occurs with direct current application to the nerve or resultant from injury potential.

> **PEARL...** It has been our clinical experience that a reduction of greater than 50% of the initial stimulus amplitude between proximal and distal nerve strongly suggests postoperative weakness or dysfunction.

INTRAOPERATIVE MONITORING OF OTHER CRANIAL NERVES

CRANIAL NERVE V– THE TRIGEMINAL NERVE

The bulk of the fibers of cranial nerve V are sensory in nature, transmitting information regarding pain, temperature, proprioception, and touch to the face. Afferent fibers pass through the superior orbital fissure (V1), foramen rotundum (V2), and foramen ovale (V3) to the trigeminal ganglion entering the brainstem at the level of the middle cerebellar peduncle (lateral midpontine level).

Fibers from the trigeminal motor nucleus originate in the region of the rostral pons, passing to the foramen ovale, and joining the mandibular division (V3) to innervate the masseteric muscles. Because the trigeminal nerve has both motor and sensory component fibers that can be monitored, several schemes may be employed in assessing neural integrity. Motor function may be studied by electromyogram (EMG) compound muscle action potential (MAP) or nerve action potential (NAP).

In apposition, the somatosensory cortical evoked potential may be used to assess sensory activity. Stimulating cranial nerve V results in antidromic action potentials directed to the contralateral parietal lobe. While several schemes have been suggested, Richmond et al suggest a 10- to 20-electrode placement system with electrodes set at FPZ and either C3 or C4. Twenty-millisecond time windows at two per second stimulus rate with an intensity of 1.0 mA with stimulus duration of 150 microseconds

with filters set at 30 to 3000 Hz will provide an optimal environment. An evoked potential signal averaging computer is needed.

> **PITFALL...** The electrode placement for the motor studies is important, as current may spread and contamination may result in an artificial response through the seventh nerve pathways.

CRANIAL NERVE VII— THE FACIAL NERVE

By receiving input from both cortices, the facial nucleus, which is in the pontine-tegmentum, sends out axons that loop the cranial nerve VI nucleus (internal genu) and exits the ventral brainstem at the pontomedullary junction. The nerve traverses the cerebellopontine angle and passes with the eighth nerve complex through the porous acousticus and the internal auditory canal. The nerve occupies the anterior-superior compartment of the canal, where at the level of the fundus it is noted to be anterior to the superior vestibular nerve separated by Bill's bar above the falciform crest. The nerve passes through the narrow labyrinthine segment to the geniculate ganglion where the greater superficial petrosal branch exits. The nerve then travels anteriorly at the first genu and folds backward above the cochleariformis process passing in a horizontal segment to the second genu, where it is directed inferiorly to the mastoid compartment to its exit at the stylomastoid foramen.

In its vertical segment the nerve gives off branches to the chordae tympani nerve, which enters into the middle ear at the iter chordae posterius, and the stapedius branch, which supplies the stapedius muscle. The extratympanic seventh nerve divides at the pes into five major components, which subtend the muscles of mimetic expression.

Once the electrodes are set at both the orbicularis oculi and marginal mandibular, the tap test developed by Beck and Benicki is employed. The face is gently tapped at the electrode insertion sites and a mechanical-audio response is observed. This results in a display on the EMG of less than 5000 ohm, with the interelectrode difference being less than 1000 ohms.

Recording Montage

Monopolar or bipolar recording arrays may be employed. This arrangement is referred to as the recording montage. A bipolar montage employs paired inputs from the same muscle.

PITFALL••• While minimizing the chance for contamination from adjacent musculature, the bipolar montage may at times result in a distorted wave form wherein the two source inputs effectively cancel each other out.

The monopolar montage has one dedicated electrode with the silent electrode placed away from the index muscle. This setup allows for the potential of artifact intrusion, however, and must be accounted for. The signal picked up by the electrodes must be filtered and amplified to develop a clear EMG signal response. Most EMG responses are low frequency, and thus a low-frequency "high-pass" filter should be employed. By using high-frequency cutoffs, DC line noise can be filtered out.

CONTROVERSY

There has been a significant debate about the optimal technique to employ in the stimulation of the facial nerve. During tumor extirpation Moore has advocated a constant voltage stimulus even with shunting, whereas Prass and Liiders (1985) recommend tip stimulation.

Stimulators may be either monopolar or bipolar. With the monopolar stimulator the signal is generated from a catheter tip and a distally placed grounding anode. False responses can occur when tumors investing the nerve give an artificial response as the signal is propagated from the index nerve. The bipolar stimulator in contradistinction, has the cathode and anode together in the stimulator tip end. With the distance between the two being less than 1 mm, there is a very low likelihood of artifact. The probe, however, is physically larger than the monopolar Prass stimulator.

Generic stimulus parameters to the facial nerve include a two- to five- pulse burst per second stimulus threshold with intensity varying between 0.05 and 2 mA. Inadvertent stimulation of cranial nerve V has been noted to occur as stimulus thresholds have been raised.

SPECIAL CONSIDERATION

Mechanical stimulation will generate two distinct patterns of signal response as described by Prass and Liiders (1985). These are referred to as trains and bursts. Trains are described as asynchronous repetitive EMG firings that suggest injury to the nerve, while a burst is a discrete potential response following stimulation.

CRANIAL NERVE VIII—
THE COCHLEOVESTIBULAR NERVE

The auditory brainstem response (ABR) is a highly selective method of giving feedback regarding the integrity of both the brainstem and auditory systems during skull base surgical procedures. The principles of ABR testing do not vary in the intraoperative modality and in the office setting.

The auditory nerve contains about 30,000 myelinated fibers that join to form a common cochlear nerve within the brainstem prior to its exit at the pontomedullary junction adjoined to the vestibular nerves. Within the confines of the internal auditory canal, the cochlear nerve comes to occupy a position in the anterior-inferior compartment before it enters the modiolus through the habenula perforata to connect to the receptor end-organ.

The ABR is a far-field measure of activity within the auditory system, and is less reliable than direct eighth nerve stimulus response. By means of filtered amplification, the ABR generates a stable signal consisting of five identifiable wave forms that can be retrieved during a procedure to compare signal characteristics such as inter- and intra-aural latencies, intensity, or amplitude response. There are a number of commercially available insert stimulus devices that are currently on the market. Irrespective of the delivery system chosen, the earpiece plug must be firmly applied to the conchal bowl and the ear canal to avoid displacement during the operative procedure. Presently, we use bone wax and a paraffin cover to keep the plug sterile and dry.

> **PEARL•••** It is important to establish a baseline study at the inception of the surgical procedure before any manipulation has been undertaken.

If the signal generated is not clear, the rate of stimulus intensity can be reduced to obtain a clearer signal. Another technique to optimize the development of a clear signal is to increase the sample size. Furthermore, by increasing the loudness of the signal, it can often be cleaned up, as there is an inverse relationship between loudness and latency.

CRANIAL NERVE X—THE VAGUS NERVE

Morbidity from violation of the vagus nerve, especially when the lesion is high, can be quite significant. This is of particular importance during removal of tumors from the jugular foramen.

The nucleus ambiguus of the medulla, located between the cerebellar peduncle and the

> **PITFALL•••** The major problem with monitoring cranial nerve X (recurrent laryngeal nerve) is establishing the accuracy of needle electrode placement. While percutaneous placement may result in inferior localization and result in a poor signal, direct endolaryngeal placement while more accurate is not foolproof.

inferior olive, is the site of origin for the vagus nerve. It leaves the brainstem below the cerebellopontine angle and exits the skull shortly thereafter through the pars nervosa of the jugular foramen to innervate the laryngopharynx. Most recently Teflon-coated wires have been replaced by modified endotracheal tubes that have bipolar stainless steel wires affixed to their external surface. The presence of these wires intimately juxtaposed to the vocal fold provides a direct contact point for feedback from cranial nerve X.

CRANIAL NERVE XII— THE HYPOGLOSSAL NERVE

This nerve takes origin from the hypoglossal nucleus located in the floor of the fourth ventricle. Coursing in a ventral direction, the nerve passes out of the brainstem in a series of rootlets between the olive and medullary pyramid. The nerve passes through the hypoglossal canal between the carotid artery and jugular vein.

> **PEARL•••** Monitoring the twelfth nerve is fairly easy with two stainless steel direct electrodes placed into the oral cavity and into the body of the tongue. Maintenance of fixed nonmobile position is most important. Either monopolar or bipolar delivery systems can provide feedback.

CONCLUSION

The utility of intraoperative monitoring has enjoyed success recently.

> **PEARL•••** The individual doing the monitoring must converse with the surgeons as well as be able to troubleshoot problems in the operating room.

The systems employed, however, should never be a substitute for direct visualization of the cranial nerves. Ultimately, the microdissection of neural structure with minimal trauma will ensure a good outcome.

SUGGESTED READINGS

Bankaitis A, Keith R. Cranial nerve monitoring beyond the facial and auditory nerves. *Semin Hearing* 1993;14(2):161–169.

Barber H, Stockwell C. *Manual of Electronystagmography.* St. Louis: CN Mosby; 1980.

Beck DL. *Handbook of Intraoperative Monitoring.* San Diego: Singular; 1994.

Carl J. Practical anatomy and physiology of the oculomotor system. In: Jacobson G, Newman C, Kartush J, eds. *The Handbook of Balance Function Testing.* St. Louis: CV Mosby; 1993:53–68.

Gutnick HN, Kelleher M, Prass RL. A model for waveform reliability in facial nerve electroneurography. *Otolaryngology Head Neck Surg* 1990;103:344–350.

Harner SG, Daube JR, Beatty CW, Ebersold MJ. Intraoperative monitoring of the facial nerve. *Laryngoscope* 1988;98:209–212.

Hilger J. Facial nerve stimulator. *Trans Am Acad Ophthalmol Otolaryngol* 1964;68:74–76.

Jacobsen G, Tew J Jr. Intraoperative evoked potential monitoring. *J Clin Neurophysiol* 1987; 4:145–176.

Kartush JM, Bouchard KR. *Neuromonitoring in Otology and Head and Neck Surgery.* New York: Raven Press; 1992.

Kartush JM, Prass RL. Facial nerve testing: electroneurography and intraoperative monitoring. In: *Instructional Courses.* Vol 1. St. Louis: CV Mosby; 1988:231–247.

Kwartler J, Luxford W, Atkins J, Shelton C. Facial nerve monitoring. *Otolaryngol Head Neck Surg* 1991;103:681–684.

Lipton TJ, McCaffrey TV, Litchy WJ. Intraoperative electrophysiologic monitoring of laryngeal muscle during thyroid surgery. *Laryngoscope* 1988;98:1292–1296.

Little JR, Lesser RP, Leuders H, et al. Brain stem auditory evoked potentials in posterior circulation surgery. *Neurosurgery* 1983;12:496–502.

Moller AR, Jannetta PJ. Monitoring auditory functions during cranial nerve microvascular decompression operations by direct recording from the eighth nerve. *J Neurosurg* 1983; 59:493–499.

Moller AR, Jannetta PJ. Preservation of facial function during removal of acoustic neuromas: use of monopolar constant voltage stimulation and EMG. *J Neurosurg* 1984;62:757–760.

Moller AR, Moller MB. Does intraoperative monitoring of auditory evoked potentials reduce the incidence of hearing loss as a complication of microvascular decompression of cranial nerves? *Neurosurgery* 1989;24:257–316.

Prass RL, Liiders H. Constant-current versus constant-voltage stimulation. *J Neurosurg* 1985; 62: 622–623.

Schwaber MK, Netterville JL, Maciunas R. Microsurgical anatomy of the lower skull base—a morphometric analysis. *Am J Otol* 1990;11:401–405.

Spahn JG, Bizal J, Ferguson S, Lingeman RE. Identification of the motor laryngeal nerves—a new electrical stimulation technique. *Laryngoscope* 1981;91:1865–1868.

Chapter 83

NEOPLASMS AND CYSTS

Myles L. Pensak

Tumors of the temporal bone and skull base not infrequently grow insidiously and are discovered after they have achieved considerable size (Fig. 83–1). In contradistinction, however, small lesions of the external auditory canal, which often mimic infectious processes and are commonly treated as such, continue to grow until suspicion is raised and a biopsy or definitive treatment is undertaken. This chapter reviews the lesions found in the temporal bone and skull base and discusses management options. Table 83–1 lists common lesions found in the temporal bone.

BENIGN LESIONS OF THE EXTERNAL AUDITORY CANAL

Lesions of the external auditory canal often do not clinically manifest until they cause obstruction or lead to infection. Aural fullness, pressure, tinnitus, hearing loss, and otalgia can be noted. With a secondary infection aural discharge may present. It is not uncommon that a patient has been treated with several courses of antibiotics and drops for the secondary infection when the underlying tumor mass has not been appreciated.

Benign adematous lesions of the ear canal are rare. Inasmuch as cerumen glands are found only in the outer (cartilaginous) third of the ear canal, these lesions manifest by obstructing the auditory canal.

PEARLS... Benign adenoma, ceruminoma, cystadenoma, and pleomorphic adenoma need only be fully excised to be treated. It is important to establish that these lesions have not grown into the canal, in particular from the parotid region. Neuroradiographic studies with either high-resolution computed tomography (CT) scan or magnetic resonance imaging (MRI) provide anatomic detail that should clear or implicate the parotid gland.

Another class of benign lesions that may impact the ear canal are skin adnexal lesions including papilloma and fibroma. An uncommon lesion that may intimately involve the facial nerve as well as the external canal is the plexiform neurofibroma. This lesion is notoriously difficult to fully extirpate, and debulking of the ear canal on a periodic basis will limit morbidity.

Bony and fibrous lesions may involve the canal. The two most commonly noted osseous lesions are the osteoma and the exostosis. Osteoma is a true neoplasm. Found most commonly as a narrow-based lateral external canal lesion, it represents a variant of the fibro-osseous lesion that includes monostotic and polyostotic fibrous dysplasias. The osteoma can obstruct and be readily drilled out or curetted away. Exostoses represent new bone formation and are found most commonly in the medial aspect of the bony external canal. The lesions are frequently multiple and bi-

559

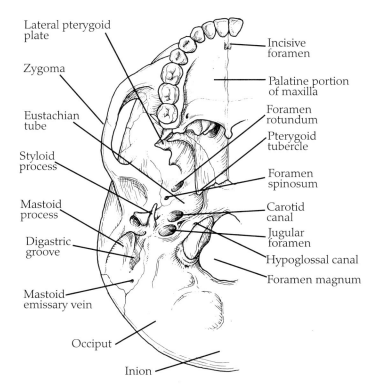

Lateral pterygoid plate
Zygoma
Eustachian tube
Styloid process
Mastoid process
Digastric groove
Mastoid emissary vein
Occiput
Inion

Incisive foramen
Palatine portion of maxilla
Foramen rotundum
Pterygoid tubercle
Foramen spinosum
Carotid canal
Jugular foramen
Hypoglossal canal
Foramen magnum

FIGURE 83–1 Anatomically, the skull base is divided into three constituent fossae. Generally, tumors of the sinonasal tract, pituitary, and optic tract invade the anterior fossae. The middle fossa and infratemporal fossa are invaded by lesions of the petrous bone as well as tumors extending from the clival region. The posterior fossa, the largest of the three areas, contains the widest array of skull base tumors.

lateral. The deposition of squamous elements and subsequent irritation leads to an inflammatory otitis externa and secondary infection. When noninflamed, these lesions are asymptomatic. If surgical removal is required, generally a postauricular approach is advocated as the lesions can distort the local anatomy, and, because drilling is done, the facial nerve may be at risk as the annular margin is approached.

TABLE 83–1 BENIGN AND MALIGNANT TUMORS OF THE TEMPORAL BONE

Benign	Malignant
Meningioma	Squamous cell
Schwannoma	Basal cell
Glomus tumor	Ceruminous gland tumor
Osteoma	Rhabdomyosarcoma
Adenoma	Melanoma
Chordoma	Adenoid cystic carcinoma
Hemangiopericytoma	Chondrosarcoma
Lipoma	Glioma
	Astrocytoma
	Medulloblastoma
	Neuroblastoma
	Choroid plexus tumors

Fibrous dysplasia uncommonly encompasses the temporal bone.

> **PITFALLS...** Remodeling of the external auditory canal and the temporomandibular joint may lead to entrapment of squamae as a canal stenosis manifests. Surgical management is often resorted to when conservative means of aural hygiene are not effective.

When a canaloplasty is performed, care needs to be taken to identify the tympanic annulus, the facial nerve, and the limits of the glenoid fossa. Following a widening of the canal, the raw surface must be covered by a skin graft. A complementary meatal opening must be performed to accommodate the newly enlarged ear canal.

MALIGNANT LESIONS OF THE EXTERNAL AUDITORY CANAL

Malignant tumors of the ear canal may be of primary origin, regionally invasive (parotid malignancy), or metastatic. In most reported series squamous cell carcinoma (SCC) represents the most commonly encountered lesion. Unlike its auricular counterpart, this lesion does not arise due to solar exposure but arises in an environment of chronic inflammation. Table 83–2 lists all the signs and symptoms found in a recently published report describing malignancy of the temporal bone. Not uncommonly, patients report a significant antedating history of intermittent or chronic aural drainage and irritation that have been treated by recurrent administration of topical aural drops and antibiotics.

> **PEARL...** It is incumbent upon the treating physician to be highly suspicious of and biopsy any ear canal lesion that does not respond to aggressive treatment.

Prior to definitive treatment radiographic studies with CT and MRI will help to determine the extent of growth.

> **PITFALL...** The physician and patient should be aware that subtle changes on a scan may not reflect the extent of tumor invasion, and both parties need to be prepared for a major extirpative endeavor.

Lesions confined to the canal may be treated with en bloc lateral temporal bone resection. If the mastoid or middle ear is invaded, a subtotal temporal bone resection must be done with selective sparing of the facial nerve and cochleovestibular end-organ if these anatomic sites are free of disease. Invasion of either structure would necessitate resection. Gross invasion of the temporal lobe or internal carotid artery is a contraindication to radical surgery (Fig. 83–2).

Reconstruction of the operative site is predicated on the defect size, medial extent, and potential for acoustic rehabilitation. Split-thickness skin grafts, local and regional flaps, myocutaneous flaps, and free vascular flaps have all been successfully employed. For most patients, with the exception of lesions that are discovered when they are quite small, a full course of radiation therapy is advocated (5000–7000 cGy), depend-

TABLE 83–2 TEMPORAL BONE MALIGNANCY: INCIDENCE OF OCCURRENCE

Signs		Symptoms	
Canal mass or lesion	88%	Pain	74%
Aural drainage	84%	Hearing loss	62%
Periauricular swelling	25%	Pruritis	40%
Facial paralysis	18%	Bleeding	28%
Neck nodes	8%	Headache	18%
Temporal mass	8%	Tinnitus	18%
		Facial numbness	12%
		Vertigo	10%
		Hoarseness	4%

ing on the extent of the patient's overall medical condition.

In contrast to the rapid and highly aggressive nature of SCC, basal cell carcinoma of

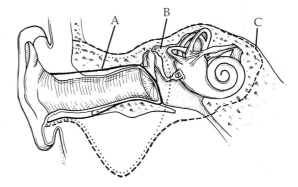

FIGURE 83–2 Malignant tumors of the temporal bone (TB) need to be treated aggressively. Small tumors confined to the lateral portion of the canal may be treated by sleeve resection. Invasion to the bony cartilaginous interface or medially are treated with a lateral temporal bone resection. Gross invasion to the mastoid air cells, middle ear, or juxtaposing air-cell regions requires both anterior and posterior petrousectomies, whereas direct invasion of the cochleovestibular end-organ, facial canal, or internal auditory canal requires a subtotal TB resection. A, sleeve resection; B, lateral TB resection; C, subtotal TB resection.

the ear canal is rather indolent. Often resulting from the auricular invasive route, basal call carcinomas that arise de novo in the ear canal are quite rare. Frequently presenting as a painful ulcer that has been refractory to conventional treatment, there is often a long history of aural symptoms. Interestingly, many of these lesions may be associated with rather extensive periauricular growth patterns without deep tissue invasion. As with SCC, wide excision is often followed by radiation therapy.

Malignant glandular tumors may arise within the canal or be associated with extension from local salivary glands, primarily parotid tumors. Mucoepidermoid, adenocarcinoma, cylindroma, and acinic cell carcinoma have all been observed. Surgical excision and radiation constitute the general approach to these lesions.

Rhabdomyosarcoma is uncommonly found invading the temporal bone and accounts for between 4 and 7% of reported head and neck cancers.

SPECIAL CONSIDERATION

Frequently diagnosed as chronic otitis because of the friable granulation encountered in the ear canal, the lesion remains unresponsive to antibiotic therapy.

Following diagnosis, although surgery may play an adjunctive role, chemotherapy is the principal mode of treatment.

Table 83–3 lists those tumors that have been identified with metastasis to the temporal bone. Because of the wide range of lesions noted, the clinician when taking a history should always inquire about previous treatment for malignancy

TABLE 83–3 TUMORS METASTATIC TO THE TEMPORAL BONE

Breast
Renal
Lung
Adrenal
Gastrointestinal

as well as general symptoms that may suggest a systemic process or a debilitating state resulting from an unrecognized tumor.

BENIGN TUMORS OF THE MIDDLE EAR

The most common tumor found in the middle ear space is the glomus tumor or paraganglioma. The glomus bodies are found in multiple sites about the head and neck but are frequently found along Jacobson's and Arnold's nerves, the jugular foramen, and the promontory. Epidemiologically, the tumors are found with a higher frequency in females, and there appears to be a genetic basis for their development as patients who develop these lesion sporadically often have a family history of these tumors. Table 83–4 outlines two commonly employed classification systems.

Histologically, the lesions are noted to be lobulated vascular masses that contain the pathognomonic chief cells (Zellbellin) in clusters enveloped in a highly vascular stoma. Neural elements and sustentacular supporting cells commonly found in paragangliomas are frequently absent in these tumors.

SPECIAL CONSIDERATION

The chief cells have the capacity to secrete catecholamines; although quite uncommon, the sudden release of these chemicals can lead to severe cardiac and hemodynamic consequences. If thresholds are elevated on preoperative assessment, both alpha and beta blockage are advisable.

Clinically paragangliomas manifest in a number of ways, often reflecting their growth patterns and degree of invasion.

Glomus jugulare tumors take origin from glomus bodies juxtaposing the jugular bulb or from the proximal segments of the nerves of Arnold or Jacobson. As the tumor extends superiorly, hearing loss, pulsatile tinnitus, or aural

TABLE 83–4 CLASSIFICATION SCHEMES FOR GLOMUS TUMORS

Glasscock/Jackson classification of glomus tumors

Glomus tympanicum

Type I	Small mass limited to the promontory
Type II	Tumor completely filling the middle ear space
Type III	Tumor filling the middle ear and extending into the mastoid
Type IV	Tumor filling the middle ear, extending into the mastoid or through the temporal bone to fill the external auditory canal; ±internal carotid artery involvement

Glomus jugulare

Type I	Small tumors involving the jugular bulb, middle ear, and mastoid
Type II	Tumor extending under the internal auditory canal; might have intracranial extension
Type III	Tumor extending into petrous apex; might have intracranial extension
Type IV	Tumor extending beyond petrous apex into clivus or infratemporal fossa; might have intracranial extension

Fisch classification of glomus tumors

Type A	Tumors limited to the middle ear cleft (glomus tympanicum)
Type B	Tumors limited to the tympanomastoid area with no bone destruction in the infralabyrinthine compartment of the temporal bone.
Type C	Tumors involving the infralabyrinthine compartment with extension in the petrous apex
Type D1	Tumors with intracranial extension $\leqq$2 cm in diameter
Type D2	Tumors with intracranial extension >2 cm in diameter

Adapted from Jackson CG. Skull base surgery. *Am J Otol* 1981;3:161–171 and Oldring D, Fisch U. Glomus tumors of the temporal region: surgical therapy. *Am J Otol* 1979;1:7–18.

fullness may manifest. As the lesion encroaches upon the jugular foramen, the lower cranial nerves may be affected (IX–XI). If the fallopian canal or the otic capsule is violated, seventh and eighth nerve dysfunction become pronounced. Intracranial extension is not uncommonly found at the time of diagnosis. Extension inferiorly along the jugular vein may cause compression or the presence of an overt neck mass.

Glomus tympanicums arise from the promontory. As the tumors expand, the patient be-

PEARLS... To differentiate the underlying pathology, the diagnostic study of choice is the CT scan (high-resolution, high bone density windows). Here the bony separation between the jugular bulb and the carotid may be visualized as well as the bony plate that separates the hypotympanum from the dome of the jugular bulb. MRI may enhance the radiographic features of the lesion, and in particular help to define the extent of the intracranial growth.

comes aware of pulsatile tinnitus and a progressive hearing loss. As the lesion grows it may infrequently disrupt the facial nerve or otic capsule. More commonly with the glomus jugulare, the annular margin is violated and the lesion presents in the ear canal as a friable, bleeding, polypoid mass.

Angiographic studies will clearly define the feeding vessels as well as attendant venous channels. Moreover, with extensive anterior growth the internal carotid artery is at risk of invasion. Angiographic studies will help define the pathway. Often during the preoperative period, selective embolization will be performed to reduce blood loss during the definitive surgical extirpation. The surgical removal may be done via a transcanal, transmastoid, or infratemporal fossa route, depending on the extent of tumor present (Fig. 83–3).

Radiation therapy has been quite successful in controlling tumors that are incompletely excised or in cases where surgery is not done. A long-term follow-up study from the M. D. Anderson Hospital suggests that there may a role

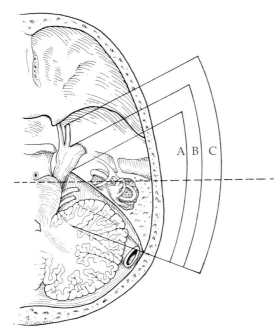

FIGURE 83–3 Fisch has described a series of progressively enlarging infratemporal fossa dissections for skull base lesions. The type A approach is generally employed for glomus tumors invading the infratemporal fossa, type B dissection allows access to the clivus, and type C exposure accesses the nasopharynx.

for radiation therapy as the primary mode of therapy.

The second most common tumor of middle ear origin is the adenoma. This slow-growing lesion presents as conductive hearing loss. There is generally limited vascularity, and simple surgical excision is required. Because the lesion may pass into the protympanum or the posterior recesses, complete removal is required to avoid recurrence. Other uncommon tumors present and are mapped in similar fashion.

MALIGNANT TUMORS OF THE MIDDLE AND INNER EAR

Malignant tumors of the middle ear generally result from extension of SCCs that have originated within the external auditory canal.

Tumors that involve the inner ear are generally benign, except for the spread of malignancy from the lateral temporal bone or the rare malignancy that has metastasized to the internal auditory canal (IAC) or the cerebellopontine angle (CPA). The one exception to this is the highly aggressive papillary adenoma of the endolymphatic sac. Although histologically benign, this lesion grows quite aggressively. The lesion may manifest with hearing loss, vertigo, facial paralysis, or, once invading the jugular foramen, may cause lower cranial neuropathy. These tumors may readily extend intracranially.

Malignant lesions require radical surgical removal.

CONTROVERSY

The use of radiation therapy is controversial, but it appears to play a role in management in cases where lesions may not have been fully excised.

Table 83–4 defines a commonly employed classification system for staging temporal bone malignancy.

BENIGN TUMORS OF THE INNER EAR AND SKULL BASE

Schwannomas involving the inner ear generally take origin within the IAC, although there have been isolated reports of primary schwannomas taking origin within the inner ear. As with intracanalicular acoustic neuroma, the lesions present with hearing loss, tinnitus, and balance dysfunction. Diagnosed with gadolinium-enhanced MRI scanning, the primary treatment is surgical extirpation.

TABLE 83–4 STAGING GUIDELINE

Grade 1	Tumor in a single site ≤1 cm
Grade 2	Tumor in a single site >1 cm
Grade 3	Transannular tumor extension
Grade 4	Mastoid or petrous air cell invasion
Grade 5	Periauricular or contiguous extension (extratemporal)
Grade 6	Neck adenopathy, distant anatomic site, or infratemporal fossa extension

Schwannomas of the IAC and CPA are the most common tumors of the temporal bone. In general, these lesions take origin from the vestibular divisions of cranial nerve VIII; however, they are still referred to as acoustic neuromas.

> **PEARL...** Acoustic neuromas (vestibular schwannomas) are derived from schwannoma cells at the Obersteiner-Redlich zone. Arising equally from the superior/inferior vestibular nerves, true vertigo is rarely a clinical symptom, whereas most patients experience balance dysfunction.

Clinically, schwannomas present with a number of features including tinnitus, aural fullness, hearing loss, and gait and postural instability. True vertigo is uncommon. However, patients may present with symptoms reflecting trigeminal involvement, facial nerve dysfunction, or sudden sensorineural hearing loss.

Historically, audiometric studies raised suspicion with reduced speech discrimination scores, along with asymmetric sensorineural thresholds.

> **PITFALL...** Recently, the ABR has been shown to have a high false-negative rate of 12 to 18% so that presently if the clinical suspicion for an acoustic neuroma is high the patient is probably best served by undergoing a gadolinium-enchanted MRI scan.

Fast spin echo MRI with high-resolution T2-weighted images outline the contents of the IAC by enhancing the bright signal of the cerebrospinal fluid (CSF) T1 contrast against a lesion. For individuals who cannot undergo MRI scanning, contrast-enhanced CT scanning will define all but the smallest lesion.

> **PEARL...** CSF leak is more common in patients undergoing translabyrinthine removal of acoustic neuromas. Headache, however, is more commonly reported with suboccipital removal.

Grossly, schwannomas are smooth globular tumors with variable vascularity and fatty content. Morphologically, two types of patterns are described. Tumors with a predominant Antoni A pattern are densely packed with palisades of cells. The whorled pattern described is called a Verocay body. The Antoni B is loosely arranged with a greater degree of cellular pleomorphism. The biology of these tumors, however, does not differ.

> **PEARL...** Jugular foramen schwannomas are noted to be smooth walled on scan, whereas glomus tumors tend to have an irregular contour. Jugular foramen lesions, in particular glomus tumors that extend anteriorly to the internal carotid artery (vertical segment), will require rerouting of the seventh nerve to safely extirpate the lesion.

Removal of acoustic neuroma is the treatment of choice. For small lesions within the IAC and up to 1 cm growth in the CPA, the middle fossa is an optimal approach for hearing preser-

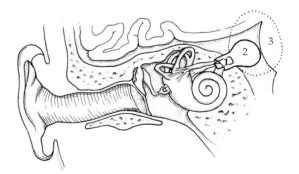

FIGURE 83–4 Acoustic neuromas may be located within the internal auditory canal (1), within the cistern (2), or filling the cerebellopontine angle (CPA), encroaching upon the brainstem (3). Small intracanalicular lesions may be approached via a middle fossa or suboccipital transmeatal route to remove the tumor and preserve hearing. As tumors grow into the CPA, the likelihood of hearing preservation diminishes and either a translabyrinthine or suboccipital route will allow access for removal. The translabyrinthine route affords the optimal view of the lateral portion of the canal and the facial nerve.

vation. For larger lesions where hearing preservation is not feasible, the translabyrinthine removal is generally preferred. For large lesions or tumors that are greater than 1 cm and when there is an attempt at hearing preservation, a suboccipital transmeatal approach is generally employed (Fig. 83–4).

There has been a recent debate about the effectiveness of gamma knife radiosurgery. The data available suggest that it is an excellent approach for small tumors when surgery is not the strategy of choice. However, there is still insufficient data to make definitive recommendations on the role of gamma knife radiosurgery.

FACIAL NERVE TUMORS

The two benign tumors associated with the facial nerve are schwannomas and osseous hemangiomas of the geniculate ganglion. The latter lesion is not specifically a lesion of the facial nerve but takes origin from the plexus of vessels that intimately juxtapose the geniculate ganglion. As the tumor expands, it compresses the nerve and causes bony destruction in the perigeniculate bone.

> **PEARL...** Facial neuromas may have skip lesions and present as a multifocal tumor along substantial portions of the nerve.

In contradistinction, the schwannoma will expand with the fallopian canal, often causing a fusiform tumor mass to develop with skip lesions. The tumors are variably vascular.

Clinically, the most common presenting history is one of progressive facial paresis. Rarely, due to sudden vascular compromise, there may be a paroxysmal onset of facial paralysis. Paradoxically, twitch or spasm may herald the onset of dysfunction due to a tumor. As the tumor mass expands, violation of the middle ear will cause a conductive loss, whereas growth within the IAC will compress the eighth nerve, resulting in retrocochlear findings not dissimilar

to that of a classic acoustic neuroma. Diagnostic radiology includes the utilization of CT scanning to assess the subtle changes in petrous bony architecture as well as MRI with contrast, which will give soft tissue definition of the expansile mass.

Generally, management involves surgical removal. It is possible to extirpate either a hemangioma or schwannoma without compromise of the nerve; however, as the facial nerve dysfunction is increased preoperatively, it is less likely that the nerve can be preserved. Removal is done generally via a transmastoid middle fossa approach to give full visualization to the nerve while preserving cochleovestibular function. Depending on the extent of nerve resection, reanimation can be accomplished either with a VII–XII anastomosis or cable graft. Static reanimation with Gore-Tex and gold weight to the eye will provide satisfactory cosmetic results.

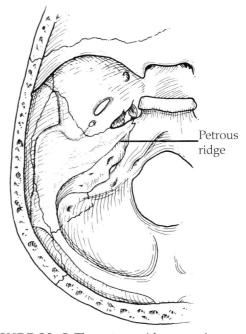

Petrous ridge

FIGURE 83–5 The petrous ridge occupies a central position in the skull base. Lesions may expand medially to the clivus, anteriorly toward the sphenoid, inferiorly to the infratemporal fossa, and posteriorly into the posterior fossa.

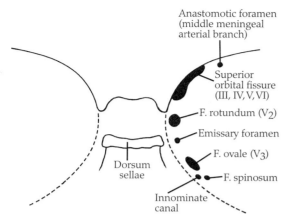

Anastomotic foramen
(middle meningeal
arterial branch)

Superior
orbital fissure
(III, IV, V, VI)

F. rotundum (V₂)

Emissary foramen

F. ovale (V₃)

F. spinosum

Dorsum
sellae

Innominate
canal

FIGURE 83-6 Extensive growth of skull base tumors may result in the compromise of neural structures within the confines of the cavernous sinus. Contemporary skull base procedures allow for the extirpation of lesions involving this heretofore inaccessible region. F., foramen.

PETROUS APEX LESIONS AND SKULL BASE

Tumors of the apex are uncommon (Fig. 83–5). Most frequently the apical cells become involved due to direct extension of neighboring lesions.

Meningiomas, trigeminal schwannomas, chondromas, chordomas, paragangliomas, and, uncommonly, space-occupying lesions such as cholesterol granuloma are noted. Malignant lesions including chondrosarcoma may extend from the clival region.

> **PITFALL···** Total tumor removal for large petroclival meningiomas is rare without the sacrifice of cranial nerves, especially in cases where the tumor extends into the cavernous sinus. Cytoreductive surgery followed by radiation therapy appears to be a successful method of containment with minimal morbidity.

Metastases have been reported from kidneys, breast, and lungs. For the latter group, a high degree of suspicion as well as radiographic evidence of aggressive bone destruction along with the patient's history will suggest the diagnosis.

The surgical approach to these lesions involves a variety of combined neurotologic and neurosurgical strategies that employ a transtemporal-transcranial access (Fig. 83–6 to 83–8).

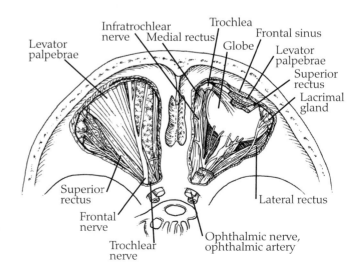

Infratrochlear
nerve

Trochlea

Medial rectus

Globe

Frontal sinus

Levator
palpebrae

Levator
palpebrae

Superior
rectus

Lacrimal
gland

Superior
rectus

Frontal
nerve

Trochlear
nerve

Ophthalmic nerve,
ophthalmic artery

Lateral rectus

FIGURE 83-7 Trauma, infection, or tumor may invade directly into the orbital contents. Moreover, excision of tumors from the petroclival region and apex may violate ocular function.

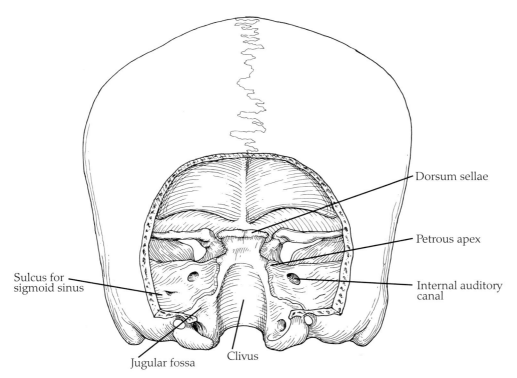

FIGURE 83–8 Lesions involving the jugular foramen may expand superiorly, involving the temporal bone structures, posteriorly into the posterior fossa, or medially and anteriorly to the clivus. Extensive growth may manifest before diagnosis is made, requiring radical removal for treatment.

Suggested Readings

Alford BR, Guilford FR. A comprehensive study of tumors of the glomus jugulare. *Laryngoscope* 1962;72:765–787.

Arena S, Keen M. Carcinoma of the middle ear and temporal bone. *Am J Otol* 1988;9(5):351–356.

Arriaga S, Keen M. Carcinoma of the middle ear and temporal bone. *Am J Otol* 1988;9(5):351–356.

Batsakis JG. Adenomatous tumors of the middle ear. *Ann Otol Rhinol Laryngol* 1989;98:749–752.

Benecke JE, Noel FL, Carberry JN, House JW, Patterson M. Adenomatous tumors of the middle ear and mastoid. *Am J Otol* 1990;11:20–26.

Bressler K, Shelton C. Ear foreign-body removal: a review of 98 consecutive cases. *Laryngoscope* 1993;103:367–370.

Cannon CR, McLean WC. Adenoid cystic carcinoma of the middle ear and temporal bone. *Otolaryngol Head Neck Surg* 1983;91:96–99.

Carrasco V, Rosenman J. Radiation therapy of glomus jugulare tumors. *Laryngoscope* 1993;103(11 pt 2, suppl):23–27.

Chandler JR. Malignant external otitis. *Laryngoscope* 1968;78:1257–1294.

Conley J, Schuller DE. Malignancies of the ear. *Laryngoscope* 1976;86:1147–1163.

Fisch U, Ruttner J. Pathology of intratemporal tumors involving the facial nerve. In: Fisch U, ed. *Facial Nerve Surgery.* Birmingham, England: Aesculapius; 1977:448–456.

Fisher EW, McManus TC. Surgery for external canal exostoses and osteomata. *J Laryngol Otol* 1994;108:106–110.

Gacek RP. Pathology of jugular foramen neurofibroma. *Ann Otol Rhinol Laryngol* 1983;92:128–133.

Glasscock ME, Minor LB, McMenomey SO. Meningiomas of the cerebellopontine angle. In: Jackler RK, Brackmann DE, eds. *Neurotology.* St. Louis: CV Mosby; 1994:795–821.

Goodwin WJ, Jesse RH. Malignant neoplasms of the external auditory canal and temporal bone. *Arch Otolaryngol* 1980;106(11):675–679.

Graham MD, Sataloff RT, et al. Total en bloc resection of the temporal bone and carotid artery for malignant tumors of the ear and temporal bone. *Laryngoscope* 1984;94(4):528–533.

Gulya AJ. Paraneoplastic disorders. In: Jackler RK, Brackmann DE, eds. *Neurotology.* St. Louis: CV Mosby; 1994:535–542.

Gulya AJ, Glasscock ME, Pensak ML. Neural choristoma of the middle ear. *Otolaryngol Head Neck Surg* 1987;97(1):52–56.

Holt JJ. Ear canal cholesteatoma. *Laryngoscope* 1992;102:608–613.

House WF, Glasscock ME. Glomus tympanicum tumors. *Arch Otolaryngol* 1968;87:124–128.

Jackler RK. Acoustic neuroma (vestibular schwannoma). In: Jackler RK, Brackmann DE, eds. *Neurotology.* St. Louis: CV Mosby; 1994:729–785.

Jackler RK, Pitts LH. Selection of surgical approach to acoustic neuroma. *Otolaryngol Clin North Am* 1992;25:361–387.

Jackson CG. Neurotologic surgery for skull base tumors: diagnosis for treatment planning and treatment options. *Laryngoscope* 1993;103(11 pt suppl):17–27.

Jackson CG. Skull base surgery. *Am J Otol* 1981;3:161–171.

Jackson CG, Cueva RA, Thedinger BA, Glasscock ME. Cranial nerve preservation in lesions of the jugular fossa. *Otolaryngol Head Neck Surg* 1991;105:687–693.

Kinney SE, Wood GB. Malignancies of the external ear canal and temporal bone: surgical techniques and results. *Laryngoscope* 1987;97(2):158–164.

Krouse JH, Nadol JB, Goodman ML. Carcinoid tumors of the middle ear. *Ann Otol Rhinol Laryngol* 1990;99:547–552.

Laird FJ, Harner SG, Laws ER, Reese JDF. Meningiomas of the cerebellopontine angle. *Otolaryngol Head Neck Surg* 1985;93:163–167.

Lalwani AK, Jackler RK. Preoperative differentation between meningioma of the cerebellopontine angle and acoustic neuroma using MRI. *Otolaryngol Head Neck Surg* 1994;109(1):88–95.

Lewis JS. Surgical management of tumors of the middle ear and mastoid. *J Laryngol Otol* 1983;97:299–311.

Lewis JS. Temporal bone resection: review of 100 cases. *Arch Otolaryngol* 1975;101:23–25.

Lustig LR, Jackler RK. Benign tumors of the temporal bone. In: Hughes GB, Pensak ML, eds. *Clinical Otology.* New York: Thieme; 1997:313–334.

Maddox HE III. Metastatic tumors of the temporal bone. *Ann Otol Rhinol Laryngol* 1967;76:149–165.

Mirimanoff RO, Dosoretz DE, Linggood RM, Ojemann RG, Martuza RL. Meningioma: analysis of recurrence and progression following neurosurgical resection. *J Neurosurg* 1985;62:18–24.

Nedzelski JM, Schessel DA, Pfleiderer A, Kassel EE, Rowed DW. Conservative management of acoustic neurons. *Otolaryngol Clin North Am* 1992;25:691–705.

O'Donoghue GM. Tumors of the facial nerve. In: Jackler RK, Brackmann DE, eds. *Neurotology.* St. Louis: CV Mosby; 1994:1321–1331.

Oldring D, Fisch U. Glomus tumors of the temporal region: surgical therapy. *Am J Otol* 1979;1:7–18.

Parisier SC, Kimmelman CP, Hanson MB. Diseases of the external auditory canal. In: Hughes GB, Pensak ML, eds. *Clinical Otology.* New York: Thieme; 1997:191–203.

Pensak ML. Alford and Guilford: a comprehensive study of tumors of the glomus jugulare. A review. *Laryngoscope* 1996;106:83–86.

Pensak ML, Gleich LL, Gluckman JL, Shumrick KA. Temporal bone carcinoma—contemporary perspectives in the skull base surgical era. *Laryngoscope* 1996;106:1234–1237.

Pensak ML, Willging JP. Tumors of the temporal bone. In: Jackler R, Brackmann D, eds. *Neurotology.* New York: CV Mosby; 1994:1049–1057.

Schramm VL. Temporal bone resection. In: Sekhar LN, Schramm VL, eds. *Tumors of the Cranial Base: Diagnosis and Treatment.* Mount Kisco, NY: Futura; 1987:683–698.

Selesnick SH, Jackler RK, Pitts LW. The changing clinical presentation of acoustic tumors in the MRI era. *Laryngoscope* 1993;103:431–436.

Spector JG. Management of temporal bone carcinomas: a therapeutic analysis of two groups of patients and long term follow-up. *Otolaryngol Head Neck Surg* 1991;104:58–66.

Wiatrak BJ, Pensak ML. Rhabdomyosarcoma of the ear and temporal bone. *Laryngoscope* 1989;99:1188–1192.

Wiet RJ, Teixido M, Liang JG. Complications in acoustic neuroma surgery. *Otolaryngol Clin North Am* 1992;25:389–412.

Wiet RJ, Zappia JJ, Hecht CS, O'Connor CA. Conservative management of patients with small acoustic tumors. *Laryngoscope* 1995;105 (8 pt 1):795–800.

Chapter 84

TRAUMA
Myles L. Pensak

Temporal bone trauma rarely occurs as an isolated event when the bone of the skull base is disrupted. High-speed motor vehicle accidents account for the vast majority of injuries seen. However, interpersonal violence is not infrequently the cause of substantial injury.

PEARL... The temporal bone is very dense, requiring a great force to incur a fracture, suggesting the degree of trauma that needs to be inflicted to cause neural disruption.

In contradistinction, acoustic, thermal, or barometric trauma may result in significant disability affecting the cochleovestibular end-organ without concomitant craniofacial disability.

TEMPORAL BONE FRACTURES

Many temporal bone fractures are complex, and although convention dictates that they be named, it is often best to describe the disability encountered rather than just identify a violated anatomic structure.

LONGITUDINAL TEMPORAL BONE FRACTURES

In longitudinal temporal bone fractures, the fracture line is noted to extend along the long axis of the petrous bone due to a direct insult to the temporal or parietal region of the skull (Fig. 84–1A). This fracture is most commonly seen extending down the posterior-superior wall of the external auditory canal, across the pars flaccida and the tegmen tympani, to end at the petrous apex or the level of either the foramen lacerum or foramen ovale.

The patient presents with bloody otorrhea, hearing loss due to disruption of the drum or ossicles, and, less frequently, vestibular problems or facial paralysis. The latter, however, is most commonly associated with longitudinal temporal bone fracture due to the higher incidence of this injury. Overall, facial paralysis occurs in approximately 15% of cases of longitudinal temporal bone fracture. Bilateral fractures have been reported in upwards of 30% of basal skull fractures.

PEARL... Facial paralysis occurs most frequently with transverse temporal bone fractures; however, because longitudinal fractures are more common, more cases of facial paralysis are due to longitudinal fractures.

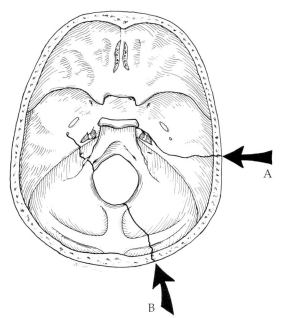

FIGURE 84–1 (A) Classically, skull base fractures involving the temporal bone are described as longitudinal or transverse. The fracture line of a longitudinal fracture is most commonly observed to extend down the posterior-superior wall of the external auditory canal (EAC), across the pars flaccida and the tegmen, ending at the petrous apex. The transverse fracture begins in the posterior fossa, bisects the bony axis of the petrous ridge, and ends commonly at the foramen spinosum. (B) Multiple neural and vascular structures traverse the irregular and complex osteology of the skull base.

TRANSVERSE TEMPORAL BONE FRACTURES

Transverse temporal bone fractures begin in the posterior fossa and generally bisect the long axis of the petrous ridge, ending most commonly in the region of the foramen spinosum (Fig. 84–1B). It is not uncommon for these fractures to either pass through the otic capsule itself or disrupt the internal auditory canal with the fracture line ending at either the oval or round windows.

> **PEARL...** Few temporal bone fractures are pure fractures; in fact, the majority are mixed (longitudinal and transverse components).

Patients presenting with transverse temporal bone fractures generally are more debilitated than those with longitudinal temporal bone fractures.

> ## SPECIAL CONSIDERATION
>
> Violation of the otic capsule or the internal auditory canal generally results in profound sensorineural hearing loss with severe disabling vertigo.

In 50% of cases the facial nerve is disrupted either within the IAC or at the geniculate ganglion manifesting with facial paralysis.

Because the lesion occurs medial to the annular margin, patients do not present with otorrhea but may, in fact, manifest cerebrospinal fluid (CSF) rhinorrhea and/or the presence of a hemotympanum.

OTHER INJURIES OF THE TEMPORAL BONE DUE TO TRAUMA

Penetrating wounds of the temporal bone may occur from projectile insults that may be incurred as a result of industrial accidents, gunshot wounds, or direct violation due to bludgeoning or stabbing wounds.

> **PEARL...** Low-velocity gunshot wounds account for the majority of penetrating temporal bone traumatic injuries.

Depending on the degree and caliber of the insulting weapon, there may be concomitant fracture of the petrous bone or direct violation of attendant anatomic structures.

Other injuries that result from direct contact with the temporal bone may not, in fact, be associated with fractures. Included among these are concussive injury, barometric trauma injury, thermal injury, and the introduction of foreign bodies such as hairpins or toothpicks. In the latter disruption of the canal, the drum, or the ossicles may occur, which results in hearing loss or vertigo.

> **PEARL...** With an antedating history of temporal bone trauma, if a patient develops a soft pulsatile external canal mass, an encephalocele should be considered.

With regard to slag burns and thermal injuries, severe injury can result in the disruption of the skin of the ear canal, the drum, and the middle ear. Slag burns can result in both total perforation and scarring of the ear canal. These cases can represent the most difficult of tympanoplastic reconstructions.

Injuries sustained in which there is a failure of equilibration of pressure between the ambient environment and the middle ear space may result in either implosive or explosive injury, resulting in violation of either the oval or round window niches. Patients may experience a paroxysmal degradation in auditory acuity, the potential for fluctuant hearing loss, and/or severe vestibulopathy. On rare occasion, a perilymphatic fistula may manifest.

DISABILITIES ASSOCIATED WITH TEMPORAL BONE TRAUMA

Hearing loss associated with trauma to the temporal bone may manifest with a conductive loss, a sensorineural hearing loss, or a mixed loss. The conductive hearing loss may obtain due to obstruction of the sound-conducting mechanism beginning at the level of the auricle and extending down the ear canal and across the eardrum to involve the middle ear space. Blood, foreign bodies, squamae, cerumen, or hematoma may obstruct the air-conducting mechanism of the external auditory canal. Disruption of the bone and/or skin in the canal itself may in fact result in a conductive hearing loss. Medially, disruption of the eardrum and/or the ossicular chain will manifest with a conductive hearing loss. Perforation of the drum may in fact only manifest with a slight conductive component.

It is possible, however, not to have violation of the ear canal or the drum and still sustain injury to the conductive mechanism. The middle ear, filled with blood, spinal fluid, serous fluid, or reactive mucus, may manifest with a conductive hearing loss. Concussive injury may manifest with disarticulation of the ossicular chain resulting, with an intact drum, in a maximal conductive hearing loss. In the latter case, should the drum itself be disrupted, direct passage of sound to the oval and/or round window would optimize hearing.

Sensorineural hearing loss may obtain with violation of either the endolymphatic or perilymphatic spaces. In cases where there is violation of the IAC with transection of cranial nerve VIII or disruption of the internal auditory artery, profound anacusis may result.

On occasion, perilymphatic fistula may manifest with waxing and waning sensorineural hearing loss. In addition, with an antedating history of temporal bone trauma, delayed endolymphatic hydrops may manifest with classic signs associated with those of Meniere's syndrome, including fluctuant sensorineural hearing loss, episodic vertigo, tinnitus, and aural fullness.

> **PEARL...** At times it is difficult to differentiate a delayed endolymphatic hydrops from a perilymph fistula if the patient has a history of temporal bone trauma. Symptoms provoked by the Valsalva maneuver should suggest a perilymphatic fistula.

Vestibular manifestations due to trauma may manifest with acute vertigo with the concomitant constitutional symptoms of nausea, diaphoresis, and emesis. Violation of the labyrinth and/or cranial nerve VIII will lead to the paroxysmal onset of debilitating vertigo and associated nystagmus. Over a period of weeks there will be a quieting of symptoms, but depending on the degree of vestibular deficit and the patient's age as well as proprioceptive and ophthalmologic conditions, the extent of rehabilitation varies.

Posttraumatic cupulolithiasis or benign positional vertigo may manifest with classic signs associated with that of gravity-dependent postural vertigo. Often, the patient has both latency and fatigability of symptoms, and the vast majority of cases resolve within 6 to 8 weeks of the onset of symptoms.

Posttraumatic hydrops is recognized as a cause of recurrent episodes of vertigo.

In cases where the stapes footplate is either subluxed or disarticulated with resultant perilymphatic leakage, episodes of vertigo that are related either to barotrauma or to the continued leak of perilymph fluid may manifest. In addition, patients may go on to develop a labyrinthitis of a serous nature. On rare occasion, with violation of the tympanic membrane there may in fact develop a bacterial labyrinthitis with significant vestibular sequelae.

Other intraaural symptoms that may manifest include the feeling of fullness or pressure, associated tinnitus, suppuration, or drainage.

Cranial neuropathy and intracranial complications are uncommon. As cited earlier, temporal bone fracture may manifest with facial paralysis, and presently electroneuronography and electromyography are employed to establish the degree of disability. In cases of immediate-onset facial paralysis, there is general consensus that the nerve needs to be explored when the patient is medically stable.

> **PEARLS...** For a patient with an anacusic ear, a transmastoid, translabyrinthine exploration of the facial nerve will optimize visualization. For patients who have preservation of sensorineural levels, we combine a transmastoid middle fossa approach to allow for visualization of the facial nerve.

For those individuals with delayed onset of facial paralysis beginning at the third day, serial electroneuronography is undertaken. It is generally felt that with degeneration of greater than 95% and with electromyographic evidence of denervation potentials, optimal long-term recovery will be obtained when the facial nerve is explored surgically.

In cases where the nerve has been partially transected and the edges are freshened, the nerve may be coapted. In cases where there is a complete sectioning of the nerve or a severe concussive injury to the nerve, either primary, tension-free anastomosis or a short cable graft will optimize the chance for reanimation.

Injuries along the floor of the hypotympanum and base of the skull may manifest with violation of the pars nervosa affecting cranial nerves IX, X, and XI. Usually there is significant vascular injury attendant to this type of a lesion. In cases where the hypoglossal canal is violated, isolated injuries to cranial nerve XII, though rare, have been observed.

Neurovascular complications have been reported and have included aneurysms, pseudoaneurysms, and lacerations of both the internal carotid artery and the neighboring venous structures, including the petrosal sinuses and the sigmoid and transverse sinus.

CSF otorrhea and rhinorrhea are not infrequent complications associated with temporal bone fracture. The leak in most cases is noted to spontaneously stop, and packing is discouraged.

> ## SPECIAL CONSIDERATION
>
> Although some authors have advocated the use of prophylactic antibiotic, in general the area is clean and there is no evidence of a breach in sterility, so careful observation is recommended.

Other neural complications from temporal bone fracture have included arteriovenous fistula, encephalocele and meningocele, pneumocephalitis, and otitic meningitis.

> **PEARL...** Recurrent meningitis may present years after a temporal bone fracture with no evidence of a CSF leak. Pneumococcus is the most common causative organism.

ASSESSMENT AND MANAGEMENT OF TEMPORAL BONE TRAUMA

All patients sustaining a temporal bone fracture, once stable, should undergo a complete otorhinolaryngologic examination. As pertains to the ear, otomicroscopic debridement will optimize the efficiency of evaluation. The canal is to be assessed for laceration, and ceruminous material and squamous debris should be carefully removed.

The auricle is examined and it is noted whether or not a Battle's sign is present. The patient should have temporomandibular joint function assessed in both a closed- and an open-bite position. The patient undergoes both tuning fork confirmation for hearing status as well as formal audiometric studies.

> **PEARL...** Delayed ocular and orbital symptoms, including proptosis, lid edema, orbital bruit, and ophthalmoplegia with or without epistaxis, should suggest a carotid-cavernous fistula.

If possible, a formal neurotologic test is undertaken. Postural and positional testing is performed to assess the presence or absence of nystagmus. It is encouraged that the patient be tested utilizing Frenzel glasses to minimize the degree of visual fixation suppression. Tandem posturing and Romberg positioning, likewise, may be performed. Cranial nerve testing is undertaken as part of a neurologic examination, with particular attention being paid to the lower cranial nerves including those of the jugular foramen as well as the seventh nerve.

CSF otorrhea and/or rhinorrhea may be definitively assessed by collecting samples and examining for β_2 transferrin.

> **PEARL...** Most CSF leaks spontaneously resolve within 3 to 5 days. Antibiotic coverage is generally not employed so as not to mask an early meningitis.

From a neuroradiographic perspective high-resolution, high-density computed tomography (CT) scanning with a bone window of 1 to 1.5 mm will give the best evidence for the pathway of a temporal bone fracture.

Once the patient is stable, the only indications for emergent surgery are in situations

where a suspected subluxation of the stapes with perilymph fistula manifests, or in patients in whom an immediate-onset facial paralysis is noted.

> ## SPECIAL CONSIDERATION
>
> Patients with longitudinal temporal bone fractures without vertigo may be followed conservatively to assess long-term the results of both the healing of the tympanic membrane and the potential ossicular dissociation. It is important, however, to identify the presence of entrapped skin prior to the development of a cholesteatoma.

Patients may ultimately undergo an exploratory tympanotomy with ossicular reconstruction or may be fitted for amplification. For those patients with sensorineural hearing loss, often accompanied by rather debilitating tinnitus, amplification may obviate both problems. For patients with profound anacusis, contralateral routing of signal (CROS) amplification and tinnitus counseling may be appropriate.

As for management of vertigo, vestibular suppressant medication should generally be employed during the acute phase; Valium, Xanax, Buspar, Meclizine, and Dramamine have proven quite efficacious.

For stabilized patients with benign paroxysmal positional vertigo (BPPV), both Semont maneuvers and Cawthorne exercises have been effective in helping with vestibular rehabilitation. Most recently outstanding results obtained with the Eply maneuver have been demonstrated. For the rare refractory case, singular neurectomy or posterior canal occlusive procedures have proven successful.

The patient who develops posttraumatic Meniere's vertigo may be controlled medically or with conventional surgical therapies. Patients who have a severe injury to the labyrinth that is uncompensated may undergo transmastoid labyrinthectomy.

SUGGESTED READINGS

Adour K, Boyajean J, Kahn Z, Schneider GS. Surgical and nonsurgical management of facial paralysis following closed head injury. *Laryngoscope* 1977;87:380–390.

Andrews JC, Canalis RF. Otogenic pneumocephalus. *Laryngoscope* 1986;96:521–528.

Atthous SR. Perilymph fistulas. *Laryngoscope* 1981;91:538–562.

Barrs DM. Facial nerve trauma: optimal timing for repair. *Laryngoscope* 1991;101:835–848.

Bayliss GJA. Aural barotrauma in naval divers. *Arch Otolaryngol* 1968;88:141–147.

Cannon CR, Jahrsdoerfer RA. Temporal bone fractures. *Arch Otolaryngol* 1983;109:285–288.

Coker NJ. Management of traumatic injuries to the facial nerve. *Otolaryngol Clin North Am* 1991;24:215–227.

Duncan NO III, Coker NJ, Jenkins HA, Canalis RF. Gunshot injuries of the temporal bone. *Otolaryngol Head Neck Surg* 1986;94:47–55.

Fee GA. Traumatic perilymphatic fistulas. *Arch Otolaryngol* 1968;88:477–480.

Fisch U. Facial paralysis in fractures of the petrous bone. *Laryngoscope* 1974;84:2141–2154.

Freeman J. Temporal bone fractures and cholesteatoma. *Ann Otol Rhinol Laryngol* 1983;92:558–560.

Ghorayeb BY, Yeakley JW. Temporal bone fractures: longitudinal or oblique? The case for oblique temporal bone fractures. *Laryngoscope* 1992;102:129–134.

Goodhill V. Leaking labyrinth lesions, deafness, tinnitus and dizziness. *Ann Otol Rhinol Laryngol* 1981;90:99–106.

Goodhill V. Traumatic fistulae. *J Laryngol Otol* 1980;94:123–128.

Grove WE. Skull fractures involving the ear. A clinical study of 211 cases. *Laryngoscope* 1939;49:678–706, 833–867.

Huang MY, Lambert PR. Temporal bone trauma. In: Hughes GB, Pensak ML eds. *Clinical Otology*. New York: Thieme Medical Publishers; 1997:251–268.

Makishima K, Snow JB. Pathogenesis of hearing loss in head injury; studies in man and experimental animals. *Arch Otolaryngol* 1975;101:426–432.

May M, Klien SR. Facial nerve decompression complications. *Laryngoscope* 1983;93:299–305.

McGuit WF Jr, Stool S. Temporal bone fractures in children: a review with emphasis on long-term sequelae. *Clin Pediatr* 1992;31:12–18.

Orobello P. Congenital acquired facial nerve paralysis in children. *Otolaryngol Clin North Am* 1991;24:647–652.

Podoshin L, Fradis M. Hearing loss after head injury. *Arch Otolaryngol* 1975;101:15–18.

Pullen FW II, Rosenberg GJ, Cabeza CH. Sudden hearing loss in divers and fliers. *Laryngoscope* 1979;89:1373–1377.

Roberto M, Hamernik RP, Turrentine GA. Damage of the auditory system associated with acute blast trauma. *Ann Otol Rhinol Laryngol Suppl* 1989;98:23–24.

Schuknecht HF. Mechanism of inner ear injury from blows to the head. *Ann Otol Rhinol Laryngol* 1969;78:253–362.

Schuknecht HF, Davison RC. Deafness and vertigo from head injury. *Arch Otolaryngol* 1956;63:513–528.

Selzer S, McCabe BF. Perilymph fistula: the Iowa experience. *Laryngoscope* 1986;94:37–49.

Spector G, Pratt LL, Randall G. A clinical study of delayed reconstruction in ossicular fractures. *Laryngoscope* 1873;83:837–851.

Tos M. Prognosis of hearing loss in temporal bone fractures. *J Laryngol Otol* 1971;85:1147–1159.

Weisman JL, Curtin HD. Pneumolabyrinth: a computed tomographic sign of temporal bone fracture. *Clin Radiol* 1992;13:113–114.

Ylikoski J, Palva T, Sanna M. Dizziness after head trauma; clinical and morphologic findings. *Am J Otol* 1982;3:343–352.

FLAP
RECONSTRUCTION
IN HEAD AND
NECK SURGERY

Chapter 85

Basic Principles

Allen M. Seiden

Advances in anesthesia and refinements in surgical instrumentation have facilitated more aggressive surgical approaches to head and neck malignancies. But such extensive resections cannot be performed without innovative reconstructive efforts that address both form and function. The development of alloplastic materials notwithstanding, perhaps nothing has furthered our reconstructive efforts more than the use of flaps.

Flaps satisfy a number of reconstructive requirements. They can be used to resurface large skin or mucosal defects and can provide often-needed soft tissue bulk, which can provide a more natural contour and facilitate prosthetic rehabilitative efforts. They also provide coverage and protection for major vascular structures. As opposed to skin grafts, the viability of a flap is ensured by its pedicled blood supply, and therefore is relatively independent of conditions in the recipient bed. This makes it better suited to cover bone, nerves, scarred areas, and previously irradiated areas.

When determining the most appropriate reconstructive approach, factors other than the wound defect need to be considered. The age and general health of the patient may preclude extensive flap repair. In certain situations it may be preferable not to place a thick tissue flap into a

defect where the likelihood of recurrence is very high, thereby impeding early detection. In terms of flap selection, certain donor-site characteristics may be desirable, whereas any associated donor-site morbidity is undesirable. Sometimes multiple flaps will do the job better than one.

The difficulty in flap reconstruction lies not in the surgical technique but in preoperative planning and judgment. It is important to understand the ramifications of flap selection and to maintain a variety of options in case the defect is altered at the time of surgery or other unanticipated factors arise.

FLAP HEMODYNAMICS

Every flap has a vascular pedicle that ensures its survival, although the nature of this vascular supply will vary. The successful design and execution of flap reconstruction are dependent on a thorough understanding of this underlying blood supply.

VASCULAR ANATOMY

Segmental vessels are large, named vessels that arise from the aorta and run deep to the muscle, providing branches to the muscle and overlying

579

skin. Each segmental branch has an associated vein and nerve. The perforators connect the deep segmental vessels with the overlying cutaneous circulation, while at the same time being responsible for supplying the muscles through which they pass. An example would be the pectoral branch (perforator) arising from the thoracoacromial artery (segmental), supplying the pectoralis muscle and communicating with the overlying cutaneous vessels. The intercostal perforators arise from the internal mammary artery (segmental) to supply the medial portion of the pectoralis major muscle, as well as providing cutaneous vessels to the deltopectoral flap.

The cutaneous circulation consists of both musculocutaneous and direct cutaneous arteries. The former pass perpendicularly from the muscle through the subcutaneous fat to terminate in the subdermal plexus. This type predominates and is scattered throughout the body where skin overlies muscle, although each vessel supplies only a small surface area. Direct cutaneous arteries run parallel to the skin surface and also terminate in the subdermal plexus, individually providing vascularity to a much larger area of skin. A rich anastomotic network exists between these two types of vessels, fulfilling both a nutritional and thermoregulatory function.

Based on the underlying vascular anatomy, three kinds of flaps can be developed: a random pattern flap, such as local facial skin flaps that depend on musculocutaneous arteries at their base for survival; flaps having a direct cutaneous artery, such as the deltopectoral flap; and flaps that have a segmental arterial supply, such as the pectoralis major myocutaneous flap.

SPECIAL CONSIDERATION

An axial pattern flap is based on an anatomically recognized arteriovenous circulation that includes a segmental artery following the long axis of the flap. Its survival is therefore based on the distribution of this vessel. On the other hand, a random pattern flap derives its blood supply solely from the dermal-subdermal plexus.

PEARL••• Flat muscles, such as the pectoralis major, trapezius, and latissimus dorsi, generally have axial blood supplies. Round muscles, such as the sternocleidomastoid, tend to have a more random blood supply without an axial segmental vessel.

The difference between axial and random blood supplies becomes very important when considering flap design, although the two are not necessarily mutually exclusive. For example, the thoracoacromial artery runs axially along the undersurface of the pectoralis major muscle, providing perforator vessels along its course. A skin island overlying this muscle has an axial pattern blood supply derived from these perforators and as such is very dependable. However, any part of this skin island extending beyond the muscle has a random pattern blood supply and therefore its survival is less predictable.

The oxygen demand of a random pattern flap depends on its surface area, whereas the oxygen supply depends on the width of the pedicle as well as perfusion pressure. As already stated, random pattern flaps depend on musculocutaneous arteries that penetrate perpendicularly into the base and then perfuse the flap through the interconnecting dermal-subdermal plexi. The mean arterial pressure in segmental vessels is approximately 90 to 100 mm Hg, which drops to 80 mm Hg in the musculocutaneous and direct cutaneous vessels and then to 30 mm Hg in the distal arterioles. That point at which the perfusion pressure drops below vascular resistance represents the line of demarcation for flap survival.

FLAP DELAY

Various techniques to enhance flap survival have included hypertensive perfusion, dextran, cooling, hyperbaric oxygen, and pharmacologic manipulation. None has been sufficiently consistent or clinically practical to have met with widespread success. On the other hand, it has been known for over a century that delayed harvesting of a flap will tend to augment survival.

Delaying a flap involves making the outlining incisions, elevating it in the appropriate plane, and then laying it back down to be lightly sutured. This initial elevation was shown by Reinisch (1974) to cause sympathetic denervation that allows arteriovenous shunts to open. Such shunts normally divert large amounts of blood to the superficial venous plexi for the purpose of thermoregulation and thereby bypass the nutrient capillary bed. This would impair flap circulation during primary transfer. Over a period of 14 to 21 days spontaneous closure of these shunts seems to occur as sympathetic tone is regained, and flap perfusion is enhanced. It therefore follows that the optimum time for transfer of a flap following delay should be approximately 2 to 3 weeks.

Patients with advanced age, arteriosclerosis, diabetes, malnutrition, or previously irradiated tissue may warrant delay. It is also possible to delay a myocutaneous or axial pattern flap when incorporating a large skin paddle that has a significant random component.

ASSESSMENT OF FLAP VIABILITY

Flap necrosis may occur from errors in design, improper elevation, poor tissue handling, and inadequate postoperative care. Ultimately, the most common event causing failure is venous occlusion. Significant morbidity results. Therefore, the earlier flap compromise is recognized, the better the chance of salvage and avoidance of further complications.

> **PEARL...** Skin flaps and free flaps can tolerate up to 8 hours of ischemia before irreversible tissue damage occurs, whereas myocutaneous flaps can tolerate only 4 hours. This is largely due to the higher metabolic demand of skeletal muscle.

The color of a flap is the most obvious way to judge its viability. If venous outflow is obstructed, for example, from tension or constriction of the vascular pedicle, then the flap will appear blue. On the other hand, if arterial flow becomes obstructed, the flap will appear white and feel cool to the touch.

> **PEARL...** After blanching the distal end of a flap by finger pressure, the rate of capillary filling or color return can be compared to surrounding skin, but it should occur within 4 seconds.

Generalized oozing of bright red blood from the edges of a flap, or after pricking the skin surface, indicates a good blood supply. If the blood appears dark or bleeding is irregular, vascularity is likely compromised.

More objective methods to evaluate flap viability have been described and have focused on blood flow, oxygenation, and energy metabolism. Fluorescein is a nontoxic dye that is injected intravenously as a 5% solution at a dose of 15 mg/kg body weight. If the flap is well vascularized, the fluorescein rapidly diffuses into the extracellular space. Maximal fluorescence occurs at 15 to 20 minutes, and this will stain the flap yellow when viewed with an ultraviolet light. Although the fluorescein test is simple and fairly reliable, studies have shown that the surviving area of a flap is generally greater than its staining area. To serially monitor flap perfusion, various methods to quantify uptake and elimination of fluorescein over time have been described. Other methods to assess flap viability include:

▼ The elimination of various radioisotopes from the skin of the flap has been used to measure circulatory flow with mixed success.

▼ Oxygen tension, which would reflect the adequacy of the underlying blood supply, can be measured transcutaneously by either a gas analyzer or mass spectrometry. If the blood supply is compromised and oxygen concentration decreases, anaerobic metabolism results with an increase in lactic acid. This would be reflected in pH measurements.

▼ Skin temperature can be measured as an estimation of blood flow, primarily by the use of either thermoelectric thermometers and infrared thermometry or thermography.

▼ Photoplethysmography has been described as a technique to monitor pulsatile blood flow. However, it does not distinguish nutrient from nonnutrient flow.

▼ Perhaps the most widely utilized noninvasive technique for detecting blood flow is the ultrasound or laser Doppler flowmeter. Although it too does not distinguish between nutrient and nonutrient flow, it is relatively simple to perform and is sensitive to hemodynamic changes. It can be used to continuously monitor flaps postoperatively.

▼ Other more recent, noninvasive techniques have included magnetic resonance spectroscopy, positron emission tomography, and optical methods that use near-infrared spectrophotometry. Most of these, at this point, remain experimental and not widely utilized clinically.

SALVAGING FLAP FAILURE

In the postoperative period, if a flap demonstrates signs of impending failure, then technical factors should be sought. Excessive stretching or kinking of the flap or improper positioning of the patient can compromise blood supply. The release of some sutures can sometimes help to relieve excessive tension. Dressings that inadvertently place pressure on the base of the flap should be avoided, including tightening of tracheotomy umbilical tape.

Hematoma formation can distend the flap to the point of interrupting the vascular supply and is a common cause of flap morbidity. If present, it needs to be evacuated emergently and its recurrence prevented by maintaining closed suction drainage and adequate hemostasis.

Agents such as dextran, heparin, aspirin, and vasodilators have all been tried with little success. Local hypothermia has shown some ability to delay and reduce the severity of ultimate necrosis, although not salvaging the flap entirely. Hyperbaric oxygen can enhance flap survival provided it is given as soon after surgery as possible, preferably within 48 hours. Theories to explain its effectiveness include heightened fibroblastic activity that increases the collagen matrix necessary for capillary ingrowth, and the vasoconstrictive properties of oxygen that selectively close arteriovenous shunts, thereby allowing greater flow to the nutrient capillary bed.

SUGGESTED READINGS

Baker SR. Local cutaneous flaps. *Otolaryngol Clin North Am* 1994;27:139–159.

Hayden RE, Tavill MA, Nioka S, et al. Oxygenation and blood volume changes in flaps according to near-infrared spectrophotometry. *Arch Otolaryngol Head Neck Surg* 1996;122: 1347–1351.

Hjortdal VE, Hansen ES, Hauge E. Myocutaneous flap ischemia: dynamics following venous and arterial obstruction. *Plast Reconstr Surg* 1992;89:1083–1091.

Milton SH. Pedicled skin-flaps: the fallacy of the length-width ratio. *Br J Surg* 1970;57:502–508.

Reinisch JF. The pathophysiology of skin flap circulation. The delay phenomenon. *Plast Reconstr Surg* 1974;54:585–598.

Seiden AM. Flap reconstruction in head and neck surgery. In: Lee KJ, ed. *Otolaryngology and Head and Neck Surgery.* New York: Elsevier; 1989:861–888.

Chapter 86

SKIN FLAPS

Allen M. Seiden

Skin flaps are created by the transfer of skin and subcutaneous tissue from a donor to a recipient site, the vascular pedicle generally remaining attached during transfer. Because they bring their own nourishment, such flaps are useful for coverage when the recipient bed has a compromised blood supply or when there are exposed blood vessels, bone, or cartilage. In contrast to skin grafts, the underlying pad of fatty areolar tissue incorporated into the flap maintains its pliancy, prevents shrinkage, and provides a modest amount of bulk.

Skin flaps can have either a random vascular pattern or a specific axial pattern. The foremost example of random skin flaps is local flaps developed adjacent to the defect, which are utilized to resurface relatively small or moderately sized areas of skin loss.

> **PEARL...** Donor site scars can usually be camouflaged in natural creases or junctions of anatomic landmarks.

LOCAL SKIN FLAPS

Local flaps are designed immediately adjacent to the defect and can be broadly divided into three types.

ADVANCEMENT FLAPS

An advancement flap is any design in which the skin edges of the defect are undermined and simply advanced to be closed over the open wound. This includes the fusiform excision of small lesions, which is perhaps the most often utilized flap technique (Fig. 86–1). It is best utilized in areas where there is an excess of skin.

> **PEARL...** It is important to remember three points when performing a fusiform excision: (1) the line of excision should fall along relaxed skin tension lines, (2) the angles at each end should be less than 30 degrees to avoid tissue protrusions or dog ear deformity, and (3) the flaps should be closed without tension.

Another type of advancement flap is the rectangular, single-pedicle advancement flap, in which parallel incisions allow a sliding movement of tissue into the defect (Fig. 86–2). The long axis of the flap should be designed along relaxed skin tension lines. Tissue protrusions on either side may be removed by excision of Burrow triangles (Fig. 86–2), or Z-plasties.

A special application of the advancement flap is the V-Y technique. This is particularly useful when lengthening or release from contracture is required.

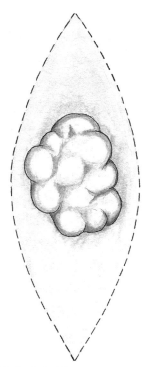

FIGURE 86–1 A fusiform excision.

ROTATION FLAPS

A rotation flap is rotated about a fixed pivot point adjacent to the defect. It has a curvilinear configuration and is most effective for closing triangular defects. Its broad base ensures a reliable blood supply.

Large rotation flaps are useful for closing large cheek and neck defects. The curvilinear in-

cision may be concealed at the border between aesthetic units but requires extensive undermining.

TRANSPOSITION FLAPS

A transposition flap is one in which the flap is transposed over a bridge of intervening normal tissue before being placed into the defect (Fig. 86–3). The advantage of this particular flap is its ability to bring tissue from an adjacent area where the skin may be more redundant, as well as being able to distribute wound tension over a wide area. This minimizes distortion and scar deformity.

There are many different types of local transposition flaps, including the rhomboid and bilobe flap, as well as a Z-plasty, but Figure 86–3 demonstrates a typical example. The flap is transposed over the tissue marked by the arrow and placed into the defect after the lesion is excised. PV marks the pivot point and is the point of greatest tension. The length from PV to point C

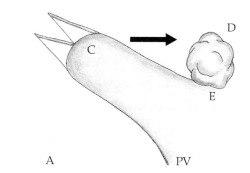

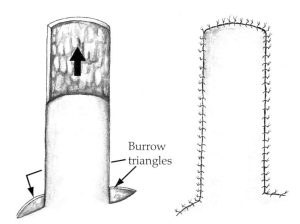

FIGURE 86–2 A rectangular advancement flap.

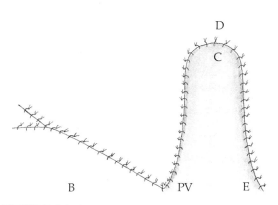

FIGURE 86–3 A transposition flap.

must equal PV to point D. If possible, the donor site is closed primarily.

Transposition flaps are perhaps the most widely utilized cutaneous flaps in head and neck reconstruction for small and moderately sized defects. Although most are random flaps, the rich vascularity of the face and scalp allows versatile design and application.

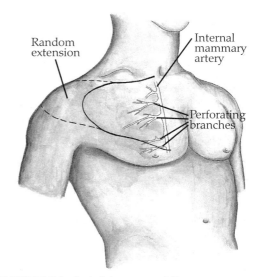

FIGURE 86–4 A deltopectoral flap.

THE DELTOPECTORAL FLAP

Described by Bakamjian in 1965, the deltopectoral flap was for many years the workhorse for head and neck reconstruction. It utilizes chest skin overlying the pectoralis major and deltoid muscles and is an axial pattern flap relying primarily on the internal mammary artery (Fig. 86–4). Within the upper five or six intercostal spaces, about 1.5 cm lateral to the sternal border, this artery gives off perforators that ultimately give way to direct cutaneous vessels that supply the skin over the pectoralis major. However, the deltoid portion lateral to the deltopectoral groove remains random in its blood supply, relying upon the dermal-subdermal plexus.

The base of the deltopectoral flap is designed to incorporate the first four intercostal spaces. The appropriate length depends on the size and location of the defect, but if extra length over the deltoid portion is needed, delay should be considered. Flap elevation is performed deep to the fascia that covers the pectoralis major and deltoid muscles in order to protect the vascular supply.

The deltopectoral flap can be rotated to cover a wide variety of defects, extending as far as the skull base, and can be used for both extraoral or intraoral reconstruction. The length required is determined by measuring the distance from the pivot point of the flap to the defect.

If the defect is not adjacent to the flap, then the flap must be transposed over an intervening bridge of normal skin. This may be handled in one of three ways: (1) the skin may be excised; (2) the pedicle of the flap may be tubed, which then would require a second stage at 17 to 21 days, at which point the pedicle is divided and repositioned into the donor site; and (3) the pedicle may be de-epithelialized and then buried beneath the intervening skin. Although this reduces the procedure to a single stage, care must be exercised to avoid injury to the vascular supply. The defect is then covered with a split-thickness skin graft, which presents little cosmetic or functional difficulty.

The deltopectoral flap is reliable and generally provides healthy, nonirradiated tissue with a good blood supply. It provides relatively little bulk, but as a result it can be contoured easily to fit a variety of cervicofacial defects.

Partial necrosis of the tip may occur when the flap has been lengthened without prior delay. The dependent position of the base facilitates venous drainage, but gravitational pull and the weight of the tissue may lead to wound separation. Close postoperative monitoring is essential to prevent such complications that will jeopardize flap survival.

THE NAPE OF THE NECK FLAP

The nape of the neck or posterior neck flap is based essentially over the posterior occiput and mastoid region, directed laterally over the shoulder (Fig. 86–5). Although it receives blood supply from branches of the occipital and posterior auricular arteries, it nevertheless remains

primarily a random pattern flap, particularly in its distal portion. It can be used to resurface large defects on the side of the face or neck.

The flap generally measures 10 to 12 cm wide at its base and 30 cm in length, although the actual design will depend on the size of the defect. The anterior incision descends along the anterior border of the trapezius muscle, while the posterior incision begins across the midoccipital line and curves down the neck to lie over the scapular spine. Elevation should be deep to the underlying muscular fascia. Following transfer, the donor site is generally covered with a split-thickness skin graft.

THE FOREHEAD FLAP

The forehead flap was first introduced in the early 1800s and is one of the oldest flaps utilized for facial reconstruction. McGregor popularized it in the 1960s by demonstrating its versatility. It is generally based either laterally on the superficial temporal artery or medially on both supratrochlear arteries (Figs. 86–6 and 86–7).

The laterally based forehead flap is an axial-pattern flap and therefore is very reliable. The entire forehead skin can be utilized. The incisions are generally placed along the frontal hairline and brow for better concealment and may extend to the contralateral temple. Proximally, to avoid injury to the frontal branch of the facial nerve, the incision should not come beyond the level of the lateral canthus. The superior incision curves toward the ear to incorporate the anterior branch of the superficial temporal artery, the main axial vessel of the flap. Elevation should be deep to the frontalis muscle but superficial to the pericranium.

The laterally based flap can be used to resurface external defects on the face and can

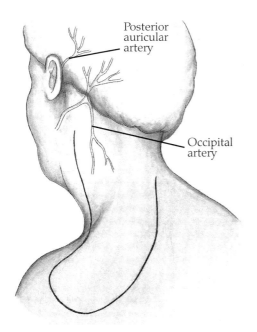

Posterior auricular artery

Occipital artery

FIGURE 86–5 A nape of the neck flap.

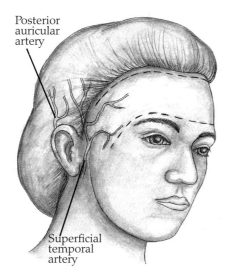

FIGURE 86–6 A laterally based forehead flap.

also be utilized for intraoral reconstruction, which would require tunneling through the defect or a separate incision. More recent options in flap design have largely superseded this latter application. The primary drawback in using the laterally based forehead flap is the large donor site defect that necessarily must be skin grafted; its adynamic nature and poor color match giving a poor cosmetic result. The deformity is

minimized by using the entire forehead, but it relegates this flap to one that is used when there are few other alternatives.

> **PITFALL...** If the ipsilateral external carotid artery has been previously ligated, such as during a radical neck dissection, the blood supply to this flap will be compromised.

The midline forehead flap remains more actively utilized. It too is an axial-pattern flap, based on both supratrochlear arteries with lesser contributions from the dorsal nasal artery (Fig. 86–7). It is useful for smaller midfacial defects and has been most widely described for reconstructing the caudal two-thirds of the nose. The distal undersurface of the flap can be lined with a split-thickness skin graft for repairing full-thickness defects.

The flap is outlined in a vertical direction and can be extended as far as the hairline when necessary. Elevation is superficial to the periosteum and must be done bluntly below the nasofrontal angle to avoid injury to the pedicle. The flap is then rotated 180 degrees to the defect.

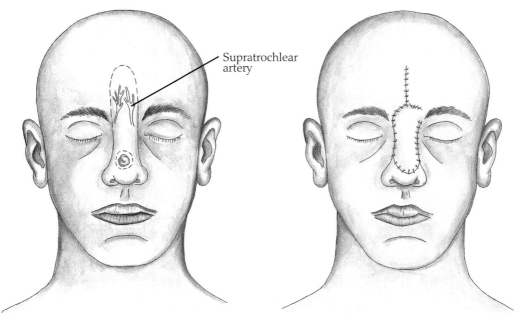

FIGURE 86–7 A midline forehead flap.

The donor site can generally be closed primarily with adequate undermining, although if not it can be allowed to heal secondarily with very little scar deformity. One of the disadvantages of this flap is its need for a second stage, the pedicle being taken down at approximately 3 weeks. At that time only the proximal portion of the pedicle is returned to its original position.

SUGGESTED READINGS

Bakamjian VY. A two-stage method for pharyngoesophageal reconstruction with a primary pectoral skin flap. *Plast Reconstr Surg* 1965;36: 173–184.

Baker SR. Local cutaneous flaps. *Otolaryngol Clin North Am* 1994;27:139–159.

Baker SR, Swanson NA, eds. *Local Flaps in Facial Reconstruction.* St. Louis: CV Mosby; 1995.

Becker FF. *Facial Reconstruction with Local and Regional Flaps.* New York: Thieme-Stratton; 1985.

McGregor IA. The temporal flap in intra-oral cancer: its use in repairing the post excisional defect. *Br J Plast Surg* 1963;16:318–335.

Price JC, Davis RK. The deltopectoral flap vs. the pectoralis major myocutaneous flap. *Arch Otolaryngol* 1984;110:35–40.

Seiden AM. Flap reconstruction in head and neck surgery. In: Lee KJ, ed. *Otolaryngology and Head and Neck Surgery.* New York: Elsevier; 1989:861–888.

Chapter 87

MUSCLE AND MYOCUTANEOUS FLAPS

Allen M. Seiden

MUSCLE FLAPS

Muscle flaps were first widely described for lower extremity reconstruction in the 1970s, and were subsequently adapted to other areas. For a given skeletal muscle to be used as a flap, it must have a dependable blood supply that can be easily preserved during transfer. Flat muscles have a single vascular pedicle supplying the entire muscle and therefore are the most reliable. So-called round muscles have multiple vascular pedicles that provide a segmental blood supply, and as a result their use is more limited.

> **PEARL...** The arc of rotation for each muscle flap is determined by the distance from the flap tip to the origin of the vascular pedicle, the latter being the pivot point.

Excessive tension on the pedicle must be avoided.

Muscle flaps are typically used to augment regional deficiencies when there is no skin or mucosal defect, and therefore an additional skin island is not needed. On the other hand, when a skin paddle would be too bulky such as for oral reconstruction, they provide a good bed for skin grafting. They serve to provide good coverage when major vessels are exposed and may be compounded with bone when mandibular re-construction is required. Preservation of neural input has been described when used for facial reanimation.

TEMPORALIS MUSCLE FLAP

The temporalis is a broad, fan-shaped muscle arising from the periosteum of the temporal fossa (Fig. 87–1). It descends deep to the zygomatic arch to insert onto the coronoid process and anterior mandibular ramus. It relies on the anterior and deep temporal arteries for its vascular supply. These arteries arise from the internal maxillary artery and enter the muscle on its deep surface at the level of the zygoma. The middle temporal artery, off of the superficial temporal artery, provides a lesser contribution. However, this latter vessel is usually sacrificed during elevation of the flap. Innervation of the flap is from branches of the mandibular division of the trigeminal nerve.

> **PEARL...** The dominant blood supply to the temporalis filters through the muscle in such a fashion that it can be divided coronally or sagittally, depending on the reconstructive needs. The overlying temporalis fascia may be incised and reflected, leaving it attached to the tip of the muscle and thereby extending the flap as a musculofascial unit.

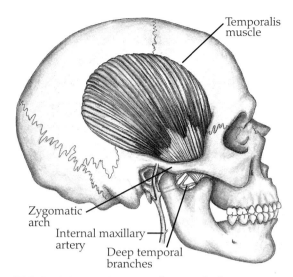

FIGURE 87–1 A temporalis muscle flap.

The temporalis muscle is usually approached via an incision along the superior temporal line or a unilateral coronal incision. Injury to the vascular pedicle at the level of the zygomatic arch must be avoided. The flap is then inverted to pass either superficial or deep to the zygoma. Some recommend removing the arch to technically facilitate transfer and allowing the rolled edge of the muscle to provide contour.

The temporalis muscle flap can be used to augment defects of the upper two-thirds of the face, orbit, and anterolateral skull base, which may be difficult to reach with more inferiorly based flaps. It may be used to restore facial contour following radical parotidectomy and partial mandibulectomy. For facial reanimation, the flap may be divided into strips to facilitate both eye closure and oral commissure support, with the potential to provide both static and dynamic support. The main advantage of this flap is that it can provide a considerable amount of tissue, but the donor site is within the same operative field as these defects and is seldom compromised by prior resection. It is well vascularized and versatile, although its range is somewhat limited.

Donor-site morbidity includes a hollowed appearance of the temporal fossa, which can be augmented with a synthetic implant if the patient finds it objectionable. The most common complication of the flap is paralysis of the frontal branch of the facial nerve. Subsequent difficulties with occlusion or mastication rarely if ever occur.

MASSETER MUSCLE FLAP

The masseter muscle is a relatively short, flat muscle arising from the anterior two-thirds of the zygomatic arch and extending to the lateral surface of the mandibular ramus and angle. It receives an axial pattern blood supply from the masseter artery, which branches from the internal maxillary artery and passes through the coronoid notch to penetrate the deep surface of the muscle. Innervation is provided by the mandibular division of the trigeminal nerve.

This flap has traditionally been used primarily for facial reanimation but can be used to augment regional defects. In the former instance, it is used to rehabilitate the oral commissure and nasolabial fold. It can be approached either extraorally, through a submandibular incision, or intraorally, through a gingivobuccal incision. It is elevated in a subperiosteal plane from the mandible, while avoiding injury to the vascular pedicle. A nasolabial incision usually needs to be made to complete the transfer.

MYOCUTANEOUS FLAPS

Myocutaneous flaps are composite flaps of skeletal muscle and skin in which the underlying muscle pedicle provides vascular support to the overlying skin island. Generally, the muscle receives its blood supply from a dominant vascular pedicle that contains a segmental artery, vein, and nerve. The artery gives rise to perforators that actually supply the muscle, and in turn form musculocutaneous vessels that supply the overlying skin or myocutaneous territory. The size and shape of the skin island are determined by the underlying skeletal muscle but is not limited to conventional length-width ratios. In addition, the size of the skin island can be extended to include a random portion, the survival of which may be enhanced by delay maneuvers when necessary.

Myocutaneous flaps have several advantages over skin flaps. Generally they are more reliable because of the secure vascular supply. They can usually be performed in a single stage because there is rarely a need for delay and the muscular pedicle can be buried. The pedicle provides bulk that helps to restore contour and provide protection for the carotid artery. Lastly, due to the strong blood supply, a segment of bone to which the muscle is attached can be harvested as an osseomyocutaneous flap to enhance reconstruction of mandibular defects.

PECTORALIS MAJOR MYOCUTANEOUS FLAP

In 1977 Ariyan was the first to describe this flap for use in head and neck reconstruction, and it subsequently has become one of the most versatile and reliable flaps at our disposal. It provides a generous amount of soft tissue and skin, is relatively easy to harvest, and results in minimal donor-site morbidity.

The pectoralis major muscle is a flat, fan-shaped muscle that arises from the medial half of the clavicle, the lateral half of the sternum, and the upper adjacent six or seven costal carti-

lages. It inserts onto the crest of the greater tubercle of the humerus (Fig. 87–2). The sternocostal portion is a powerful adductor of the arm, whereas the clavicular portion medially rotates the humerus. Innervation is provided by the medial and lateral pectoral nerves.

The dominant vascular pedicle is the pectoral branch of the thoracoacromial artery. The thoracoacromial artery branches from the first part of the axillary artery just proximal to the insertion of the pectoralis minor muscle into the coracoid process of the scapula, and descends between the pectoralis major and minor muscles. Here, under the clavicle, it gives off the pectoral branch.

PEARL... Once exiting from beneath the clavicle, the pectoral branch turns obliquely to lie approximately along a line from the acromion to the xiphoid process. This is a useful landmark to remember during flap elevation.

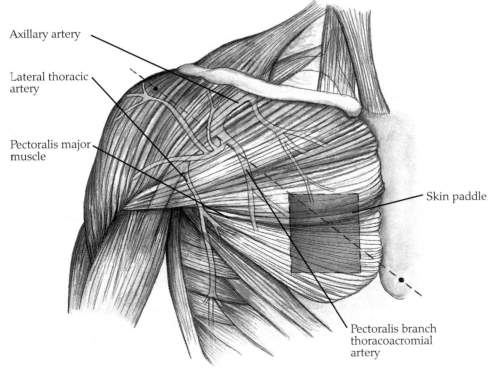

Axillary artery

Lateral thoracic artery

Pectoralis major muscle

Skin paddle

Pectoralis branch thoracoacromial artery

FIGURE 87–2 A pectoralis major myocutaneous flap.

The vascular pedicle travels deep to the muscle and is protected within the clavipectoral fascia that envelopes the muscle's undersurface.

A second blood supply comes from the lateral thoracic artery. This artery typically leaves the second portion of the axillary artery from beneath the pectoralis minor and pierces the clavipectoral fascia lateral to this muscle. In less than 10% of cases it may arise from a common trunk with the thoracoacromial artery. It descends along the lateral border of the pectoralis minor muscle but within the fascial envelope of the pectoralis major. Several studies have demonstrated a co-dominance between the lateral thoracic and pectoral branch of the thoracoacromial artery: the former seems to perfuse the lateral and inferior portions of the muscle, whereas the latter perfuses the clavicular and sternal portions.

Sasaki et al (1986) found that the cutaneous territory of the pectoral artery was essentially limited to skin overlying the pectoralis major muscle, whereas the lateral thoracic actually supplied skin beyond the border of the muscle, that is, below the nipple. The lateral thoracic artery is usually sacrificed when the horizontal fibers of the pectoralis major muscle are cut at their humoral attachment, because preservation limits upward rotation to about the level of the tonsillar fossa. However, if a significant portion of random skin is utilized, it may be wise to try to preserve this contribution.

The size of the defect determines the size of the skin paddle. The more superior the defect, the more inferiorly placed the skin paddle needs to be, the pivot point for the flap being the emergence of the vascular pedicle from beneath the clavicle. A rectangular paddle is generally adequate, with that area of skin over the most medial and inferior portion of the muscle having the furthest arc of rotation.

If the pectoralis major muscle is freed up to the clavicle, including release of its humoral attachment, it may reach defects as high as the skull base, temporal fossa, and orbit. Its versatility is such that it can be applied to almost any defect with which the head and neck surgeon is confronted. The skin island allows for a good watertight mucosal closure, and the underlying subcutaneous tissue and muscle pedicle provide bulk for contour and protection to the carotid artery. It is generally accomplished as a single stage, and this is important when postoperative adjuvant therapy is required. For through-and-through defects, the cutaneous portion may be split to provide both intraoral and skin closure, or the skin can be used for intraoral closure while a split-thickness skin graft is applied externally to the exposed muscle. For lateral mandibular defects, occasionally the bulk of the flap is enough to restore some contour and reduce mandibular drift. Following extensive mandibular resections, a segment of attached rib can be transferred for osteomyocutaneous reconstruction.

Perhaps the flap's greatest advantage is its reliability, with complete necrosis occurring in less than 5% of cases. The patient can remain supine without the need for repositioning. Finally, with proper undermining, the donor site can usually be closed primarily.

Despite these advantages, the pectoralis major myocutaneous flap does have certain limitations that need to be addressed relative to the reconstructive demands of each patient. Although the bulk of the flap is usually helpful, in some situations it is undesirable. The thickness is dependent on the muscle mass and subcutaneous fat. This fat cannot be manipulated without risking injury to the musculocutaneous nutrient

SPECIAL CONSIDERATION

Extension of the paddle can usually be made to the costochondral junction without the need for delay, recognizing that the portion below the border of the pectoralis major muscle has a random blood supply.

PITFALLS... The bulkiness of the muscle pedicle makes it more difficult to examine these patients in follow-up, that is, to detect recurrent disease. It also makes the flap very difficult to use if a neck dissection has not been performed or if the sternocleidomastoid muscle has been saved in a modified neck dissection.

vessels to the skin. This thickness restricts the ability of the flap to be contoured to some defects.

Other less significant shortcomings include the potential transfer of hair-bearing skin to the oral cavity or pharynx, and closure of the donor site causing significant breast distortion in women. The functional loss associated with elevation of the pectoralis major muscle may be objectionable, particularly when combined with resection of the spinal accessory nerve. However, the latissimus dorsi remains a powerful adductor of the arm and compensates to some degree.

TRAPEZIUS MYOCUTANEOUS FLAP

The trapezius is a flat, triangular muscle that, when right and left are joined, forms a trapezoid shape. It originates from the external occipital protuberance, the nuchal ligament, and the spinous processes of the seventh cervical and all thoracic vertebrae. The occipital and upper cervical fibers insert onto the lateral third of the clavicle, whereas the lower cervical and upper thoracic fibers insert onto the acromion and crest of the scapular spine. Its function is to assist in the elevation and rotation of the shoulder.

Innervation of the trapezius muscle is by the spinal accessory nerve, which enters the muscle 5 cm above its attachment to the clavicle. In addition, fibers from C3 and C4 may provide motor innervation. The blood supply can be somewhat confusing because it can be somewhat variable. The dominant blood supply is provided by the transverse cervical artery, with additional contributions by the occipital artery superiorly, the dorsal scapular artery at the shoulder tip, and perforating branches of the posterior intercostal arteries medially.

The transverse cervical artery most commonly branches off the thyrocervical trunk but may also branch off the suprascapular artery or the dorsal scapular artery, or directly off the subclavian artery. It then travels to the posterior triangle, superficial to the phrenic nerve and brachial plexus, and deep to the omohyoid muscle. At the anterior border of the levator scapulae muscle, it divides into a superficial and deep branch, with the superficial branch passing deep to the anterior border of the trapezius muscle. In 25% of cases, this superficial branch will arise separately from the subclavian.

The superficial branch is the dominant pedicle, dividing into an ascending and descending branch. The descending branch passes along the undersurface of the trapezius muscle down the upper back between the spine and scapula, reaching the lower fibers of the trapezius muscle.

The occipital artery courses beneath the mastoid to supply the skin overlying the superior medial trapezius fibers. The dorsal scapular artery originates from the second or third portion of the subclavian artery, passes under the middle trunk of the brachial plexus, and descends along the medial border of the scapula to supply the lower third of the trapezius.

Recognizing the extent and variation of blood supply to the trapezius, several flaps can be designed that can be useful in head and neck reconstruction. The superior trapezius flap is based on the occipital artery and paraspinous muscle perforators. The anterior incision is made along the anterior border of the trapezius, whereas the posterior incision follows in a parallel fashion approximately 10 cm behind, very much like the nape of the neck (Fig. 87–3). A random portion of skin extending up to 10 cm beyond the muscle may be included without delay. Elevation incorporates the trapezius muscle and its underlying fascial envelope without necessarily identifying the vascular pedicle. The transverse cervical and dorsal scapular arteries are ligated unless, in rare circumstances, they do not interfere with flap rotation. Following transfer, the donor defect will usually need to be closed with a split-thickness skin graft.

A modification of this flap, utilizing the myocutaneous territory over the superior lateral trapezius fibers, but based on the superficial branch of the transverse cervical artery, is known as the lateral island flap (Fig. 87–4). The skin paddle can be centered over the acromion process and does not need to lie entirely over the trapezius muscle. The transverse cervical artery and vein must be delineated prior to rotation of this flap.

> **PITFALL...** These vessels are often sacrificed during a radical neck dissection, and this must be considered if a patient has had a prior neck dissection or will be needing a neck dissection.

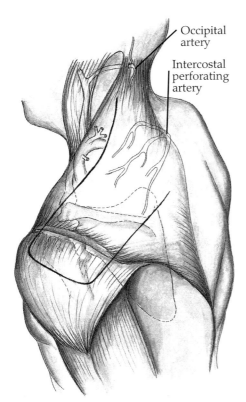

FIGURE 87–3 An upper trapezius myocutaneous flap.

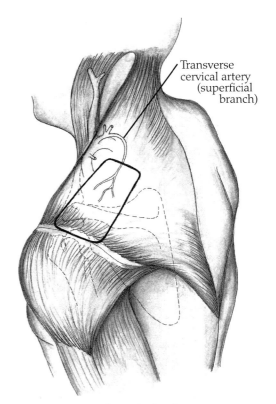

FIGURE 87–4 A lateral island trapezius myocutaneous flap.

The trapezius muscle is transected medial to the vascular pedicle and the origin of the transverse cervical artery and vein become the pivot point. The flap is then tunneled beneath the neck skin to the defect. The donor site can usually be closed primarily.

The last potential flap utilizing the trapezius muscle is the lower or inferior trapezius myocutaneous flap. This requires rotation of the patient into the lateral decubitus position, which is cumbersome, but it does achieve a wider arc of rotation. The skin paddle is centered between the scapula and spine and may extend 10 to 15 cm caudal to the tip of the scapula (Fig. 87–5). As the muscle is elevated, the descending branch of the transverse cervical artery should be identified on its undersurface and mobilized under direct vision. Preserving the contribution of the dorsal scapular artery as well improves the flap's reliability. The donor defect may be closed primarily, and the patient returned to the supine position to complete the reconstruction.

The upper trapezius flap has a range and utility similar to the nape of neck flap. It is particularly useful for upper neck and posterior mandibular defects and fistulas. The lateral island flap has a wider arc of rotation, and because of the thin subcutaneous tissue in this area, it is more supple and more easily contoured. It can reach the lower face, anterior floor of mouth, oropharynx, and hypopharynx, for both lining and coverage. The lower trapezius flap will reach almost any area in the head and neck, although its color match with facial skin is poor.

The main advantage of the trapezius myocutaneous flaps are their lesser bulk, particularly in comparison to the pectoralis major myocutaneous flap, when bulk is not required. The secondary donor scar may be preferable to some women as well. The flaps are generally hairless and are locally available outside the field of irradiation.

The main disadvantage is in the case of the lower trapezius flap, which requires reposition-

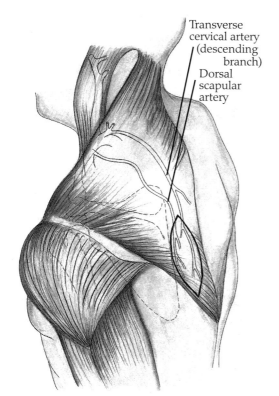

FIGURE 87-5 A lower trapezius myocutaneous flap.

The latissimus dorsi is a flat, triangular muscle that originates from the lower six thoracic, lumbar, and sacral vertebrae and the posterior iliac crest (Fig. 87–6). Its fibers converge to form a flat tendon that inserts into the intertubercular groove of the humerus. Its function is to extend, medially rotate, and adduct the arm. Innervation is provided by the thoracodorsal nerve, a branch of the posterior cord of the brachial plexus.

The subscapular artery is the largest branch off of the third portion of the axillary artery. It quickly divides into the circumflex scapular, which courses posteriorly around the scapula, and the thoracodorsal artery. The latter vessel descends deep to the latissimus dorsi to enter the undersurface of that muscle 8 to 12 cm proximal to the muscle's tendinous insertion into the humerus. Along with the thoracodorsal vein and nerve, it forms the dominant neurovascular pedicle to the latissimus dorsi muscle.

Once entering the muscle, the thoracodorsal artery bifurcates, with an upper branch coursing transversely across the muscle and a lower branch descending toward the iliac crest.

ing of the patient. In addition, the transverse cervical vessels may be variably placed and may be deep to vital structures such as the brachial plexus, which would severely limit the arc of rotation. It may also be difficult to preserve these vessels during a neck dissection, and a history of previous head and neck surgery may require a preliminary angiogram. Certainly metastatic disease in the posterior triangle would limit the feasibility of using the lateral island or lower trapezius flaps.

LATISSIMUS DORSI MYOCUTANEOUS FLAP

The latissimus dorsi is perhaps the oldest of the myocutaneous flaps, having been described for breast reconstruction around the turn of the century. Quillen, in 1978, first described its use in head and neck reconstruction.

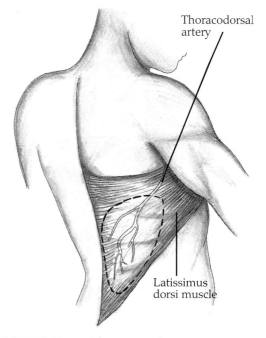

FIGURE 87-6 A latissimus dorsi myocutaneous flap.

This design makes it possible to split the muscle and the overlying skin paddle into two separate units.

Use of this flap requires that the patient be placed in the lateral decubitus position with the ipsilateral arm draped in a sterile stockinette across the shoulder. Care must be taken to properly cushion the axilla to avoid excessive traction and subsequent injury to the brachial plexus.

A skin island corresponding in size to the defect is then designed, lying within the boundaries of the latissimus dorsi muscle, usually over the sixth to tenth ribs. For superior defects, the cutaneous paddle may be extended 2 to 4 cm beyond the iliac crest, recognizing that the density of perforators to the skin and therefore its reliability decreases as one moves inferiorly.

SPECIAL CONSIDERATION

The potential donor area for this flap is the largest of any flap used in head and neck reconstruction and may reach 40×25 cm^2 in size.

The donor site may occasionally be closed primarily but usually will require skin grafting.

During flap elevation the tendinous humeral attachment of the latissimus is cut so that the skin muscle flap becomes tethered only by the vascular pedicle, which should be freed up to the axilla. The flap is transferred into the neck through a tunnel created either subcutaneously above the pectoralis major muscle or between the pectoralis major and minor muscles.

The main advantage of the latissimus dorsi flap is the large surface area of skin it can provide, which generally has been free of radiation exposure. The intramuscular vascular anatomy is such that the flap can be readily folded or even split for internal and external closure. The wide arc of rotation allows coverage of almost any site in the head and neck. Donor-site morbidity, both aesthetic and functional, is minimal. There is no alteration in breast position, and the scar is unobtrusive. Although shoulder function is certainly affected, other muscles of the shoulder girdle help to compensate.

PEARL••• When a radical neck dissection has been performed and the spinal accessory nerve sacrificed, use of an ipsilateral latissimus dorsi flap should probably be avoided due to the resulting compromise of shoulder function.

The primary disadvantage in using this flap is the need to reposition the patient, which adds both time and expense to the procedure. There is also a risk of injury to the brachial plexus. For these reasons, this flap is generally reserved for those situations when more local, simpler flaps are unavailable or have failed or when the substantial amount of tissue it offers is required.

STERNOCLEIDOMASTOID MYOCUTANEOUS FLAP

Being a round muscle, there is no axial distribution of vessels along the undersurface of the sternocleidomastoid as is seen with the flat muscle group. A muscular branch from the occipital artery enters the superior portion of the muscle, whereas a branch from the thyrocervical trunk enters the inferior portion (Fig. 87–7). The midportion is supplied by one or more small branches of the superior thyroid, the inferior thyroid, or directly from the carotid artery. Ariyan (1979) demonstrated that the muscle can be safely rotated on any one or more of these vascular pedicles. In practice, this means a myocutaneous flap can be designed such that it is based superiorly or inferiorly, with a paddle of skin pedicled on the length of the muscle.

The sternocleidomastoid arises from the medial third of the clavicle and manubrium of the sternum. It inserts by an aponeurosis onto the lateral occipital and mastoid bones, as well as interdigitating with the dermal and subdermal tissues around the mastoid tip. It receives its innervation from the spinal accessory nerve.

Depending on the location of the defect, the flap may be based superiorly or inferiorly, and the skin paddle outlined over either the mastoid tip area or the supraclavicular area. The muscle is mobilized from beneath the skin pad-

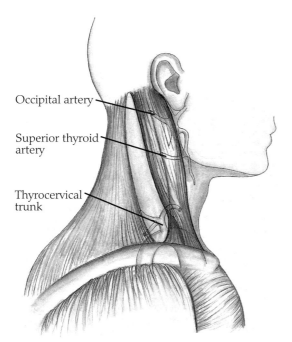

Occipital artery

Superior thyroid artery

Thyrocervical trunk

FIGURE 87–7 A sternocleidomastoid myocutaneous flap.

dle, and the opposite vascular bundle as well as the midportion vascular supply are preserved. The maximum safe diameter for the skin paddle has been reported to be 6 cm.

The sternocleidomastoid myocutaneous flap is used primarily to reconstruct moderate intraoral defects, whether from trauma or following tumor resections. It is best tunneled beneath the mandible and can extend from the anterior floor of the mouth to the pharynx. The donor site can usually be closed primarily, if not by simple advancement, then by a variety of simple transposition flaps.

There does not seem to be any significant difference in reliability with an inferiorly based as opposed to a superiorly based flap. Previous radiation therapy does not seem to adversely affect the flap provided there is no significant induration or edema of the skin paddle. On the other hand, an unusually high incidence of necrosis of the skin paddle has been reported, especially when compared to other myocutaneous flaps, indicating that it is less reliable. In most cases the muscle remains viable and will allow for remucosalization.

The primary advantage of this flap is that it does allow for single-stage reconstruction of moderate oropharyngeal defects by employing local tissues, regardless of previous exposure to radiation. Donor-site morbidity, both functional and cosmetic, is minimal.

> **PITFALLS...** This flap's main disadvantage, when compared to other myocutaneous flaps, is its unreliability due to its random pattern blood supply. The high incidence of skin slough and necrosis prevents its utilization as a flap of first choice.

Oncologically, this flap is acceptable in properly selected patients, when a modified neck dissection is being considered.

PLATYSMA MYOCUTANEOUS FLAP

The platysma muscle is a broad, thin, quadrangular muscle that originates from the clavicle and extends obliquely across the mandibular border to insert into the chin, corner of the mouth, and lower part of the cheek. Its fibers interdigitate with the muscles of the lower lip and with its opposite across the chin, but is deficient in the midline of the neck. It is intervated by the cervical branch of the facial nerve and, when contracted, pulls the corner of the mouth downward to create an expression of sadness, fright, or other unpleasantries.

The platysma gets its blood supply from essentially two sources, one being superiorly and the other inferiorly (Fig. 87–8). The submental branch of the facial artery is the largest cervical branch of the facial and seems to be the dominant source. The flap is more conveniently based superiorly for head and neck reconstruction, so this is the most frequently utilized pedicle. The superficial branch of the transverse cervical artery seems to supply the lower portion of the muscle.

Technically, the first step is to design the skin island. This may be placed virtually anywhere over the muscle but should be provided with a long enough pedicle to reach the defect. In the superiorly based flap, the pivot point will

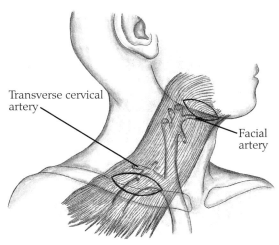

Transverse cervical
artery

Facial
artery

FIGURE 87–8 A platysma myocutaneous flap.

be the mandible. In males, the lower non–hair-bearing cervical skin in the supraclavicular area will generally be preferred for intraoral reconstruction.

> **PEARL...** The patient can be asked to grimace preoperatively to allow outlining of the muscle.

The platysma myocutaneous flap has been largely utilized to provide intraoral lining in the buccal and mandibular alveolar ridge area. Its pliability and thinness make it particularly well suited for these areas. It can be used to replace skin, with reasonable color match and mucosa. It cannot be used for very extensive defects, but it has been used following floor of mouth, tongue, and oropharyngeal resections.

The advantages of this flap are its proximity and thinness. Its thinness allows reasonable contour and closely approximates the thickness of oral mucosa and underlying soft tissue. Again, the skin provides a good color match, and the donor site is usually closed primarily with little cosmetic deformity.

The flap's biggest drawback is its relatively tenuous blood supply. Conley et al (1986) emphasized the importance of incorporating the facial artery in this flap, noting that when it is ligated, all or part of the flap will be lost in 40% of the cases. Still, this is not an axial blood supply, and the muscular base will need to be left broad to en-

sure survival. Previous irradiation seems to be a relative contraindication due to secondary skin changes and postradiation arteritis with compromise of the vascular supply. A previous neck dissection also contraindicates the use of this flap because of secondary scarring and fibrosis and usual ligation of the facial artery. Certainly if significant bulk is required, this flap is not appropriate. Of the myocutaneous flaps described, the platysma is probably the least utilized, but it still may be very useful in specific situations.

SUGGESTED READINGS

Ariyan S, Krizek TJ. Reconstruction after resection of head and neck cancer. Cine clinics. Dallas: Clinical Congress of the American College of Surgeons, October, 1977.

Ariyan S. One-stage reconstruction for defects of the mouth using a sternocleidomastoid myocutaneous flap. *Plast Reconstr Surg* 1979; 63:618–625.

Ariyan S, Cuono CB. Myocutaneous flaps for head and neck reconstruction. *Head Neck Surg* 1980;2:321–345.

Bakamjian V, Littlewood M. Cervical skin flaps for intraoral and pharyngeal repair following cancer surgery. *Br J Plast Surg* 1964;17:191–210.

Conley JJ, Lanier DM, Tinsley P. Platysma myocutaneous flap revisited. *Arch Otolaryngol* 1986;112:711–713.

Freeman JL, Walker EP, Wilson JSP, et al. The vascular anatomy of the pectoralis major myocutaneous flap. *Br J Plast Surg* 1981;34:3–10.

McGraw JB, Dibbell DG. Experimental definition of independent myocutaneous vascular territories. *Plast Reconstr Surg* 1977;60:212–220.

McGraw JB, Dibbell DG, Carraway JH. Clinical definition of independent myocutaneous vascular territories. *Plast Reconstr Surg* 1977; 60:341–352.

Moloy PJ, Gonzales FE. Vascular anatomy of the pectoralis major myocutaneous flap. *Arch Otolaryngol* 1986;112:66–69.

Price JC, Davis RK. The deltopectoral flap vs. the pectoralis major myocutaneous flap. *Arch Otolaryngol* 1984;110:1035–1040.

Quillen CG, Shearing JG, Georgiade NG: Use of the latissimus dorsi myocutaneous island flap for reconstruction in the head and neck area. *Plast Reconstr Surg* 1978;62:113–117.

Sasaki CT, Gardiner LJ, Carlson RD, et al. The extended pectoralis major flap in head and neck reconstruction. *Otolaryngol Head Neck Surg* 1986;94:274–278.

Schuller DE. Limitations of the pectoralis major myocutaneous flap in head and neck cancer reconstruction. *Arch Otolaryngol* 1980;106: 709–714.

Seiden AM. Flap reconstruction in head and neck surgery. In: Lee KJ, ed. *Textbook of Otolaryngology and Head and Neck Surgery.* Elsevier; New York: 1989:861–888.

Shindo ML, Sullivan MJ. Muscular and myocutaneous pedicled flaps. *Otolaryngol Clin North Am* 1994;27:161–172.

Surkin MI, Lawson W, Biller HF. Analysis of the methods of pharyngoesophageal reconstruction. *Head Neck Surg* 1984;6:953–970.

Chapter 88

MICROVASCULAR FREE FLAPS

Allen M. Seiden

Through the 1970s and 1980s soft tissue defects in the head and neck were reconstructed largely with local and regional pedicled flaps. These flaps dramatically enhanced our ability to handle these complex reconstructive problems. However, several limitations remained, including a frequently limited arc of rotation, bulky skin paddles, and donor-site morbidity. Microvascular free flaps offered a way to circumvent these problems. The fixed pivot point is eliminated, and the donor flap can be more appropriately customized to fit the defect. The donor site is generally distant, concealed, and usually associated with less morbidity.

Although the first microvascular free flap in the head and neck region was described in 1976, the technique was slow to catch on. First, not many such flaps were available at the time, and most had relatively small vascular pedicles. Second, microsurgical expertise was required and reliability was less predictable as compared to regional flaps. Cost and surgical time were also greatly increased.

Interest in this technique was renewed in the 1980s as new flaps were introduced and experience increased, with success rates increasing steadily over the last 15 years. Utility was increased by incorporating skin, muscle, bone, or a combination of these tissues. A recently published multicenter, prospective survey examined factors affecting outcome, looking at a variety of free flaps not limited to reconstruction in the head and neck. A total of 493 microvascular free flaps were reported, with a failure rate of 4.1%. Use of a muscle flap covered by a skin graft had a higher failure rate as compared to myocutaneous free flaps. This is believed to relate to the difficulty in recognizing thrombosis of a muscle flap and the subsequent need for early intervention, whereas a skin paddle generally displays early indications of venous congestion or arterial insufficiency.

CONTROVERSY

This survey found a higher failure rate occurred when the recipient bed had been previously irradiated. Other studies have failed to demonstrate a similarly negative effect. Nevertheless, caution should be exercised in these cases.

In the aforementioned study, postoperative thrombosis was more common when vein grafts were used and when the flap was used to repair an existing wound rather than a primary defect. The overall rate of return to the operating room for thrombosis was 9.9%, with a salvage rate of 69%, suggesting that early reexploration is indicated in such cases. Surprisingly, a number of factors were found not to significantly affect the outcome of the flap, including the patient's age, a history of smoking, diabetes, or whether the arterial anastomosis was performed with an end-to-end or end-to-side technique.

SPECIAL CONSIDERATION

Despite a variety of antithrombotic regimens that were reported, only subcutaneous heparin given postoperatively significantly lowered the postoperative incidence of thrombosis.

A variety of free flaps are favored for head and neck reconstruction and can be classified based on the tissues they incorporate or the nature of their blood supply. For defects that require only skin, cutaneous free flaps avoid the need to sacrifice muscle at the donor site, which would be necessary in a pedicled myocutaneous flap. This provides a more pliable, thinner flap and decreases donor-site morbidity. Cutaneous free flaps commonly used include the radial forearm, lateral arm, lateral thigh, parascapular, and scapular flaps. When more soft tissue bulk is required, the rectus abdominis and latissimus dorsi flaps are the most commonly used myocutaneous free flaps.

RADIAL FOREARM FLAP (FIG. 88–1)

Advantages

This flap is very reliable and not technically difficult to harvest. It has a long vascular pedicle that makes it useful, for example, if contralateral neck vessels must be utilized. The tissue provided is thin and pliable, making it ideal for those defects that do not require very much bulk, such as the floor of the mouth. Bone may be incorporated when necessary.

Disadvantages

The major disadvantage of this flap involves potential complications to the donor site. The hand

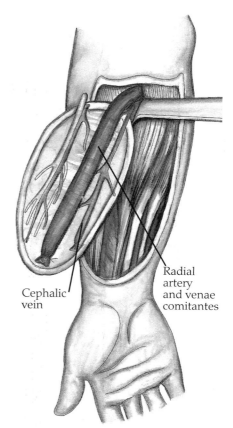

FIGURE 88–1 The radial forearm flap.

may become ischemic, which may be avoided by preoperative use of the Allen test to assess adequate perfusion based on the ulnar artery.

PEARL... In the Allen test, the radial and ulnar arteries are digitally occluded at the wrist while the patient opens and closes the hand, which then becomes pale within 20 seconds. The patient is asked to relax, and pressure is released from the ulnar artery. Capillary blush should appear within the thumb and index finger within 5 seconds. The flap should not be used if refill takes longer than 10 seconds.

Tendon exposure may occur, which may be avoided by not using the most distal third of the forearm skin, meticulous skin grafting, and postoperative immobilization of the arm. Some object to the postoperative cosmetic appearance

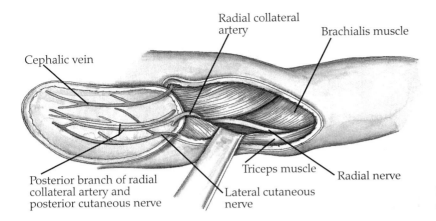

Cephalic vein

Radial collateral artery

Brachialis muscle

Posterior branch of radial collateral artery and posterior cutaneous nerve

Lateral cutaneous nerve

Triceps muscle

Radial nerve

FIGURE 88–2 The lateral arm flap.

of the donor site as well. The nondominant arm should be utilized.

LATERAL ARM FLAP (FIG. 88–2)

Advantages

This flap is relatively thin and pliable and can be effectively used for small to medium-sized defects that do not require much bulk, although it provides more bulk than the radial forearm flap and has been described for repair of the base of tongue. It has a long vascular pedicle, and the skin paddle is usually devoid of hair. The donor site can be closed primarily and is therefore cosmetically more acceptable. Sensation can be restored by incorporating the lateral cutaneous nerve of the arm. Morbidity is typically limited to anesthesia along the posterolateral aspect of the forearm.

Disadvantages

The donor vessels tend to be of small caliber. The flap is technically more difficult than the radial forearm flap and takes longer to raise.

LATERAL THIGH FLAP (FIG. 88–3)

Advantages

The distant location of the donor site allows this flap to be raised during tumor resection. It is a moderately thick flap that is useful for large defects that require some bulk. The donor site can be closed primarily and has very little morbidity.

Disadvantages

In obese individuals this flap may be too thick to provide a good functional result.

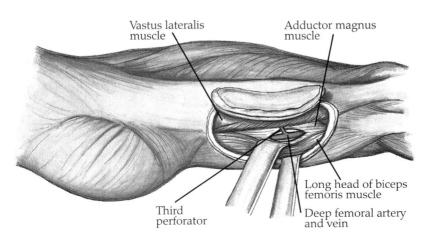

Vastus lateralis muscle

Adductor magnus muscle

Third perforator

Long head of biceps femoris muscle

Deep femoral artery and vein

FIGURE 88–3 The lateral thigh flap.

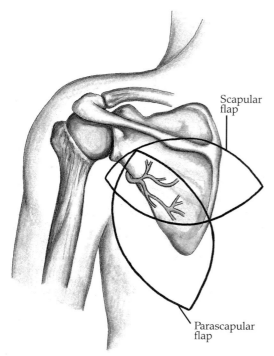

FIGURE 88–4 Scapular and parascapular flaps.

SCAPULAR AND PARASCAPULAR FLAPS (FIG. 88–4)

Advantages

The circumflex scapular artery is a terminal branch of the subscapular artery that in turn arises from the third portion of the axillary artery. The circumflex scapular artery divides into the cutaneous scapular artery and the cutaneous parascapular artery, each of which gives off small perforators to supply the overlying skin. This allows the development of two adjacent skin paddles based on the same vascular pedicle, which may be an advantage when the defect requires coverage of two surfaces. Thickness of the flap depends on the thickness of the back skin and subcutaneous tissue, but it tends to be rather bulky and is best for larger defects.

Disadvantages

The patient generally needs to be repositioned for harvesting of the flap. The tissue provided may be too bulky for some defects.

INFERIOR RECTUS ABDOMINIS MYOCUTANEOUS FLAP (FIG. 88–5)

Advantages

Based on the deep epigastric artery and vein, this flap is extremely reliable and versatile. Skin paddles may be designed in various patterns and orientations in order to better fit the defect. The flap may be harvested during tumor resection by a second team. A large volume of tissue is provided that has generally been used to re-

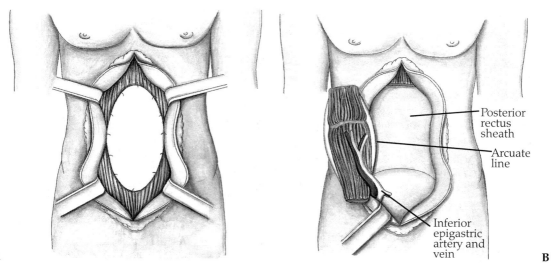

FIGURE 88–5 Dissection of the inferior rectus myocutaneous flap. (A) Exposure of the inferior rectus with preservation of a skin paddle. (B) Elevation of the myocutaneous flap with identification of the vascular pedicle.

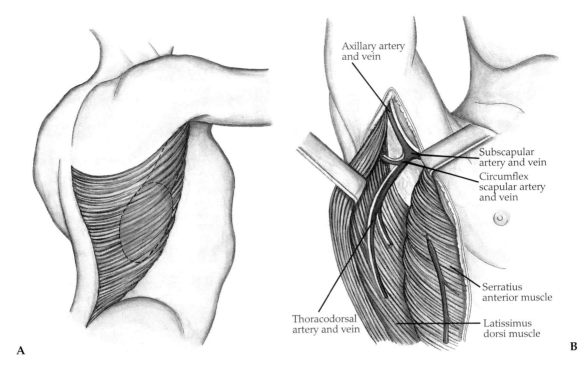

A

B

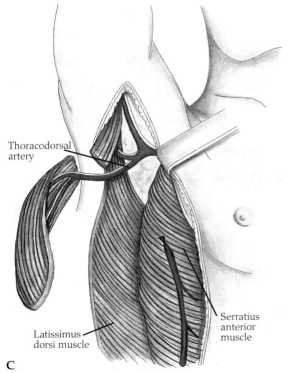

C

FIGURE 88–6 The latissimus dorsi myocutaneous flap. (A). Flap design. (B). Initial flap dissection anteriorly and exposure of the thoracodorsal artery. (C). The flap is elevated and ready for transfer.

construct very large head and neck defects such as following total glossectomy and extensive skull base resections. In the latter instance it has been particularly useful in preventing postoperative cerebrospinal fluid leaks.

Disadvantages

This flap cannot be used in patients who have had previous abdominal, pelvic, or inguinal hernia surgery. The flap may be particularly bulky in obese individuals. The donor site may potentially develop a ventral hernia.

Latissimus Dorsi Myocutaneous Flap (Fig. 88–6)

Advantages

This is a reliable flap that provides a large amount of soft tissue. The broad, thin muscle provides a large surface area that allows effective closure of extensive scalp, orbitomaxillary, and skull base defects. The vascular pedicle is long and the vessels of large caliber. Bone may be incorporated when required.

Disadvantages

The patient needs to be repositioned for harvesting of the flap. Arm and shoulder weakness may result but is generally minimal. Nevertheless, this flap should be avoided when the ipsilateral spinal accessory nerve has been sacrificed in a prior neck dissection.

Perhaps the most challenging defects facing the reconstructive surgeon are those following resection of the anterior mandible and following a laryngopharyngoesophagectomy. Nowhere else are proper form and function so difficult to achieve, and it is these two areas that have largely fueled the increased enthusiasm for free flaps in head and neck reconstruction.

Oromandibular Reconstruction

The ideal reconstructive technique should restore preoperative appearance as well as oral compe-

tence, the ability to chew, swallow, speak, and allow for dental rehabilitation. Over the years, a variety of approaches have been described.

Osteomyocutaneous flaps are rarely used for this purpose today, as proficiency with free flaps has increased. Those most frequently used were the pectoralis osteomyocutaneous flap with rib graft, the trapezius osteomyocutaneous flap with rib graft, the sternocleidomastoid osteomyocutaneous flap with clavicle, and the latissimus osteomyocutaneous flap with scapula. The bone transferred with these flaps generally had a random blood supply and was therefore unreliable, leading to low success rates. The arc of rotation and pedicle length also presented technical problems.

Reconstruction plates are another option for oromandibular repair, generally considered when patients are poor candidates for a free flap, such as when the disease is extremely advanced or there are contrary coexistent medical conditions. Plates have the advantages of no donor-site morbidity and require less time and expense than free flaps. However, they frequently fail due to fistula, plate exposure, or loosening and fracture of the plate. Although adequate contour may be achieved, acceptable function has been more elusive. Plates are more often utilized for lateral mandibular defects, but must be provided with adequate soft tissue coverage.

The first composite free flap for oromandibular reconstruction was described in 1970. However, there was concern about the viability and stability of the bone graft, particularly in view of the typically contaminated field and the need for adjunctive radiation therapy.

Fluorochrome marker studies have shown that vascularized bone grafts maintain their regenerative capacity, whereas nonvascularized bone grafts do not. This capacity has correlated with more predictable healing, callus formation, and solid union at 7 weeks. The graft's independent blood supply appears to promote healing regardless of whether the recipient bed has been previously irradiated or there is oral contamination.

Success rates with nonvascularized bone grafts or pedicled osteomyocutaneous flaps ranged from 40 to 70%. This rate improved to 80 to 90% when reconstruction was delayed. However, secondary reconstruction is ham-

---

pered by fibrosis and contracture, and this leads to poor functional results. Primary reconstruction can be completed with free vascularized bone grafts, and comparable technical results can be achieved with the potential for excellent functional rehabilitation. Urken (1991) reviewed 322 cases reported in the literature from 1986 to 1990 and found a 96% success rate in terms of graft survival. This success has enabled the placement of endosteal dental implants that facilitate denture fittings, improve cosmesis, and restore the potential to maintain a normal diet.

The most commonly used sites for vascularized bone grafts that are appropriate for mandibular reconstruction include the iliac crest, the scapula, and the fibula. Factors that determine donor-site selection derive from an assessment of the defect requirements and the potential for donor-site morbidity in each patient. The donor site should offer bone that has a contour similar to the mandible but that can be shaped without compromise to its vascularity. In addition, it should be substantial enough to allow the placement of dental implants. The soft tissue component should be thin and pliable. Unfortunately, the transplanted skin generally remains insensate, and this greatly inhibits masticatory function and swallowing. Work continues to provide more adaptive sensory reinnervation to such flaps. In addition, interposition nerve grafts to the inferior alveolar

nerve have been described to reestablish sensation to the lower lip.

PHARYNGOESOPHAGEAL RECONSTRUCTION

The goal of pharyngoesophageal reconstruction is to restore a conduit from the oral cavity to the esophagus or stomach that allows for trouble-free swallowing and vocal rehabilitation. This is particularly problematic when the defect is circumferential. For partial defects, there are many more options, including pedicled cutaneous and myocutaneous flaps. However, these tend to be too bulky to tube for circumferential defects.

It is of historical interest that one of the first methods for pharyngoesophageal reconstruction utilizing laterally based cervical skin flaps was popularized by Wookey in 1942. Although limited success was reported, a requisite three or more procedures, prolonged hospitalization, and a postoperative complication rate of 94% have left little role for this approach today.

GASTRIC PULL-UP

When there is significant extension of tumor into the cervical esophagus, skip lesions may be present, and an oncologic resection must include a total esophagectomy. In these cases, a microvascular free flap is not an option, and a gastric pull-up becomes the technique of choice. The stomach and duodenum are mobilized and a primary anastomosis is performed in the neck.

The advantages of this technique are that there is but one suture line and that it occurs high in the neck at the base of the tongue where stenosis is unlikely. Speech is possible through a tracheogastric puncture. The primary disadvantage is the potential for thoracic and abdominal complications, occurring in as many as 50% of patients. The incidence of necrosis is 3%, with a mortality of 10 to 15%. Regurgitation of gastric contents as well as dumping syndrome are common. Unless an esophagectomy needs to be performed, the significant morbidity and mortality associated with this procedure preclude its use.

FREE JEJUNAL FLAP

This flap incorporates a segment of the second loop of jejunum, which closely approximates the diameter of the pharynx and is mucosally lined. Once revascularized it is a very reliable flap and offers much less donor-site morbidity than a gastric pull-up, without the need to violate the thoracic cavity. It has been suggested that the inherent peristaltic capability of the jejunum would be of benefit, but this has not been clearly demonstrated. It has also been suggested that mucus production by the jejunal segment would be helpful, but it can be excessive and problematic.

This flap can be irradiated postoperatively without untoward effect. Speech is possible through a puncture, although limited by excess mucus and the folds of mucosa. Stricture at the distal anastomosis may occur, as may intraabdominal adhesions.

This flap is the choice of many reconstructive surgeons when confronted by a circumferential pharyngoesophageal defect. It is the method of choice in an obese patient in whom cutaneous free flaps would be less effective.

Several sites within the colon are also available for free bowel transfer. The sigmoid colon has been most often utilized, but in comparison to jejunum it has a number of distinct disadvantages. The diameter is not a good match for the esophageal anastomosis, and the blood supply is not as reliable. Although long segments of jejunum may be harvested without a deleterious effect upon the digestive system, this is not the case with colon. Finally, colonic transfer carries a much higher risk of postoperative complications.

CUTANEOUS FREE FLAPS

Another option for closing a circumferential defect is to use one of the cutaneous free flaps described above. In the nonobese patient these flaps are thin and pliable and can be effectively tubed to fit the defect. This approach is becoming increasingly popular because a laparotomy is avoided. Although theoretically the peristaltic capability of jejunum may be an advantage, in reality this has not been observed. The success

and stricture rate with cutaneous flaps seems to be comparable to that of jejunal grafts, but further experience is needed. The two favored flaps are the lateral thigh flap and the radial forearm flap.

SUGGESTED READINGS

Burkey BB. The evolving role of sensate flaps in head and neck reconstruction. *Curr Opin Otolaryngol Head Neck Surg* 1996;4:259–261.

Burkey BB, Coleman JR. Current concepts in oromandibular reconstruction. *Otolaryngol Clin North Am* 1997;30:607–630.

Civantos FJ, Burkey B, Lu FL, et al. Lateral arm microvascular flap in head and neck reconstruction. *Arch Otolaryngol Head Neck Surg* 1997;123:830–836.

Evans GRD, Schusterman MA, Kroll SS, et al. The radial forearm free flap for head and neck reconstruction: a review. *Am J Surg* 1994;168: 446–450.

Haller JR. Concepts in pharyngoesophageal reconstruction. *Otolaryngol Clin North Am* 1997; 30:655–661.

Kelly KE, Anthony JP, Singer M. Pharyngoesophageal reconstruction using the radial forearm fasciocutaneous free flap: preliminary results. *Otolaryngol Head Neck Surg* 1994;111:16–24.

Khouri RK, Cooley BC, Kunselman AR, et al. A prospective study of microvascular free-flap surgery and outcome. *Plast Reconstr Surg* 1998; 102:711–721.

Markowitz BL, Calcaterra TC. Preoperative assessment and surgical planning for patients undergoing immediate composite reconstruction of oromandibular defects. *Clin Plast Surg* 1994;21:9–14.

Panje WR, Moran WJ. *Free Flap Reconstruction of the Head and Neck.* New York: Thieme; 1989.

Shindo ML, Sullivan MJ. Soft-tissue microvascular free flaps. *Otolaryngol Clin North Am* 1994;27:173–194.

Stepnick DW, Hayden RE. Options for reconstruction of the pharyngoesophageal defect.

Otolaryngol Clin North Am 1994;27:1151–1158.

Urken ML. Composite free flaps in oromandibular reconstruction. *Arch Otolaryngol Head Neck Surg* 1991;117:724–732.

Urken ML, Buchbinder D, Constantino PD, et al. Oromandibular reconstruction using microvascular composite flaps: report of 210 cases. *Arch Otolaryngol Head Neck Surg* 1998; 124:46–55.

Urken ML, Buchbinder D, Weinberg H, et al. Functional evaluation following microvascular oromandibular reconstruction of the oral cancer patient: a comparative study of reconstructed and nonreconstructed patients. *Laryngoscope* 1991;101:935–950.

Wookey, II. The surgical treatment of carcinoma of the pharynx and upper esophagus. *Surg Gynec Obstet* 1942;75:499.

SECTION XV

AESTHETIC SURGERY OF THE FACE

Chapter 89

Aesthetic Surgery of the Face

Kevin A. Shumrick

The human desire to project a normal or even attractive appearance is far older than the specialty of facial plastic surgery. An appearance that projects youth and vigor not only enhances one's chances of being accepted, but also raises the individual's status within the group. Contrasted with this desire to appear normal or attractive is an underlying current of conservatism, left over from a more repressive era that had frowned on aesthetic surgery, considering it a sign of vanity. Within the last 20 years, the stigma associated with aesthetic surgery of the face has significantly diminished and individuals are seeking elective facial surgery at increasing rates. With these increasing numbers of individuals seeking facial surgery comes the inevitable increase in individuals seeking surgery for primarily psychological issues.

SPECIAL CONSIDERATION

It is incumbent on the surgeon to try to screen surgical candidates who are unlikely to be satisfied with the surgery regardless of the result.

Some patient traits that should raise red flags when considering an individual for cosmetic surgery are the following:

Exaggerated or unrealistic expectations

Excessive demands

Excessive indecision

Immaturity

An inflated sense of self-importance

Secretiveness

The wish to have surgery to make someone else happy

The expectation that surgery will enhance the person's career or social life

An additional warning sign is that the patient has had multiple previous procedures.

Experienced surgeons develop a sense of which patients will respond well to an appropriate surgical procedure and which patients will never be satisfied regardless of the outcome. In the meantime, it is wise to avoid the patient types mentioned above.

RHINOPLASTY

When questioned with regard to what they feel is the most demanding procedure in facial plastic surgery, most surgeons routinely respond that rhinoplasty poses their biggest challenge. The reason lies with the complex anatomy of the nose, with interfaces between cartilage and bone, the influence of the septum, and the wide variations of the enveloping skin. Add to these challenges the fact that many of the changes made to the nasal skeleton must be made while performing surgical maneuvers under the overlying nasal skin, and it is apparent that considerable experience and judgment are required to achieve consistently good results.

ANATOMY

The external nose is a topographically complex structure with a pyramidal form (Fig. 89–1). Its apex projects anteriorly and the base is attached to the facial skeleton. The external nasal pyramid is composed of three distinct, interrelated triangular structures: the bony pyramid, the cartilaginous vault, and the lower lateral cartilages.

The bony pyramid is made up of the paired nasal bones and the ascending process of the maxilla upon which they rest. The nasal bones fuse in the midline with a distinct suture. They attach to the frontal bone superiorly and the upper-lateral cartilages inferiorly.

The cartilaginous vault consists of the upper lateral cartilages, which, although spoken of separately, are actually a single structure fused with the underlying septum. Laterally, the cartilages approximate the piriform aperture, and superiorly they attach to the undersurface of the nasal bones.

The lower lateral cartilages are paired, free-floating structures that support the lower third of the nose. They come into close proximity to the upper lateral cartilages via a scroll arrangement, which provides support to the lower lateral cartilages, yet allows them to move independently. The lower lateral cartilages have three distinct portions: the lateral crus, the middle crus, and the medial crus.

SPECIAL CONSIDERATION

The point at which the lateral crus turns inferiorly is termed the dome, and this dome is usually, but not always, responsible for determining the most anteriorly projecting portion of the nose, also referred to as the nasal tip.

The muscles of the nose are supplied by the seventh nerve and serve to assist in opening and closing the nasal aperture as well as facial expression. The degree of activity of the nasal muscles can vary tremendously from individual to individual, with some people showing active changing of the nasal shape; in others the muscles are virtually dormant. The main nasal muscles are the procerus, nasalis (transverse and alar) levator labii superior isalaeque nasi, depressor septi, and anterior and posterior dilator naris (Fig. 89–2). The procerus elevates the skin over the dorsum of the nose and depresses the medial eyebrow. The nasalis acts to compress the nostril. Dilatation of the nostrils takes place through the action of the dilators and the levator labii superioris alaeque, which is part of the quadratus labii. The depressor septi originate from the nasal spine and insert into the lower portion of the columella. They function to depress the nasal tip and may be quite active, causing significant tip ptosis with smiling.

The arterial supply to the nose is rich and derived from several sources. The angular vessel (the continuation of the facial artery) gives off a lateral nasal artery inferiorly, and superiorly the ophthalamic artery gives off the dorsal nasal artery. There is also a consistent, but unnamed, artery running the length of the columella, which is routinely encountered during open rhinoplasty.

Sensory innervation of the nose is supplied by the first and second divisions of the trigeminal nerve. The skin of the root, bridge, and upper part of the side of the nose is supplied by twigs from the supratrochlear and infratrochlear branches of the ophthalmic division. The skin of the lower lateral nose is supplied by the infraorbital branch of the maxillary division. The skin of the lower dorsum and nasal tip is supplied by the anterior ethmoidal nerve, which emerges between the nasal bone and the upper lateral cartilages.

TERMINOLOGY

Rhinoplasty terminology is extensive, inconsistent, and confusing. The following are the most commonly and consistently used terms. There are several different rhinoplasty terms used to denote direction: *cephalic* means toward the head (superior) and *caudal* means toward the

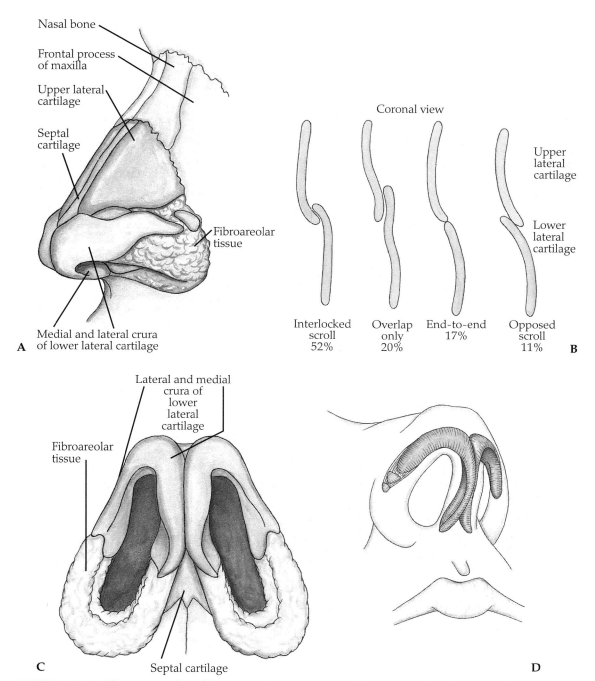

Nasal bone

Frontal process of maxilla

Upper lateral cartilage

Septal cartilage

Fibroareolar tissue

Medial and lateral crura of lower lateral cartilage

A

Coronal view

Upper lateral cartilage

Lower lateral cartilage

Interlocked scroll 52%

Overlap only 20%

End-to-end 17%

Opposed scroll 11%

B

Lateral and medial crura of lower lateral cartilage

Fibroareolar tissue

C

Septal cartilage

D

FIGURE 89–1 The topography of the external nose structure. (A). Bony and cartilaginous framework of the nose. (B). Relationship of upper and lower cartilages. (C,D). Caudal views of lower lateral cartilages.

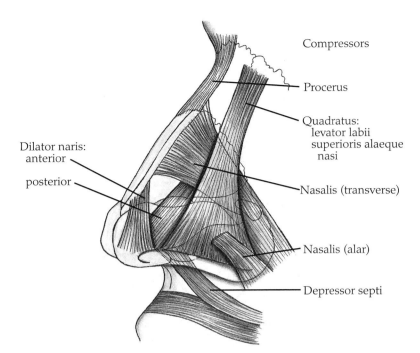

Compressors

Procerus

Quadratus:
  levator labii
  superioris alaeque
  nasi

Dilator naris:
  anterior

  posterior

Nasalis (transverse)

Nasalis (alar)

Depressor septi

FIGURE 89–2 The muscles of the nose.

feet (inferior) (Fig. 89–3A, B). These terms replace the more commonly used anatomic terms *superior* and *inferior*. *Anterior* and *posterior* refer to movement relative to the plane of the nasal dorsum and are frequently replaced with *dorsal* and *ventral*.

The nasion is located at the junction of the nasal and frontal bones at the frontonasal suture, typically the deepest portion of the nasofrontal angle (Fig. 89–3C). The rhinion is the junction of the upper lateral cartilages and the nasal bones in the mid-dorsum. This is the most common site for location of a dorsal hump. The nasal tip is the most anteriorly projecting portion of the lower third of the nose. This typically, though not always, corresponds to the domes of the lower lateral cartilages. The supratip depression is the subtle indentation cephalic to the nasal tip. This often corresponds to the underlying anterior septal angle.

The nasal tip rotation is the movement of the nasal tip along an arc that is a constant distance from the facial plane. Nasal tip projection is a measurement of the distance of the nasal tip from the facial plane. The soft tissue triangle is a triangular portion of skin lying just superior to the superior medial nostril margin. It corresponds to the area of the nostril inferior to the inferior border of the lower lateral cartilage. Its importance lies in the fact that there is no cartilage to support it, and any scarring will result in notching of the nostril margin. The anterior septal angle is the portion of the cartilaginous septum that underlies the supratip depression. It corresponds to the most anterior inferior portion of the septal cartilage.

The nasal lobule is defined as the rounded prominence over the lower anterior portion of the nose. The lobule is made up mostly of the underlying lateral crura and domes of the two tip cartilages. It is bounded superiorly by the supratip depression and laterally by the depression between the tip and ala.

AESTHETICS

Despite the trend toward equality of the sexes, there remain definite facial characteristics that are considered masculine and feminine. This is also true with regard to the nose. The typical male nose is somewhat larger than the female and has thicker skin. The lower nasal skin is more sebaceous, and therefore has more pores and irregular texture. The male dorsum tends to

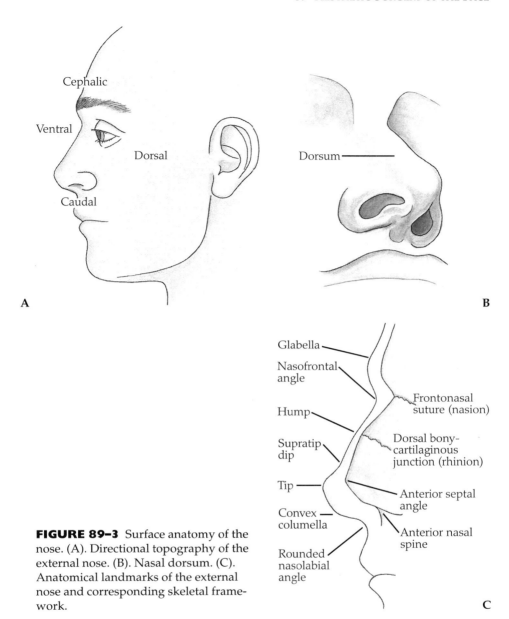

FIGURE 89–3 Surface anatomy of the nose. (A). Directional topography of the external nose. (B). Nasal dorsum. (C). Anatomical landmarks of the external nose and corresponding skeletal framework.

be relatively wider, and a dorsal prominence or even slight hump is felt to add character to a man's face. The nasal lobule, alae, and nares are relatively more prominent but still harmonious with the male face. The male nasal tip typically is not as rotated as the female's, with a rotation of 90 to 105 degrees.

The ideal female nose is relatively smaller than the male nose, with thinner, smoother, less sebaceous skin. The dorsum is narrower, and

a hump is definitely not felt to be aesthetic. A more rotated nasal tip is generally preferred for women with ideal angles between 105 and 120 degrees.

BODY TYPE

Indirectly, body type relates to age and sex characteristics. Three basic body types are recognized: (1) slender and slight of frame (ectomorph); (2) square and athletic (mesomorph); (3) heavy and rounded (endomorph). When considering rhinoplastic changes, the nose must be considered not only as part of the face, but also in relation to the rest of the patient's body. For example, giving a tall person a rotated nasal tip would induce increased exposure of the nostril, and would be undesirable.

RACE

Interracial variation with regard to nasal anatomy is significant and surgical techniques must be adjusted to accommodate these variations. Typically, Asian and African noses lack a strong dorsum and often require augmentation. Mediterranean noses often have poor tip support and require tip augmentation as well as dorsal lowering. Northern European noses frequently have prominent nasal humps that require resection.

> **PITFALL...** Regardless of the nasal anatomy, the surgeon should be conservative with regard to changing an individual's nasal appearance if the results are not in keeping with their ethnic origin. Not infrequently these individuals will regret their decision at a later date when they feel a loss of identity at having changed their appearance.

Of course, these ideals are just that, and are rarely found in nature. They are even more difficult to create surgically. However, they do serve as guidelines to help direct surgical endeavors. In the end it is the patient who must live with the nose, and a detailed consultation is required so that the patient's desires and expectations are fully appreciated.

NASAL APPEARANCE BASED ON VIEWS (FIG. 89–4)

Side View

The commonly accepted ideal nose for Western societies has a dorsal projection of roughly 30 degrees from the facial plane. The nasofrontal angle should be sufficiently distinct to separate the dorsum from the glabella. In men, a suggestion of a dorsal hump at the rhinion is acceptable. A supratip depression (greater in women than men) is desirable. The nasal tip should be the leading or most anterior point of the profile. The tip should also curve into a convex columella. The nasolabial angle should be obtuse and gently curved.

Base View

On the base view the nasal collumellar length should be approximately twice the length of the lobule (Fig. 89–5). The shape of the nasal base

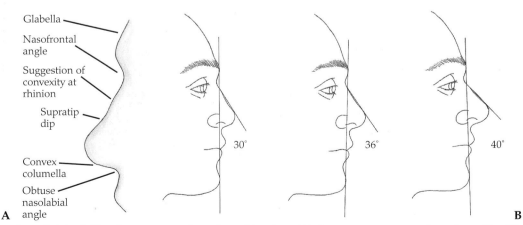

Glabella
Nasofrontal angle
Suggestion of convexity at rhinion
Supratip dip
Convex columella
Obtuse nasolabial angle

30°

36°

40°

A

B

FIGURE 89–4 Nasal appearance based on side view. (A). Important aspects of nasal profile. (B). It is important to consider nasal profile in relation to projection of the forehead and chin.

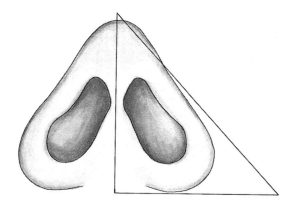

FIGURE 89–5 The base of the nose can roughly be circumscribed by an equilateral triangle.

should approximate an isosceles triangle with the lobule being neither too broad nor too narrow.

Surgical Techniques

Perhaps no other surgical procedure has as many variations and competing techniques as does rhinoplasty. This section outlines the major goals of most rhinoplasties being performed today, recognizing that there are different techniques for achieving each goal. Before discussing specific surgical techniques, it is appropriate to consider the various surgical approaches to the nose. Basically there are two methods of modifying the nasal structures during rhinoplasty—closed and open approaches. Closed rhinoplastic techniques are performed with strictly intranasal incisions, whereas open rhinoplasties are performed with a combination of intranasal incisions and an incision across the columella.

The advantage of the closed approach is the avoidance of a potential external scar. The disadvantage is restricted visualization of nasal structures and the necessity of manipulating structures off the midline (due to the fact that the columella is intact). The open rhinoplasty approach provides unparalleled exposure of the nasal tip and dorsum and the ability to work on nasal structures in their normal midline positions. The disadvantage of an open rhinoplasty approach is the necessity of a columellar scar. It has also been noted that open rhinoplasties typically take longer than closed rhinoplasties,

and nasal tip edema may persist for a longer period of time.

CONTROVERSY

In the 1980s and early 1990s, a debate raged over which approach, open or closed, should be used for rhinoplasty, with adherents in each camp stating that all rhinoplasties should be carried out by only one or the other approach. It is now recognized that each approach has merits and should be tailored to the needs of the patient and the experience and expertise of the surgeon. An open approach is generally recommended for more complex cases as well as for inexperienced surgeons.

Within the realm of rhinoplasty surgery there are two distinct patient groups—primary rhinoplasty and secondary (or posttraumatic) rhinoplasty. For purposes of this discussion we will be covering only the standard techniques for primary rhinoplasty via an open or external approach.

The external rhinoplasty incision is performed by making intranasal incisions along the inferior (caudal) border of the lower lateral cartilage. These incisions are continued on to the columella. At approximately the midpoint of the columella an inverted-V incision is made across the columella, joining the intranasal incisions of both nostrils. The skin of the nose is then lifted off the medial crura of the lower lateral cartilages and dissection continues onto the nasal tip and dorsum. This gives a clear and unobstructed view of the nasal bones, upper lateral cartilages, and lower lateral cartilages.

The next step in most rhinoplasties is to remove the hump, which is typically composed of the osseocartilaginous junction of the nasal bones and upper lateral cartilages. It should be noted that when the dorsal hump has been removed, the configuration of the nasal dorsum is similar to removing the apex of a triangle. The side walls will not be touching and there will be a palpable and visible gap between them. This is referred to as the "open book," and it needs to be closed by lateral osteotomies (which are typically performed as the last step in a rhinoplasty).

The next step in most primary rhinoplasties is to address the nasal tip. The most common perceived aesthetic deficiency of the nasal tip is lack of projection and excessive width. The only way to truly increase nasal tip projection is to increase the distance between the nasal tip and facial plane. This may be done by augmenting the nasal tip with tip grafts. However, the most common method is to create the illusion of increased tip projection by rotating the nasal tip superiorly.

> **PEARL•••** Nasal tip rotation is most commonly accomplished by resecting the cephalic portion of the lateral crus of the lower lateral cartilage, a procedure referred to as a "complete strip"; only the superior portion of the lateral crus is resected, leaving an intact (or complete) strip of cartilage inferiorly.

> **PITFALL•••** It is important to maintain the integrity of the lower lateral crus so that the tip does not collapse or become excessively pinched. Overresection of the lateral crus leads to collapse and tip pinching, both of which will give poor aesthetic results and nasal obstruction.

Generally, it is felt that the amount of minimal lateral crus necessary to maintain tip support is 5 mm in females and 7 mm in males (Fig. 89–6).

> # CONTROVERSY
>
> There are several tip procedures that compromise the integrity of the lateral crus, such as the rim strip, lateral crural flap, and dome division (or Goldman tip). They all have in common that the structural integrity of the inferior portion of the lateral crus is cut or excised. These techniques have generally fallen out of favor with most rhinoplasty surgeons due to the difficulty in predicting outcome and propensity to produce aesthetic and functional difficulties.

The final maneuver for most rhinoplasties is the lateral osteotomies, which are performed to "close the book" left by reduction of the dorsal hump. Remember that the nose has a roughly pyramidal shape and when the superior portion is removed the nasal bones will remain (with the attached upper-lateral cartilages) positioned laterally, resulting in a flat nasal dorsum with the septum in the middle—the so-called open book (Fig. 89–7).

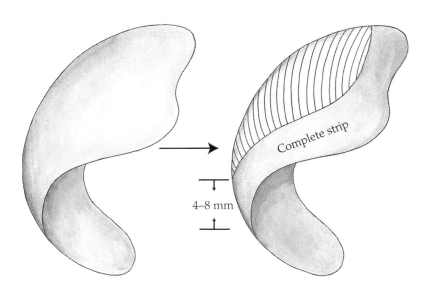

Complete strip

4–8 mm

FIGURE 89–6 Maintenance of a complete strip of cartilage after volume reduction is desirable. At least 4 to 8 mm of uninterrupted latera crus in vertical dimension should be preserved to ensure long-term support and natural contouring.

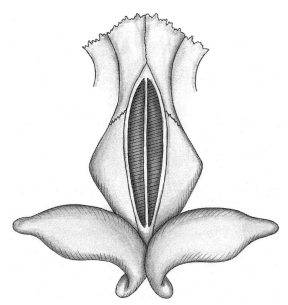

FIGURE 89–7 Removal of a bony hump partially separates the nasal bones from each other and from the nasal septum.

The lateral osteotomies close the book by making incisions along the inferior portion of the ascending process of the maxilla and repositioning it medially, thereby restoring the pyramidal shape of the nose (Fig. 89–8). Note that the osteotomies do not pass through the nasal bones themselves, but more inferiorly through

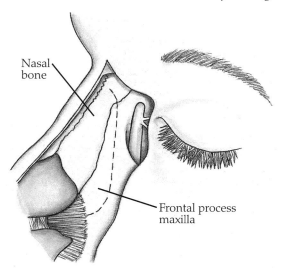

Nasal bone

Frontal process maxilla

FIGURE 89–8 The incision along the frontal process of the maxilla made by a lateral osteotomy.

the ascending process of the maxilla (to which the nasal bones are attached).

> **PITFALL...** If the osteotomies pass through the nasal bones or the suture with the maxilla, the osteotomized segments will lack sufficient length to form a stable side wall and will collapse into the nasal cavity.

The process of performing the lateral osteotomies at the base of the ascending process of the maxilla is referred to as a "low to high osteotomy." This is to distinguish it from special situation osteotomies where the nasal bones themselves are osteotomized.

Patients are counseled that changes following rhinoplasty will continue for at least 6 months, and there will still be subtle changes taking place at 1 year postoperatively. Therefore, any revision procedures should be delayed until at least 6 months postoperatively to avoid the situation in which surgery is being performed on tissues that have not completely recovered from the previous procedure.

FACE-LIFT

Rhytidectomy is the technical term for the facial cosmetic procedure commonly referred to as the face-lift. Although there are a variety of rhytidectomy procedures, they all have in common the goal of reversing the sagging face commonly associated with the aging process. In the past, a rhytidectomy consisted of simple subcutaneous undermining with excision of excess skin. Recent advances in facial plastic surgery enable the surgeon to lift the underlying muscle and fat, reposition these structures, excise excess adipose tissue, and reposition the overlying skin. The combination of these modalities results in a more youthful appearance that reportedly lasts longer than conventional rhytidectomy.

PATIENT SELECTION

Perhaps the single most important element responsible for a successful rhytidectomy is patient selection. Patient selection includes not only anatomic and physiologic considerations, but also the patient's psychological status.

Psychological Considerations

The surgeon must be a good listener and be insightful as to the motivation and expectations of the patient. The surgeon must (1) be able to recognize those patients with overly high expectations who may be completely unsatisfied with an excellent surgical result, and (2) successfully communicate the surgical limitations or tactfully refuse surgery if necessary. A motivated patient with realistic expectations and suitable anatomy can be almost guaranteed a successful rhytidectomy in experienced surgical hands.

Physical Considerations

> **PEARL...** The anatomic features associated with a good patient outcome include good skin elasticity, lack of solar damage, and an attractive angular facial skeleton.

The overlying facial skin should slide over the skeletal features easily. Although chronologic age is an unreliable indicator, most ideal patients are between 45 and 60 years of age. Ideally, the patient's facial features have not been overwhelmed by the aging process and only early changes are apparent and bothersome.

> **SPECIAL CONSIDERATION**
>
> Smoking is well known to contribute to complications from rhytidectomy, including flap necrosis and hematoma. Patients who smoke should be counseled accordingly.

Less than ideal anatomic features include excessive facial adipose tissue, deep nasolabial folds, severe actinic damage, a low hyoid, and poorly developed or asymmetric skeletal features.

Anatomy

The external skin is the most obvious structure affected by aging, but there is also coincident progressive degeneration and stretching of the underlying connective tissue and fascia, which allows drooping of the facial muscles, fat, and salivary glands. Modern face-lift surgery requires a thorough understanding of the anatomy of these structures to properly restore them to their original position and provide adequate support for long-lasting results. Also, a firm understanding of the anatomic course and distribution of the facial nerve and facial vasculature allows for safer and more consistent face-lift surgery.

Muscles of the Face

The muscles of facial expression are paired, originate from major facial bones, act on skin, and are innervated by the seventh cranial nerve.

The facial muscles are generally subdivided into five groups according to their anatomic location: oral (upper and lower), nasal, orbital, auricular, and scalp. The cheek muscles all converge to intermingle with the orbicularis, and this allows coordination of lip and cheek movements.

The facial muscles are unique in the body because their primary site of action is on the skin by way of attachments to the dermis.

> **SPECIAL CONSIDERATION**
>
> The muscles of facial expression are ensheathed by an anterior extension of the superficial musculoaponeurotic system (SMAS), and it is through these attachments to the skin that SMAS suspension places traction on the anterior facial skin.

Fascia of the Face

With aging the supporting fasciae of the face tend to elongate and stretch, resulting in sagging anteriorly and inferiorly. It has long been recognized that simple excision of lax skin gives good

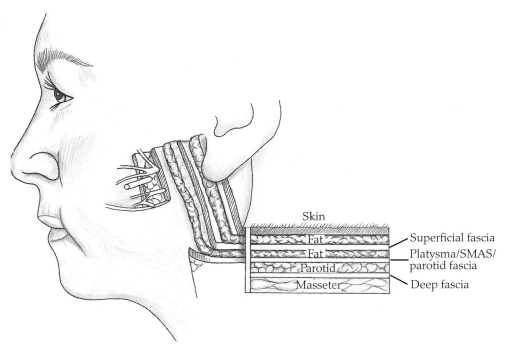

FIGURE 89–9 Diagram of the various layers in the cheek region with relation to the superficial musculoaponeurotic system (SMAS).

short-term results but does not provide long-lasting improvement. To achieve lasting results in face-lift surgery, the surgeon must also reposition and support the underlying muscles, adipose tissue, and salivary glands and secure them in some fashion. To accomplish this, repositioning and suspension of the underlying facial units requires a structure with considerable strength, and this has prompted intense study of the facial and cervical fasciae.

The SMAS layer has been found to meet many of these requirements and is noted to have the following characteristics (Fig. 89–9): (1) It is a distinct fibrous sheath lying deep to the first layer of subcutaneous fat. (2) It is in continuity with the posterior part of the frontalis muscle and superior portion of the platysma. (3) It is densely adherent to, but separate from, the parotid fascia. (4) It extends from the parotid area to encircle the muscles of facial expression, and at the same time it sends attachments to the dermis. These connections with the dermis and muscles of facial expression are the factors that allow suspension of the SMAS to exert a pull on the facial skin in areas well anterior to the cheek. (5) The sensory nerves of the parotid area (great auricular, greater occipital, lesser occipital) lie superficial to the SMAS. (6) The motor fibers of the seventh cranial nerve run deep to the SMAS. (7) The main facial vessels (the facial artery and vein) lie deep to the SMAS and send perforating vessels through the SMAS to reach the subdermal plexus.

Recognition of the SMAS as a distinct anatomic unit was a major advance in face-lift surgery. Previously, face-lift surgery consisted simply of widely undermining the facial skin with posterior, superior traction and then simply excising the excess skin. This technique effected only short-term improvement and was associated with a higher incidence of complications such as hematomas, flap necrosis, and injury to the seventh cranial nerve. Since recognition of the SMAS, it has become possible to literally resuspend the soft tissues of the face and secure them with sutures through the SMAS, providing more secure and long-lasting face lifts.

The Facial Nerve in Face-Lift Surgery

After the SMAS, the structure that most directly affects face-lift surgery is the facial nerve. The facial nerve is a major concern in any type of surgery in this area, and fear for its safety is often a limiting factor in the amount of dissection that may be safely performed. Knowledge of the anatomy of the facial nerve has become particularly important with the more recent innovations in face-lift surgery such as sub-SMAS and subplatysmal flaps, because the plane of dissection is deeper than that utilized in simple skin elevation and there is no doubt that the facial nerve is at increased risk in these types of procedures.

As the facial nerve travels anteriorly, it becomes more superficial owing to the thinning of the parotid. At the anterior portion of the parotid, the facial nerve lies under only a thin sheet of connective tissue corresponding to the SMAS, and is lateral to the masseter muscle and parotid duct.

As the nerve approaches the muscles of facial expression, it enters them from the deep side and then courses through the muscle to provide innervation. The following are pertinent observations with regard to the anatomy of the facial nerve: (1) the main branch of the nerve and most of its anastomoses are contained within the substance of the parotid gland and will not be injured unless the parenchyma of the gland itself is violated; (2) a dissection that stays lateral to the SMAS, muscles of facial expression, or platysma will be superficial to the plane of the facial nerve; and (3) if the parotid fascia is violated or the plane of dissection is deep to the SMAS, platysma, or muscles of facial expression, there is a danger of injury to the facial nerve.

It is extremely rare to encounter an injury to the entire nerve; rather, the most common scenario is to injure a branch or branches. Although injury to the zygomatic and buccal branches of the facial nerve cause the most deleterious effects due to paralysis of the periocular or perioral muscles, this rarely occurs because there are considerable anastomotic connections between branches, and the nerve is usually able to compensate for injuries to distal, small, individual branches.

PITFALL... The temporal and marginal mandibular branches have virtually no interbranch connections, and thus recovery is usually much less complete. In addition, the marginal and temporal branches occupy the most superficial portions of the nerve's course and are at greatest risk of injury.

SURGICAL TECHNIQUES

Considerable dogma and controversy focus on face-lift surgery techniques. The classic rhytidectomy consisting of just a skin flap elevation and skin excision has largely been replaced by skin flap elevation in combination with SMAS techniques. Within the last several years there have been a number of techniques designed to be performed under the SMAS, which have been called deep-plane rhytidectomies and even subperiosteal face-lifts. These techniques are still evolving and represent a greater risk for complications, particularly to the facial nerve. Therefore, this section focuses on the most commonly performed face-lift technique using a skin flap with SMAS plication.

Incisions for Face-Lift

There are many variations in the type of incision used for rhytidectomy, and they differ for male and female patients. In the past, the anterior incision was brought into the temporal region, but this has the disadvantage that with flap rotation and skin excision non–hair-bearing skin is brought into the temple region. For this reason we now place the temple incision just at the inferior border of the sideburn. The incision is then brought inferiorly in the preauricular crease until the tragus is reached, and then curved into the ear canal just behind the tragus. At the inferior border of the tragus it is brought back into the preauricular crease and around the inferior border of the lobule. Posteriorly, the incision runs in the postauricular sulcus until the level of the superior border of the external canal is reached. At this point the incision is brought straight back into the hairline for 6 to 7 cm. An inferior back cut is then made to accommodate redundant tissue. In males the incision is basically the same except that anteriorly the incision is not brought behind the tragus because advancement of facial skin would place hair-bearing skin in the ear.

Skin Flap Elevation

The skin flap is elevated by creating tunnels with blunt scissor dissection and then connecting the tunnels. The flaps are elevated in a subdermal plane with approximately 4 mm of subcutaneous tissue left attached to preserve the subdermal vasculature of the skin flap.

Length of Flap Elevation

The amount of subcutaneous undermining and length of the flap needs to be tailored to the anatomy of each patient. In general, the more skin laxity, platysmal bands, and jowling that is present, the longer the flap required to bring about significant changes. The average flap length is 5 to 7 cm and stops short of the melolabial crease.

SMAS Plication

SMAS plication consists of advancing the SMAS upon itself, without incising it, and then securing it with sutures. Imbrication consists of incising the SMAS and removing a portion and then sewing the two edges together. Because plication does not require dissecting underneath the SMAS or platysma, the chances of injuring a branch of the facial nerve are lower. For this reason SMAS plication is the most commonly performed method of suspending the SMAS.

Skin Excision

Once the SMAS has been plicated, the skin flap can be advanced superiorly and posteriorly and the redundant skin marked and trimmed. The ideal amount of skin tension at closure depends on the patient's tissue, the area of closure, and surgical judgment. As a general rule, most of the tension needed to elevate the face should be

taken up by the SMAS plication, and little, if any, tension is placed along the incision. Particular attention should be given to avoiding tension on portions of the ear that are mobile such as the lobule or tragus.

Complications

Although face-lift surgery is generally a safe and well-tolerated procedure, there are several potential complications that should be kept in mind while performing the surgery. The most common complication is hematoma under the skin flap. Minor hematomas require only suction aspiration and pressure dressing. Major hematomas require reelevation of the flap and evacuation of the clot, usually in the operating room under general anesthesia. Elevated blood pressure; increased intrathoracic pressures from coughing, straining, or vomiting; antiplatelet drugs; and cigarette smoking all may contribute to the formation of hematomas.

> **SPECIAL CONSIDERATION**
>
> Men are believed to have a somewhat higher incidence of hematoma formation than women.

The next most common complication is necrosis of a portion of the skin flaps as a result of compromised skin vascularity. This usually occurs as a result of excess tension on the wound closure. Additional causes of skin necrosis are extensive hematomas, postoperative infection, and cigarette smoking.

Injury to the facial nerve is catastrophic for the patient as well as the surgeon. Although this complication is standardly addressed during the informed consent, the actual incidence of facial nerve injuries is quite low—less than 1%. Causes of facial nerve paralysis are (1) transection of a branch (most commonly temporal or marginal); (2) cautery heat trauma; (3) plication or suspension suture entrapping a branch of the nerve; (4) inadvertent clamping of the nerve; (5) postoperative edema causing nerve compression; (6) coincidental facial nerve palsy such as

TABLE 89–1 POSSIBLE COMPLICATIONS FOLLOWING RHYTIDECTOMY

Immediate	Delayed
Hematoma	Hematoma
Facial nerve injury	Hypertrophic scars
Infection	Alopecia
Hypesthesia	Facial asymmetry
Wound dehiscence	Earlobe distortion
Flap necrosis	
Hairline change	
Depression	

Bell's palsy, Melkersson-Rosenthal syndrome, or Ramsay Hunt syndrome.

Other potential complications associated with face-lift surgery are noted in Table 89–1.

BLEPHAROPLASTY

Changes related to aging often present in the periorbital region, and blepharoplasty can address many of these changes with a dramatic restoration of a more youthful appearance. Due to the eyelids' high visibility and distinct anatomy, errors in surgical technique during eyelid surgery can have significant psychological impact and physical morbidity.

ANATOMY

As with surgery anywhere on the body, a firm comprehension of the regional anatomy is mandatory. The orbicularis oculi is a circular muscle located directly beneath the eyelid skin and is divided into the palpebral (lying anterior to the orbital septum) and orbital portions (Fig. 89–10). The palpebral portion is further subdivided into the pretarsal and preseptal muscles. The preseptal muscle elevates the lower lid through its circular contraction.

Both the upper and lower lids contain tarsal plates, which are composed of dense fibrous connective tissue (Fig. 89–11). The tarsal plates act as support to the eyelids and are attached to medial and lateral canthal ligaments. Support for the superior tarsus is provided by the levator palpebrae superioris muscle and its aponeurosis. The inferior tarsus gains support from the orbital septum. The orbital septum originates from the inferior border of the inferior tarsus and incorporates fascia from the inferior oblique muscle.

The position of the orbital fat pads has been a subject of much discussion. The fat pads are often said to reside within five distinct compartments in each eye—two in the upper lid and three in the lower lid (Fig. 89–12). Orbital fat is thought to be different from fat elsewhere because it does not appear to be directly related to body weight. The orbital fat is most noticeable in the medial canthal area of the upper lid and in the central compartment of the lower lid.

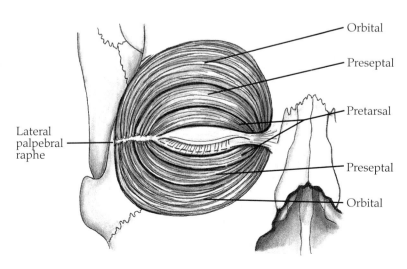

Lateral palpebral raphe

Orbital

Preseptal

Pretarsal

Preseptal

Orbital

FIGURE 89–10 Divisions of the orbicular muscle of the eye.

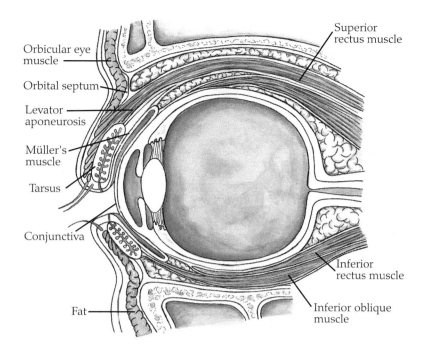

FIGURE 89–11 Cross section of orbit and eyelids.

Orbicular eye muscle
Orbital septum
Levator aponeurosis
Müller's muscle
Tarsus
Conjunctiva
Fat
Superior rectus muscle
Inferior rectus muscle
Inferior oblique muscle

SPECIAL CONSIDERATION

Although these prominent fat pads are often referred to as herniated, this is incorrect because the orbital septum is intact but relaxed.

PITFALLS... It should be noted that the inferior oblique courses between the medial and central fat pads of the lower lid. As such, this muscle is at high risk for injury during fat pad resection. It should also be noted that the lacrimal gland occupies the lateral compartment of the upper lid, and there is no consistent lateral fat pad of the upper lid. Occasionally the lacrimal gland will become ptotic and be mistaken for a fat pad. Fullness in the lateral area of the upper eyelid should raise suspicion of a malposition of the larimal gland, and surgery in this area should be undertaken with extreme care.

TERMINOLOGY

Blepharochalasis is a term that has been used as a generic description for any amount of excess skin of the upper eyelid. However, *blepharocha-*

lasis should be reserved for a relatively uncommon variant of angioneurotic edema, which occurs in young women with swelling and edema of the lids, leading to progressive tissue breakdown. *Dermatochalasis* refers to relaxation of

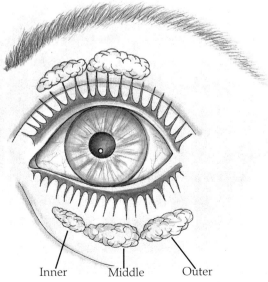

Inner   *Middle*   *Outer*

FIGURE 89–12 Five separate compartments for periorbital adipose tissue.

skin and probably best describes the changes of the aging process.

Blepharoptosis (or simply *ptosis*) describes a condition in which the inferior position of the upper eyelid margin sits over the iris. The normal position of the upper lid margin is at or just above the margin of the iris.

> **PITFALL•••** Blepharoptosis (or simply ptosis of the upper lid) occurs due to levator muscle dysfunction and is not caused by excess tissue or fat herniation and thus will not be corrected with conventional blepharoplasty techniques.

Pseudoptosis occurs when the upper lid margin remains in the proper position relative to the iris, but excess lid skin hangs down below the lid margin, giving the appearance of ptosis. *Lagophthalmos* or *upper lid retraction* occurs when the upper lid margin is positioned above the iris and the white of the sclera is seen between the lid and the iris.

WORKUP AND EVALUATION

Due to the significant functional issues related to the eyes, patients being considered for blepharoplasty should have a complete ophthalmologic exam and be screened for systemic conditions that may affect the eyes. In particular the surgeon should be alert for the following conditions: thyroid disease (hypo- and hyper-), renal disease, coagulopathies, diabetes, cardiac disease, chronic steroid use, allergies to various medications, and nervous disorders with spasms or tics. A detailed ophthalmologic history is also important and should include any history of visual abnormalities or orbital trauma. A search should be made for a personal or family history of glaucoma. The patient should also be questioned with regard to the presence of dry eyes or chronically irritated eyes.

PHYSICAL EXAMINATION

Many surgeons feel that it is important for patients about to undergo blepharoplasty to obtain a preoperative ophthalmologic evaluation to es-

tablish baseline eye function and uncover any conditions that may contraindicate surgery. The following parameters are generally felt to be important: visual acuity, extraocular muscle function, visual fields, glaucoma evaluation, Schirmer test, funduscopic exam, and corneal evaluation.

The surgeon should evaluate the following physical parameters relevant to blepharoplasty: brow position, laxity of upper and lower eyelid skin, periorbital skin pigmentation, presence of ptotic lacrimal glands (which may be mistaken for fat pads), proptosis, enophthalmos, exophthalmos, blepharoptosis, entropion, and ectropion. Additionally, the upper lid should be evaluated for the presence of ptosis. Ptosis is identified if the upper lid margin sits below the superior border of the iris. This is important to document preoperatively because, if noted postoperatively, may be assumed to have been caused by the surgery.

Special attention should be given to the lower lids with regard to their tone and whether they are excessively lax. Lower lid tone is important because any resection of skin or postoperative scarring may result in lower lid retraction and resultant ectropion.

> **PEARL•••** A useful test to gauge the lower lid tension is the "snap test," which is performed by pinching the lower lid between the fingers and pulling the lid away from the globe. When released the lid should briskly snap back into position. Any delay or prolonged wrinkling of the lid should raise concerns about possible lid laxity, which may require a lid-tightening procedure to avoid lower lid ectropion.

SURGICAL TECHNIQUES

Upper Lid Blepharoplasty

Prior to administration of any sedation, the patient is evaluated in a sitting position and surgical marking performed. The medial point of the incision is 4 mm medial and 4 mm cephalad to the medial canthal tendon. The lower incision is planned along the tarsal crease, approximately 9 mm from the lid margin (Fig. 89–13A). A smooth forceps is used to imbricate the skin until the eye just begins to open. The most cephalic mark is made at the upper forceps position. The lateral point of the incision is 3 to 4 mm past the lateral canthal tendon. An incision is then planned between the four points with tapering medial and lateral extensions—basically an ellipse. The upper lid skin encompassed by the ellipse is elevated off the underlying orbicularis with scissor dissection. A strip of orbicularis is then elevated off the underlying orbital septum and resected to help define the supratarsal crease (Fig. 89–13B). The next step is to remove the middle and medial fat pads (remember that laterally the major structure is the lacrimal gland) by opening the septum and ex-

pressing the fat by gentle pressure on the lid. The fat pad is amputated with incremental cuts and appropriate bipolar cautery (Fig. 89–13C). The skin is then closed in a single layer with a fine running suture of the surgeon's choice.

Lower Lid Blepharoplasty

There are two possible surgical approaches for performing lower lid blepharoplasty: subciliary (with an external incision just below the eye lashes) and transconjunctival (with an incision on the inner aspect of the eyelid). The indications for these approaches have been evolving, but the most common indications at present are

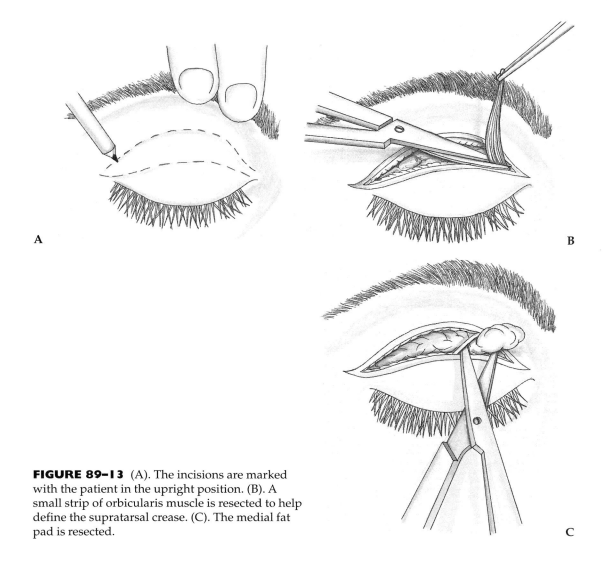

FIGURE 89–13 (A). The incisions are marked with the patient in the upright position. (B). A small strip of orbicularis muscle is resected to help define the supratarsal crease. (C). The medial fat pad is resected.

to utilize the subciliary approach when skin and fat are to be removed and the transconjunctival approach when just orbital fat is to be resected.

The subciliary incision is made 1 to 2 mm below the lower eyelashes and carried laterally into a skin fold. A plane is developed deep to the orbicularis and a skin muscle flap elevated off the orbital septum (Fig. 89–14). With the transconjunctival approach, an incision is made on the inner aspect of the lower lid through the conjunctiva to expose the orbital septum. Once the septum is exposed, small openings are made in it overlying the medial, middle, and lateral fat pads. If skin is to be excised, it should be removed conservatively and only from the lateral portion of the subciliary incision (Fig. 89–15).

COMPLICATIONS

Dry Eyes

Postblepharoplasty dry eyes with recurring bouts of irritation, burning, and itching may occur due to increased conjunctival exposure. Patients at risk for this situation should be identified preoperatively. Conservative therapy is usually indicated, with methylcellulose eyedrops by day and taping by night. More severe cases may require Lacri-Lube and a plastic moisture-retaining eye dressing at night.

Hyperpigmentation

Increased pigmentation of the blepharoplasty scar occurs most frequently in the lower lid sub-

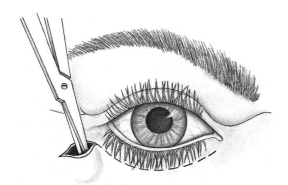

FIGURE 89–14 A submuscular plane is established and carried across the lower eyelid in the premarked subcilliary incision.

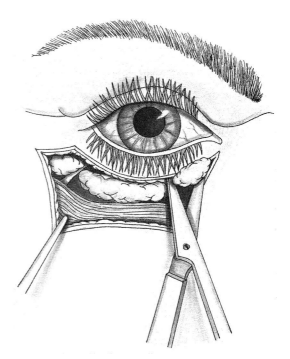

FIGURE 89–15 With the skin muscle flap retracted inferiorly, gentle pressure on the globe reveals the fat pads bulging deep to the orbital septum. Small openings are made in the septum and the fat pads are dissected out. They are then cauterized at their base and resected. Again, it should be emphasized that the medial rectus runs between the middle and medial fat pads and should be identified before resecting the tissue.

ciliary scar. It is usually self-limiting and resolves with simple observation. Dark circles of the lower eyelid may be seen, particularly in Asian or dark-skinned patients, and they are usually self-limited and resolve within 6 months.

Ptosis

An evaluation for ptosis should be part of the surgeon's preoperative evaluation to rule out preexisting conditions. Temporary ptosis may result postoperatively secondary to edema, and this will resolve with time. However, if the levator muscle (or its aponeurosis) has been damaged, then a permanent ptosis may result. If the ptosis persists past 3 months, then it is likely to be permanent and probably warrants subspecialty consultation.

Incomplete Removal of Herniated Orbital Fat

Residual visible orbital fat pads are not a true complication of surgery; rather, they are a manifestation of incomplete surgical technique. The most common site for residual fat pads is in the lateral compartments. A conservative approach should be employed, and any revisional surgery put off for at least 4 months. If the problem is isolated to the lateral fat pad, a limited transconjunctival approach may be employed.

Ectropion

Ectropion of the lower lid is one of the most frequent and the most serious (other than blindness) complications of lower lid blepharoplasty. The most common cause of lower lid ectropion is generally felt to be excessive skin removal. However, if the lower lid is lax, ectropions may occur even when no skin has been excised. This highlights the need for careful preoperative evaluation of lower lid tone. Ectropions can be graded on a scale of I to IV, with grade I being the least severe and grade IV being the most severe. Often grade I to III ectropions will improve over time with massage and squinting exercises. Grade IV ectropions are frequently associated with corneal ulcerations due to the patient's inability to completely close the eyes. If the ectropion persists, then a combination of lid tightening and possibly skin grafting may be required.

Lagophthalmos

Inability to completely close the upper lid is common in the immediate postoperative period following blepharoplasty. However, it usually corrects itself within the first 24 to 36 hours. Persistence of lagophthalmos usually indicates excessive skin removal, but scarring of the levator aponeurosis may also cause upward retraction of the lid margin. The initial management should be careful observation with gentle lid traction exercises. If the problem persists and is due to excessive lid resection, then a thin full-thickness graft to the area may be required. Scarring of the levator aponeurosis may require grafting as well.

Hollow Eye Syndrome

Excessive removal of orbital fat may result in the eye having a sunken or hollow appearance. Treatment of this condition is very difficult and is best avoided by removing only the fat that freely protrudes into the surgical field. Excessive dissection of orbital fat or undue pressure on the globe can result in over-resection of fat and an unnatural sunken-appearing eye.

Hematoma, Orbital Hemorrhage

Small, superficial hematomas may occur under the skin closure lines and may be managed by careful opening and massage of the clot. These superficial hematomas must be distinguished from retrobulbar or diffuse orbital hemorrhage. In these situations the globe bulges anteriorly and the patient experiences significant discomfort. Orbital hemorrhage with a retrobulbar hematoma is a true emergency, and blindness is a possibility. It is generally recommended that the surgical incisions be opened to allow the blood to egress, but usually these bleeds are occurring deep in the orbit and the blood does not have an easy route to escape. As the bleeding continues, pressure within the orbit and globe will increase. When the pressure within the globe reaches systolic levels, the flow of the central retinal artery will slow or stop and the retina will be rendered ischemic. The retina is sensitive to decreased blood flow and permanent injury or blindness may result from as little as 6 minutes of complete lack of blood flow. Therefore, the primary goal is to reduce the intraorbital pressure and allow perfusion of the retina. It is now felt that the most efficacious means of decreasing orbital pressure is to remove the restraining influence of the lower lid by releasing its lateral attachment at the lateral canthus. This is accomplished by means of a lateral canthotomy and inferior cantholysis, which essentially disinserts the lateral eyelid and allows the globe to move forward and relieve pressure on the central retinal artery. When the acute episode has passed, the tendon can be reattached with little residual morbidity. Ancillary measures such as mannitol infusion and anterior chamber paracentesis have been mentioned as theoretically helpful but should not be used in lieu of orbital decompression and should only be done with experienced ophthalmologic consultation.

SUGGESTED READINGS

Beeson WH, McCollough EG. Blepharoplasty. In: Beeson WH, McCollough EG, eds. *Aesthetic Surgery of the Aging Face.* St. Louis: CV Mosby; 1986:22–70.

Cotton JH, Beekkuis GJ. Blepharoplasty. In: Cummings CW, Korause CJ, eds. *Otolaryngology–Head and Neck Surgery.* St. Louis: CV Mosby; 1993:566–587.

Heinze JB, Hueston JT. Blindness after blepharoplasty. *Plast Reconstr Surg 1978;* 61:347–354.

Johnson C, Toriumi D. *Open Structure Rhinoplasty.* Philadelphia: WB Saunders; 1990.

Rees TD, Baker DC, Tabbal N. *Rhinoplasty Problems and Controversies.* St. Louis: CV Mosby; 1988.

Sheen J, Sheen A. *Aesthetic Rhinoplasty.* St. Louis: CV Mosby; 1987.

Shumrick KA, Mandell-Brown M. Rhytidectomy and coronal forehead lift. In: Paparella M, Shumrick D, Gluckman J, Meyerhoff W, eds. *Otolaryngology.* 3d ed. Philadelphia: WB Saunders; 1990:2733–2757.

Webster RC, Beeson WH, McCollough EG. Face-lift. In: Beeson WH, McCollough EG, eds. *Aesthetic Surgery of the Aging Face.* St. Louis: CV Mosby; 1986:71–128.

Wienberg MS, Becker DG, Toriumi DM. Rhytidectomy. In: *Otolaryngology–Head and Neck Surgery.* Vol 2. St. Louis: CV Mosby; 1998:648–659.

SECTION XVI

SKIN
LESIONS

Chapter 90

CUTANEOUS MALIGNANCY

Allen M. Seiden

Skin cancer is the most common form of malignancy in humans, resulting in over 800,000 cases annually. Sun-exposed areas of the head and neck are the most frequently involved sites, accounting for roughly 85 to 90% of all lesions. Estimates suggest that 60% or more are basal cell tumors and 30% are squamous cell tumors, with melanoma being the least common.

RISK FACTORS

Ultraviolet radiation is the most important cause of both premalignant and malignant epithelial lesions. The ultraviolet B band, in the range of 280 to 320 nm, has the most carcinogenic potential and causes the common sunburn.

Patient factors that predispose to the development of skin cancer include a fair complexion; fair hair; blue, green, or gray eyes; and a history of multiple or severe sunburns particularly before the age of 20. Prior trauma resulting in burns and scars, a history of radiation to the skin, and immunosuppression are also associated with a higher incidence of cutaneous malignancy. Indirect factors include an outdoor occupation, frequent sessions in a tanning booth, and living in sun-drenched regions. Age is also a factor, with 50% of patients presenting after the age of 65.

Exposure to certain industrial products and chemicals has been associated with a higher risk of skin cancer. These include tar, polycyclic aromatic hydrocarbons, creosote, and inorganic arsenic compounds, the latter being found still in herbicides, pesticides, and pharmaceutical products.

Xeroderma pigmentosum and nevoid basal cell carcinoma syndrome are two genetic syndromes associated with an increased risk of developing multiple basal cell carcinomas, beginning at an early age.

PEARL... Regardless of risk factors, a lesion that persistently bleeds or does not heal should be presumed to be malignant and requires a biopsy.

PREMALIGNANT LESIONS

ACTINIC KERATOSES

Actinic (solar, senile) keratosis is the most common premalignant skin lesion. It is induced by sun exposure and therefore occurs on sun-exposed areas of the skin, particularly the face, dorsal surfaces of the hands and forearms, and the scalp. It appears as a well-circumscribed, scaly lesion typically 3 to 6 mm in diameter. When inflamed it is pink or red, but otherwise it is generally flesh-colored or brown. Occasionally a marked hyperkeratosis may be present.

PEARL... On clinical examination, the most distinctive feature of these lesions is a gritty, sandpaper-like scale that can be detected on palpation.

These lesions may not be well demarcated and can spread peripherally but are superficial without evidence of infiltration.

The differential diagnosis should include seborrheic keratosis, benign lentigo, squamous cell carcinoma, and basal cell carcinoma. Seborrheic keratosis develops as an elevated plaque that appears stuck on the skin, and has a more waxy rather than gritty feel. It is unrelated to sun exposure and has no malignant potential. Benign lentigo or "liver spot" occurs on sun-exposed skin areas but is a flat, pigmented, non-scaly lesion. Differentiation of actinic keratosis from early basal cell or squamous cell carcinoma may be difficult and generally requires a biopsy.

The incidence of progression of actinic keratosis to invasive squamous cell carcinoma is approximately 12 to 25% and therefore most recommend surgical excision.

CONTROVERSY

There is disagreement as to whether treatment of actinic keratoses truly reduces patient morbidity. Nevertheless, the risk from excision is generally low, and malignant potential is real enough that treatment is usually recommended.

Excision may be accomplished by elliptical removal, although curettage or cryosurgery may be just as effective, with a 99% success rate having been reported. For patients with numerous lesions, application of a 1 to 5% 5-fluorouracil solution topically once or twice a day for 4 to 6 weeks may also be effective, although inflammatory side effects and irritation may occur. Caustic agents such as 35 to 50% trichloroacetic acid may also be used.

Patients should be followed for the development of additional lesions and should be instructed on proper protection from the sun.

BOWEN'S DISEASE

Bowen's disease is an in situ squamous cell carcinoma. It appears as a well-demarcated, scaly, red plaque frequently misdiagnosed as a benign dermatologic lesion, such as psoriasis. It occurs most often in white adults of middle-age or older. Although it has been linked to sun exposure, it may also occur on nonexposed skin areas.

Treatment is complete excision, which, as with any early-stage cutaneous malignancy, may include surgical excision, curettage with electrodesiccation, or cryosurgery.

KERATOACANTHOMA

Although this is not truly a premalignant lesion, it is often confused with squamous cell carcinoma on both clinical and histologic examination. There are those who claim that malignant transformation to squamous cell carcinoma may occur, although others insist that such lesions were likely squamous cell carcinoma from the beginning.

It is more common in older men and presents with a history of rapid growth over 6 to 8 weeks. The most frequently involved sites are on the head, neck, arms, and hands; the nose is the most commonly affected site in the head and neck. It begins as a smooth rounded nodule, but as it enlarges the center ulcerates and becomes filled with a keratinous material. Histologically, it is an exophytic and endophytic cup-shaped growth with a central, well-defined, keratin-filled crater that is lined by a well-differentiated squamous epithelium. Most involute spontaneously within 6 to 12 months, leaving a depressed scar. Nevertheless, complete surgical excision is usually recommended, largely to exclude malignancy. A 5% recurrence rate has been reported, particularly around the lips and nose. Intralesional injection with cytotoxic agents, including 5-fluorouracil and methotrexate, has also been described.

Hutchinson's Melanotic Freckle

This is a spreading, macular pigmentation that most often develops in the skin of the head and neck in elderly patients. It is most common on the temple and cheek, although it may also occur on other sun-exposed areas. It has a smooth surface with irregular borders. The development of an elevated nodule within the freckle is indicative of malignant degeneration into lentigo maligna melanoma, with invasion. The risk of malignant degeneration is less than 5% but increases with increasing size of the freckle.

Basal Cell Carcinoma

Basal cell carcinoma is the most common cutaneous malignancy, with 85% occurring on the head and neck. Fortunately, it is the slowest growing and least likely to metastasize, and therefore generally has the best prognosis.

> **PEARL...** Patients typically present with a sore that tends to crust or bleed and fails to heal.

There are essentially five clinical forms of basal cell carcinoma. The nodular or noduloulcerative lesion is the most common type and generally appears as a small, raised pink and waxy nodule with a rolled border. Overlying telangiectasias are often present, and central ulceration with crusting ("rodent ulcer") may develop as the lesion grows. It generally has a well-defined border, making it easier to treat.

Superficial basal cell carcinoma appears as a red, scaly plaque with an irregular waxy border. It frequently presents as multiple red patches and typically grows peripherally, although over time it may become nodular and ulcerate. It is more common on the trunk and extremities rather than the head and neck. It may be mistaken for eczema, psoriasis, tinea, or Bowen's disease.

The sclerosing or morpheaform basal cell carcinoma is a less common but more dangerous variant. It often has the appearance of a scar, presenting as a yellowish-white plaque with ill-defined borders, and rarely ulcerates. Therefore, it may go unnoticed until reaching a considerable size. There are often subclinical extensions that make complete removal difficult, resulting in higher rates of recurrence. It occurs largely on the face.

The pigmented basal cell carcinoma is not common and is characterized by its brown pigmentation. It behaves and appears just as the nodular type except for its pigmentation.

> **PITFALL...** The pigmented basal cell carcinoma may be mistaken for seborrheic keratosis, a pigmented nevus, dermatofibroma, or melanoma.

Lastly, fibroepitheliomas present as firm, pedunculated lesions that most often occur on the back.

Aside from the clinical type of basal cell carcinoma, the anatomic location also affects behavior.

SPECIAL CONSIDERATION

Those basal cell carcinomas occurring along embryonic fusion planes (e.g., the preauricular area, the nasolabial fold, and the inner and outer canthus of the eye) tend to invade multiple tissue planes and are associated with higher rates of recurrence.

The most common site of recurrence is the nose, followed by the ears, the periorbital areas, the remainder of the face, the neck and scalp, the trunk, and then the upper extremities. Lesions larger than 2 cm are more likely to recur. These factors determine the most appropriate form of therapy. Two-thirds of recurrent lesions develop within 3 years of the initial diagnosis.

Metastases rarely occur with basal cell carcinoma, but cases have been reported. There seems to be no correlation with the site of the primary tumor, histologic type, or underlying immunosuppression. In descending order of frequency, the sites of metastasis include the regional lymph nodes, lung, bone, skin, and liver. The interval from the discovery of the primary tumor to the development of metastatic disease has ranged from 1 to 45 years.

Histology

The characteristic cell in basal cell carcinoma resembles the basal cell of the epidermis but lacks intercellular bridges. There is a large, oval, blue-staining nucleus with minimal cytoplasm, giving the tumor a basophilic appearance. Mitotic figures are rarely seen. At the periphery of tumor nests, the cells are arranged with their long axis perpendicular to the edge of the nest, creating a "picket fence" appearance. A connective tissue stroma proliferates and is often mucinous, oriented in parallel bundles around the tumor nests. Mucin shrinks with dehydration and fixation of the specimen, and therefore the stroma often shows retraction from the tumor islands. This is referred to as "clefting" and is helpful in making the diagnosis.

Depending on the degree of differentiation, basal cell tumors may be divided into different histologic patterns. The solid type demonstrates no differentiation and may be further categorized as circumscribed or infiltrative. The keratotic type differentiates toward hair structures, the cystic type toward sebaceous structures, and the adenoid type shows some glandular formation. When there is considerable differentiation toward keratinous cysts, the appearance is similar to epithelial pearls of squamous cell carcinoma. This has been referred to as basosquamous cell or keratotic basal cell carcinoma and is believed by some to be more aggressive.

CONTROVERSY

Some suggest that the greater differentiation seen in basosquamous cell carcinoma is a sign of decreased aggressiveness, whereas others consider it a sign of greater aggressiveness due to the similarity in appearance with squamous cell carcinoma. Some studies report a higher rate of metastases, whereas others do not.

Treatment

Treatment is complete excision. For small, early lesions, curettage with electrodesiccation is the most common mode of therapy, although cryosurgery and surgical excision are also effective. For larger tumors, over 2 cm, surgical excision or Mohs' micrographic surgery is preferred. Appropriate margins for a nodular basal cell carcinoma range from 2 to 4 mm; however, this becomes more difficult to define in a sclerosing type or infiltrating tumor. The indications for Mohs' micrographic surgery are listed in Table 90–1. Mohs' surgery has demonstrated close to a 99% success rate for the treatment of basal cell carcinoma.

For primary lesions less than 2 cm in size, surgical excision with a 4-mm margin can achieve a 98% cure rate. This drops down to 85% and 75%, respectively, for 3-mm and 2-mm margins.

TABLE 90–1 Indications for Mohs' Micrographic Surgery

Sclerosing or morpheaform type of basal cell carcinoma

Ill-defined margins

Recurrent lesions

Locations associated with higher rates of recurrence, e.g., nose, ear, periorbital region

Locations where 4 mm margin would compromise cosmesis or function

Large size
    Basal cell carcinoma greater than 2 cm
    Squamous cell carcinoma greater than 1 cm

For morpheaform lesions, if Mohs' surgery is not available, a 7- to 10-mm margin is recommended. Although not as accurate as the Mohs' technique, frozen section control should be utilized. If subsequent histologic examination demonstrates a positive margin, recurrence rates as high as 82% around the nose, ears, and eyes, and 25% elsewhere have been reported. Therefore, reexcision should be performed rather than watchful waiting. Bone or cartilage invasion requires full-thickness excision.

Irradiation is generally reserved for patients in poor health or for large lesions in difficult-to-treat areas, or if free margins cannot be achieved.

SPECIAL CONSIDERATION

It has been found that 40% of patients with basal cell carcinoma will develop a new basal cell lesion within 5 years, and therefore they need to be followed for new lesions as well as recurrence.

SQUAMOUS CELL CARCINOMA

Squamous cell carcinoma typically presents as an erythematous, ulcerated lesion with associated crusting, although it may also present as a thickened, hyperkeratotic patch. Its base tends to be granular and quite friable, and the lesion is often surrounded by induration. It generally lacks the telangiectasias typical of basal cell carcinoma, with more scaling and ulceration.

As with most skin cancers, squamous cell carcinoma tends to arise most commonly in sun-damaged skin. Metastases occur at a rate of generally less than 1%, usually within the first 2 years, and most often to regional lymph nodes, although distal spread to bone, lung, and brain may occur. Squamous cell carcinoma may also develop de novo in nonexposed areas. The latter tend to be more aggressive and are more likely to metastasize, at a rate of approximately 2 to 3% to both regional and distant sites. Lesions may also arise in areas of previous trauma, burns, or old scar, known as Marjolin's ulcer. These tend to be most aggressive, frequently

demonstrating a spindle cell configuration and metastatic rate reported between 10 and 40%. Carcinoma of the lip, because it is a mucosal variant, also tends to be more aggressive, with a metastatic potential of 11 to 12%. In general, lesions larger than 2 cm are more apt to metastasize, although this may be reflective of depth of invasion. It has been reported that 70 to 85% of local recurrences and metastases occur within the first 2 years. Once metastases have occurred, prognosis is poor, with an overall 5-year survival rate of approximately 25%.

HISTOLOGY

The histologic appearance of cutaneous squamous cell carcinoma is that of irregular masses of epidermal cells proliferating downward to invade the dermis. It may be classified qualitatively based on the degree of differentiation, or quantitatively based on the depth of invasion.

In 1921 Broders proposed a system of classification based on the degree of differentiation: grade I tumors have more than 75% well-differentiated cells, grade II 50 to 74%, grade III 25 to 49%, and grade IV less than 25%. The well-differentiated tumors generally have a better prognosis.

PEARL••• Differentiated tumors tend to demonstrate evidence of keratinization, specifically keratin pearls.

Tumor thickness and the depth of invasion have also been shown to correlate with aggressiveness, with tumors measuring more than 6 mm in thickness considered to be high risk.

Cutaneous squamous cell carcinoma can be further subdivided into five histologic types. The generic type displays actinic changes. Adenoid squamous cell carcinoma has a pseudoglandular appearance, with alveolar formations resulting from dyskeratosis and acantholysis. The bowenoid type appears histologically similar to Bowen's disease, but there is evidence of invasion through the basement membrane. Verrucous carcinoma is uncommon on the skin and appears as a whitish, cauliflower lesion that invades by blunt pseudopod-like growth. Lastly, the spindle type shows the least differentiation with little keratinization and is the least common.

A recent prospective study by Breuninger and associates (1997) suggests that desmoplasia is a highly significant negative prognostic factor for squamous cell carcinoma of the skin; 44 of 594 tumors were desmoplastic, defined as those tumors with fine branches of tumor cells at the periphery and a surrounding desmoplastic stromal reaction. These tumors tend to be more undifferentiated with less keratinization and are more advanced at the time of diagnosis. Local recurrences were ten times more common, and the rate of metastatic spread was six times greater than observed for the other tumors.

Treatment

Surgical excision with primary closure is ideal for most early squamous cell carcinomas of the skin. It offers the advantages of histologic control and rapid healing and usually results in superior functional and cosmetic results. A 4- to 6-mm margin is usually recommended for primary lesions. Advanced lesions may also be approached surgically, although some situations may warrant consideration for Mohs' micrographic surgery or radiation. Postoperative radiation may be considered when margins are indistinct or there is evidence of perineural invasion. For advanced or recurrent lesions, margins of 1 to 2 cm are required, and any involved bone or cartilage must be resected. Table 90–2 lists those characteristics associated with more aggressive lesions. The 5-year cure rate for advanced lesions is approximately 95 to 97% with Mohs' surgery and 85 to 87% with standard surgical excision. For recurrent lesions, the literature suggests a 5-year cure rate of 90% with Mohs' surgery but only 50 to 75% with other techniques.

In contrast to basal cell carcinoma, attention must often be given to regional lymph nodes. However, neck dissection is rarely indicated unless palpable nodes are present. If the primary site includes the temple or preauricular area, and the patient presents with a cervical

TABLE 90–2 Squamous Cell Carcinoma of the Skin: Factors Associated with Higher Risk

Recurrence

Thickness greater than 6 cm (invasion to the reticular dermis or adipose)

Size greater than 2 cm

Poorly differentiated

Immunocompromised host

Anatomic site: ear, lip

Perineural invasion

Tumor arising in scar, radiated skin, or chronic ulcer

metastasis, the neck dissection should include a superficial parotidectomy so that all of the at-risk nodes are removed. Postoperative radiation should be considered when multiple nodes are involved, if a single lymph node is larger than 2.5 cm, if there is evidence of extracapsular invasion, or if there is histologic evidence of neural, vascular, or lymphatic invasion.

MALIGNANT MELANOMA

It is reported that the incidence of malignant melanoma is rising faster than any other human cancer, having more than doubled in the United States within the past 30 years. This has been attributed to increased recreational sun exposure and depletion of the earth's ozone layer. Approximately 38,000 new cases develop annually in the United States, resulting in 7,300 deaths. The overall 5-year survival rate has improved from 60% in 1963 to 81% currently.

SPECIAL CONSIDERATION

By far the most important determinant of survival is early diagnosis.

Approximately 25 to 30% of primary melanomas occur in the head and neck. The cheek and scalp are more common because the density of epidermal melanocytes is much greater in these locations. There is a slight male preponderance, most likely due to occupational exposure. The average age at presentation is within the sixth decade, but it may rarely occur in children as well.

Lesions of the scalp are frequently discovered late and tend to be aggressive. Lymphatic drainage is based on location: anterior to a coronal plane through the external ear canals would drain to parotid, submandibular, submental, and upper jugular lymph nodes, whereas posterior to this line would drain to occipital, suboccipital, postauricular, and posterior cervical nodes.

Surprisingly, the auricle is a relatively uncommon site for melanoma, with an incidence of roughly 10 to 15%. The helical rim is most frequently involved. Lesions of the canal, concha, tragus, and antitragus have a worse prognosis due to the difficulty in obtaining adequate margins. The nose is also an uncommon site, accounting for 2 to 5% of head and neck melanomas. Drainage is to facial, parotid, or cervical lymph nodes and may be bilateral.

> **PEARL•••** The earliest sign of melanoma is an increase in size or change in color of a preexisting or new pigmented lesion that occurs over a period of months.

Persistent itching, and subsequent bleeding, tenderness, and ulceration are suggestive symptoms that would warrant a biopsy. Clinical criteria include the ABCD's:

A—Asymmetry

B—Border: a poorly circumscribed or irregular border

C—Color: varied, nonuniform color is characteristic, including black, blue (dermal melanin), red (inflammation), and white (regression)

D—Diameter: larger than 6 mm is generally suspicious

A melanoma may spread within the adjacent skin, to regional lymph nodes, or distantly. The organs most frequently involved are the liver, lung, bone, and brain. The lifetime risk of developing a second primary in those patients with melanoma is roughly 6% but increases to 30% in those with familial melanoma.

DIFFERENTIAL DIAGNOSIS

Approximately half of melanomas arise from preexisting benign nevi, whereas the remainder arise de novo, there being no apparent prognostic significance to either situation. The differential diagnosis must include a variety of benign and malignant pigmented lesions (Table 90–3).

Common acquired nevi are generally round or oval with smooth, regular borders and measure less than 6 mm. The color tends to be uniform, from tan to brown. Junctional nevi tend to be macular and nonpalpable, uniform in color from pale to dark brown, and smaller than 1 cm. Compound nevi are papular and hair-bearing, and darkly pigmented but not black. They may have a depigmented halo. Dermal nevi tend to be pink or flesh-colored and dome-shaped and may be hair-bearing.

An atypical or dysplastic nevus is generally larger than a common mole, measuring up to 15 mm in diameter. It demonstrates an irregular border, with irregular coloration including tan,

TABLE 90–3 DIFFERENTIAL DIAGNOSIS OF CUTANEOUS MALIGNANT MELANOMA

Seborrheic keratosis—multiple, waxy

Nevi

  Junctional—macular, nonpalpable, usually less than 1 cm, pale to dark brown

  Compound—palpable, dark brown, may have depigmented halo

  Dermal—dome shaped, lacks pigment

Hemangioma—blue-black to red, usually blanches with pressure

Blue nevus—usually less than 0.5 cm, blue-black, palpable, rarely becomes malignant

Pyogenic granuloma—similar to hemangioma with surrounding inflammation

Spitz nevus—less than 2 cm flat, reddish

Pigmented basal cell carcinoma—biopsy required to differentiate from melanoma

Squamous cell carcinoma—nonpigmented and rarely confused with melanoma

Adapted from Clevens RA, Johnson TM, Wolf GT. Management of head and neck melanoma. In: Cummings CW, Fredrickson JM, Harker LA, Krause CJ, Schuller DE, eds. *Otolaryngology—Head and Neck Surgery.* St. Louis: Mosby Year Book; 1998:502–526. Reprinted by permission of the publisher.

brown, or pink. The surface is usually a combination of macular and papular elements. Such lesions should be followed, and the development of black or friable areas should signal the need for biopsy.

Most Caucasians have anywhere from 10 to 40 nevi that develop during early childhood. The presence of an unusually large number of pigmented nevi increases the risk for developing melanoma. This is particularly true on the legs where the presence of 20 or more common nevi increases the risk 12-fold. Giant congenital nevi, larger than 20 cm, also place the patient at increased risk. The incidence of melanoma in such lesions ranges from 5 to 20%, leading many to recommend prophylactic resection during childhood.

FOUR COMMON VARIATIONS OF MELANOMA

Superficial Spreading Melanoma

This type is the most common, accounting for roughly 75% of melanomas. It begins as a superficial spreading pigmentation, and this radial growth phase may last 1 to 7 years, but rarely does the lesion get larger than 2 cm before invasion occurs. This is generally heralded by ulceration and bleeding.

> **PEARL...** The characteristic clinical feature of a superficial spreading melanoma is a kaleidoscopic variety of colors, including tan-black, brown, blue-gray, and violaceous pink.

If diagnosed during this early period of radial growth, the lesion remains highly curable. The average age at diagnosis is 40 to 50.

Lentigo Maligna Melanoma

This type makes up 6 to 10% of melanomas. It generally appears as an irregularly pigmented flat lesion that grows slowly over several years, and as such is slow to invade. This purports a slightly better prognosis. During this prolonged radial growth phase it is known as lentigo ma-

ligna or Hutchinson's freckle (see above), but once the vertical phase begins and invasion occurs, it is considered a melanoma. It is most common on the malar region of the cheek and temple, and the average age at diagnosis is 70.

Nodular Melanoma

Nodular melanoma accounts for approximately 10% of melanomas and has the worst prognosis. There is no radial growth phase, but only early vertical invasion. The coloration is characteristically a shade of blue, and ulceration is common. It may occur on both sun-exposed and -unexposed skin surfaces. The age at diagnosis is generally 40 to 50.

Acral Lentiginous Melanoma

This type accounts for 5 to 7% of melanomas and is the most common form seen in blacks. It occurs on the palm, sole, nail bed, and mucous membranes. It has a variable radial and vertical growth phase, but it has a poor prognosis due to an associated rich vascular supply with early spread and delayed diagnosis. The average age at diagnosis is 60.

Histology

Melanomas arise from melanocytes. These cells produce the pigment melanin and are located along the basal layer of the epidermis. A melanoma typically has an initial radial growth phase, characterized by superficial spread, followed by a nodular or vertical growth phase, when invasion occurs.

> **PEARL...** An increase in the lesion's height correlates with deeper penetration into the skin (vertical growth phase) and is a sign of more advanced disease.

Clark discovered that the level of invasion was an important prognostic variable in assessing melanoma and described levels to correspond to this invasion. Breslow further refined this classification, relating prognosis to the actual measured depth or thickness of invasion (Fig. 90–1).

Clark levels

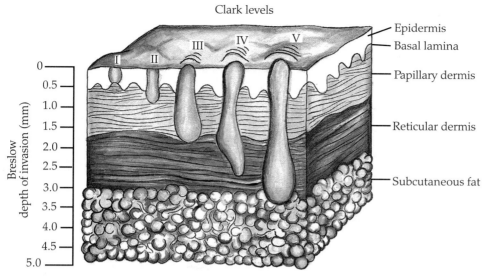

FIGURE 90–1 Revised Clark classification of melanomas.

SPECIAL CONSIDERATION

Lesions are thus characterized as thin (less than 1 mm), intermediate (1 to 4 mm), and thick (more than 4 mm), and this is the most important independent factor influencing survival.

Thin lesions are not likely to metastasize, whereas intermediate lesions are associated with a 25 to 50% risk of regional metastasis and a 10 to 20% risk of distant metastasis. Thick lesions have a distant metastatic rate of 60%. The American Joint Committee on Cancer staging for melanoma is based on the level of invasion (Table 90–4).

TREATMENT

Effective treatment for melanoma depends on early diagnosis and accurate surgical resection. The extent of surgery depends on the size and location of the lesion, the type of melanoma, regional lymphatic drainage, and the general health of the patient.

Shave excision and curettage as a biopsy technique for pigmented lesions should be

CONTROVERSY

Traditional approaches to surgical excision have recommended wide margins of 3 to 5 cm; however, more recent data suggest that narrow margins of 1 cm do not alter the prognosis. It has been recommended that surgical margins correlate with the thickness and thus the risk of the lesion, such that 1-cm margins are adequate for lesions less than 1 mm thick, 1- to 2-cm margins for lesions 1 to 2 mm thick, progressing to 3-cm margins for lesions more than 4 mm in thickness.

avoided. To adequately stage melanoma, a full-thickness biopsy into the subcutaneous tissue needs to be obtained. Thickness should be measured at the point of maximal elevation, through the point of maximal pigmentation, or from the base of an ulcer. Frozen section is unreliable.

There is little argument that patients with palpable adenopathy require a regional lymph

TABLE 90–4 AMERICAN JOINT COMMITTEE ON CANCER STAGING FOR MELANOMA

T0:   No evidence of primary tumor

Tis: In situ, not an invasive lesion (Clark's level 1)

T1:   Invades papillary dermis (level II) or 0.75 mm thick or less

T2:   Invades papillary-reticular dermis interface (level III) or 0.76 to 1.5 mm thick

T3:   Invades reticular dermis (level IV) or 1.51 to 4.0 mm thick

T4:   Invades subcutaneous tissue (level V) or more than 4.0 mm thick

N0:   No regional lymph node involvement

N1:   Metastasis 3 cm or less

N2:   Metastasis greater than 3 cm

M0:   No distant metastasis

M1:   Distant metastasis

    M1a: In skin or subcutaneous tissue, lymph nodes beyond regional nodes

    M1b: Visceral metastasis

node dissection. Nevertheless, the prognosis is extremely poor, as 70 to 85% of such patients will die of distant disease. On the other hand, a 25% 5-year survival rate is better than can be achieved with either radiation or chemotherapy.

When regional adenopathy is not clinically apparent, there is much argument as to whether an elective or delayed neck dissection is more beneficial. The literature presents data to support either approach. Wilmes and Bujia (1993) found a significant survival advantage when a prophylactic neck dissection was performed for lesions 0.75 to 1.5 mm in thickness. However, for lesions with invasion deeper than 1.5 mm, the outcome was unchanged. Nevertheless, most authors suggest basing the decision on the likelihood of occult metastases. Therefore, wide local exicision alone should be adequate for thin lesions and for lentigo maligna melanoma. Otherwise, elective neck dissection is indicated for (1) lesions 0.75 to 1.49 mm in thickness (risk of regional metastases 25%) only if the lesion is ulcerated or involves a high-risk site, or if the primary is a nodular melanoma; (2) lesions 1.5 to 4.0 mm in thickness (risk of regional metastases approaches 57%) if the lymphatic drainage is predictable; (3) lesions more than 4.0 mm in thickness, largely for local and regional control; and (4) for any lesion when poor patient follow-up is anticipated.

The scalp, posterior lateral neck, and skin over the mandible are at greater risk for metastases as compared to the face and anterior neck. Ulcerated lesions metastasize more readily and require more aggressive treatment. In the presence of palpable parotid lymph nodes, a neck dissection should include a total parotidectomy with preservation of the facial nerve, whereas an elective neck dissection would generally include only a superficial parotidectomy.

Due to the sometimes uncertain lymphatic drainage patterns for sites on the face, scalp, and neck, various investigators have attempted to better define the likelihood of occult nodal disease. Intradermal injection of a blue dye at the primary site at the time of surgery has been performed to try to identify the sentinel node, which can then be sent for frozen section analysis. When properly performed, this technique can predict the presence of metastatic disease with a better than 96% accuracy. However, this accuracy depends on intact dermal lymphatics and therefore is not reliable when a previous resection has been performed. Positron emission tomography scanning using various dyes is under investigation as a tool to reveal subclinical regional and distant metastases.

Historically, melanoma has been considered to be radioresistant. However, although melanoma cells appear to be able to repair sublethal radiation damage, more recent investigations have suggested that large dose per fraction regimens may be more effective. Nevertheless, there is generally no role for primary radiotherapy in the treatment of melanoma unless the patient is not a surgical candidate.

Radiation can provide effective palliation for metastatic disease.

Chemotherapy offers no survival advantage, and even in the presence of advanced disease should not be considered unless the patient is symptomatic.

Unlike squamous cell carcinoma of the upper aerodigestive tract, melanoma carries a high risk of recurrence for 15 years or more after initial diagnosis. These patients need to be followed accordingly, with particular reference to the development of metastatic disease.

Immune factors seem to play a role in controlling tumor growth, and there has been recent work looking at various immunotherapeutic approaches. Although it remains experimental, the most promising approach thus far is active immunization with specific melanoma vaccines. Intralesional injection with α-interferon has also been attempted with temporary improvement in regression rates.

MUCOSAL MELANOMA

Mucosal melanoma represents less than 2% of malignant melanomas diagnosed in the United States each year, but the prognosis is universally very poor, with 5-year survival ranging from 10 to 15%. Approximately 25% of mucosal melanomas occur in the head and neck. Based on a recent review, the most common site is the nasal cavity, followed by the oral cavity, maxillary antrum, oropharynx, hypopharynx, and ethmoid sinus. The most favored therapeutic approach is generally surgery followed by adjuvant radiotherapy. However, even if local disease can be controlled, failure generally occurs from distant metastases.

SUGGESTED READINGS

Breslow A. Thickness, cross-sectional areas, and depth of invasion in the prognosis of cutaneous melanoma. *Ann Surg* 1970;172:902.

Breuninger H, Schaumburg-Lever G, Holzschuh J, Homy HP. Desmoplastic squamous cell carcinoma of skin and vermillion surface: a highly malignant subtype of skin cancer. *Cancer* 1997;79:915–919.

Cady B. Prophylactic lymph node dissection in melanoma: does it help? *J Clin Oncol* 1988;6:2.

Clevens RA, Johnson TM, Wolf GT. Management of head and neck melanoma. In: Cummings CW, Fredrickson JM, Harker LA, Krause CJ, Schuller DE, eds. *Otolaryngology—Head and Neck Surgery.* St. Louis: Mosby Year Book; 1998:502–526.

Fisher SR. Cutaneous malignant melanoma of the head and neck. *Laryngoscope* 1989;99:822.

Lever WF, Schaumburg-Lever G. *Histopathology of the Skin.* Philadelphia: JB Lippincott; 1983.

Loree TR, Mullins AP, Spellman J, North JH, Hicks WL. Head and neck mucosal melanoma: a 32-year review. *Ear Nose Throat J* 1999;78:372–375.

Loree JR, Spiro RH. Cutaneous melanoma of the head and neck. *Am J Surg* 1989;158:388.

Morton DL, Wen D, Wong JH, et al. Technical details of intraoperative lymphatic mapping for early stage melanoma. *Arch Surg* 1992; 127:392–399.

Seung LM, Rivlin D, Moy RL. Premalignant and malignant epithelial tumors. In: Cullen JP, ed. *Current Practice of Dermatology.* Philadelphia: Current Medicine; 1995:37–42.

Sober AJ, Barnhill RL. Benign and malignant pigmented lesions. In: Cullen JP, ed. *Current Practice of Dermatology.* Philadelphia: Current Medicine; 1995:43–49.

Stucker FJ, Nathan CA. Cutaneous malignancy. In: Bailey BJ, ed. *Head and Neck Surgery—Otolaryngology.* 2nd ed. Philadelphia: Lippincott-Raven; 1998:1415–1438.

Stucker FJ, Shockley WW. Skin cancer of the head and neck. In: Paparella MM, Shumrick DA, Gluckman JL, Meyerhoff WL, eds. *Otolaryngology.* 3rd ed. Philadelphia: WB Saunders; 1991:2599–2616.

Suffin SC, Waisman J, Clark WH, Morton DL, Clark WH Jr. Comparison of the classification by microscopic level (stage) of malignant melanoma by three independent groups of pathologists. *Cancer* 1977;40:3112–4.

Trotti A, Peters LJ. Role of radiotherapy in the primary management of mucosal melanoma of the head and neck. *Semin Surg Oncol* 1993; 9:246.

Urist MM, et al. The influence of surgical margins and prognostic factors predicting the risk of local recurrence in 3445 patients with primary cutaneous melanoma. *Cancer* 1985;55:1398.

Veronesi U, Cascinelli N. Narrow excision (1 cm margin). *Arch Surg* 1991;126:438.

Weiss RL. Melanoma of the head and neck. In: Bailey BJ, ed. *Head and Neck Surgery—Otolaryngology.* 2nd ed. Philadelphia: Lippincott-Raven; 1998:1439–1443.

Wilmes E, Bujia J. Recommendations for therapy of head and neck cutaneous melanoma. *Am J Otolaryngol* 1993;14:267.

SECTION XVII

SYNDROMES
AND
EPONYMS

Chapter 91

SYNDROMES AND EPONYMS

Myles L. Pensak

ABRIKOSSOFF'S TUMOR (GRANULAR CELL TUMOR) A benign neoplasm most frequently observed in the tongue. It usually presents as a small, firm, circumscribed nodule.

ABRUZZO-ERICKSON SYNDROME Characteristics of this syndrome included (1) probable X-linked inheritance; (2) coloboma of iris, choroid, and retina; (3) cleft palate; (4) short stature; (5) radial synostosis; (6) hypospadias; and (7) sensorineural hearing loss.

ACHONDROPLASIA Characteristics include (1) autosomal-dominant inheritance, although about 80% of cases represent new mutations; (2) short-limbed dwarfism; (3) enlarged head; (4) short trident hands; (5) lordotic spine; (6) skeletal changes; and (7) hearing loss.

ACKERMAN TUMOR Verrucous carcinoma.

ACRICRANIOFACIAL DYSOSTOSIS The characteristics of this syndrome include (1) autosomal-recessive transmission; (2) malformation of the auricles with narrow external auditory canals and preauricular pits; (3) characteristic craniofacial anomalies, short stature, and developmental delay; and (4) moderately severe, nonprogressive, sensorineural, and conductive hearing loss.

ADAMS-STOKES DISEASE Paroxysmal changes in cardiac output due to atherosclerotic heart disease.

ADDISON'S DISEASE Hypofunction of the adrenal cortex.

ADIE'S SYNDROME This syndrome is characterized by decreased pupillary reaction and deep tendon reflexes.

ADULT RESPIRATORY DISTRESS SYNDROME (ARDS) Characteristics include hypoxia and pulmonary infiltrates secondary to increased pulmonary vascular permeability and/or microvascular hemorrhage. This syndrome generally presents 12 to 24 hours following shock trauma or injury.

ALBERS-SCHÖNBERG DISEASE The major characteristics are (1) autosomal-recessive inheritance; (2) otosclerotic involvement of all bones of the skeleton; (3) facial palsy and visual loss; and (4) mild to moderate mixed hearing loss.

ALBRIGHT'S SYNDROME Characterized by polyostotic fibrous dysplasia, scattered melanotic macular spots, and, in females, precocious puberty. The bony lesions may occasionally occur in single bones. There is often an elevation of the serum alkaline phosphatase due to abnormal bone metabolism.

ALDRICH'S SYNDROME Thrombocytopenia, eczema, and recurrent infections occur during the first year of life. It is inherited through a sex-linked recessive gene. The bleeding time is prolonged, the platelet count is decreased, and the bone marrow megakaryocytes are normal in number.

ALEXANDER SYNDROME   An autosomal-dominant syndrome that consists of progressive glomerulonephritis and sensorineural hearing loss. The auditory deficit is symmetric, worse in the high frequencies, and primarily due to a loss of hair cells.

ALPORT SYNDROME   Characteristics of this syndrome include (1) genetic heterogeneity with X-linked dominant inheritance being most common; but autosomal-dominant or -recessive inheritance has been noted in some kindreds; (2) progressive nephritis with uremia; (3) lens abnormalities including lenticonus or cataracts in those with early-onset, end-stage renal disease; (4) leiomyomatosis of the esophagus and vulva occasionally; and (5) progressive sensorineural hearing loss beginning during the first or second decades and showing variable expressivity.

ALSTRÖM SYNDROME   Characteristics of this syndrome include (1) autosomal-recessive inheritance; (2) onset of atypical retinal degeneration with loss of central vision in infancy; (3) onset of diabetes mellitus in childhood; (4) transient obesity; (5) onset of posterior cortical cataract in second decade; (6) onset of nephropathy in the third decade; (7) acanthosis nigricans; and (8) onset of progressive sensorineural hearing loss in late childhood.

AMALRIC'S SYNDROME   Granular macular pigment epitheliopathy (foveal dystrophy) is associated with sensorineural hearing loss. Visual acuity is usually normal. This syndrome may be a genetic disorder, or it may be the result of an intrauterine rubella infection.

ANNULUS OF ZINN   The fibrous ligament that encircles the contents of the optic foramen.

ANTONI TYPE A TUMOR   Schwannoma with a picket-fence or palisade arrangement of the Schwann cells. The formation results in a Verocay body pattern with the intertwined connective tissue and reticular fibrils forming a regular pattern.

ANTONI TYPE B TUMOR   Schwannoma with irregular loosely packed arrangement. There is no clinical difference from Antoni type A tumors.

APERT SYNDROME   Characteristics include (1) autosomal-dominant inheritance; (2) craniosynostosis; (3) soft tissue syndactyly and progressive synostosis of hands and feet; (4) midfacial hypoplasia; (5) hypertelorism; (6) mental retardation; and (7) mild conductive hearing loss.

ARNOLD-CHIARI SYNDROME   Cerebellar tonsillar herniation through the foramen magnum region, which may result in balance dysfunction as well as lower cranial nerve entrapment.

ARNOLD'S NERVE   The auricular branch of the vagus. It arises from the jugular ganglion, passes through the temporal bone via the mastoid canaliculus, and exits the skull through the tympanomastoid fissure. It supplies the skin of the posterior external auditory canal and posterior auricle.

ASCHER SYNDROME   A rare possibly autosomal-dominant disorder. Manifestations are a loss of elasticity in the skin of the eyelids (blepharochalasis), goiter, edema, and thickening of the gingivobuccal mucosa, which gives the appearance of double lips.

AUERBACH'S PLEXUS   The myenteric plexus of the esophagus.

AUTOSOMAL-DOMINANT PIEBALDISM AND SENSORINEURAL HEARING LOSS   Telfer syndrome. This syndrome is characterized by (1) autosomal-dominant inheritance; (2) congenital piebaldism; (3) ataxia; (4) mental retardation in about 80%; and (5) variable, sometimes asymmetric, sensorineural hearing loss in about 60%.

AVELLIS SYNDROME   Thrombosis of the vertebral artery results in disruption of blood to the spinothalamic tract, the nucleus ambiguus, and the bulbar nucleus of the accessory nerve. Ipsilateral paralysis of the soft palate, larynx, and pharynx. Contralateral loss of pain and temperature is noted in the trunk and extremities.

BABINSKI-NAGEOTTE SYNDROME   This syndrome is caused by multiple or scattered lesions, chiefly in the distribution of the vertebral artery. Ipsilateral paralysis of the soft palate, larynx, pharynx, and sometimes tongue occurs. There is also ipsilateral loss of taste on the posterior third of the tongue, loss of pain and temperature sensation around the face, cerebellar asynergia, Horner's syndrome with contralateral spastic hemiplegia, and loss of proprioceptive and tactile sensation.

BALEZ SYNDROME Characterized by onset in childhood or early adolescence of thickening of the lower lip and hyperplasia of the minor salivary glands in this region. Papules sometimes form at the duct openings, and saliva can be easily expressed. Some forms may predispose toward an increased risk of squamous cell cancer.

BARAKAT SYNDROME Characteristics of this syndrome include (1) recessive inheritance, either X-linked or autosomal; (2) nephrotic syndrome with rapidly progressive renal insufficiency; (3) anatomic defects of the parathyroid, producing hypoparathyroidism; and (4) sensorineural hearing loss.

BARANY SYNDROME A combination of unilateral headache in the back of the head, periodic ipsilateral deafness (alternating with periods of unaffected hearing), vertigo, and tinnitus.

BARCLAY-BARON DISEASE Vallecular dysphagia.

BARRE-LEIOU SYNDROME Occipital headache, vertigo, tinnitus, vasomotor disorders, and facial spasm due to irritation of the sympathetic plexus around the vertebral artery in rheumatic disorders of the cervical spine. It is also known as cervical migraine.

BARRETT'S ESOPHAGITIS Replacement of the squamous epithelium of the distal esophagus by columnar epithelium, similar to that which lines the stomach. The most common cause is chronic gastroesophageal reflux; 2 to 5% of cases may progress to adenocarcinoma.

BARSONY-POLGAR SYNDROME A diffuse esophageal spasm caused by disruption of the peristaltic waves by an irregular contraction resulting in dysphagia and regurgitation is evidence for this syndrome.

BARTHOLIN'S DUCT The major duct of the sublingual gland. It is formed by the confluence of several of the more anterior small sublingual ducts (ducts of Rivinus) and empties into the submandibular duct.

BASAL CELL NEVOID SYNDROME This familial syndrome, non–sex-linked, autosomal dominant with high penetrance and variable expressivity manifests early in life. It appears as multiple nevoid basal cell epitheliomas of the skin, cysts of the jaw, abnormal ribs and metacarpal bones, frontal bossing, and dorsal scoliosis. Endocrine abnormalities have been reported and it has been associated with medulloblastoma.

BATTLE'S SIGN Ecchymosis over the mastoid process indicative of a temporal fracture.

BAYFORD AUTENRIETH DYSPHAGIA (ARKIN'S DISEASE) Dysphagia lusoria is said to be secondary to esophageal compression from an aberrant right subclavian artery.

BECKWITH'S SYNDROME This is a congenital disorder characterized by macroglossia, omphalocele, hypoglycemia, pancreatic hyperplasia, noncystic renal hyperplasia, and cytomegaly of the fetal adrenal cortex.

BEGEER SYNDROME This disorder is characterized by (1) autosomal-recessive inheritance; (2) cataracts; (3) mental retardation; (4) ataxia; (5) motor and sensory neuropathy; and (6) sensorineural hearing loss.

BEHÇET SYNDROME A symptom complex consisting of oral ulcers, genital ulcers, and iritis.

BERK-TABATZNIK SYNDROME Characteristics include (1) unknown inheritance; (2) congenital optic atrophy; (3) cervical kyphosis; (4) spastic quadriparesis; (5) brachytelephalangy; (6) short stature; and (7) sensorineural hearing loss.

BERMAN SYNDROME This syndrome is characterized by (1) autosomal-recessive inheritance; (2) ataxia; (3) mental retardation; (4) spastic diplegia; (5) motor and sensory neuropathy; and (6) sensorineural hearing loss.

BESNIER-BOECK-SCHAUMANN SYNDROME Systemic sarcoidosis.

BEZOLD'S ABSCESS A subperiosteal abscess of the temporal bone, most commonly found in the region just anterior to the mastoid tip. The cause is usually a mastoiditis with extravasation through the inner bony table into the digastric fossa.

BOERHAAVE SYNDROME   Spontaneous rupture of the esophagus, usually due to severe vomiting.

BOGORAD SYNDROME (CROCODILE TEAR SYNDROME)   Profuse lacrimation during eating. It is usually the result of faulty regeneration of autonomic nerves after facial trauma, with parasympathetic fibers originally intended for the salivary glands reinnervating the lacrimal gland.

BOHN'S NODULES   See Epstein's pearls.

BOLTSIEAUSER SYNDROME   This syndrome is characterized by (1) autosomal-dominant inheritance; (2) mild motor neuropathy; (3) vocal cord paralysis; and (4) sensorineural hearing loss.

BONES OF BERTIN   Scroll-like bones (sphenoid concha) at the base of the sphenoid osteum.

BONNET SYNDROME   Tic douloureux and Horner's syndrome.

BONNIER'S SYNDROME   This syndrome is caused by a lesion of Deiters' nucleus and its connection. Its symptoms include ocular disturbances, deafness, thirst, anorexia, as well as other symptoms referable to involvement of the vagal centers, cranial nerves VIII, IX, X, and XI, and the lateral vestibular nucleus.

BOROUD SYNDROME   This disorder is characterized by (1) maternal (mitochondrial) inheritance; (2) ataxia; (3) cardiomyopathy; (4) mitochondrial myopathy; (5) myoclonic jerks; (6) peripheral neuropathy; (7) pigmentary retinopathy; and (8) sensorineural hearing loss.

BOURNEVILLE-PRINGLE SYNDROME   Eponym for tuberous sclerosis, a neurocutaneous disease characterized by epilepsy, mental retardation, and adenoma sebaceum of the face and oral mucosa.

BOWEN'S DISEASE   A variant of squamous cell cancer characterized by a full-thickness dysplasia of the epidermis. It is by definition noninvasive, but it can progress to invasive carcinoma. Its appearance is that of a red, scaly patch in sun-exposed areas, which can be confused with psoriasis.

BRANCHIO-OCULO-FACIAL (BOF) SYNDROME   The syndrome is characterized by (1) autosomal-dominant inheritance; (2) cleft lip and/or palate or pseudocleft of the upper lip; (3) nasolacrimal duct obstruction; (4) prematurely gray hair; (5) cervical thymus; (6) malformed pinnae; and (7) conductive hearing loss.

BRANCHIO-OTO-RENAL (BOR) SYNDROME   Characteristics of this syndrome include (1) autosomal-dominant transmission with variable expressivity; (2) unilateral or bilateral preauricular pits; (3) unilateral or bilateral bronchial fistulas; (4) hearing loss that may be sensorineural, conductive, or mixed; (5) anomalies of the external ear; and (6) renal abnormalities of varying severity.

BRANCHIO-OTO-URETERAL SYNDROME   Characteristics of this syndrome include (1) autosomal-dominant inheritance; (2) duplication of the renal collecting system; (3) a preauricular pit or tag; and (4) mild to severe unilateral or bilateral sensorineural hearing loss.

BRIQUET'S SYNDROME   Briquet's syndrome is characterized by a shortness of breath and aphonia due to hysterical paralysis of the diaphragm.

BRISSAUD-MARIE SYNDROME   Hysterical unilateral paralysis or spasm of the tongue and lips.

BROWN-SÉQUARD SYNDROME   Transverse myelopathy.

BROWN-VIALETTO–VAN LAERE SYNDROME   This disorder is characterized by (1) probably autosomal-dominant inheritance; (2) pontobulbar paralysis; (3) motor neuron disease, predominantly affecting the cervical cord; and (4) sensorineural hearing loss.

BROWN'S SIGN   Blanching of a red or blue mass juxtaposing the tympanic membrane when air pressure is applied by pneumo-otoscopy. It is indicative of a glomus tympanicum tumor.

BROYLE'S LIGAMENT   Anterior commissure ligament of the larynx.

BRUDZINSKI'S SIGN   Flexion movement of the neck produces flexion movement of the knee, hip, and ankle due to meningeal irritation.

BRUNNER'S ABSCESS   Abscess of the posterior floor of the mouth.

BRUNS' SYNDROME   Vertigo, headache, vomiting, and visual disturbances due to an obstruction of cerebrospinal fluid (CSF) flow during positional changes of the head. Obstruction of the ventricular system due to mass lesions or inflammatory changes are implicated.

Burckhardt's dermatitis An eruption of the external ear consisting of red papules and vesicles that appear after exposure to sunlight. The rash usually resolves spontaneously.

Burton's line A dark line that follows the margins of the gingiva. It is caused by the deposition of insoluble lead sulfide in the capillary endothelial cells and histiocytes. Burton's line is not seen in edentulous patients.

Caffey's disease (infantile cortical hyperostosis) It is characterized by hyperirritability, fever, and hard nonpitting edema that overlies the cortical hyperostosis. Pathologically, it involves the loss of periosteum with acute inflammatory involvement of the intratrabecular bone and the overlying soft tissue. Treatment is supportive, consisting of steroids and antibiotics. The mandible is the most frequently involved site.

Caisson disease Failure to equilibrate pressure when there is a rapid change in environmental pressure related to body tissue and fluid dynamic pressure. Nitrogen bubbles may encapsulate within the cardiopulmonary system leading to pain, headache, vertigo, dizziness, and in rare occurrence, circulatory collapse.

Caldwell-Luc procedure Traditional external approach in creating a maxillary antrostomy.

Campbell-Clifton syndrome This disorder is characterized by (1) autosomal-dominant inheritance; (2) meningitic migraine; (3) arthropathy; (4) chorioretinitis; (5) rash; and (6) sensorineural hearing loss—all possibly related to peripheral arterial disease.

Camptomelic syndrome Characteristics include (1) autosomal-recessive inheritance; (2) relatively frequent sex reversal; (3) frequent lethality; (4) bent femora and tibiae; (5) conductive hearing loss; and (6) craniofacial anomalies.

Camurati-Engelmann syndrome The characteristics of the condition include (1) autosomal-dominant inheritance; (2) sclerosis and hyperostosis of skull and long bones; (3) weakness and reduction in muscle mass; (4) leg pain and abnormal gait; and (5) mixed hearing loss and vestibular disturbances.

Canal of Huguier The space within the petrotympanic fissure containing the chordae tympani nerve.

Cannon's nevus An autosomal-dominant disorder characterized by asymptomatic white nevoid lesions of the oral mucosa. The lesions are found from the newborn period until adolescence and do not require treatment.

Carcinoid syndrome A constellation of vasomotor and neurogenic symptoms including flushing, tachyarrhythmia, and ascites resultant from a neuroendocrine tumor that can secrete serotonin. The tumor may give a positive dihydroxyphenylalanine (DOPA) reaction on immunochemical analysis.

Carotid sinus syndrome (Charcot-Weiss-Baker syndrome) When the carotid sinus is abnormally sensitive, pressure may cause a paroxysmal fall in blood pressure due to vasodilation and cardiac slowing.

Carraro syndrome Characteristics include (1) probable autosomal-recessive inheritance; (2) significant shortening of the tibiae; and (3) congenital profound hearing loss.

Cavernous sinus syndrome Cavernous sinus syndrome results from obstruction of the cavernous sinus due most commonly to tumor or infection. Symptoms include orbital pain with venous congestion of the retina, lids, and conjunctiva. The eyes are proptosed with exophthalmos. The patient has photophobia and involvement of nerves III, IV, V, and VI.

Cestan-Chenais syndrome Occlusion of the vertebral artery below the posterior-inferior cerebellar artery (PICA), resulting in ipsilateral paralysis of the soft palate, larynx, and pharynx associated with cerebellar dysfunction and Horner's syndrome.

Champion-Gregah-Klein syndrome A familial syndrome associated with popliteal webbing, cleft lip, cleft palate, lower lip fistula, syndactyly, onychodysplasia, and pes equinovarus.

CHAPPLE'S SYNDROME Unilateral facial weakness or paralysis seen in the newborn, in conjunction with weakness or paralysis of the contralateral vocal cord and/or muscles of deglutition due to lateral flexion of the head in utero, injuring the recurrent or superior laryngeal nerve, or both.

CHARCOT-MARIE-TOOTH SYNDROME This disorder is characterized by (1) autosomal-dominant inheritance; (2) hereditary motor and sensory neuropathy; and (3) sensorineural hearing loss.

CHARGE ASSOCIATION CHARGE: C, coloboma; H, heart defects; A, atresia of chonae; R, retarded growth and development; G, genital hypoplasia; E, ear anomalies and/or deafness. Some patients with manifestations of the VATER association (V, vertebral defects; A, imperforate anus; T, tracheoesophageal fistula; R, radial and renal dysplasia) have features that overlap with the CHARGE association.

CHÉDIAK-HIGASHI SYNDROME Autosomal-recessive syndrome of granulocyte defects, partial albinism, photophobia, and abnormalities in platelet and coagulation function.

CHIME SYNDROME CHIME: C, coloboma; H, heart defect; I, ichthyosis; M, mental retardation; E, ear anomalies.

CHONDRODYSPLASIA, TYPE KHALDI Retinitis pigmentosa and marked sensorineural hearing loss.

CHONDRODYSPLASIA, TYPE NANCE-SWEENEY Slowly progressive mixed hearing loss, more severe at high frequencies.

CHONDRODYSPLASIA, TYPE TEMTAMY Severe congenital hearing loss.

CHVOSTEK'S SIGN Tapping over the facial nerve results in spasm of the facial muscles in tetany.

COCKAYNE SYNDROME This disorder is characterized by (1) autosomal-recessive inheritance; (2) severe growth failure; (3) mental retardation; (4) dementia; (5) spastic quadriplegia; (6) ataxia; (7) motor and sensory neuropathy; (8) pigmentary retinopathy; (9) optic atrophy; (10) cataracts; (11) photodermatitis; (12) decreased subcutaneous tissue; (13) abnormal facial appearance;

(14) defective DNA repair; and (15) sensorineural hearing loss.

COFFIN-LOWRY SYNDROME Characteristics include (1) X-linked inheritance with milder expression in female heterozygotes; (2) characteristic facies; (3) short stature; (4) large soft hands; (5) pectus and scoliosis; (6) variable mental retardation; and (7) sensorineural hearing loss.

COGAN'S SYNDROME Nonsyphilitic interstitial keratitis with vestibular and auditory symptoms of probable autoimmune etiology.

COLLET-SICARD SYNDROME Similar to Villaret's syndrome in the absence of Horner's syndrome.

COOPER-JABS SYNDROME Characteristics of this syndrome include (1) autosomal-recessive transmission; (2) bilateral auricular deformities; (3) associated physical findings of short stature, developmental delay, ventriculoseptal defect, and anterior placement of the anus; (4) atresia of the external auditory meatus; and (5) mixed hearing loss.

COPPETO-LESSELL SYNDROME This disorder is characterized by (1) autosomal-recessive inheritance; (2) dystonia including blepharospasm; (3) pigmentary retinopathy; (4) possible dementia; and sometimes (5) sensorineural hearing loss.

COSTEN SYNDROME A symptom complex consisting of pain in the temporomandibular joint (TMJ) area, hemicranial pain, tinnitus, and vertigo.

COTTLE'S SIGN Movement of the cheek draws the upper lateral cartilage outward, relieving nasal obstruction due to collapse of the nasal valve.

CRI DU CHAT SYNDROME Characteristics include mental retardation, respiratory stridor, microcephaly, hypertelorism, midline oral clefts, and laryngomalacia with poor approximation of the posterior vocal cords.

CROUZON SYNDROME Characteristics include (1) autosomal-dominant inheritance; (2) premature variable craniosynostosis; (3) ocular hypertelorism, midface hypoplasia, and ocular proptosis; (4) variable mandibular prognathism; (5) atresia of auditory canals in about 15%; and (6) conductive hearing loss in about 50%.

CRUSE SYNDROME This syndrome consists of (1) autosomal-dominant inheritance; (2) motor and sensory neuropathy (most similar to hereditary motor and sensory neuropathy [HMSN] type 1) with onset in childhood; (3) trigeminal neuralgia; and (4) sensorineural hearing loss.

CRYPTOPHTHALMUS SYNDROME (FRASER SYNDROME) Cryptophthalmos syndrome is characterized by (1) autosomal-recessive inheritance; (2) unilateral or more often bilateral extension of skin of the forehead to completely cover the eye or eyes; (3) variable soft tissue syndactyly of fingers and/or toes; (4) coloboma of nasal alae; (5) various urogenital anomalies; and (6) mixed hearing loss and atresia of external auditory canals.

CURTIUS SYNDROME Hypertrophy of one entire side of the body or a single part. When it occurs in the face, it is known as congenital hemifacial hypertrophy.

DANDY SYNDROME Oscillopsia caused by bilateral loss of vestibular function.

DAVENPORT SYNDROME The major phenotypic features include (1) autosomal-dominant inheritance; (2) hypopigmentation of skin, hair, and eyes; (3) joint contractures; (4) psoriasiform lesions of the skin; (5) abnormal chemotaxis, and (6) sensorineural hearing loss with onset in early childhood.

DEJEAN SYNDROME Characterized by exophthalmos, diplopia, superior maxillary pain, and numbness along the route of the trigeminal nerve. It is classically caused by a nasal tumor that involves the pterygopalatine fossa and floor of the orbit.

DEJERINE'S ANTERIOR BULBAR SYNDROME Thrombosis of the anterior spinal artery resulting in either an alternating hypoglossal hemiplegia or an alternating hypoglossal hemianesthetic hemiplegia.

DELPHIAN NODE Cricothyroid lymph node, suggesting extralaryngeal spread of carcinoma.

DEMARQUAY-RICHET SYNDROME Characteristics include cleft lip, cleft palate, lower lip fistulas, and progeria facies. Defective dentition, heart defects, dwarfism, and digital abnormalities may be seen.

DE QUERVAIN'S DISEASE Subacute thyroiditis.

DIDMOAD SYNDROME An autosomal-recessive disorder including *diabetes insipidus*, *diabetes mellitus*, *optic atrophy*, and *deafness*.

DIGEORGE SYNDROME This condition is characterized by (1) various chromosomal and single gene disorders; (2) hypoplasia or aplasia of parathyroid glands and thymus; (3) interrupted aortic arch or truncus arteriosus; and (4) conductive hearing loss.

DOWN SYNDROME (TRISOMY 21) Hearing loss is variable and is reflected by conductive, sensorineural, and mixed hearing loss. Other common craniofacial abnormalities include macroglossia, narrow ear canals, epicanthus, and broadened nasal bridge.

DYCK SYNDROME This disorder is characterized by (1) autosomal or X-linked recessive inheritance; (2) motor and sensory neuropathy; (3) adrenocortical insufficiency; (4) hepatosplenomegaly; (5) optic atrophy; (6) pigmentary retinopathy; and (7) sensorineural hearing loss.

DYSPHAGIA LUSORIA This condition is secondary to an abnormal right subclavian artery. The right subclavian arises abnormally from the thoracic aorta by passing behind or in front of the esophagus, causing compressive symptoms.

EAGLE'S SYNDROME An elongated styloid process causes dysphagia, otalgia, and a foreign body sensation in the throat.

ECTODERMAL DYSPLASIA An x-linked recessive syndrome consisting of hypodontia, hypotrichosis, and hypohidrosis. Aplasia of the eccrine sweat glands may lead to severe hyperpyrexia.

EDWARDS SYNDROME Characteristics of the syndrome include (1) autosomal-recessive inheritance; (2) onset in infancy of nystagmus, photophobia, and progressive blindness; (3) developmental delay and mild to moderate mental retardation; (4) childhood-onset obesity; (5) sometimes acanthosis nigricans, diabetes mellitus, and male hypogonadism; and (6) onset in late childhood of progressive sensorineural hearing loss.

EHLERS-DANLOS SYNDROME (GENERAL) A collagen disorder with multiple system involvement.

EHLERS-DANLOS SYNDROME (VARIANT VI) The characteristics of the syndrome include (1) autosomal-recessive inheritance; (2) keratoconus or keratoglobus with thin, fragile cornea; (3) blue sclerae; (4) loose ligaments; and (5) mixed hearing loss.

18Q-SYNDROME This syndrome consists of psychomotor retardation, hypotonia, short stature, microcephaly, hypoplastic midface, epicanthus, ophthalmologic abnormalities, cleft palate, congenital heart disease, abnormalities of the genitalia, tapered fingers, aural atresia, and conductive hearing loss.

EISENLOHR'S SYNDROME Numbness and weakness in the extremities associated with paralysis of the lips, tongue, and palate.

ELSCHING'S SYNDROME Extension of the palpebral fissure laterally, displacement of the lateral canthus, ectropion of the lower lid, and lateral canthus are observed. Hypertelorism, cleft palate, and cleft lip are commonly described.

EMPTY SELLA SYNDROME Primary empty sella syndrome is due to the congenital absence of the diaphragm sella, with gradual enlargement of the sella secondary to pulsations of the brain. Secondary empty sella syndrome may be due to necrosis of the pituitary due to surgery, radiation therapy, or pseudotumor.

EPSTEIN SYNDROME Epstein syndrome is characterized by (1) autosomal-dominant inheritance; (2) nephropathy similar to classic Alport syndrome; (3) giant platelets with thrombocytopenia; and (4) moderate to severe sensorineural loss.

EPSTEIN'S PEARLS Multiple small white keratin nodules on the palate and oral mucosa of newborns.

ESCHERICH'S SIGN Action of protrusion of the lips caused by percussion of the inner surface of the lips or tongue. It is seen in hypoparathyroidism.

EWALD'S LAW (OF CANAL FUNCTION) Based on the application of positive and negative pressures to each semicircular canal membrane to cause ampullopetal or ampullofugal endolymph flow, the following observations may be noted: (1) the eye and head movement occur in the plane of the canal being stimulated and the direction of endolymph flow; (2) ampullopetal endolymph flow in the horizontal canal causes a greater response than does ampullofugal flow; and (3) ampullofugal endolymph flow in the vertical canals causes a greater response than ampullopetal flow.

FABRY DISEASE The characteristics of this syndrome include (1) X-linked inheritance with partial expression in female carriers; (2) cutaneous angiokeratomata; (3) paresthesia or burning pain in fingers and toes; (4) cataracts; and (5) high-tone sensorineural hearing loss.

FACIOSCAPULOHUMERAL MUSCULAR DYSTROPHY This disorder is characterized by (1) autosomal-dominant inheritance with high penetrance and marked variability in expression; (2) weakness in face and shoulder girdle with spread to other muscle groups; (3) retinal telangiectasia; (4) occasional mental retardation; and (5) sensorineural hearing loss.

FANCONI'S ANEMIA Aplastic anemia with skin pigmentation, skeletal deformities, renal anomalies, and mental retardation. The disorder rarely occurs in adults. The bleeding time is prolonged, the platelet count is decreased, and the bone marrow megakaryocytes vary from decreased to absent.

FECTNER SYNDROME The syndrome is characterized by (1) autosomal-dominant inheritance; (2) nephropathy in males that is more variable than in classic Alport syndrome; (3) giant platelets with thrombocytopenia; (4) leukocyte inclusion, which is characteristic for this syndrome; and (5) mild to moderate sensorineural hearing loss.

FELTY'S SYNDROME Leukopenia, arthritis, splenomegaly, and enlarged lymph nodes.

FIRST AND SECOND BRACHIAL ARCH SYNDROMES (HEMIFACIAL MICROSOMIA, LATERAL FACIAL DYSPLASIA) Craniofacial malformations characterized by asymmetric facies with unilateral abnormalities. Characteristics include hypoplastic mandible or absent ramus and condyle, aural atresia, skin tags from the tragus to the oral commissure, coloboma of the upper eyelid, malar hypoplasia, and cleft palate. Cardiovascular, renal, and nervous system abnormalities have been noted in association with this disorder.

FLYNN-AIRD SYNDROME This disorder is characterized by (1) autosomal-dominant inheritance; (2) ataxia; (3) cataracts; (4) motor and sensory neuropathy that results in neuropathic pain; (5) myopia; (6) pigmentary retinopathy; (7) skeletal abnormalities such as kyphoscoliosis; (8) skin atrophy; and (9) sensorineural hearing loss.

FORDYCE'S DISEASE A developmental anomaly characterized by enlarged, ectopic sebaceous glands (Fordyce's spots) in the oral mucosa. These glands appear as numerous small yellowish-white granules.

FOSTER KENNEDY SYNDROME Anterior (frontal skull base) meningioma produces anosmia and personality changes. As the tumor expands pressure or invasion cause optic atrophy and papilledema.

FOTHERGILL'S DISEASE Tic douloureaux and angiose scarlatina.

FOVILLE SYNDROME Facial paralysis, para abducens paralysis causing loss of conjugate gaze, and contralateral hemiplegia.

FREY'S SYNDROME (AURICULOTEMPORAL SYNDROME) Following parotidectomy parasympathetic reinnervation causes an aberrant innervation of the sweat glands. When a stimulus for salivary flow occurs, sweating over the anterior skin flap area also occurs.

FRIEDRICH'S ATAXIA This disorder is characterized by (1) autosomal-recessive inheritance; (2) onset before 25 years of age; (3) progressive ataxia; (4) absent tendon reflexes in legs; and (5) mild motor and sensory neuropathy. Later manifestations include (6) mild spastic diplegia; (7) scoliosis; (8) infrequent optic atrophy; and (9) infrequent sensorineural hearing loss.

GARCIN'S SYNDROME Paralysis of cranial nerves III to X due to extensive invasion of nasopharyngeal or retropharyngeal tumors.

GARD-GIGNOIX SYNDROME Cranial nerve X and XI paralysis due to a lesion below the jugular foramen.

GARDNER'S SYNDROME Characterized by multiple osteomas that develop in the skull and facial bones, including the mandible. It is an autosomal-dominant disease; other symptoms include multiple epidermoid cysts of the skin and polyposis of the colon and rectum. There is a tendency for these polyps to become malignant.

GEMIGNANI SYNDROME The syndrome is manifested by (1) autosomal or X-linked recessive inheritance; (2) ataxia; (3) localized amyotrophy of hands; (4) spastic paraparesis; (5) hypogonadism; (6) short stature; and (7) sensorineural hearing loss.

GERNET SYNDROME Characteristics of this syndrome include (1) autosomal-dominant transmission; (2) progressive optic atrophy; and (3) congenital, generally severe, sensorineural hearing loss.

GILLES DE LA TOURETTE'S SYNDROME See Tourette's Syndrome.

GLANDS OF EBNER Minor salivary glands in the posterior part of the tongue near the circumvallate papillae.

GOLDENHAR SYNDROME The syndrome is characterized by (1) usually sporadic but rare autosomal-dominant inheritance (1 to 2% of cases); (2) anomalies of aural, oral, and mandibular development, generally unilateral but occasionally bilateral, and of varying severity; (3) congenital heart defects; (4) anomalies of cervical spine; (5) mental retardation in 5 to 15% of cases; and (6) conductive or occasionally sensorineural hearing loss.

GORDON'S SYNDROME This disorder is characterized by (1) autosomal-recessive or X-linked inheritance; (2) spastic quadriparesis; (3) both mental retardation and dementia; (4) optic atrophy; (5) pigmentary retinopathy; and (6) sensorineural hearing loss.

GRADENIGO'S SYNDROME   Suppurative otitis followed by pain in the distribution of the ophthalmic branch of the trigeminal nerve and paralysis of the abducens nerve caused by an extradural abscess involving the petrous apex.

GRIESINGER'S SIGN   Thrombophlebitis of the mastoid emissary veins resulting in pain and edema over the mastoid.

GRISEL'S DISEASE   Atlantoaxial dislocation secondary to infection. Tonsillectomy, sinus pathology, or nasopharyngeal infection may antedate the process.

GROLL-HIRSCHOWITZ SYNDROME   This syndrome is characterized by (1) autosomal-recessive inheritance; (2) sensory and autonomic neuropathy; (3) cardiac rhythm disturbances due to loss of autonomic regulation; (4) intestinal pseudo-obstruction; (5) small bowel diverticulitis; and (6) sensorineural hearing loss.

GUILLAIN-BARRÉ SYNDROME   Polyneuritis of probable viral etiology causing marked paresthesias of the limbs, muscular weakness, or a flaccid paralysis.

HAJDU-CHENEY SYNDROME   Characteristics include (1) autosomal-dominant inheritance; (2) dissolution of terminal phalanges; (3) dolichocephaly with occipital prominence; (4) short stature; (5) premature loss of teeth; and (6) conductive or sensorineural hearing loss.

HALLER CELL   The expansion of ethmoid cells along the orbital floor into the medial and posterosuperior aspect of the maxillary sinus.

HALLERMANN-STREIFF SYNDROME   Characteristics include (1) hypoplastic mandible; (2) brachycephaly; (3) a characteristic beak-like nose (parrot-nose); and (4) hypotrichosis.

HARBOYAN SYNDROME   Major features of this syndrome include (1) autosomal-recessive inheritance; (2) congenital corneal dystrophy with slow progression; and (3) childhood onset of slowly progressive sensorineural hearing loss.

HEERFORDT'S SYNDROME   Uveoparotid fever associated with sarcoidosis.

HEFTER-GANZ SYNDROME   Characteristics include (1) autosomal-dominant inheritance; (2)

meatal atresia; and (3) hearing loss, largely conductive.

HENNEBERT'S SIGN   A positive fistula test resulting in vertigo with or without nystagmus with the application of either positive or negative pneumatic pressure to the tympanic membrane.

HERRMANN'S SYNDROME   This disorder is manifested by (1) probably maternal (mitochondrial inheritance); (2) progressive myoclonic epilepsy; (3) ataxia; (4) dementia; (5) diabetes mellitus; (6) nephropathy; (7) possible neuropathy; and (8) sensorineural hearing loss.

HERSH SYNDROME   Characteristics of this syndrome include (1) autosomal-recessive inheritance; (2) mental retardation; (3) unusual facies; (4) pigmentary retinopathy; (5) mild hypogonadism; (6) hypotonia; and (7) marked sensorineural hearing loss.

HESS-OPITZ SYNDROME   This disorder is characterized by (1) x-linked recessive inheritance; (2) mental retardation; (3) multiple congenital anomalies; (4) growth deficiency; (5) spastic quadriplegia; (6) visual loss; (7) susceptibility to neoplasia, especially hematologic; (8) increased chromosomal breakage; and (9) hearing loss.

HICK'S SYNDROME   This disorder is characterized by (1) autosomal-dominant inheritance; (2) sensory and autonomic neuropathy; (3) dementia; and (4) sensorineural hearing loss.

HIPPEL-LINDAU DISEASE   Angioma of the cerebellum, usually cystic, associated with like lesions of the retina and polycystic kidneys.

HIXLER SYNDROME   The characteristic features of the syndrome include (1) autosomal-recessive inheritance; (2) microtia and meatal atresia; (3) ocular hypertelorism; (4) cleft lip and palate; (5) renal anomalies; (6) growth retardation; and (7) conductive hearing loss.

HOLLANDER SYNDROME   Appearance of a goiter during the third decade of life related to a partial defect in the coupling mechanism in thyroxine biosynthesis. Deafness due to cochlear abnormalities is usually related.

HOLMES-SCHEPENS SYNDROME   The syndrome is characterized by (1) autosomal-recessive inheritance; (2) hypertelorism and prominent brows; (3) myopia, choroidal atrophy, cataract, iris stroma hypoplasia, and possibly retinal detachment; and (4) congenital profound sensorineural hearing loss.

HOMOCYSTINURIA A recessive hereditary syndrome secondary to a defect in methionine metabolism with resultant homocystinemia, mental retardation, and sensorineural hearing loss.

HORNER'S SYNDROME Ptosis, miosis, anhidrosis, and enophthalmos due to paralysis of the cervical sympathetic nerves.

HORTON'S NEURALGIA Classic cluster headache.

HUTCHINSON'S TEETH Characterized by small and widely spaced permanent, not deciduous teeth (especially the upper incisors) with notches on their biting surfaces. It is a characteristic sign of congenital syphilis.

HYPERPHOSPHATASEMIA (JUVENILE PAGET'S DISEASE) Characteristics include (1) autosomal-recessive inheritance; (2) fever, bone pain, and selling during early years; (3) enlargement of the calvaria; (4) frequent pseudoxanthoma elasticum; (5) radiographic changes similar to those of Paget's disease; (6) elevated serum alkaline and acid phosphatase; and (7) progressive mixed hearing loss.

IMMOTILE CELIA SYNDROME A congenital defect in the ultrastructure of cilia that renders them incapable of movement. Clinical manifestations include bronchiectasis, sinusitis, male sterility, situs inversus, and otitis media.

IVIC (INSTITUTE VENEZOLANA DE INVESTIGACIONES CIENTIFICAS) SYNDROME A syndrome of radial ray hypoplasia, external ophthalmoplegia, thrombocytopenia, and congenital mixed hearing loss.

JACKSON SYNDROME Paralysis of cranial nerves X, XI, and XII due to nuclear or radicular lesions.

JACOBSON'S NERVE The tympanic branch of the ninth cranial nerve, which supplies sensory fibers to the mucosa of the middle ear; running with it are preganglionic parasympathetic fibers that leave the middle ear as the lesser superficial petrosal nerve to eventually innervate the parotid.

JACOD'S SYNDROME Total ophthalmoplegia, optic tract lesions with unilateral amaurosis, and trigeminal neuralgia. It is caused by a middle cranial fossa tumor involving cranial nerves II through VI.

JENSEN SYNDROME This disorder is characterized by (1) X-linked recessive inheritance; (2) optic atrophy; (3) dementia; and (4) profound sensorineural hearing loss.

JEQUIER-DEONNA SYNDROME This disorder is characterized by (1) autosomal-recessive inheritance; (2) optic atrophy; (3) polyneuropathy in the teen years; and (4) progressive sensorineural hearing loss in childhood accompanied by (5) vestibular dysfunction.

JERVELL AND LANGE-NIELSEN SYNDROME The major features of this syndrome include (1) autosomal-recessive transmission; (2) prolonged electrocardiographic Q-T intervals; (3) recurrent Stokes-Adams attacks beginning in early childhood and occasionally resulting in sudden death; and (4) congenital severe sensorineural hearing loss.

JEUNE-TOMMASI SYNDROME This disorder is characterized by (1) autosomal-recessive inheritance; (2) progressive ataxia; (3) childhood-onset dementia; (4) myocardial fibrosis associated with cardiac conduction abnormalities; (5) skin pigmentary changes; (6) possible retinitis pigmentosa; and (7) sensorineural hearing loss.

JOB'S SYNDROME This syndrome is one of the group of hyperimmunoglobulin E (IgE) syndromes that are associated with defective chemotaxis. The clinical picture includes (1) fair skin; (2) red hair; (3) recurrent staphylococcal skin abscesses; and (4) chronic purulent pulmonary infections.

KALLMANN SYNDROME The syndrome is characterized by (1) genetic heterogeneity; (2) hypogonadism; (3) anosmia; (4) occasionally cleft lip or palate; and (5) sensorineural occasionally mixed, hearing loss.

KAPOSI'S SARCOMA Recently associated with human immunodeficiency virus (HIV) infection, patients have multiple idiopathic, hemorrhagic sarcomatosis, particularly of the skin and viscera.

KARTAGENER'S SYNDROME Characteristics include (1) complete situs inversus associated with (2) chronic sinusitis and (3) bronchiectasis.

KEARNS-SAYRE SYNDROME This disorder is characterized by (1) sporadic occurrence or maternal (mitochondrial) inheritance; (2) progressive external ophthalmoplegia and ptosis; (3) atypical pigmentary retinopathy; (4) mitochondrial myopathy with ragged-red fibers; (5) ataxia; (6) mental retardation or dementia; (7) cardiac conduction defects; (8) growth deficiency; (9) delayed sexual development; (10) vestibular abnormalities; (11) elevated cerebrospinal fluid (CSF) protein; and (12) sensorineural hearing loss.

KEIPERT SYNDROME Characteristics include (1) autosomal or X-linked recessive inheritance; (2) unusual facies; (3) broad terminal phalanges; and (4) sensorineural hearing loss.

KELLIAN'S AREA Area of muscular weakness in the posterior pharyngeal wall juxtaposing the cricopharyngeus muscle resulting in a hypopharyngeal diverticulum (Zenker's).

KEUTEL SYNDROME Characteristics include (1) autosomal-recessive inheritance; (2) brachytelephalangy; (3) calcification and/or ossification of cartilages of nose, auricles, trachea, bronchi, and ribs; (4) multiple peripheral pulmonary stenoses; (5) recurrent otitis media, sinusitis, and bronchitis; and (6) mixed hearing loss.

KIESSELBACH'S PLEXUS An area in the anterior septum in which the capillaries merge. It is often the site of anterior epistaxis. It also has been referred to as Little's area.

KILLIAN-JAMESON SPACE Area between the cricopharyngeus and the upper esophagus that may result in Zenker's diverticulum.

KLEINSCHMIDT'S SYNDROME Symptoms include influenzal infections resulting in (1) laryngeal stenosis; (2) suppurative pericarditis; (3) pleuropneumonia; and (4) occasionally meningitis.

KLINKERT'S SYNDROME Paralysis of the recurrent and phrenic nerves due to a neoplastic process in the root of the neck or upper mediastinum. It can be a part of Pancoast's syndrome.

KNIEST DYSPLASIA Characteristics include (1) autosomal-dominant inheritance; (2) disproportionate short stature; (3) round flattened face with short neck; (4) enlarged stiff joints; (5) myopia; (6) spondyloepimetaphyseal bone dysplasia; (7) cleft palate; and (8) mixed hearing loss.

KOPLIK'S SPOTS Pale round spots on the oral mucosa and conjunctiva that are seen in the early stages of measles.

KÖRNER'S SEPTUM A remnant of the petrosquamous suture line, which may persist as a plate of bone separating the central tract of mastoid air cells from the antrum.

KRABBE DISEASE Characteristics of this syndrome include (1) severe spasticity; (2) optic atrophy; (3) profound deafness; and (4) autosomal-recessive inheritance.

KRAUSE'S NODES Lymph nodes in the region of the jugular foramen.

LADD SYNDROME (LEVY-HOLLISTER SYNDROME) The syndrome is characterized by (1) autosomal-dominant inheritance; (2) cup-shaped ears; (3) nasolacrimal duct obstruction and hypoplasia of the lacrimal puncta, with occasional lack of tear formation; (4) various preaxial ray/radial anomalies; (5) peg-shaped or missing teeth with mild amelogenesis imperfecta; and (6) mixed hearing loss with a large sensorineural component.

LANGER'S LINES Tension lines in the skin.

LARSEN SYNDROME This syndrome is characterized by (1) flat facies; (2) multiple congenital joint dislocations; and (3) frequently cleft palate. Hearing loss is uncommon but has been reported to be conductive, mixed, or sensorineural.

LATHAM-MUNRO SYNDROME This disorder is characterized by (1) autosomal-recessive inheritance; (2) progressive myoclonic epilepsy; (3) dementia; and (4) profound congenital sensorineural hearing loss.

LEMIEUX-NEEMEH SYNDROME The syndrome is characterized by (1) probable autosomal-dominant inheritance with variable expression and incomplete penetrance; (2) nephropathy consisting of nephrotic syndrome; (3) progressive neuropathy similar to heredity motor and sensory neuropathy, type I (Charcot-Marie-Tooth syndrome); and (4) variable presence of sensorineural hearing loss beginning in childhood.

LENZ-MAJEWSKI SYNDROME Characteristics include (1) macrocephaly; (2) loose skin and prominent veins; (3) progressive sclerosis of skull; (4) mental retardation; and (5) hearing loss.

LEOPARD SYNDROME LEOPARD is an acronym for the following phenotypic features: *l*entigines, *e*lectrocardiographic defects, *o*cular hypertelorism, *p*ulmonary stenosis, *a*bnormalities of genitalia, *r*etardation of growth, and sensorineural *d*eafness.

LERMOYEZ SYNDROME Paroxysmal attacks of tinnitus and loss of auditory acuity followed by vertigo that often relieves the vestibuloacoustic symptoms. It is considered a Meniere's variant.

LICHTENSTEIN-KNORR SYNDROME This syndrome is characterized by (1) autosomal-recessive inheritance; (2) ataxia; (3) scoliosis and pes cavus, and (4) sensorineural hearing loss.

LÖFFLER'S SYNDROME Pneumonitis characterized by eosinophilic infiltration.

LOUIS-BAR SYNDROME Characterized by ataxia during early childhood associated with telangiectasias of the orbit, face, or neck. It is better known as ataxia-telangiectasia. Affected patients lack immunoglobulin A (IgA) and often have recurrent pulmonary and sinus infections.

LUDWIG'S ANGINA Submandibular space infection that penetrates the mylohyoid muscle to invade the submaxillary space and neck.

MADELUNG'S DEFORMITY Deformity of the distal radius, ulna, and proximal carpal bones associated with mesomeric dwarfism and bilateral conductive hearing loss.

MAFFUCCI SYNDROME Cavernous hemangiomas of the head and neck. Affected patients also have multiple end chondromas with the potential for malignant transformation.

MANDIBULOFACIAL DYSOSTOSIS (TREACHER COLLINS SYNDROME) Facial abnormalities include bilateral, hypoplastic supraorbital rims, and hypoplastic zygomas. The face is narrow. Downward-sloping palpebral fissures, depressed cheekbones, malformed pinnae, receding chin, and a large down-turned mouth are characteristic. The palpebral fissures are short and slope laterally downward and, often (75%) there is a coloboma in the outer third of the lower lid. Choanal atresia has been reported, and microtia is noted in 60% of cases. Ear tags and blind fistulas may occur anywhere between the tragus and the angle of the mouth. The palate is cleft in about 35%.

MARFAN SYNDROME Marfan syndrome is characterized by (1) arachnodactyly; (2) scoliosis; (3) joint hypermobility; (4) dislocated lenses; and (5) cardiac anomalies. Hearing loss has rarely been associated.

MARIE-STRÜMPELL DISEASE Rheumatoid arthritis of the spine.

MARSHALL SYNDROME Characteristics of this syndrome include (1) autosomal-dominant transmission; (2) short stature; (3) severe myopia; (4) congenital and juvenile cataracts; (5) saddle-nose defect; (6) various skeletal abnormalities; and (7) early-onset progressive moderate sensorineural hearing loss.

MAY-WHITE SYNDROME This syndrome is characterized by (1) autosomal-dominant inheritance; (2) ataxia; (3) myoclonic and other seizures; and (4) sensorineural hearing loss.

MEISSNER PLEXUS Submucous neural plexus containing autonomic fibers to the esophagus.

MELKERSSON-ROSENTHAL SYNDROME Characterized by manifestations in childhood or early adolescence as recurring attacks of unilateral or bilateral facial paralysis with concomitant swelling of the lips and tongue. Affected patients also have a fissured tongue that becomes more prominent with age. Genetically, it is transmitted as an autosomal-dominant disease with variable penetrance.

MELLER SYNDROME (GENEE-WEIDEMANN SYNDROME) The major characteristics of this syndrome include (1) probable autosomal-recessive inheritance; (2) craniofacial dysostosis, including malar hypoplasia with ectropion, long philtrum, micrognathia, and cleft palate; (3) postaxial limb anomalies affecting all four limbs; (4) cupped simple ears; and (5) occasional conductive hearing loss.

MICHEL'S APLASIA   Complete arrest of inner ear development.

MICHEL'S SYNDROME   Characteristics of this condition include (1) autosomal-recessive inheritance; (2) blepharophimosis-ptosis; (3) inverse epicanthus; (4) mental retardation; (5) cleft lip and palate; and (6) mixed hearing loss.

MIDDLE LOBE SYNDROME   This syndrome results from a chronic atelectatic process with fibrosis (bronchiectasis) in one or both segments of the middle lobe. It is most commonly due to obstruction of the middle lobe bronchus by hilar adenopathy.

MIKULICZ DISEASE   Bilateral, recurrent swelling of the lacrimal and salivary glands, resultant from systemic pathology that may be inflammatory or infectious (TB). Pathology shows a diffuse lymphocytic infiltrate.

MIKULICZ'S CELLS   Pathognomonic altered histiocytes with clear empty cytoplasm found in rhinoscleroma.

MILLARD-GUBLER SYNDROME   Lateral rectus palsy and ipsilateral facial paralysis with contralateral hemiplegia.

MÖBIUS SYNDROME   Facial weakness and paralysis associated with extraocular motor disorders.

MONDINI DYSPLASIA   Mondini dysplasia is characterized by one and one-half turns of the bony cochlea forming a common cavity.

MORGAGNI-STEWARD-MOREL SYNDROME   This syndrome occurs in menopausal women and is characterized by obesity, dizziness, psychological disturbances, inverted sleep rhythm, and hyperostosis frontalis interna.

MOTT CELLS   Transformed plasma cells found in scleroma.

MUCKLE-WELLS SYNDROME   Characteristics of this syndrome include (1) autosomal-dominant transmission with variable expressivity; (2) adolescent onset of recurrent episodes of urticaria, fever, and limb and joint pain; (3) amyloidosis resulting in nephropathy and uremia; and (4) childhood onset of progressive sensorineural hearing loss.

MUCOPOLYSACCHARIDOSES (HUNTER SYNDROME, HURLER SYNDROME, HURLER-SCHEIE SYNDROME, MAROTEAU SYNDROME, MORQUIO SYNDROME, SANFILIPPO SYNDROME, SCHEIE SYNDROME, SLY SYNDROME)   In general, the characteristics of these syndromes include (1) autosomal-recessive inheritance, except for mucopolysaccharide (MPS) II (X-linked Hunter syndrome); (2) coarsening of facial features and dysostosis multiplex, except in MPS IV (Morquio syndrome); (3) storage and urinary excretion of one or more specific mucopolysaccharides; and (4) hearing loss, varying in type and degree with the specific mucopolysaccharidosis.

MULTIPLE ENDOCRINE ADENOMATOSIS (MEA)   MEA type IIA Sipple's syndrome is a familial syndrome associated with medullary carcinoma of the thyroid, hyperparathyroidism, and pheochromocytoma. The MEA type II variant consists of multiple mucosal neuromas, pheochromocytoma, medullary carcinoma of the thyroid, and hyperparathyroidism. This syndrome is inherited in an autosomal-dominant pattern.

MUNCHAUSEN'S SYNDROME   Psychiatric patients with dramatic presentation of symptoms with no defined organic pathology.

MYENBURG'S SYNDROME   This syndrome is a disease in which the striated muscles are replaced by fibrosis. Fibrosarcoma rarely occurs.

NAGER ACROFACIAL DYSOSTOSIS SYNDROME   Characteristics of this syndrome include (1) usually sporadic with occasional autosomal-dominant and perhaps autosomal-recessive inheritance; (2) malformations of the external ear; (3) abnormalities of the radial ray, particularly thumb aplasia or hypoplasia and radial aplasia or hypoplasia; (4) characteristic facial appearance with down-slanting palpebral fissures malar and zygomatic hypoplasia, cleft palate, and retromicrognathia; and (5) conductive hearing loss.

NAGER–DE REYNIER SYNDROME   Hypoplasia of the mandible with abnormal implantation of teeth associated with aural atresia.

NATHALIE SYNDROME This disorder is characterized by (1) autosomal-recessive inheritance; (2) spinal muscular atrophy; (3) cardiac conduction abnormalities; (4) cataracts; (5) hypogonadism; (6) osteochondrosis; and (7) sensorineural hearing loss.

NEUROFIBROMATOSIS (VON RECKLINGHAUSEN'S DISEASE) Characteristics of neurofibromatosis (NF) include (1) autosomal-dominant inheritance; (2) bilateral vestibular schwannomas (acoustic neuromas); (3) schwannomas involving other nerves; (4) brain tumors, especially meningiomas and gliomas; (5) juvenile posterior subcapsular cataracts; (6) sometimes café-au-lait spots and subcutaneous neurofibromas (but fewer than in NF-1); and (7) neural hearing loss and altered vestibular function.

NORRIE SYNDROME Characteristics of this syndrome include (1) X-linked recessive transmission; (2) eye changes, including retinal glial proliferation, complicated cataract, and phthisis; (3) mild to severe mental deficiency in about two-thirds of patients; and (4) mild to severe sensorineural hearing loss in about one-third of patients.

NOTHNAGEL SYNDROME Ipsilateral third nerve palsy and contralateral cerebellar ataxia caused by tumors of the midbrain involving the area juxtaposing the red nucleus. The most common cause is a pineal body tumor.

OCULODENTODIGITAL SYNDROME The syndrome is characterized by (1) autosomal-dominant inheritance; (2) typical facies showing thin nose with hypoplastic alae; (3) microcornea; (4) enamel hypoplasia; (5) bilateral camptodactyly and often syndactyly of the fourth and fifth fingers; (6) poor modeling of metaphyseal area of long bones; and (7) conductive hearing loss.

ODINES' CURSE Also known as the alveolar hypoventilation syndrome, it may be associated with increased appetite and transient central diabetes insipidus. Hypothalamic lesions are thought to be the cause of this disorder in which central respiratory apnea occurs.

OHDO SYNDROME The characteristics of this disorder include (1) possible autosomal-recessive inheritance; (2) blepharophimosis-ptosis; (3) mental retardation; (4) dysmorphic pinnae with auricular stenosis; and (5) hearing loss, possibly conductive.

OHNGREN'S LINE Imaginary line drawn between the medial canthus of the eye and angle of the mandible, dividing the maxillary antrum into the infrastructure (anteroinferior) and suprastructure (posterosuperior).

OLIVER'S SIGN A pulling sensation felt in the larynx and trachea due to an aortic arch aneurysm. It is most evident when the head is extended.

ONODI CELL (SPHENOETHMOID CELL) Cellular variation where a posterior ethmoid cell grows laterally around the passage of the optic nerve.

OPJORDSMOEN-NYBERG-HANSEN SYNDROME This disorder is characterized by (1) autosomal-dominant inheritance; (2) spastic paraplegia; (3) syndactyly; and (4) sensorineural hearing loss.

ORAL-FACIAL-DIGITAL SYNDROME, TYPE I Characteristics include (1) X-linked dominant (lethal in the male inheritance); (2) pseudocleft in the midline of the upper lip; (3) mild mental retardation in about 40%; (4) bifid, trifid, or tetrad tongue with hamartomata; (5) asymmetric cleft palate; (6) hyperplastic frenula; (7) various hand anomalies including brachydactyly, clinodactyly, and occasionally polydactyly; (8) adult polycystic disease of kidneys; and (9) occasional decreased hearing.

ORAL-FACIAL-DIGITAL SYNDROME WITH TIBIAL DYSPLASIA, TYPE IV Characteristics include (1) autosomal-recessive inheritance; (2) bifid tongue with hamartomata; (3) mild mental retardation; (4) various digital anomalies; (5) shortened tibiae; and (6) occasional conductive hearing loss.

ORBITAL APEX SYNDROME This syndrome involves the nerves and vessels passing through the superior orbital fissure and the optic foramen with paresis of cranial nerves III, IV, and VI. The optic nerve usually is also involved.

ORTNER SYNDROME A rare cause of hoarseness in infants with congenital cardiac disease. Compression of the left recurrent laryngeal nerve between the aorta and a dilated pulmonary artery results in paralysis of the left vocal cord.

OSLER-WEBER-RENDU DISEASE (HEREDITARY HEM-ORRHAGIC TELANGIECTASIA) Characterized by punctate hemangiomas usually developing around puberty and commonly seen in the oral and nasal mucosa as well as the tongue. Other common sites include the gastrointestinal tract, bladder, and liver. It is inherited as an autosomal-dominant disease.

OSTEOGENESIS IMPERFECTA Osteogenesis imperfecta is a disorder of connective tissue characterized by bone fragility. Associated features variably include blue sclerae, dental abnormalities, hearing loss, deformity of the long bones and spine, and joint hyperextensibility.

OTO-FACIO-CERVICAL SYNDROME The syndrome is characterized by (1) autosomal-dominant inheritance; (2) prominent auricles with deep chordae; (3) preauricular pits; (4) lateral cervical fistulas; (5) hypoplasia and weakness of the cervical musculature with abnormal range of movement at the shoulders; (6) characteristic radiographic abnormalities; and (7) moderate to severe conductive hearing loss.

OTOPALATODIGITAL SYNDROME The characteristics of this condition include (1) X-linked inheritance with expression in many female heterozygotes; (2) characteristic facies having large supraorbital ridges, broad nasal bridge, downslanting palpebral fissures; (3) cleft palate; (4) subluxation of radial heads; (5) wide space between abbreviated halluces and the other toes; (6) other radiographic changes; and (7) conductive hearing loss.

PAGET'S DISEASE Characteristics include (1) onset in middle age; (2) macrocephaly; (3) bending of weight-bearing bones; (4) involvement of sacrum, pelvis, vertebrae, long bones, and skull; (5) neurologic deficits and/or spinal cord compression; (6) elevated alkaline phosphatase; and (7) mixed hearing loss.

PANCOAST SYNDROME Tumor in the apex of the lung that eventually invades the brachial plexus causing sensory symptoms in the upper extremity. Horner's syndrome, indicating involvement of the cervical sympathetic chain, may also be present.

PARINAUD SYNDROME Bilateral palsy of the third and fourth nerves, leading to decreased upward gaze and ptosis. It is caused by compression of the nuclei of the third and fourth nerves in the tectum and is most frequently due to intracranial tumors.

PATERSON–BROWN KELLY SYNDROME See Plummer-Vinson syndrome.

PAULI SYNDROME This disorder is characterized by (1) autosomal-dominant inheritance; (2) motor and sensory neuropathy; (3) pigmentary retinopathy; and (4) sensorineural hearing loss.

PENDRED SYNDROME Characteristics of this syndrome include (1) autosomal-recessive transmission; (2) goiter developing in most cases prior to adolescence; (3) positive perchlorate discharge test; (4) symmetric, generally severe, congenital sensorineural hearing loss; and (5) frequent disturbed vestibular function.

PERRAULT SYNDROME Characteristics include (1) autosomal-recessive inheritance; (2) primary amenorrhea and streak gonads; (3) deficiency of breast and pubic hair; (4) elevated urinary gonadotropins; (5) sensorineural hearing loss as the only expression in males; and (6) possibly diminished vestibular function.

PEUTZ-JEGHERS SYNDROME An autosomal-dominant disorder characterized by benign polyps of the intestinal tract and mucocutaneous melanotic macules.

PIERRE ROBIN SYNDROME This syndrome consists of (1) glossoptosis; (2) micrognathia; (3) cleft palate; (4) chronic otitis; (5) auricular abnormalities; (6) ocular pathology; and (7) occasional mental retardation. There is no sex predilection.

PLUMMER-VINSON SYNDROME Characterized by pale skin, dysphagia, atrophy of the tongue papillae, and sometimes oral leukoplakia or angular cheilosis, found almost exclusively in middle-aged women. This condition is primarily due to iron-deficiency anemia. The dysphagia is attributed to the formation of an esophageal web. There also may be an increased risk of postcricoid cancer in these patients.

POLIEP SYNDROME   This disorder is characterized by (1) autosomal-recessive inheritance; (2) chronic intestinal pseudo-obstruction; (3) motor and sensory neuropathy (most similar to hereditary motor and sensory neuropathy [HMSN] type 1) with associated cranial neuropathy; (4) ophthalmoplegia and ptosis; (5) asymptomatic leukoencephalopathy; and (6) sensorineural hearing loss.

PRUSSAK'S POUCH   A space defined by the pars flaccida laterally, short process of the malleus caudally and superiorly by the lateral mallear fold.

RAMSAY HUNT SYNDROME   Classically described as a unilateral otalgia and facial paralysis accompanied by a vesicular rash involving the external ear resultant from a herpetic infection. Evidence of a polyneuropathy is often elicited.

RASMUSSEN SYNDROME   The major characteristics of this syndrome include (1) autosomal-dominant inheritance; (2) bilateral clubfeet and vertical talus; (3) atresia of the external auditory canals with normal pinnae; and (4) conductive hearing loss.

RATHKE'S POUCH   A diverticulum of mucosa that develops into the anterior lobe of the hypophysis and the pars intermedius. The path that this diverticulum takes during development may persist as the craniopharyngeal canal.

REFSUM SYNDROME   The syndrome is characterized by (1) autosomal-recessive inheritance; (2) progressive atypical retinitis pigmentosa with constricted visual fields and night blindness; (3) mild cerebellar ataxia and nystagmus; (5) increased plasma phytanic acid; and (6) progressive sensorineural hearing loss.

REICHERT'S SYNDROME   Neuralgia of the glossopharyngeal nerve.

REITER'S SYNDROME   Arthritis, urethritis, and conjunctivitis.

REYE'S SYNDROME   Pediatric encephalopathy and fatty metamorphosis of the liver. Morphologic abnormalities have been observed in the labyrinth and cochlea.

RICHARDS-RUNDLE SYNDROME   This syndrome is characterized by (1) autosomal-recessive inheritance; (2) ataxia; (3) distal amyotrophy; (4) mental retardation; (5) diabetes mellitus; (6) absent development of secondary sex characteristics; and (7) sensorineural hearing loss.

RIEDEL'S STRUMA (REIDEL'S THYROIDITIS)   An uncommon form of chronic thyroiditis in which a fibrotic reaction of unknown etiology replaces most thyroid tissue and frequently extends out of the thyroid capsule to compress adjacent structures. Patients are usually middle-aged women and may present with a painless neck mass, dysphagia, or hoarseness.

ROLLET'S SYNDROME   Mass effect from tumor or infection results in compression at the orbital apex resulting in paralysis of cranial nerves III, IV, and VI. This syndrome is characterized by (1) ptosis; (2) diplopia; (3) ophthalmoplegia; (4) optic atrophy; (5) hyperesthesia or anesthesia of the forehead, upper eyelid, and cornea; and (6) retrobulbar neuralgia. Exophthalmos and papilledema may occur.

ROSENBACH'S SIGN   Fine tremor of the closed eyelids, which is seen in both hysteria and hyperthyroidism.

ROSENBERG-CHUTORIAN SYNDROME   This disorder is characterized by (1) X-linked recessive inheritance with partial expression in carrier females; (2) motor and sensory neuropathy (most similar to hereditary motor and sensory neuropathy [HMSN] type 1); (3) optic atrophy; and (4) sensorineural hearing loss.

ROSENBERG SYNDROME   This disorder is characterized by (1) X-linked semidominant inheritance; (2) ataxia; (3) gout; (4) hyperuricemia related to overactivity of phosphoribosyl pyrophosphate (PRPP) synthetase; (5) possible renal and cardiovascular dysfunction; (6) sensorineural hearing loss; and (7) abnormal vestibular function.

RUSSELL BODIES   Coalescence of globules and inclusion bodies found in scleroma.

RUTHERFORD'S SYNDROME   A familial oculodental syndrome characterized by (1) corneal dystrophy; (2) gingival hyperplasia; and (3) failure of tooth eruption.

SAETHRE-CHOTZEN SYNDROME Characteristics include (1) autosomal-dominant inheritance; (2) variable craniosynostosis; (3) eyelid ptosis; (4) facial asymmetry; (5) straight nasofrontal angle; (6) brachydactyly and occasional mild syndactyly; and (7) occasional conductive hearing loss.

SAMTER'S SYNDROME A clinical triad consisting of sensitivity to aspirin, nasal polyposis, and asthma.

SCHÄFER'S SYNDROME This syndrome is characterized by (1) mental retardation; (2) sensorineural hearing loss; (3) proteinemia; (4) hematuria; and (5) photogenic epilepsy. It is due to a deficiency of proline oxidase with resultant buildup of the amino acid proline.

SCHAUMANN'S SYNDROME Systemic sarcoidosis.

SCHEIBE'S APLASIA The pars inferior (cochlear duct and saccule) remain undifferentiated.

SCHMIDLEY SYNDROME This syndrome is characterized by (1) X-linked recessive inheritance; (2) onset in infancy with subsequent progression; (3) discrete episodes of neurologic deterioration; (4) ataxia; (5) dysphagia and choking; (6) early hypotonia and later spasticity and areflexia; (7) mental retardation; (8) seizures; (9) esotropia that evolves to ophthalmoplegia; (10) optic atrophy; and (11) sensorineural hearing loss.

SCHMIDT'S SYNDROME Paralysis of cranial nerves X and XI due to lesions of the nucleus ambiguus, bulbar, and spiral nuclei.

SCLEROSTEOSIS Characteristics include (1) autosomal-recessive inheritance; (2) generalized osteosclerosis with hyperostosis of calvaria, mandible, clavicles, and pelvis; (3) syndactyly of the second and third fingers; (4) increased height; (5) increased intracranial pressure; (6) cranial nerve dysfunction; and (7) mixed hearing loss.

SHEEHAN'S SYNDROME Ischemic necrosis of the anterior pituitary associated with postpartum hypotension.

SHY-DRAGER SYNDROME Progressive systemic dysfunction of the autonomic nervous system beginning in middle age. Clinical abnormalities reflect atrophy of the corticospinal and cerebellar pathways as well as the basal ganglia. Initial symptoms include postural hypotension, impotence, sphincter dysfunction, and anhydrosis with later progression to panautonomic failure.

SJÖGREN SYNDROME (SICCA SYNDROME) Defined by the presence of two or more of the following symptoms: (1) dry eyes (keratoconjunctivitis sicca); (2) dry mouth (xerostomia); (3) painless swelling of the parotid glands; and (4) polyarthritis.

SLUDER'S NEURALGIA Similar to Horton's neuralgia (cluster headache) and also known as sphenopalatine neuralgia. A unilateral headache felt to be due to pressure on the middle turbinate by a nasal septal spur.

SPRINTZEN SYNDROME Characteristics include (1) autosomal-dominant inheritance; (2) characteristic facies; (3) congenital heart anomalies; (4) mild mental retardation; (5) absent tonsils and/or adenoids; (6) cleft palate or velopharyngeal insufficiency; and (7) conductive hearing loss.

STEWART-BERGSTROM SYNDROME This disorder is characterized by (1) autosomal-dominant inheritance; (2) congenital hand deformity; and (3) congenital sensorineural hearing loss.

STICKLER SYNDROME Characteristics include (1) autosomal-dominant inheritance; (2) ossification disturbances, including epiphyseal abnormalities, diaphyseal narrowing, and platyspondylia; (3) joint hypermobility; (4) hypoplastic midface; (5) severe myopia and often retinal detachment; (6) occasionally cleft palate; and (7) mixed hearing loss.

STROMGREN SYNDROME This disorder is characterized by (1) autosomal-dominant inheritance; (2) posterior polar cataracts appearing during the third decade; (3) intrabulbar hemorrhage; (4) late-onset ataxia; (5) later onset of paranoid psychosis and dementia; (6) late-onset, severe sensorineural hearing loss; and (7) loss of vestibular function.

STURGE-WEBER SYNDROME Characterized by a unilateral port-wine stain within the distribution of the trigeminal nerve. Clinically, angioma of the leptomeninges, orbit, mouth, and nasal mucosa may occur. Intercerebral calcifications are noted radiographically.

SUPERIOR ORBITAL FISSURE SYNDROME   There is involvement of cranial nerves III, IV, V, VI, the ophthalmic veins, and the sympathetic branches of the cavernous sinus. The syndrome can be caused by sphenoid sinusitis or regional tumor mass. Symptoms include paralysis of the upper lid, orbital pain, photophobia, and paralysis of the above noted nerves. The optic nerve may become involved as a lesion expands or causes neural or vascular compression.

SUPERIOR VENA CAVA SYNDROME   This syndrome is characterized by obstruction of the superior vena cava or its main tributaries by bronchogenic carcinoma, mediastinal neoplasm, or lymphoma. Edema and upper respiratory obstructive symptoms may manifest.

SYLVESTER SYNDROME   This disorder is characterized by (1) probable autosomal-dominant inheritance; (2) ataxia; (3) variable spasticity and amyotrophy; (4) optic atrophy; and (5) sensorineural hearing loss.

TAPIA'S SYNDROME   Paralysis of cranial nerves X and XII due to tegmental lesions of the lower medulla.

TAY-SACHS DISEASE   Characteristics include (1) autosomal-recessive inheritance; (2) progressive mental and motor retardation; (3) enlarged head circumference; and (4) seizures, blindness, deafness, and death before 3 years of age.

TIETZE'S SYNDROME   Costal chondritis, presenting with pain, tenderness, and swelling of one or more of the upper costal cartilages.

TOLOSA-HUNT SYNDROME   Unilateral retro-orbital pain and ophthalmoplegia that is either progressive or recurrent. It is thought to be due to inflammation or pseudotumor involving the cavernous sinus.

TOURETTE SYNDROME   A disorder of the central nervous system, characterized by the appearance of involuntary tic movements such as rapid eye blinking, facial twitches, head jerking, or shoulder shrugging. Involuntary sounds, such as repeated throat clearing, nervous coughing, or coprolalia, are noted.

TOWNES-BROCK'S SYNDROME   This syndrome is characterized by (1) autosomal-dominant inheritance with variable expressivity; (2) satyr ears, often accompanied by preauricular tags and occasional pits; (3) imperforate anus with rectovaginal or rectoperineal fistula; (4) various bony anomalies; (5) renal anomalies; (6) congenital heart defects; and (7) sensorineural hearing loss.

TREACHER COLLINS SYNDROME   This syndrome is characterized by (1) bilateral mandibular hypoplasia; (2) macrostomia; (3) downward sloping palpebral fissures; (4) stapes fixation; (5) axial loss; (6) microtia; (7) atresia; (8) clefting of the lip/palate; and (9) flat mid-face with broad nasal root.

TREFT SYNDROME   This disorder is characterized by (1) autosomal-dominant inheritance; (2) ataxia; (3) ptosis and ophthalmoplegia; (4) optic atrophy; (5) mild mitochondrial myopathy; and (6) sensorineural hearing loss.

TROTTER SYNDROME (SINUS OF MORGAGNI SYNDROME)   This syndrome may be seen with tumors of the nasopharynx that block the eustachian tube and produce a conductive hearing loss secondary to middle ear fluid. Other symptoms may be pain in the distribution of the ophthalmic branch of the trigeminal nerve, decreased mobility of the soft palate, and possibly trismus.

TROUSSEAU'S SIGN   Tetany caused by a tourniquet placed around the arm of a patient with hypocalcemia.

TULLIO'S PHENOMENON   Loud noise precipitates vertigo. Fibrosis within the vestibule attached to a mobile footplate accounts for the symptom.

TURNER SYNDROME   Gonadal dysgenesis found in an XO karyotype. Clinical features include (1) growth retardation; (2) webbed neck; (3) cardiac and ocular abnormalities; (4) amenorrhea; (5) middle ear infections; and (6) possible defect of the organ of Corti.

TURPIN'S SYNDROME   This syndrome is characterized by (1) congenital bronchiectasis; (2) megaesophagus; (3) tracheoesophageal fistula; (4) vertebral deformities; (5) rib malformations; and (6) a heterotopic thoracic duct.

UMITA SYNDROME   Characteristics of this syndrome include (1) autosomal-recessive inheritance; (2) variable signs of hypoparathyroidism; and (3) moderate to severe sensorineural hearing loss.

USHER SYNDROME   This syndrome is characterized by retinitis pigmentosa and sensorineural hearing loss. Three variants are recognized: type I—congenital, severe to profound, hearing loss with development of retinitis pigmentosa by 10 years and absent vestibular responses; type II—congenital moderate to severe stable hearing loss with onset of retinitis pigmentosa from late teens to early twenties and normal vestibular responses; and Type III—progressive hearing loss with variable onset of retinitis pigmentosa.

VAIL'S SYNDROME   This syndrome consists of unilateral, nocturnal, vidian neuralgia that may be associated with sinusitis.

VALVE OF BAST   Located between the utricle and the utricular duct, this valve may limit communication between the utricle, utricular duct, and endolymphatic and saccular ducts.

VAN DUCHEM DISEASE   Characteristics include (1) autosomal-recessive inheritance; (2) hyperostosis and osteosclerosis of the skeleton; and (3) mixed hearing loss.

VERNET'S SYNDROME   Cranial nerve IX, X, and XI paralysis due to lesions of the jugular foramen.

VILLARET'S SYNDROME   Paralysis of cranial nerves IX, X, XI, and XII due to a lesion in the retropharyngeal or retroparotid space. Horner's syndrome is also noted.

VINCENT'S ANGINA   Gram-negative bacterial pharyngitis presenting with a fetid ulcerative lesion of the oral cavity.

VIRCHOW'S NODE   A palpable lymph node in the left supraclavicular triangle indicating metastatic carcinoma.

WAARDENBURG SYNDROME   Major characteristics of this syndrome include (1) autosomal-dominant inheritance with variable expressivity; (2) lateral displacement of medial canthi; (3) high broad nasal root; (4) hyperplasia of medial eyebrows; (5) heterochromia (hypoplasia) irides and loss of pigment epithelium of optic fundis; (6) white forelock; (7) skin pigmentary changes, including piebaldism or spotty hyperpigmentation; (8) cleft lip and/or palate (in less than 5%); (9) vestibular hypofunction; and (10) congenital mild to severe unilateral or bilateral sensorineural hearing loss.

WALDEYER'S RING   The lymphoid tissue that surrounds the oropharyngeal and nasopharyngeal inlets.

WALLENBERG'S SYNDROME   Thrombosis of the posterior inferior cerebellar artery resulting in vertigo, paresthesia, dysphagia, Horner's syndrome, and incoordination. Contralateral hypesthesia over trunk and limbs is noted.

WILDERVANCK SYNDROME   Characteristics include (1) doubtful genetic etiology; (2) fused cervical vertebrae; (3) abducens palsy with retracted globe; and (4) hearing loss—sensorineural, conductive, or mixed.

WINKELMANN SYNDROME   Characteristics of the syndrome include (1) autosomal-recessive inheritance; (2) somatic and sexual infantilism due to deficiency of growth hormone and gonadotropins; (3) normal intelligence; and (4) sensorineural hearing loss, appearing at about 6 to 8 years of age and progressing rapidly to complete hearing loss.

WINKLER'S DISEASE (CHONDRODERMATITIS NODULARIS CHRONICA HELICIS)   One or more painful nodules involving the helix in older men.

WINTER SYNDROME   This syndrome is characterized by (1) autosomal-recessive transmission; (2) unilateral or bilateral renal hypoplasia or agenesis; (3) variable involvement of the genital system with occasional hypoplastic ovaries, tubes, or vagina; and (4) moderate to severe conductive hearing loss with malformation of the ossicles.

WOODHOUSE-SAKATI SYNDROME   The syndrome is characterized by (1) autosomal-recessive inheritance; (2) mental retardation; (3) alopecia; (4) diabetes mellitus; (5) hypogonadism; (6) ECG abnormalities; and (7) sensorineural hearing loss.

XERODERMA PIGMENTOSUM   Photosensitive skin with multiple basal cell epitheliomas. Squamous cell carcinoma or malignant melanoma can result from it.

Zimmermann pericyte   A round cell capable of malignant transformation identified with hemangiopericytoma.

Zonula of Zinn   Suspensory ligament of the crystalline lens.

Suggested Readings

Cummings CW, Fredrickson JM, Harker LA, Krause CJ, Schuller DE, eds. *Otolaryngology Head and Neck Surgery.* 2nd ed. St. Louis: Mosby Yearbook, 1993.

Gorlin RJ, Toreillo HC, Cohen MM Jr, eds. *Hereditary Hearing Loss and Its Syndromes.* New York: Oxford University Press; 1995.

Hughes GB, Pensak ML, eds. *Clinical Otology.* 2nd ed. New York: Thieme; 1997.

Lee KJ. Syndromes and eponyms. In: Lee KJ, ed. *Essential Otolaryngology Head and Neck Surgery.* 5th ed. New York: Elsevier; 1987:645–682.

APPENDICES

CRANIAL NERVES

I. OLFACTORY

Origin: Olfactory neuroepithelium in the nasal vault.

Course: Through cribriform plate to olfactory bulb. Central projections occur along medial branch ending in subcallosal gyrus and the paraolfactory area, and lateral branch ending in uncus and hippocampal gyrus.

Function: Smell.

II. OPTIC

Origin: Ganglion cells of retina.

Course: Through optic foramen to optic chiasm, then along optic tract to lateral geniculate body. Second-order neuron goes to visual center in the cuneus.

Function: Vision.

III. OCULOMOTOR

Origin: Floor of cerebral aqueduct.

Course: Emerges at upper pons, proceeds lateral to posterior clinoid, in lateral wall of cavernous sinus, through superior orbital fissure into the orbit.

Function: Motor to all ocular muscles except the lateral rectus and superior oblique. Also provides parasympathetic fibers to pupillary sphincter and ciliary muscle.

IV. TROCHLEAR

Origin: Floor of cerebral aqueduct.

Course: Emerges between upper pons and cerebral peduncle, proceeds lateral to posterior clinoid, in lateral wall of cavernous sinus, crosses oculomotor nerve, and enters orbit through superior orbital fissure.

Function: Motor to superior oblique muscle (rotates eyeball outward and downward).

V. TRIGEMINAL

Origin: Floor of fourth ventricle, with a large sensory and small motor root.

Course: Emerges at lateral pons and passes over petrous apex to form gasserian ganglion. Here divides into three branches:

1. Ophthalmic: Enters superior orbital fissure, yielding the lacrimal, frontal (supraorbital, supratrochlear), and nasociliary (anterior ethmoid, external nasal, posterior ethmoid, infratrochlear, long ciliary) nerves.

2. Maxillary: Through foramen rotundum, across the pterygopalatine fossa where it gives off the posterior superior alveolar nerve and enters the orbit through inferior orbital fissure, along infraorbital groove to infraorbital foramen, yielding the infraorbital (middle and anterior

superior alveolar), zygomaticofacial, and zygomaticotemporal nerves.

3. Mandibular: Through foramen ovale, then splitting into anterior (masseteric nerve, deep temporal nerves, nerve to medial pterygoid, nerve to lateral pterygoid, nerve to tensor veli palatini, and buccal [sensory] nerve) and posterior (auriculotemporal, lingual [joined from behind by chorda tympani branch of facial], and inferior alveolar nerves) divisions. The inferior alveolar nerve gives off the motor nerve to mylohyoid before entering the mandibular canal, exiting as the mental nerve.

Function:

1. Ophthalmic: Sensation to skin of nose, upper eyelid, eyebrow, forehead, and scalp as far back as lambdoid suture, and to conjunctiva, cornea, lacrimal gland.

2. Maxillary: Sensation to skin of lower lid, side of nose, cheek, upper lip, anterior temple, and to the nasal mucosa, palatal mucosa, and upper gums.

3. Mandibular: Motor to muscles of mastication (medial and lateral pterygoid, masseter, temporalis), and to tensor veli palatini; sensation to skin over mandible, lower part of cheek and zygomatic arch, middle third of temporal fossa, upper part of external ear, and floor of mouth and lower gums.

VI. ABDUCENS

Origin: Lower portion of pons.
Course: Passes through aperture of petrous apex, then lateral portion of cavernous sinus, into orbit through superior orbital fissure.
Function: Motor to lateral rectus (rotates eyeball outward).

VII. FACIAL

Motor Division

Origin: Lower portion of pons.
Course: Passes through internal acoustic meatus along facial canal, giving off chorda tympani above oval window, exits temporal bone through stylomastoid foramen, passing through parotid gland to divide into frontal, zygomatic, buccal, marginal mandibular, and cervical branches.
Function: Motor to facial muscles, scalp, auricle, buccinator, platysma, stapedius, stylohyoid, and posterior belly of digastric.

Sensory Division (Nervus Intermedius)

Origin: Geniculate ganglion.
Course: Chorda tympani to periphery, centrally through internal acoustic meatus and enters brain between inferior peduncle and olive.
Function: Taste to anterior two-thirds of tongue (chorda tympani), sensation to soft palate, parasympathetic innervation to submandibular and sublingual salivary glands (chorda tympani).

VIII. ACOUSTIC

Cochlear Division

Origin: Spiral ganglion of cochlea.
Course: From spiral ganglion peripheral fibers go to organ of Corti; central fibers go through the internal auditory meatus to enter the inferior peduncle and terminate in the ventral and dorsal cochlear nuclei.
Function: Hearing.

Vestibular Division

Origin: Vestibular (Scarpa's) ganglion.
Course: Through the internal auditory meatus to terminate in the medial, lateral, superior, and spinal vestibular nuclei and in the cerebellum.
Function: Maintenance of equilibrium.

IX. GLOSSOPHARYNGEAL

Origin: Medulla oblongata.
Course: Through the petrous temporal bone to exit the jugular foramen between the internal carotid artery and internal jugular vein. At styloid process it winds around stylopharyngeus and passes between superior and middle constrictors.
Function: Taste to posterior third of tongue. Sensation to posterior third of tongue, tonsils, pharynx, and soft palate. Sensory fibers to carotid body and carotid sinus. Motor to stylopharyngeus muscle.

X. VAGUS

Origin: Between inferior peduncle and olive.
Course: Passes through jugular foramen, continuing down the neck within the carotid sheath, giving off pharyngeal branches that run between the internal and external carotid arteries to join the pharyngeal plexus, the superior laryngeal nerve (internal and external branches), and the recurrent laryngeal nerve.
Function: Sensation to skin in back of auricle, posterior external acoustic meatus, pharynx, and larynx (internal branch to laryngeal mucosa above vocal cords, recurrent to laryngeal mucosa below vocal cords). Motor to pharynx, tongue base, and larynx (external branch to cricothyroid muscle, recurrent to all other laryngeal muscles).

XI. SPINAL ACCESSORY

Origin: Four to five rootlets at side of medulla.
Course: Passes through medial part of jugular foramen with cranial nerves IX and X, then re-verts backward across the internal jugular vein to the posterior triangle.
Function: Motor to sternocleidomastoid and trapezius muscles. Sends branches to C2, C3, and C4.

XII. HYPOGLOSSAL

Origin: Anterolateral part of medulla.
Course: Passes laterally and forward to leave skull through hypoglossal canal in occipital bone, then passes between internal carotid artery and jugular vein, loops around occipital artery, crosses both internal and external carotid arteries, receives contributions from cervical roots before giving off descending ramus to form ansa hypoglossi, then enters tongue.
Function: Motor to strap muscles (sternothyroid, thyrohyoid, sternohyoid, omohyoid), and tongue musculature (styloglossus, hyoglossus, genioglossus, and geniohyoid).

House-Brackmann Grading System for Facial Nerve Dysfunction

Grade 1: Normal movement

Grade 2: Minor abnormalities including minimal synkinesis

Grade 3: Symmetry at rest with mild disfigurement on movement, good eye closure

Grade 4: Symmetry at rest with gross disfigurement on movement, poor eye and forehead movement

Grade 5: Asymmetry at rest, minimal detectable function

Grade 6: No movement

(From House JW, Brackmann DE. Facial nerve grading system. *Otolaryngol Head Neck Surg* 1985;93:146–147. Reprinted by permission of the publisher, Mosby, St. Louis, MO.)

ANATOMIC SUBSITES FOR CERVICAL LYMPH NODES

Level I: Submental
              Submandibular

Level II: Upper jugular

Level III: Mid-jugular

Level IV: Lower jugular

Level V: Posterior triangle (spinal
              accessory)

Level VI: Prelaryngeal (Delphian)
              Pretracheal
              Paratracheal

Level VII: Upper mediastinal

Other groups: Retropharyngeal
                Buccinator (facial)
                Intraparotid
                Preauricular
                Postauricular
                Suboccipital

(From *AJCC® Cancer Staging Handbook.* 5th ed. Phila-delphia: Lippincott-Raven; 1998. Reprinted by per-mission of the American Joint Committee on Cancer [AJCC®], Chicago, IL.)

AMERICAN JOINT COMMITTEE ON CANCER (AJCC) TNM STAGING OF TUMORS OF THE HEAD AND NECK

I. LIP AND ORAL CAVITY

Primary Tumor (T)

TX: Primary tumor cannot be assessed
T0: No evidence of primary tumor
Tis: Carcinoma in situ
T1: Tumor 2 cm or less in greatest dimension
T2: Tumor more than 2 cm but not more than 4 cm in greatest dimension
T3: Tumor more than 4 cm in greatest dimension
T4: Tumor invades adjacent structures (lip: e.g., through cortical bone, inferior alveolar nerve, floor of mouth, skin of face; oral cavity: through cortical bone, into deep muscle of tongue, maxillary sinus, skin. Superficial erosion of bone or tooth socket by gingival primary does not classify as T4)

Regional Lymph Nodes (N)

NX: Regional lymph nodes cannot be assessed
N0: No regional lymph node metastasis

(From *AJCC® Cancer Staging Handbook.* 5th ed. Philadelphia: Lippincott-Raven; 1998. Reprinted by permission of the American Joint Committee on Cancer [AJCC®], Chicago, IL.)

N1: Metastasis in a single ipsilateral lymph node, 3 cm or less in greatest dimension
N2a: Metastasis in a single ipsilateral lymph node, more than 3 cm but not more than 6 cm in greatest dimension
N2b: Metastasis in multiple ipsilateral lymph nodes, none more than 6 cm
N2c: Metastasis in bilateral or contralateral lymph nodes, none more than 6 cm
N3: Metastasis in a lymph node more than 6 cm in greatest dimension

Distant Metastasis (M)

MX: Distant metastasis cannot be assessed
M0: No distant metastasis
M1: Distant metastasis

II. NASOPHARYNX

Primary Tumor (T)

TX: Primary tumor cannot be assessed
T0: No evidence of primary tumor
Tis: Carcinoma in situ
T1: Tumor confined to the nasopharynx
T2: Tumor extends to soft tissues of oropharynx and/or nasal fossa
    T2a: Without parapharyngeal extension
    T2b: With parapharyngeal extension

T3: Tumor invades bony structures and/or paranasal sinuses

T4: Tumor with intracranial extension and/or involvement of cranial nerves, infratemporal fossa, hypopharynx, or orbit

Regional Lymph Nodes (N)

NX: Regional lymph nodes cannot be assessed

N0: No regional lymph node metastasis

N1: Unilateral metastasis in lymph node(s), 6 cm or less in greatest dimension, above the supraclavicular fossa

N2: Bilateral metastasis in lymph node(s), 6 cm or less in greatest dimension, above the supraclavicular fossa

N3: Metastasis in a lymph node(s)

    N3a: Greater than 6 cm

    N3b: Extension to the supraclavicular fossa

Distant Metastasis (M)

Same as above.

III. OROPHARYNX

Primary Tumor (T)

TX: Primary tumor cannot be assessed

T0: No evidence of primary tumor

Tis: Carcinoma in situ

T1: Tumor 2 cm or less in greatest dimension

T2: Tumor more than 2 cm but not more than 4 cm

T3: Tumor more than 4 cm in greatest dimension

T4: Tumor invades adjacent structures (e.g., pterygoid muscle, mandible, hard palate, deep muscle of tongue, larynx)

Regional Lymph Nodes (N)

Same as for oral cavity.

Distant Metastasis (M)

Same as above.

IV. HYPOPHARYNX

Primary Tumor (T)

TX: Primary tumor cannot be assessed

T0: No evidence of primary tumor

Tis: Carcinoma in situ

T1: Tumor limited to one subsite of hypopharynx and 2 cm or less in greatest dimension (the subsites of the hypopharynx include the pyriform fossae, right and left, the posterior hypopharyngeal wall, and the postcricoid region)

T2: Tumor involves more than one subsite of hypopharynx or adjacent site, or measures more than 2 cm but not more than 4 cm in greatest diameter without fixation of the hemilarynx

T3: Tumor measures more than 4 cm in greatest dimension, or with fixation of hemilarynx

T4: Tumor invades adjacent structures (e.g., thyroid/cricoid cartilage, carotid artery, soft tissues of neck, prevertebral fascia/ muscles, thyroid, esophagus)

Regional Lymph Nodes (N)

Same as for oral cavity.

Distant Metastasis (M)

Same as above.

V. LARYNX

Primary Tumor (T)

TX: Primary tumor cannot be assessed

T0: No evidence of primary tumor

Tis: Carcinoma in situ

Supraglottis

T1: Tumor limited to one subsite of supraglottis with normal vocal cord mobility (the subsites of the supraglottis include the suprahyoid epiglottis, the infrahyoid epiglottis, the laryngeal surface of the aryepiglottic folds, the arytenoids, and false vocal cords)

T2: Tumor invades mucosa of more than one adjacent subsite of supraglottis or glottis or region outside the supraglottis (e.g., mucosa of base of tongue, vallecula, medial wall of pyriform sinus) without fixation of the larynx

T3: Tumor limited to larynx with vocal cord fixation and/or invades postcricoid area or preepiglottic tissues

T4: Tumor invades through the thyroid cartilage, and/or extends into soft tissues of the neck, thyroid, and/or esophagus

Glottis

T1: Tumor limited to the vocal cord(s) with normal mobility (may involve anterior or posterior commissure)

    T1a: Tumor limited to one vocal cord

    T1b: Tumor involves both vocal cords

T2: Tumor extends to supraglottis and/or subglottis, and/or with impaired vocal cord mobility

T3: Tumor limited to the larynx with vocal cord fixation

T4: Tumor invades through the thyroid cartilage and/or to other tissues beyond the larynx (e.g., trachea, soft tissues of neck, including thyroid, pharynx)

Subglottis

T1: Tumor limited to the subglottis

T2: Tumor extends to vocal cord(s) with normal or impaired mobility

T3: Tumor limited to larynx with vocal cord fixation

T4: Tumor invades through cricoid or thyroid cartilage and/or extends to other tissues beyond the larynx (e.g., trachea, soft tissues of neck, including thyroid, esophagus)

Regional Lymph Nodes (N)

Same as for oral cavity.

Distant Metastasis (M)

Same as above.

VI. Paranasal Sinuses

Primary Tumor (T)

TX: Primary tumor cannot be assessed

T0: No evidence of primary tumor

Tis: Carcinoma in situ

Maxillary Sinus

T1: Tumor limited to the antral mucosa with no erosion or destruction of bone

T2: Tumor causing bone erosion, except for the posterior antral wall, including extension into the hard palate and/or the middle nasal meatus

T3: Tumor invades bone of the posterior wall, subcutaneous tissues, skin of cheek, floor or medial wall of orbit, infratemporal fossa, pterygoid plates, ethmoid sinuses

T4: Tumor invades orbital contents beyond the floor or medial wall including the orbital apex, cribriform plate, base of skull, nasopharynx, sphenoid, or frontal sinuses

Ethmoid Sinus

T1: Tumor confined to the ethmoid with or without bone erosion

T2: Tumor extends into the nasal cavity

T3: Tumor extends to anterior orbit, and/or maxillary sinus

T4: Tumor with intracranial extension, orbital extension including apex, involving sphenoid, and/or frontal sinus, and/or skin of external nose

Frontal, Sphenoid Sinuses

Tumors are so rare that according to the AJCC staging is not warranted.

Regional Lymph Nodes (N)

Same as for oral cavity.

Distant Metastasis (M)

Same as above.

VII. MAJOR SALIVARY GLANDS (PAROTID, SUBMANDIBULAR, SUBLINGUAL)

Primary Tumor (T)

TX: Primary tumor cannot be assessed

T0: No evidence of primary tumor

T1: Tumor 2 cm or less in greatest dimension without extraparenchymal extension

T2: Tumor more than 2 cm but not more than 4 cm without extraparenchymal extension

T3: Tumor having extraparenchymal extension without seventh nerve involvement and/or more than 4 cm but not more than 6 cm in greatest dimension

T4: Tumor invades base of skull, seventh nerve, and/or exceeds 6 cm in greatest dimension

Regional Lymph Nodes (N)

Same as for oral cavity.

Distant Metastasis (M)

Same as above.

VIII. THYROID GLAND

Primary Tumor (T)

TX: Primary tumor cannot be assessed

T0: No evidence of primary tumor

T1: Tumor 1 cm or less in greatest dimension limited to the thyroid

T2: Tumor more than 1 cm but not more than 4 cm limited to the thyroid

T3: Tumor more than 4 cm limited to the thyroid

T4: Tumor of any size extending beyond the thyroid capsule

(Each T classification may be broken down into (a) solitary tumor or (b) multifocal tumor, the largest determining the classification)

Regional Lymph Nodes (N)

NX: Regional lymph nodes cannot be assessed

N0: No regional lymph node metastasis

N1: Regional lymph node metastasis

    N1a: Metastasis in ipsilateral cervical lymph node(s)

    N1b: Metastasis in bilateral, midline, or contralateral cervical or mediastinal lymph node(s)

Distant Metastasis (M)

Same as above.

INDEX

Page numbers in italics indicate the entry on that page is in a figure or a table.